THE UNSEEN
MINORITY

THE UNSEEN
MINORITY

*A Social History of Blindness
in the United States*

FRANCES A. KOESTLER

David McKay Company, Inc.

NEW YORK

THE UNSEEN MINORITY

Library of Congress Cataloging in Publication Data
Koestler, Frances A
    The unseen minority.

    Bibliography: p.
    Includes index.
    1. Blind—United States—History. I. Title.
HV1791.K64   362.4'1'0973   75-16323
ISBN 0-679-50539-3

10 9 8 7 6 5 4 3

MANUFACTURED IN THE UNITED STATES OF AMERICA

To

the memory of my parents,
Louis and Minna Adlerstein,
and of my husband,
Milton Koestler

Acknowledgments

In one of the nine file drawers of documentary material accumulated during the four years spent researching and writing this book, there is a folder labeled "Interviews." It contains notes of conversations with 37 persons who shared facts, recollections, and insights which in one way or another contributed to my knowledge and understanding of the complex subjects treated in this volume.

Many were present and former staff members of the American Foundation for the Blind. Without attempting to particularize their individual contributions, I should like to voice sincere thanks to M. Robert Barnett, John W. Breuel, Leslie L. Clark, Annette B. Dinsmore, Milton D. Graham, Arthur Helms, Ira Kaplan, John F. Likely, the late Evelyn C. McKay, Pauline M. Moor, Mary Ellen Mulholland, Eber L. Palmer, Joseph Perretto, Harold G. Roberts, Robert L. Robinson, Irvin P. Schloss, Patricia S. Smith, Susan J. Spungin, Ruth E. Wilcox, and Marion V. Wurster.

Because the bulk of the primary source material on which I drew for the compilation of this history was to be found in the extensive archives of the Foundation, very special thanks are due for the unflaggingly patient and helpful assistance of Marguerite L. Levine, supervisor of the record center and curator of the Helen Keller papers. Considerable help also came from the Foundation's librarian, Mary Maie Richardson, and her staff.

Three Foundation officers generously gave of their time to talk with me: Richard H. Migel, Jansen Noyes, Jr., and Eustace Seligman. I am also indebted to Parmenia Migel Ekstrom, daughter of the Foundation's first president, who supplied biographical and anecdotal material about her parents.

My gratitude extends as well to a number of persons associated with other major organizations in work for the blind who allowed me to consult them on their respective areas of expertise: C. Warren Bledsoe, James C. Bliss, Eric T. Boulter, Robert S. Bray, Robin C. B. Buckley, the late Ethel Everett, Howard Freiberger, Charles Galozzi, Alexander F. Handel, Marjorie S. Hooper, Arthur S. Keller, Elizabeth Maloney, Peter J. Salmon, and Henry A. Wood.

Appreciation is also expressed to five persons who, at my request, reviewed the chapters dealing with services to the war-blinded and helped bring to life a period in which they themselves played roles. In addition to Messrs. Bledsoe, Robinson, and Schloss, these were Kathern Gruber and Russell C. Williams.

In commissioning the writing of this book, the American Foundation for the Blind agreed that I, as author, would have complete latitude in determining its scope and sole power of decision in selecting and interpreting the historical data to be included. Although several persons associated with the Foundation reviewed the completed manuscript and made helpful suggestions, there was no effort to censor or control its contents. As the chapter notes and bibliography will reveal, great care was taken to document facts, dates, figures, and quotations. If, despite this care, errors have crept in, the responsibility is mine alone.

Finally, I feel compelled to acknowledge an emotional and psychological debt to the two people, both long dead, from whom I first learned about blindness. They were my father, who gradually lost his vision over a twenty-five year period and was totally blind the last eight years of his life, and my mother, who discovered for herself how to live with a blind man and give him the kind of unobtrusive help and unfaltering moral support that enabled him to live out his years in comfort and dignity.

Frances A. Koestler

BROOKLYN, NEW YORK
APRIL 1974

Contents

Foreword

In 1921 at the biennial meeting of the American Association of Workers for the Blind in Vinton, Iowa, Dr. H. Randolph Latimer spoke of the need for an American Foundation for the Blind. He spoke of the problems which faced the field. "The situation," he said, "could be overcome if there were a national body composed of three major arms. One would be a Bureau of Information to collect, codify, and disseminate the most authoritative information to be had in the world on all questions pertaining to the blind."

The foundation was formed in that year and, over the half century that followed, it established within its quarters on West 16th Street in New York City, the M.C Migel Memorial Library. In the library itself and in the adjacent archives most of the more valuable material in print about blindness has been collected. The collection, in both published and unpublished forms, covers the period from the mid-nineteenth century to the present.

At a meeting in 1970, the Foundation Board of Trustees, recognizing that there had never been a comprehensive history of the blind in the United States and the institutions that supported them, agreed that the Foundation was particularly well qualified for the task of preparing such a history. Thus, they authorized the writing and publication of a history, and suggested that the fifty-year period just ending be stressed since this was the period for which there was the most accurate information.

The publication was to commemorate the fiftieth anniversary of the Foundation but, more important, it was to help eliminate in the years ahead unnecessary replication of past errors and to bring the field a broader base of understanding so that further advances could be made with greater confidence.

Jansen Noyes, Jr.
Chairman of the Board of Trustees
The American Foundation for the
Blind, Inc.

THE UNSEEN
MINORITY

1

Myths, Taboos, and Stereotypes

They were feared, shunned, pitied, ignored. Some were thought to be blessed with magical powers, others to be accursed for their sins. They were princes and beggars, bards and soothsayers, storytellers and buffoons. Some were killed as infants, others were tolerated in youth but abandoned to die by the roadside or even buried alive when they grew old and infirm. There were those who roamed the countryside in gypsy bands, living by their wits, communicating in a secret jargon. There were others who never in their lives ventured from home and hearthside. Some came under the special protection of the church or the crown, and some were thrown into madhouses, pesthouses, almshouses, where they could be kept out of public view.

They were white, black, brown, yellow, red. They were of every race and every faith, of every class and every station, in every land under every sky.

Some were born to their fate; others came to it through caprice of accident, or in the heat of battle, or by dint of a ruler's cruel decree.

They were the blind—uncounted generations of them over the centuries, 15 million or more alive in the world today. Many, probably most, of these millions live in underdeveloped areas where they are still the victims of ignorance and superstition, still suffer the indifference, the loathing, or the casual pity of their fellow human beings. In the more civilized areas of the world, however, the past two centuries, and particularly the last fifty years, have seen the gradual emancipation of blind men, women, and children and their steady entry into the body of society.

Of all the ills and imperfections of humankind, blindness is the most universally dreaded. The deep and tangled roots of this fear have been fed through countless centuries, beginning in primeval days when early man, whose defense against his natural enemies depended largely on his ability to see and thus avoid them, felt most vulnerable in the absence of light.

Invented to explain the inexplicable, primitive mythologies often interpreted blindness as a sign of divine disfavor. Among the ancient Greeks it was thought to be a punishment imposed by the gods on mortals who had displeased them. Homer's *Odyssey* tells of Phineus, whom Jupiter deprived of sight in punishment for his cruelties; as a further torment the gods sent the harpies—hideous birds with the heads of women—to snatch whatever food was placed before the sightless victim. The soothsayer Tiresias was said to have been blinded by Minerva because he had accidentally seen the goddess at her bath. In the bloodiest legend of all, the sinning Oedipus anticipated the gods' vengeance by imposing it on himself, tearing out his eyes to assuage his incestuous and patricidal guilt.

Such sin-associated myths helped rationalize the social practices among the early Greeks that sanctioned destruction of blind infants. In Sparta newborn children were examined by a committee of elders; those deemed physically imperfect and thus unfit for future citizenship were taken to a mountain gorge and left to die. In Athens there was a period when special clay vessels were fashioned into which such luckless infants were placed before being abandoned by the wayside. The Romans maintained a similar practice; in the marketplaces, parents could buy small baskets for use in consigning their defective children to the waves of the Tiber.

In other early societies that regarded blind children as economic liabilities, parents were permitted to sell them into slavery or prostitution. Nor did those who became blind or disabled in adult life escape the harsh dictates of survival which prevailed among primitive peoples. According to Dr. Richard S. French, who made a scholarly study of the subject:

> In Wagria [Serbia] and other Wendish lands it was considered honorable for children to kill, cook and eat, or else bury alive, their aged parents and other relatives, especially all who were no longer useful for either work or war. Praetorius relates of the heathen Prussians: "Old and weak parents were killed by the son; blind, squinting and deformed children were disposed of by the father either by the sword, drowning or burning; lame and blind servants were hanged to trees. . . ."

Many centuries before barbarism receded from central and northern Europe, more humane practices were to be found in scattered centers of civilization. It may have been the fact that blindness was endemic in the tropical climate of Egypt (a fact still largely true today) that led to efforts to help rather than destroy blind people. The early Egyptian interest in medicine may also have been a factor. Egyptian documents dating back four thousand years detail the exotic medications—reinforced by spells and incantations—used in the treatment of ailing eyes. The writer Ishbel Ross described these remedies:

> Ox liver, roasted and pounded, was used for night blindness. Incantations to Isis, Osiris, Horus and Atum were helped along with honey, gum ammoniac, wax, goose fat and oil. Celery and frankincense were supposed "to expel blood in the eyes." Dry myrrh, ink powder and calamine were used for "catarrh in the eyes." Real lapis lazuli, malachite and milk were applied for cataract. Bleary eyes were treated with malachite made into a stew and applied with a vulture's feather. The treatment for trachoma was a mixture of stibium, red and yellow ocher, and gall of tortoise.

Wherever civilization began to replace primitivism, there arose a different ethos toward human life that changed social attitudes toward the disabled. In ancient China, India, and Japan the blind were not only spared automatic extinction but were helped to find constructive roles in society. In this respect the Oriental cultures were far ahead of their western counterparts, which had then advanced only to the point of tolerating blind people as charitable wards of the feudal rulers or their priesthoods.

The belief that blindness equals uselessness has prevailed so long and so firmly in western culture that its traces have yet to be fully erased. One of the factors in its perpetuation was classic literature. Factual assertions are no match for the emotional impact of poetry such as John Milton's lines from *Samson Agonistes*:

> Now blind, disheartn'd, sham'd, dishonour'd, quell'd,
> To what can I be useful, wherein serve
> My Nation, and the work from Heav'n impos'd,
> But to sit idle on the household hearth,
> A burdenous drone; to visitants a gaze,
> Or pitied object . . .

Blindness as social liability, blindness as punishment for sin, blindness as uselessness to self and others—these were but three of the strands woven into the cocoon of myths and superstitions which continue to influence modern attitudes. There were others, many of them reinforced by the Bible. The association of blindness with darkness, a common cliché which no amount of contradiction by blind people has been able to dispel, carried with it unmistakable implications of evil. "And God saw the light, that it was good," says the Book of Genesis. Was not the darkness, which was also God's creation, equally good? The Bible not only refrains from saying so but warns against the "powers of darkness." Lucifer, whose very name means light-bringer, was transformed into the Angel of Darkness when he fell from Heaven to become the embodiment of evil known as Satan.

Darkness also connoted death. The Talmud and other Hebrew commentaries referred to the blind as the living dead; there was a Talmudic command that, on encountering a blind person, one must pronounce the same benediction as was customary on the death of a near relative. Darkness as death also became part of modern psychiatric theory. One psychiatrist wrote that for a doctor "to have to tell a person that he is blind . . . is almost like condemning him to a sort of living death. At any rate, that is how we sighted people are apt to regard blindness—as a return into the black limbo out of which we came." Other psychiatrists have equated fear of blindness with fear of castration, ascribing the unconscious origin of such fears to primitive fantasies in which seeing is equated with eating or devouring. Remnants of such fantasies remain in common parlance: "He ate her up with his eyes" is a metaphor for consuming love.

Not all the fallacies and fables about blindness are negative. There are also positive images interwoven in its mystique. Chief among these is the belief that bounteous nature compensates blind people in a variety of ways: through desirable traits of character (spirituality, patience, cheerfulness); through virtuosity of accomplishment (musical talent, prophetic gifts, razor-sharp memory); or through superhuman command of the non-visual senses.

Helen Keller wrote of her surprise in finding, among otherwise well-informed persons,

> a mediaeval ignorance concerning the sightless. They assured me that the blind can tell colours by touch and that the senses they have are more delicate and acute than those of other people. Nature herself, they told me, seeks to atone to the blind by giving them a singular sensitiveness and a sweet patience of spirit. It seemed not to occur to them that if this were true it would be an advantage to lose one's sight.

Much the same idea had been expressed in 1848 by Dr. Samuel Gridley Howe, the first American educator of blind children: "To suppose there can be a full and harmonious development of character without sight is to suppose that God gave us that noble sense quite superfluously."

Despite many proofs to the contrary, the popular belief persists that blind people command a "sixth sense." This comforting thought, which helps to mitigate disquieting emotions of fear and pity, stems from the theory of a "vicariate of the senses," an arrangement whereby the four remaining senses of hearing, touch, smell, and taste automatically become vicars, or substitutes, for the absent sense of vision. Shakespeare expressed the idea very plainly in *A Midsummer Night's Dream,* although he was referring to temporary rather than permanent inability to see. When Hermia, lost in the black forest night, nevertheless locates Lysander, she explains it thus:

> Dark night, that from the eye his function takes,
> The ear more quick of apprehension makes;
> Wherein it doth impair the seeing sense,
> It pays the hearing double recompense.

What the Bard seemed not to know, and what most people continue to misunderstand, is that both acuteness of hearing and sensitivity to touch in blind people are not compensatory gifts of nature but the products of long, hard concentration and training. Scientific experiments have demonstrated that blind people do not hear better than others, they merely learn to pay more attention to the auditory cues that sighted people can afford to ignore. Similar tests dealing with the sense of touch have yielded comparable results.

For many years there prevailed, among both the sighted and the blind, a belief that it was "facial vision"—the existence of sensors in the skin—that enabled blind people to orient themselves in space, to avoid walking into trees or falling over furniture. This theory was partially demolished in 1944 when a research team reported the results of experiments conducted at Cornell University. Working with paired blind and sighted subjects, the team concluded that obstacle detection was primarily a function of the ears and not of air pressures or other sensations registered by the skin. A dozen years later the zoologist Donald R. Griffin demonstrated through his work with bats that it was "echolocation"—a kind of natural sonar that bounces sound waves off objects in the environment—that guides sightless navigation on the part of both animals and men. The same conclusion had been reached during the late eighteenth century by the Italian scientist Lazzaro Spallanzani, when he found that if bats were blinded, they could continue to function, but if their ears were plugged, these otherwise sure-flying creatures would blunder helplessly into objects in their path.

If facial vision is a myth, can fingertip vision exist? Can colors be detected, currency bills be identified, newspaper headlines be read by sensitive fingers? Most authorities tend to be skeptical about such claims, but no definitive proof has yet been evolved one way or the other. The question arises every few years when improbable feats of non-visual detection are publicly performed by blind or tightly blindfolded persons. (Curiously, but perhaps irrelevantly, virtually all such persons have been women.)

In 1922 the members of the Chicago Medical Society sat open-mouthed while Dr. Thomas J. Williams, a specialist in ophthalmology, presented the case of seventeen-year-old Willetta Huggins, a blind and deaf girl whom he had been called in to examine and treat at the Wisconsin School for the Blind. Dr. Williams climaxed his clinical report by introducing Willetta herself in a demonstration. As reported in the *Official Bulletin of the Chicago Medical Society* for June 3, 1922, and reprinted two weeks later in the *Journal of the American Medical Association (JAMA)*:

> Miss Huggins gave some remarkable demonstrations in naming colors by the sense of smell. For instance, a skein of wool composed of different colors was handed to her and she named the colors correctly by passing the skein of wool before her nose as dark blue, yellow, pink, green, blue, fiery red, brown and white.
>
> A bunch of paper flowers (colored) was handed to her and she named the colors correctly as white, yellow, pink, lavender, purple, red, tomato red, and yellow. . . . One end of a wooden pole, about 12 feet long, was placed on top of Dr. Robert H. Babcock's head, while Miss Huggins took hold of the other end, and repeated every word Dr. Babcock said to her correctly. By the sense of touch she told the denominations on a one dollar bill, a ten dollar bill, a twenty dollar bill, and a one hundred dollar bill correctly.

Although Willetta had already been certified as totally blind and totally deaf by reputable specialists, she was carefully blindfolded for her appearance before the medical society. A variety of other precautions were also taken to exclude the possibility of hoax or collusion. Several of the objects she identified with her fingers were submitted by people who had never seen or heard of her before. The paper money of various denominations, for example, came from the pockets of physicians in the audience. So did a number of newspapers, whose bolder headlines her fingers traced without difficulty.

In the same issue of the *JAMA* which reprinted the Chicago story, there appeared a challenge to the validity of the medical society demonstration by a professor of psychology who had briefly examined Willetta at her school some months earlier. Dr. Joseph Jastrow of the University of Wisconsin asserted that the physicians were victims of "the will to believe." He mentioned the possibility that the girl had some remaining sight and that it was "a slit of vision" beneath the blindfold that enabled her to see the colors of the objects she brought up to her nose. Moreover, he was of the opinion that Willetta's deafness was of a hysterical nature: "The girl deceives herself in the belief that the vibrations conveyed through her finger tips make her hear the sounds which really reach her through auditory channels."

Professor Jastrow's refutation was in turn rebutted by Dr. Williams, who charged him with "the will to believe otherwise" and urged that further scientific inquiry be made. A follow-up study was shortly undertaken by Robert H. Gault, professor of psychology at Northwestern University, whose examination of Willetta bore out at least two of the original findings. On the hypothesis that the girl's ability to distinguish colors was due to an exceptionally keen sense of smell that could differentiate among the aniline dyes used to produce colors in yarn or paper flowers, Dr. Gault made laboratory tests with 32 other persons, 10 blind and 22 sighted, and all of them blindfolded. He found that while many could smell with some accuracy whether a pair of yarns consisted of two alike or two of different colors, none could name the colors in such a test.

The claim that Willetta interpreted speech through vibrations conducted to her hand, Dr. Gault found to be indisputably so. He confirmed it by making tests with his assistant, a person of normal hearing, whose ears were stopped with soft putty and whose hand was enclosed in a soundproof box. The assistant was able, after some practice, to distinguish 35 words through vibrations against his palm sent through a speaking tube, 13 feet long and projecting through two walls and an intervening room.

As for Willetta Huggins, two years later she spontaneously recovered much of both her hearing and her sight, a change she ascribed to Christian Science, of which she subsequently became an accredited practitioner. A statement by her, attesting that through Christian Science she had been "completely and permanently healed" of blindness and deafness, was published in the "Testimonies of Healing" column of the *Christian Science Sentinel* in early 1929. Willetta later changed her name and her place of residence; in late 1970 she was living in a midwestern city, still working as a Christian Science healer and reluctant to discuss or even recall the days when she was the object of fascinated world attention.

Willetta's was not the first case of its kind, nor was it the last. Comparable wonders have been reported from time to time in medical literature over a period of several hundred years. Some were bizarre. Toward the end of the 19th century the Italian criminologist Cesare Lombroso described a case of hysterical blindness in a fourteen-year-old girl, in the course of which the child exhibited such feats of sensory transposition as smelling with her chin and, later, with her foot.

In contemporary times, a good deal of perplexed speculation was aroused in 1957 when a fifteen-year-old sighted girl, Margaret Foos, gave a demonstration of "eyeless sight" at Veterans Administration headquarters in Washington in which she read the Bible and identified various objects through a blindfold. Authorities on blindness who attended this and subsequent demonstrations dismissed them as hoaxes. Their opinion was shared by Dr. J. B. Rhine of Duke University, the recognized expert on extrasensory perception.

More serious attention was paid in 1962 to reports from the Soviet Academy of Sciences about an epileptic Russian girl, Rosa Kuleshova, whose fingertips could discriminate and identify colors and read ordinary letterpress printing. Soviet scientists who examined Rosa regarded her ability as evidence of the existence of a "dermal light sense"—a network of fine nerve endings sensitive to light. Although Rosa herself was later said to have joined a circus, subsequent reports indicated continuing investigations in Soviet scientific circles into dermal-optical sensitivity.

American interest in the subject was further stimulated in the mid-Sixties by the work of Dr. Richard P. Youtz, chairman of the psychology department of Barnard College, Columbia University. Several years of investigation led him to conclude that some people do have skin which is sensitive to electromagnetic wavelengths (similar to heat waves), among which may be the different wavelengths emitted by different colors.

Clearly, the last word has yet to be spoken on the subject of seeing fingers, and perhaps on facial vision as well.

In the popular mind, the concept of blindness simultaneously juxtaposes two contradictory notions: that loss of sight dooms most of its victims to lifelong dependence, but that it also rewards a few of them with superhuman powers. Out of these twin beliefs have grown the stereotypes of the blind beggar and the blind genius. Blind people find both labels equally irritating, for they know—as does anyone who stops to think—that they differ from others only in the single respect of visual ability.

Blindness today slices across every stratum of society. It encompasses the same proportions of the wise and the foolish, the gifted and the stupid, the efficient and the fumbling, the aggressive and the diffident, as any other random sample of the population. If there are indeed more beggars among the blind than among the sighted (not necessarily the case: the blind person is more conspicuous, and thus more easily remembered, than others who make their living in the streets), it is society and not blindness that has cast them in this role. If the accomplishments of blind men and women elicit greater praise than similar achievements by the sighted, it is once again society which has established such low standards of expectation that, as a blinded veteran of World War II once remarked, "to be able to blow your own nose without assistance" is enough to give a blind man the reputation of being exceptional.

There is sad irony in the fact that war, which has robbed so many of their sight, has often brought boons to blind people in its wake. As will be seen in later chapters, the shock of war tends to arouse the conscience of the public to needs they comfortably ignore in peacetime.

During the Middle Ages the first state-supported asylum for the blind came into being as a result of the Crusades. In 1254 l'Hôpital des Quinze-Vingts (Almshouse of the Three Hundred) was established in Paris by Louis IX (who came to be known as Saint Louis). Legend has it that the Quinze-Vingts was intended as an asylum for three hundred Crusaders who were blinded by order of the Turkish sultan when the French king, having fallen captive to the Saracens during the Seventh Crusade, was awaiting rescue by ransom. The sultan is said to have hastened the arrival of the gold by blinding 20 of Louis' men on each of the 15 days the ransom was delayed. There seems to be no historical documentation for this gory account; one scholar offers the theory "that Louis, moved probably by the misery caused by the fearful loss of sight among his crusaders in Egypt, directed his attention to the blind at home and founded the institution for the amelioration of the condition of the sightless, irrespective of the origin of their affliction."

In more modern times, war-quickened awareness of blindness and the impulse to do something for its victims reached extraordinary heights during World War I.

"Unquestionably the most worthy of all the war charities" is what its sponsors called the drive for help to blinded soldiers which was organized in England in 1915 and quickly became international in scope under the name of the American, British, French and Belgian Permanent Blind War Relief Fund.

It was more than American dollars that crossed the Atlantic for the relief of the war-blinded. Numbers of influential men and women, some operating as independent volunteers and others under the aegis of the American Red Cross, moved into the cleared battle zones of France to establish rehabilitation centers where blinded *poilus* could be helped to make a new start in life. Spurred by their personal experiences in such centers, these volunteers brought home to the States a fresh fund of zeal and determination to alleviate the miserable status which seemed to be the fate of blind people everywhere.

Some four hundred and fifty American soldiers, sailors, and marines were blinded during the 17 months of United States participation in World War I. This was an insignificant number compared with England's 3,000 or France's 2,800 (and smaller yet when measured against Germany's 7,000) war-blinded. But it was enough to give the final impetus to a movement to establish some sort of nationwide structure that could bring a degree of order and purposeful planning into services for all of America's blind men, women, and children.

In 1918 an estimated $31 million a year was already being spent on public and voluntary services for the blind in the United States, but the services were scattered, diffuse, lacking in common goals or standards. There were numerous urgent problems to be solved as well as an array of vested interests to be dealt with before solutions could even be approached.

As matters stood at the beginning of the Twenties, the major hurdles were these:

• For nearly a century, those blind children who received any sort of education had done so in state-supported residential schools where they spent their formative years physically and socially separated from their sighted peers. Beginning in 1900, a few innovative thinkers had demonstrated that it was possible for blind children to remain at home with their families and attend regular public day schools. Should this, then, be the future direction of education for blind youngsters? What special facilities and services would be needed for such schooling to be effective? How could teachers be trained to work with the blind children in their classrooms? How could parents be helped to prepare such children for educational equality? The residential schools would continue to be needed for many children; what changes should be instituted in their programs and curricula to equip their students for productive life in a sighted world? What were the possibilities for higher education, and how could these be expanded?

• Communication was a fundamental key to functioning at all stages of life. A fifty-year battle—"the war of the dots"—to arrive at a uniform system of finger-reading had finally ended in 1917 and a newly modified braille code was now accepted as the universal American standard for the written word. But no more than two hundred or three hundred books had thus far been produced in this code. Where was the money to be found to provide a decent selection of reading matter? Braille books were expensive; they cost twenty or more times as much to print as their inkprint equivalents. They were bulky; a braille edition of a four-hundred-page novel required at least three volumes, weighing more than fifteen pounds and needing fifteen or more inches of shelf space. Could ways be found to reduce both cost and bulk? How could such books be circulated? Few blind people could afford to buy their own. Their sighted neighbors could take advantage of free public libraries. Could not a similar free library system be set up for blind readers?

• Only a minority of blind persons could read braille. Persons who lost their sight in adult life found braille too taxing to learn; many who had been blind from childhood had been taught one of the other finger-reading codes. To them, mastering braille was equivalent to learning a foreign tongue. Could a way be found to deliver reading matter through a medium other than touch?

• How could blind persons be helped to earn a decent living? Could not many be trained to move out of the narrow confines of the traditional "blind trades"— broom-making, basket weaving, small handicrafts? Could sheltered workshops expand markets and develop new products so that the blind people who worked in them might achieve more than a marginal wage? And if better training and more versatile production were indeed to become realities, could the world of industry and commerce be persuaded to make room for blind workers, their services and products?

• Like every other population group, the nation's blind men and women included many who were too old or too burdened with additional physical and mental handicaps to enter the labor force. How could such persons be given a measure of financial security that would make it needless for them to choose between beggary and starvation? Poverty was not, of course, restricted to the blind, but the sighted poor were not hampered by the additional burden of immobility in their efforts to scrape together their minimal needs. Was there a way to equalize the status of blind people in their search for subsistence?

• Many blind people had worked out ingenious devices to simplify such daily routines as personal grooming, cooking, laundering, household maintenance, recreational pursuits. Could a system be established for such aids and appliances to be made known and available to all? Could engineering and scientific talent be harnessed to develop new and better tools to mitigate the handicap of blindness? Could optical aids be constructed that would enable the partially blind to make more efficient use of their residual sight? Americans prided themselves on their inventive genius. Could that genius be used to invent mobility devices that would enable the blind to move about independently?

Overriding all these specific issues was the challenge of effecting basic attitudinal change both in the sighted world and among blind people themselves. True emancipation could come about only if the community at large could be induced to give blind people a chance to demonstrate their ability to function as responsible and participating members, and for this to happen, the nation first had to be made aware of the existence of its blind citizens, of their needs and capabilities. At the same time, blind men and women needed the encouragement and support of strong and confident leadership to emerge from the personal and social isolation that had cast them in the role of an unseen minority.

Any objective observer surveying these hurdles and pitfalls dotting the road to emancipation for blind Americans might well have been dismayed by the odds against successfully negotiating such a journey. But, as has ever been the case with idealists, those who began the pilgrimage chose to forgo objective realism in favor of resolute faith. The crucial first step was the establishment of a pivotal national body that could serve as a storehouse of available knowledge, a coordinator of existing efforts, a generator of new ideas and directions, and a voice that could make itself heard in the corridors of power. Such a body came into being in 1921. It was called the American Foundation for the Blind.

The spirit of the American people was at a low ebb in 1921. The once confident hope that the sacrifice of more than a hundred thousand American lives in the "war to end war" had been worthwhile was being undermined by each day's headlines: revolution in Eastern Europe, civil ferment in Italy, national strikes in England, assassinations in newly partitioned Ireland, France suffocating in the ashes of her devastated soil and decimated population, Germany and Austria hysterical over imminent financial collapse.

Disgusted, disillusioned, the United States refused to join the League of Nations and resolutely turned its back on the endlessly quarrelsome European continent. A mere 18 months after the armistice, the nation's mood was accurately diagnosed by the Ohio senator who would shortly be chosen as the Republican Party's dark-horse candidate for the Presidency. Said Warren G. Harding:

> America's present need is not heroics, but healing; not nostrums, but normalcy; not revolution, but restoration; not agitation, but adjustment; not surgery, but serenity; not the dramatic, but the dispassionate; not experiment, but equipoise; not submergence in internationality, but sustainment in triumphant nationality. . . ."

This piece of fustian oratory, with its straining after alliteration and its unwitting coinage of a new word in place of "normality," nonetheless promised something Americans longed for: a soothing syrup to cure the throbbing headaches left by the events of the preceding half-decade.

The prescription didn't work. The Twenties were to become what one historian called "an age of rose-colored nightmares." Side by side with unprecedented economic progress and technological development were social fissures whose gravity was not detected until they gave way to the nightmare that became the depression.

Weak spots dotted the landscape of American life. The disparity between economic classes was great. A relatively narrow band of middle-class families separated the rich from the poor. With industrialization moving ahead at a gallop, the urban/rural population balance was in a state of dangerous disequilibrium. Droves of farm families left the land in search of a brighter future in the proliferating industrial factories. High tariffs, enacted to protect the swelling output of those factories, forced the American economy to turn in on itself; within less than a decade a saturated domestic market was to grow so glutted that the entire fiscal structure would collapse on a climactic day in October of 1929.

Helping to obscure these cracks in basic structure was a craving for the new and the different. The Nineteenth Amendment gave women access to the voting booth in 1920; soon the "flapper revolution" saw them bobbing their hair, smoking openly, and frequenting speakeasies. Long-established family and social patterns crumbled as women entered the labor market in record numbers and, as wage earners, demanded, and got, an unprecedented degree of freedom. Restraints were abandoned in both dress and behavior. Whalebone corsets went the way of the bustle. The use of cosmetics no longer signified harlotry. The automobile gave boys and girls undreamed-of opportunities to evade supervision.

It was not merely the young who were seeking new horizons of experience. A diet of dreams was nurtured by movies and the newly invented radio. There were fads, like mah-jongg and crossword puzzles. The new science of psychology was taking hold of the popular imagination. Educators debated John B. Watson's theory of behaviorism, while Freudianism was the latest rage in sophisticated circles.

Sophisticates and hoi polloi were as one in their heightened interest in competitive sports of all kinds. The spirit of competition found an additional outlet in land and securities speculation. But no one thought of these things as gambling fever; they were the hallmarks of the land of opportunity, the richest, fastest-growing, highest-standard nation the world had ever seen.

Were none left out in this froth of national euphoria? Decidedly yes—but little attention was paid to those not fleet enough of wit or foot to cash in on the blessings of the new age. The bonanza brought few boons to the overlooked minorities: unskilled laborers, coal miners, small farmers, sharecroppers and field hands tied to the cotton crops, American Indians languishing on their arid reservations, immigrant families held back by illiteracy and ignorance of American ways.

If hardly a thought was given to sizable population segments such as these, what consideration could be expected by an obscure minority like 100,000 blind people? Thinly sprinkled here and there across the map of the United States, blind people were unseen as well as unseeing.

A revealing index of their invisibility is the fact that the sole reference to blindness in *Middletown*, Robert and Helen Lynd's classic sociological study of American life in Muncie, Indiana, in 1924, was the following passage:

> . . . the oldest form of tax-supported charity in Middletown is the county poor asylum. . . . This institution was in 1890 the county catch-basin in which all sorts of human sediment collected: "the insane, the feeble-minded, the epileptic, the deaf, the blind, the crippled; the shiftless, the vicious, [the] respectable homeless. . . ." It was contrary to the tradition of this pioneer community that anybody should be habitually dependent upon the group; if he was, it was certainly "his own fault." Accommodations, accordingly, were not such as to encourage one to live on the county. . . . As recently as 1915 conditions [in the asylum] were described as "shocking and deplorable." . . .

The Lynds went on to say that the multiplication of new group care agencies had since "drained off from the poor asylums to special institutions many of those unable to provide for themselves." Discussing contemporaneous public attitudes toward handicapped people, they wrote that Middletown

extends ready sympathy and help to individual unfortunates whose plight is immediately before the community, and yet it is not particularly concerned with preventing the recurrence of similar situations, because there are bound to be some sick, unemployed or otherwise miserable people in the world, and no change in the present social or industrial system could presumably prevent this unfortunate condition. . . .

It was this very assumption—that nothing could change the basic plight of the "miserable people in the world"—that a handful of stubborn idealists set out to disprove one summer's day in 1921.

2

Five Days at Vinton

Vinton, Iowa (population 5,000), Thursday morning, June 23, 1921. The weather was the first thing on May Palmer's mind when she awoke just before the clock struck six. There was still a trace of morning haze over the broad meadow that lay beyond the tree-bordered lawn, but all of the omens were favorable.

Mrs. Palmer and her husband faced a busy day, with a hundred and fifty guests due to arrive for a five-day visit to the thirty-acre campus of what was then known as the Iowa College for the Blind. The occasion was the ninth biennial convention of the American Association of Workers for the Blind (AAWB), and Francis E. Palmer, just completing his third year as superintendent of the school, was eager to meet his obligations as host.

A man in his mid-fifties, Palmer was a relative newcomer to work for the blind. Before his appointment at Vinton, he had put in thirty years as teacher and principal in the Iowa public school system. Applied to his present post, his experience as an educator had brought about important changes in the curriculum and in teaching methods for the 100 blind boys and girls who lived at the school nine months of the year. Before his retirement in 1939, Superintendent Palmer was to see the school's enrollment nearly doubled and its program acknowledged to be one of the most progressive in the nation. He was also to see the inaccurate designation "college" dropped, and the name changed to Iowa School for the Blind. (Subsequent years saw yet another name change to Iowa Braille and Sight Saving School—a far remove from what the school was called when it was founded in 1853: the Asylum for the Instruction of the Blind.)

Palmer had called on all his powers of generalship to get the school's premises ready for the incoming delegates. The school's teachers, as well as its matrons, its farm hands, and its maintenance staff, had all been dragooned into service. Dormitories had been scrubbed and refurbished. Teachers had arranged to double up, or to board with families in town, so the conventioneers could use their private rooms. Classrooms had been readied for committee meetings and group sessions. The school's piano and pipe organ were freshly tuned. All the outbuildings—the gymnasium with its small swimming pool, the greenhouse, the industrial arts

13

building, the hospital, the carpentry shop—had been put in apple-pie order. Ditto the barns which housed the herd of Holsteins, the horses which worked in the grain fields, and the brood nests of the chicken flock.

Palmer and his staff were not expected to cope unassisted with the reception and registration of the delegates. Key officers of the AAWB had arrived a day earlier. The most important of these—and the man on whose shoulders rested the responsibility for leading this 1921 convention to the accomplishment of a single, overriding purpose—was a courtly southerner, Henry Randolph Latimer, then completing his first two-year term as president of the Association. The organization's first vice-president, Sherman C. Swift of Toronto, had not been able to make it to Vinton, but its second vice-president, Kate M. Foley, had come east from San Francisco, and the secretary, Charles B. Hayes, had arrived from Boston. Of the four, Hayes was the only sighted person.

At the opening session that Thursday evening Palmer made a short speech to greet the delegates; the pastor of the Vinton Presbyterian Church intoned a prayer; "America" was sung to piano accompaniment; there were welcoming addresses by the mayor of Vinton, the president of the Iowa State Board of Education and the speaker of the Iowa House of Representatives. At the reception which followed, the delegates sipped lemonade and fruit punch as they milled around, renewing old friendships and meeting some of their newer colleagues.

Attracting a major share of attention were the "Great Triumvirate" in education, the superintendents of the largest and oldest residential schools for the blind: sixty-year-old Edward Ellis Allen of the Perkins Institution for the Blind in Watertown, Massachusetts; Olin H. Burritt, fifty-four, of the Pennsylvania Institution for the Instruction of the Blind; and Edward M. Van Cleve, fifty-four, of the New York (City) Institute for the Education of the Blind.

The AAWB was not the principal power base of Allen, Burritt, Van Cleve, and their colleagues in education. They had a separate national body, the American Association of Instructors of the Blind (AAIB), which in those days met in the even-numbered years, leaving the odd-numbered years for the biennial conventions of the AAWB.

In 1921—as in the preceding decades—the AAIB (currently known as AEVH, Association for the Education of the Visually Handicapped) was the senior group in every sense. Founded in 1871, it antedated the AAWB; more important, because it had a single focus, it had been a cohesive group from the start. In an era when virtually all public expenditures for the blind were devoted to education and thus funneled through the schools for blind children, the school superintendents served as the undisputed experts on all aspects of blindness. Legislatures called upon them for counsel, the public looked to them for leadership, and the generations of blind children educated in their schools seldom wished, or dared, to challenge their authority.

The AAWB, on the other hand, had suffered several false starts before defining a workable role for itself. It had begun, in point of fact, with a purely educational goal. As described in an official history of the association:

> In 1895, at St. Louis, Missouri, the forerunner of the AAWB came into being. At that time, a group of individuals who were concerned about educational opportunities for the blind formed the American Blind People's

Higher Education and General Improvement Association, and for several years thereafter this group met to consider methods by which blind and visually impaired persons might have an opportunity to advance themselves in the society of those days. . . .

These early pioneers advocated: (1) a specialized college to serve the blind; (2) Governmental scholarships for the blind; (3) non-segregated admission to existing institutions of higher learning; and (4) the annex theory, which was a combination of the first two suggestions, namely, that scholarships be provided and a segregated unit be established in an existing college or university specifically designed to meet the needs of the blind.

By 1905, the group was ready to admit the failure of its efforts to interest federal or state officials in financing any such program. Simultaneously, however, it recognized that there were many other problems it might usefully tackle in the realm of "general improvement." At the 1905 convention the group changed its name to American Association of Workers for the Blind and formulated a new philosophy: "We ask that blind persons be given an opportunity to earn their own living. We do not approve any system to pauperize them. We are not asking for them a degrading pension, or the abstract glories of higher education."

With this broadened focus, the conferees then included on their agenda such items as industrial education, employment, standardization of a tactual reading system, the welfare of elderly blind persons, boarding homes and other housing arrangements for blind adults, nurseries for blind babies, and home teaching services for adults. At the next biennial convention, four major committees were designated to deal with the ongoing problems of higher education, federal pensions, a uniform system of embossed type, and the prevention of blindness.

Unlike the AAIB, which restricted its membership to educators, the AAWB maintained open membership rolls and encouraged the participation of interested lay persons as well as all categories of personnel engaged in all types of work for blind persons of all ages. This wide-open membership policy naturally encompassed the educators who were AAIB members; most school administrators belonged to both associations.

In a sense, the two associations constituted a kind of bicameral parliament, with the AAIB in the role of the smaller, more exclusive upper house and the AAWB in the role of the more popularly representative lower house. It became the custom for most major issues to be debated twice: one year at the AAIB convention and the next year at the AAWB meeting, or vice versa. As the mutuality of some of these issues came to be recognized, the two associations established joint committees. Notable among these was the Commission on Uniform Type, which had been in existence since 1915 to seek a solution to the troublesome question of a standardized tactual system for finger-readers.

At Vinton, that summer of 1921, the major agenda item before the AAWB had been considered by the AAIB the previous year. This was the question of forming a new kind of national organization that might be able to accomplish, in a systematic and coordinated way, those objectives that were clearly beyond the reach of loose-knit membership groups that got together for a few days every two years.

There was not a single delegate at the Vinton meeting who did not have a direct stake in the outcome of this question. Every organization engaged in work for the blind, from the long-established residential schools to the smallest and newest local voluntary agencies, stood in need of the kind of coordination and centralized research and leadership that could only be provided by a strong national body. Not too strong, some of the delegates demurred privately: there must be no interference with local dominion. But even the doubters were persuaded that, with suitable safeguards, such a national body could be servant rather than master, and that it could prove to be a convenience in many ways.

By and large, the important divisions in work for the blind were well represented at Vinton. Key school people other than the "Great Triumvirate" were on hand, among them superintendents of the schools for the blind in Jacksonville, Illinois, Baton Rouge, Louisiana, and Macon, Georgia, as well as the superintendent of one of the dual schools which still existed in various parts of the country: the Virginia School for the Deaf and Blind. And, of course, there was Francis Palmer. Latimer himself was a school man: at the time of the convention, he held the position of head teacher of the Maryland School for the Blind. His boss, Superintendent John F. Bledsoe of the Maryland School, was also there, as was Ambrose M. Shotwell, librarian of the Michigan School for the Blind, who had been a leading spirit in guiding AAWB out of its early parochialism.

Present, too, were leaders of the new and ultimately to become the dominant direction of education for blind children, the advocates of day school programs. Notable among them were fifty-year-old John B. Curtis of Chicago, who had pioneered by establishing the nation's first classes for blind children in public schools, and Robert B. Irwin, a dozen years his junior, who had introduced Curtis' methods in Cleveland and other cities in Ohio. In 1921 Irwin bore the title of supervisor, Department of the Blind, Cleveland Board of Education.

The steadily expanding diversity of work for blind adults was implicit in the range of interests represented by other delegates. There was Eben Morford, superintendent of the Industrial Home for the Blind in Brooklyn, New York, a voluntary agency specializing in vocational services through sheltered workshops and industrial placement programs. There was Charles W. Holmes, a Canadian educated at the Perkins Institution, who had left his post with the Massachusetts Commission for the Blind to organize the industrial and other service programs of the newly formed Canadian National Institute for the Blind. There was young Joseph F. Clunk, then executive secretary for the Youngstown, Ohio, Association for the Blind, who had already given a convincing preview of the extraordinary career he would pursue in placement of blind industrial workers side by side with the sighted.

The field of social work, rapidly coalescing into a profession, also drew its share of practitioners to Vinton. Prominent among the trailblazers in this area of work was Calvin S. Glover, secretary of the Cincinnati Association for the Welfare of the Blind, who was slated to report to the convention on behalf of its Legislative Committee. Present, too, were "Colonel" L.L. Watts, executive secretary of the Virginia Legislative Commission for the Blind, an acknowledged leader in demonstrating the ability of a state agency to deliver a wide range of services to blind adults and children, and Murray B. Allen, executive secretary of the newly organized Utah Commission for the Blind. Four additional state agencies were represented at Vinton: Massachusetts, California, Michigan, and Missouri. As of

1921, there existed only a handful of such state commissions; it was to take three full decades before virtually every state in the union had a comparable body.

Home teaching, which was then the major service given by most state agencies, was personified by Kate M. Foley of California, probably the nation's best-known exponent of this type of work. Miss Foley, a middle-aged woman who had been born lame as well as blind, was an eloquent writer and speaker on the subject of how significantly the visiting teacher could enrich the lives of homebound blind adults.

A number of voluntary agencies had also sent delegates to Vinton. In addition to Glover of Cincinnati and Morford of Brooklyn, program participants included both the president and executive director of the Chicago Lighthouse, the director of the Duluth Lighthouse, the executives of the Cleveland and Minneapolis Societies for the Blind, and the head of the Illinois Society for the Prevention of Blindness.

On the program to lead a round table on Embossed Literature for the Blind were two women who had already made their mark in library service and were to go on to even more notable accomplishments in the years ahead. One was Gertrude T. Rider, head of the Service for the Blind of the Library of Congress; she had initiated braille transcribing by volunteers. The other was Lucille A. Goldthwaite, in charge of the Department for the Blind of the New York (City) Public Library. It was to be ten years before the federal government would take the responsibility for supplying blind adults with reading matter; in 1921, when finger-readers were dependent on the private collections of the larger local libraries, the operation headed by Miss Goldthwaite represented a major source of embossed literature in more than a dozen states.

Three men and two women on the program at Vinton wore name badges that identified them with a new adjunct in work for the blind: the Federal Board for Vocational Education.

A year earlier, President Woodrow Wilson had signed the Smith-Fess Act which authorized the expenditure of $750,000 in the 1921 fiscal year for a joint federal-state program of vocational rehabilitation for the physically handicapped. This civilian program was put under the direction of the Federal Board for Vocational Education, which two years earlier had been given charge of similar measures on behalf of disabled veterans. The delegates were curious to hear what the board's vice-chairman, James P. Munroe, would have to say in his scheduled address: "What the United States Government Is Prepared to Do for the Civilian Blind." They would also listen with interest to the reports given at succeeding round tables by two of the federal board's vocational agents who were operating at the state level—Florence Birchard in Massachusetts and Ada Turner in Wisconsin—as well as to talks by Lewis H. Carris, the federal board's assistant director of industrial rehabilitation, and Arthur E. Holmes, supervisor for the blind in the board's Washington office.

The delegates were not overly sanguine. The Federal Board for Vocational Education's work with war-blinded soldiers had thus far been disappointing. There was little reason to think civilians would fare much better. Few states had passed the necessary legislation that would enable them to take advantage of the federal funds made available under the Smith-Fess Act. Most discouraging of all was the fact that in those states that did have enabling laws, most blinded veterans were being more or less arbitrarily classified as "nonfeasible" for vocational rehabilitation.

These doubts proved to be well founded. As it turned out, blind people profited little under Smith-Fess; it was to take 23 years and another world war before the Barden-LaFollette amendments would give the Vocational Rehabilitation Act the necessary sinews to make a real difference in their lives.

A similar time lag was to characterize the once bright hopes for the first large-scale experiment in rehabilitation of blinded soldiers at Evergreen, a handsome estate on the outskirts of Baltimore that had been loaned to the Army early in 1918 for use as a training center for war-blinded servicemen.

Although Evergreen was not phased out of existence until 1925, its fundamental weaknesses were already apparent in 1921. Nevertheless, the delegates at Vinton looked forward to the scheduled talk: "What We Have Learned from Our War-Blinded Which Can Be of Use in Our Work with Civilian Blind." It was not so much the subject that intrigued them as the speaker, Charles F.F. Campbell, easily the most colorful figure in work for the blind and one of the most popular. Anything that Charlie Campbell had to say was sure to be entertaining, challenging, perhaps even outrageous, but nonetheless worth hearing.

These, then, were among the 145 assorted personalities who, following the reception that Thursday evening in June of 1921, strolled along the well-raked gravel paths of the Iowa College for the Blind to enjoy the fresh country air before retiring for the night. We will meet most of them again as the panorama of the next fifty years unrolls.

Born in rural Prince Georges County, Maryland, in 1871, Henry Randolph Latimer came from a family whose English forebears had arrived on American shores in 1667 and had been prominent in the Maryland gentry. Henry was one of six children brought up on the family acres in an atmosphere of genteel poverty. The Latimers had lost much of their substance during the Civil War, and while they retained their land, they had little cash available. Both Henry and his sister, Lillian Emmeline, were born with poor vision. Until Henry was ten years old, however, he lived at home.

"Though I was as blind as a chicken by night," he wrote in an autobiographical sketch published in 1914,

> and had very little sight by day, I took my chances with my four brothers on the farm, doing my share of everything that came to hand, chopping wood, feeding cattle, and even rounding up stock in the pasture and milking as many as five cows at one sitting. . . . At six years of age, I entered the local public school, where, for four years, I kept abreast of my classes, leading them in mathematics. I did my work with crayon, soapstone and lead pencils, pen and ink, like other boys, with the exception that the lines on foolscap paper were made much heavier for me to see. Books in very bold print, of the pictorial type, were used to teach me to read. My lessons were regularly taught me at home by my mother or aunt, the latter being the local school teacher. Upon her removal to a school too remote for me to attend daily, my parents, with much reluctance, entered me at the Maryland School for the Blind, in Baltimore, in 1881.

At this school, which his sister soon entered as well, Latimer remained for 9 years as a student and, after graduation, for 30 years as a staff member. From his first assignment, that of foreman of the school's mattress and caning shop, he moved into teaching in the separate Department for Colored Blind and Deaf, where he served for 12 years before being transferred back to the main school. There he rose, by gradual stages, to the position of head teacher.

Simultaneously, Latimer pursued his own education. In 1892 he matriculated at Illinois Wesleyan University as a non-resident student in a correspondence course leading to a Ph.B. degree. Because he had little time to study (and also because, in 1894, he suffered an attack of typhoid fever which not only turned his hair white but destroyed his remaining vision), it took him seven years to complete the work. A year after receiving his bachelor's degree, he took a summer course at Harvard which earned him a certificate in Theory and History of Education.

The introduction to a wider world which Latimer gained through his studies led him to perceive the weaknesses that resulted from educating children in the cloistered atmosphere of the traditional school for the blind. The pattern of academic paternalism tended to stifle the impulse toward independent thought and action. Habits of dependency were hard to overcome in later life, Latimer found, when, from his base at the school, he reached out into adult work and instigated formation of the Maryland Association of Workers for the Blind to promote rehabilitation and employment of the state's blind men and women. It was his success here, added to the reputation developed out of his effective participation in several national projects, that had brought him to a major crossroads in his career. On his return home from Vinton, Latimer would pack his belongings and leave both Maryland and the field of education for Pittsburgh and full-time work for the adult blind. He would be the new executive secretary of the Pennsylvania Association for the Blind.

In his presidential address to the AAWB, Latimer presented not only a proposal but a detailed plan—complete with drafts of a certificate of incorporation, a constitution, and set of bylaws—for the creation of a new national body to be known as the American Foundation for the Blind. He asked the delegates to endorse the proposal, to enact the enabling resolution, to adopt the constitution and bylaws, and to appoint the incorporators who would bring this new body into legal existence.

Latimer had few misgivings as to the outcome. His preparatory work had been thorough. He was springing no surprises. The delegates had known for many months that this 1921 convention would center on a single theme.

"The Executive Committee of the American Association of Workers for the Blind," read the carefully phrased notice sent out with the preliminary program for the Vinton meeting,

> is responding to what it senses as the general wish of the most thoughtful workers for the blind of the United States and Canada. . . . that there should be in work for the blind some sort of General Foundation representative of and responsive to every important phase or branch of the profession. . . . It is very essential therefore that opportunity should be given for the fullest possible discussion of the question and it is to this end that the committee ventures to depart from the usual mixed program and submit one bearing almost entirely upon the topic uppermost in the public mind.

In his presidential address Latimer detailed the steps he had taken to translate these tentative ideas into concrete form, and the precautions he had observed in insuring the soundness of his proposals for such a foundation:

> We were neither reckless nor hasty in our manner of approach. In the first place, your president made it his personal business to ascertain, as far as the time and means at his disposal admitted, whether the profession generally, and certain persons in particular, would lend their support to such a program. In this connection it is gratifying to report that, while some skepticism as to the outcome was expressed, virtually everyone approved the undertaking and bade us Godspeed in the effort.
>
> In the second place, it seemed advisable that every possible precaution should be taken to avoid wrangling, destructive criticism, and other unprofitable discussion here at the convention. To this end, in assigning the topics for discussion, each speaker was asked . . . to point out in what respect his particular branch of the work could be advanced by the cooperation of a properly organized general agency in work for the blind.

Moreover, his text continued, "it seemed that something more concrete still must be done if any real organization was to result." A constitution and bylaws had therefore been drafted and circulated, first to the executive committee and then to:

> as many other persons as the time and means at hand permitted, including Messrs. E.E. Allen, Charles F.F. Campbell, W.G. Holmes, R.B. Irwin, M.C. Migel, E.P. Morford, J.F. Bledsoe, C.D. Chadwick, W.I. Scandlin, O.H. Burritt, E.H. Fowler, C.W. Holmes, E.M. Van Cleve, T.S. McAloney, G.S. Wilson, Dr. James Bordley, Miss Susan B. Merwin, and Lady Francis J. Campbell. The criticisms and suggestions received from these various sources were unusually helpful . . . and [in their light] the articles were redrafted and submitted for proper legal advice to my lawyer, Mr. W. Howard Hamilton of Baltimore.

It was Hamilton, a prominent attorney with influential business and social connections in Maryland, who had drafted the necessary papers in proper legal form, "giving free of charge both his own services and those of his office force."

In addition to all of these precautions, Latimer went on to tell the assemblage, "in order that no false step . . . should be taken, and in order that the sanest available counsels might prevail," a conference on the whole question had been held in May in New York City. He listed those in attendance, swelling the impressive roster he had already recited with additional prestigious names: Lewis H. Carris, Mrs. Rider, Miss Goldthwaite and Grace S. Harper, executive secretary of the New York State Commission for the Blind.

Latimer's peroration was characteristic of the peacemaking propensity that had won him the confidence and support of so many warring factions. It was also a fair sample of his somewhat overblown literary style:

> And now, my dear friends, why have we come to Vinton? To suspect and to discount, to wrangle and to backbite, to circumvent and to destroy? Not so, I pray you, most emphatically not so! Unless I am entirely wrong in my diagnosis of the human heart, we have come here prepared to fraternize and

to counsel, to confide and to commend, to cooperate and to construct; and, by the grace of God, we shall go forward to the consummation of one of the greatest achievements yet known to work for the blind.

The low-keyed tone of Latimer's presidential address proved to be precisely right. There had been enough rousing oratory in the past. A year earlier, at the 25th biennial convention of the AAIB, L.W. Wallace, director of the Red Cross Institute for the Blind at Evergreen, had delivered a blunt, hard-hitting address calling for the creation of a national vocational institute for the blind:

> The work being done for the blind in the United States today is sadly deficient, because of the lack of an authoritative central organization to coordinate and to crystallize and to stimulate the work. This is evidenced by the great lack of uniformity in character of and functions of the agencies dealing with the problem, and by the total absence of properly delegated agencies in some localities. . . . The majority of the agencies dealing with the question of the blind have been so limited in authority, in means and in trained personnel that they have not realized the full possibilities.

This situation, he said, could be overcome if there were a national body composed of three major arms. One would be a Bureau of Information "to collect, codify and to disseminate the most authoritative information to be had in the world on all questions pertaining to the blind." The second would be a Bureau of Research "liberally financed and . . . unhampered in scope of activity, in authority and in freedom of action," that would investigate the education of blind youth, survey the occupations already open to the blind, and identify others with practical possibilities in industry, commerce and agriculture; it would "determine, standardize, codify and disseminate" the most efficient ways for the blind to perform given operations and would, in general, serve as a living laboratory "in accord with the best practice . . . in practically every important and progressive phase of human activity." The third—and most important—arm would be a Bureau of Education responsible for educating and training workers for the blind, and blind themselves, the employer, and the public.

Special attention, he emphasized, "should be given to the training of the placement personnel. . . . Very often the placement or the employment agent has been a glaring example of misplacement himself. In many, many instances he has been a gross misfit because of the lack of proper training, unsuited personality, inexperience and limited knowledge of the factors involved."

If Wallace was hard on those who worked with and for the blind, his judgment of their clients was even harsher:

> The possibilities of vocational activity for the blind will never be realized until there is a change of attitude on the part of many of the blind themselves. . . . The attitude that many of the blind assume or acquire, or it may be a part of their natural psychology, is one of the greatest drawbacks to their development and opportunity. What do I mean? It is this, they are supersensitive, critical and unappreciative. They lack ambition and determination. They lack the spirit to will, to do. They are too prone to accept and not to earn.

But there was not much use in attempting the education of the employer or the public at large, he concluded, until "our own house is in order." This would happen when the national body acquired extensive financial backing, a sound, aggressive administration, and widespread professional support "free of unjust and destructive criticism and petty jealousy."

Perhaps it was because Wallace had stepped on so many toes. Perhaps it was because his listeners interpreted his remarks as an irked response to the criticism that had been so freely leveled at Evergreen. Perhaps it was because Wallace was an outsider (when his appointment as general manager of Evergreen was announced by the Red Cross, the *Outlook for the Blind* had blandly identified him as "late of Purdue University, and one of the best railway experts in the United States"). Whatever the reason, Wallace's speech to the AAIB's convention in 1920 had brought about passage of a resolution whose guarded wording hardly constituted a clarion call to action:

> Resolved, that this Association would welcome the cooperation of some wisely organized agency for assisting and improving the vocational education and the employment of the blind of this country, such as has been outlined at this convention by Director Wallace of the Red Cross Institute for the Blind.

What Larimer had done was to incorporate the affirmative substance of Wallace's talk while omitting the finger-pointing. The drafts circulated to the delegates of the proposed constitution and bylaws set forth an operating structure for the American Foundation for the Blind consisting of the very same three bureaus Wallace had recommended. Their scope, however, had been broadened to cover wider ground than vocational education and employment. The articles spelling out the respective functions of the three bureaus remained unchanged for thirty years. And even then, when a 1951 revision of the bylaws eliminated the provisions for specific bureaus, the substance of the foundation's purposes, although modernized and rephrased in more general terms, did not differ in essence from what was set forth in 1921.

The Bureau of Information and Publicity was charged with gathering and disseminating data on all organizations and schools in work for the blind, on existing and potential vocational pursuits, on teaching methods, on legislation, on methods of producing reading matter, and on all other subjects touching on the welfare of blind persons. The Bureau of Research was to "ascertain, develop and standardize, by comparison, experimentation and otherwise, the best methods " in these same areas, while the Bureau of Education was to "improve every facility for preparing the blind and the partially blind for the greatest possible participation in the activities and enjoyments of life" through teacher training, curriculum reform, scholarships for higher education, development of vocational instruction facilities, stimulation of better quality and greater quantity of embossed literature, and cooperation in efforts to prevent blindness.

There must have been some at Vinton who gulped a little at the vast canvas laid out for an organization that had yet to accumulate a dime's worth of assets. But of much greater interest to the delegates than what the new organization would do was the question of who would control it. This thorny issue had been carefully spelled out in Article V of the bylaws. There would be a corporate membership body which would meet annually to elect a governing body of 15 trustees, 10 of whom would be nominated by, and represent, special interest groups: residential schools, public school classes for blind and partially sighted children, librarians, embossing plants, prevention-of-blindness groups, statewide associations and commissions, workshops and industrial homes, citywide associations and clubs, direct service agencies and institutions and agencies engaged in charitable works.

As to the remaining five trustees, two were to be nominated by the membership at each convention of the AAIB and three by the membership of the AAWB.

How to structure the governing board in such a way as to satisfy all and overlook none of the major departments of work for the blind had been Latimer's most difficult problem. The two dozen people he consulted in advance had offered differing views. One of the most trenchant was voiced by Dr. James Bordley, Jr., a Baltimore ophthalmologist, who had acted as the first director of the Red Cross Institute at Evergreen while simultaneously wearing the uniform of an Army lieutenant colonel in his capacity as the U.S. Surgeon General's representative at the training center for blinded soldiers. He wrote Latimer on March 7:

> I am convinced that to succeed, a national institute must have a firm financial foundation, that that foundation must not be built up by small donations from strictly interested workers. . . . There is but one way to get the necessary money—a harmonious, generalized movement. On this point I have had experience. Believing that through certain influences we could reach a large sum of money, the Red Cross Institute undertook to gather it in for the work for the Nation's blind, only to have our efforts thwarted by certain workers for the blind. . . . You should have on your Board not only professional workers for the blind but men entirely outside of the work, men of large business experience, men who wield national influence, men who can find the money necessary to capitalize the work. . . .
>
> The great trouble with work for the blind is its restriction to its own workers. I am convinced that any movement to succeed must be a broader movement. You must encourage outside assistance, outside criticism and outside interest in your every undertaking.

As things turned out, it took very little time for the soundness of Dr. Bordley's suggestions to become evident to all. No sooner had the Foundation been incorporated, and before it even opened its offices, the bylaws were amended to enlarge the number of trustees from 15 to 25. The 10 special interest classes remained, but the remaining 15 trustees were to be "chosen from among persons of influence" by the executive committee. Thus control of the Foundation's destinies would pass out of the parochial circle of workers for the blind and into the hands of the "men of large business experience, men who wield national influence, men who can find the money necessary to capitalize the work."

On June 28, 1921, at the concluding business meeting of the ninth biennial convention of the AAWB, the delegates voted, without a dissenting voice, to adopt the enabling resolution authorizing "a properly constituted organization to cooperate with all existing agencies in work for the blind and the partially blind, and to do such other things as are not, or cannot be, done by the existing agencies."

Latimer, Campbell and Waldo Newcomer, president of the Maryland School for the Blind, were named to act as incorporators; the last-named proved unable to serve and was replaced by James H. Preston, a former mayor of Baltimore, when the corporate papers were filed in Delaware the next month.

Following adoption of the enabling resolution, the delegates proceeded to nominate and elect the first board of trustees of the American Foundation for the Blind:

> J. Robert Atkinson, Los Angeles; Mrs. Emmons Blaine, Chicago; Arthur E. Bostwick, St. Louis; George W. Brown, Boston; Olin H. Burritt, Philadelphia; Randall J. Condon, Cincinnati; (Mrs. Homer) Mabel Knowles Gage, Worcester, Mass.; W. Howard Hamilton, Baltimore; James C. Jones, St. Louis; Charles W. Lindsay, Montreal; M.C. Migel, New York; William Fellowes Morgan, New York; Prudence Sherwin, Cleveland; Felix M. Warburg, New York; Herbert H. White, Hartford, Conn.

Then, among other business, came the election of AAWB officers. Latimer won a second term as president. Joseph J. Murphy was elected treasurer, but poor health soon forced him to resign. Named to fill his unexpired term was a fast-rising star: Robert B. Irwin.

3

Talent Hunt

The American Foundation for the Blind may have been smoothly born, but it barely survived early infancy. A great many things went wrong in the first few years.

Moses Charles Migel, the man everyone had in mind for the presidency of the new organization, was out of the country when the trustees held their first meeting in New York City in November 1921. This meant that a president *pro tem* would be needed, and Olin H. Burritt accepted the post.

Lewis H. Carris, the trustees' first choice as director general of the Foundation, decided to accept another job instead; he became executive head of the National Society for the Prevention of Blindness. To keep the Foundation afloat, Henry Latimer was persuaded to become the part-time acting director.

Several trustees, nominated and elected *in absentia* at Vinton, declined to serve.

There was not even enough money for postage until, at the first meeting of the trustees, the blind Canadian piano manufacturer Charles W. Lindsay pledged $1,000, contingent on an additional $9,000 being secured. One of the two women present, Prudence Sherwin, promptly subscribed $1,000; a few days later, a check in the same amount came in the mail from the other woman, Mrs. Homer Gage. This alleviated the initial financial crisis until January 1922 when, Migel having returned to New York, the executive committee offered him the presidency and he accepted, effective on his return from another European trip. In the meantime, according to the executive committee minutes of January 23, "Mr. Migel donated $7,000 towards getting the Foundation under way" and the committee promptly voted "to inform Mr. Lindsay that the $9,000 requirement had been met and we would now appreciate his check for $1,000."

The interim period until Migel assumed the presidency on June 1, 1922, was not an idle one. Latimer lost no time in sending out feelers for staff recruits. He wrote Charles B. Hayes in Boston about his possible availability to head the proposed Bureau of Information and Publicity, and to Robert B. Irwin in Cleveland, the man who seemed the logical candidate to organize the Bureau of Research. Both men responded with guarded interest, although both demurred over the low salaries mentioned.

Simultaneously, Latimer was pursuing every lead suggested by the trustees and others for a man who might be suitable for the permanent director general's post. There were some who urged that Latimer himself should be the appointee, but Latimer knew this would put him in a ticklish position: he would be charged with having brought the Foundation into being so as to create a job for himself. There were, however, countervailing factors to be considered. These were spelled out by Irwin in a letter marked "personal" he wrote Latimer on December 12, 1921:

> I feel that it would be a fearful mistake if a man is appointed who would be subservient to the opinions of a certain small group of the present superintendents. . . . It would be infinitely better for you to remain as Director General than to have a protege of one of the leading superintendents appointed to this place.

Latimer, however, never lost sight of the fact that what the trustees were after was "a competent sighted man generally acceptable to the profession." The stumbling block was, as he put it in a confidential letter to a friend, the question of whether

> such a BIG man can be found for the money available to get him. Men really worth while . . . are usually settled in their life's work, and if they are not, there is likely some defect in them not at first apparent but which may wreck any undertaking upon which they may set out. It might be better after all . . . to build up a man rather than try to find one already full grown and full blown.

Robert Irwin's fear that the new Foundation might become the captive of the old guard led him to put in an oar where it would count—with M.C. Migel. He wrote the philanthropist a long, shrewd letter on January 17, 1922, in which he urged (perhaps gratuitously) that Migel accept the presidency because, unless the Foundation "is absolutely above all suspicion of petty politics and personal pull it can never become the factor in the work for the blind which I feel confident it can be made."

The problem Latimer had raised off the record, Irwin was bold enough to voice out loud. The Foundation would have to revise its ideas about a $6,000 salary for a director general, he wrote Migel. A figure of $10,000 would be more like it. Moreover—and here Irwin was doing some spade work concerning the job he himself had an eye on—"if you are to draw the highest type of experts in the profession to act as heads of departments you will have to pay $5,000 or $6,000."

The search for a director general proved exasperatingly elusive, even though Migel, once he assumed the presidency, took an active role in the talent hunt. He went up to Columbia University to consult President Nicholas Murray Butler concerning possible candidates. He solicited suggestions from his wide acquaintanceship in business and philanthropy. He was quite clear about his objectives. "This man need not necessarily be familiar with Blind work," he wrote to the official of a large foundation in August,

> but should be of the highest type—if possible, known throughout the coun-

try—, of good address and tact, and he should be able, in addition to his other duties, to assist in raising funds for the Foundation. A man having had experience in the latter might be of great advantage.

Our present idea of the salary for the Director General might be approximately eight thousand dollars ($8,000) annually. . . . I might be willing, personally, to guarantee the salary for several years to the *proper* man, if necessary. . . .

More than a dozen possible candidates were weighed, discreetly investigated, approached or dropped from consideration in the spring, summer, and fall of 1922. The best prospects turned the offer down. Migel found that his personal guarantee of salary did not offer sufficient assurance to men secure in good jobs. By October Migel saw the problem in broader perspective:

We have come to the conclusion that the proper method for the Foundation to function in a serious way would be to have same underwritten for a period of, say, three years, with a minimum of $25,000 yearly. Amongst ourselves, as Trustees, we have already agreed to underwrite the Foundation for practically $15,000 yearly for three years, I agreeing to subscribe $10,000 yearly. It was also agreed upon to increase our Board of Trustees with the understanding that any future Trustee would have sufficient interest in the Foundation to agree to underwrite same for a sum of not less than $1,000 yearly for a period of three years, . . .

The Foundation's archives do not reveal the precise channels which brought Dr. Joseph C. Nate into the picture, but before the end of the year he had been hired, to begin work as director general on January 1, 1923, at a salary of $8,000. Hayes and Irwin had also been engaged, at $4,800 each, as directors of the Information and Research bureaus respectively, effective February 1. A two-room office was rented on the seventh floor of the Hartford Building at 41 Union Square West in New York City, a typist and a secretary-bookkeeper were hired, and the Foundation announced that it was now formally in business.

The new director general was a complete stranger to virtually everyone in work for the blind. Joseph C. Nate had been a lawyer early in his career, and had then become a minister, entering the Methodist Episcopal Church in 1899. He had held pastorates in a number of midwestern cities, one of which was Jacksonville, Illinois, where the Illinois School for the Blind was located. His casual contacts with the school were apparently the sum total of his knowledge of work for the blind. However, in Jacksonville he had demonstrated a talent for fund-raising which had brought about the construction of an impressive new church building. This had led to a position in charge of a statewide drive to raise a million dollar fund for six church-connected educational institutions. Success in this and related promotional endeavors had then brought him into church work on a national scale. In 1920 he moved to New York City to become assistant secretary of the Board of Education of the Methodist Episcopal Church. This was the post he left to accept the job of director general of the American Foundation for the Blind.

It proved to be a sad mistake, both for Nate and for the Foundation. In less than a year, his resignation was requested at the insistence of the Foundation's president, with whom he had apparently clashed head-on.

What little is known about the exact circumstances emerges from a letter Latimer wrote on October 11, 1923, to his good friend and fellow trustee, W. Howard Hamilton:

> Mr. Nate, the Director-General of the American Foundation for the Blind, and our President, Mr. Migel, have become hopelessly involved in a controversy over the administration of the work. Mr. Nate has not measured up at all to Mr. Migel's expectations, and Mr. Migel requested his resignation. . . . I am not surprised at the outcome so far as Mr. Nate is concerned, as he has not seemed to have the capacity for bringing matters to a happy conclusion notwithstanding the reputation he seems to have enjoyed when he came to us a year ago. Mr. Migel has offered him even so much as a year's salary in advance if he will resign and leave the coast clear for another man, but Mr. Nate does not seem disposed to follow this suggestion.

The Reverend Doctor Nate had occasion to regret this refusal. Under the settlement that was ultimately arranged, his resignation took effect January 1, 1924, with his salary continued, up to a maximum of six months, until he located other work.

Perhaps it was because the Nate incident had left an unpleasant taste all around. Perhaps it was because Migel concluded that if he wanted something done right, he would have to do it himself. Whatever the reason, no further effort was made for the next four and one-half years to find a new director general. During this period Migel assumed decision-making powers in administrative as well as policy matters. The degree of control that came into his hands was seldom to slacken, even after the Foundation was being run by a fully effective executive director, until he relinquished the presidency in 1945.

One factor that certainly played a part in Migel's decision to run the Foundation himself was his satisfaction with its two bureau chiefs, Hayes and Irwin. These two had more than lived up to expectations. Even better, they made a good team, if only because they were so different from one another in background, temperament, and interests.

Charles Bishop Hayes brought to the Foundation three separate areas of relevant experience developed since graduation from Clark College in his native city of Worcester, Massachusetts.

He had been an educator—a teacher, and later the director of several private and public schools. He understood the principles of social work, having studied at the New York School of Philanthropy, forerunner of the Columbia University Graduate School of Social Work. He had amassed a good deal of organizational and administrative experience in work for the blind. For five years he had been connected with the Brooklyn Exchange and Training School for the Blind, an adjunct of the Brooklyn Association for Improving the Condition of the Poor. Thereafter, in 1917, he had been called back to his native state as general superintendent of the newly reorganized Massachusetts State Commission for the Blind. Here he had put to use not only his organizational talents but also the promotional methods tested and perfected in Brooklyn, where he had successfully organized the first of the educational exhibits known as "Weeks for the Blind."

Forty-one years old when he began work as director of the Bureau of Information and Publicity, Hayes was well known nationally. As secretary of the AAWB, he had worked hand in hand with Henry Latimer in organizing the Vinton meeting. He had as thorough an understanding as any man of the extent of public ignorance and indifference where the welfare of blind people was concerned. But he also knew there were ways to overcome this, and he was eager to demonstrate them.

Known to one and all as Charlie, Hayes was a man of jovial disposition. In his workaday life, he was apt to be seen in gartered shirt sleeves, his tie slightly askew, his glasses dangling precariously from the bridge of his nose, and his hair rumpled by the fingers he absentmindedly ran through it as he juggled the correspondence, manuscripts, and railroad timetables piled up on one of the second-hand roll-top desks with which the Foundation's early quarters were thriftily furnished.

Hayes' assignments called on the full range of his abilities, particularly his organizing skill. One of his earliest projects was to assist local communities to put on "Weeks for the Blind" of the kind that had proven so effective in Brooklyn. Henry Latimer was first in line to request Hayes' help in developing such a program for Pittsburgh. It was an unqualified success. As recounted in the Foundation's first annual report:

> Churches, Women's Clubs, Men's Clubs, Radio broadcasting stations, and countless individuals united in one splendid effort to stimulate the interest of the people of Pittsburgh in the work done for and by the Blind in that community. The President of the Board of Managers of the Western Pennsylvania School stated that this Educational Campaign which the Foundation put on, had done more in one week to show the citizens of Pittsburgh what the Blind are capable of doing, and their need of opportunity and assistance, than the Associations had been able to do in twenty years.

There were several layers of significance to this early venture, and that first annual report made a special point of the most telling: "It is one of the important purposes of the Foundation to be of service to states wishing to develop plans for improving the condition of their blind population. . . . The Foundation is in a position to bring to such states the fruits of the experience of other sections of the country which have developed splendid agencies for the Blind after many years of study and experimentation."

What underlay this statement was the recognition that the Foundation's existence was viewed with trepidation in many places. A speech made to the Indiana Association for the Blind by Latimer, when he was still the acting director general, faced this issue frankly:

> There is a more or less ill defined fear in some quarters that any country-wide organization, such as the Foundation, is likely to interfere unduly, by overstandardization of method and practice, with the special interests of particular localities. . . . There is little, if any, [such] danger. . . . So far as local and state organizations are concerned, it will be a matter of their own individual choice whether and to what degree they follow the lines which may be laid down by the Foundation as the wisest and the best in any given case.

Hayes bore this factor constantly in mind as he went about his work with local agencies. His instinctive tact and sensitivity to local pride were largely responsible for the success with which, over the years, he staged "Weeks for the Blind" in dozens of communities. One of the earliest, in Newark, New Jersey, attracted more than 25,000 people. An account of this event made careful note that "the receipts of the sale of articles went to the blind workers who had produced them. In addition, all demonstrators were paid for their services, and each child of the blind and low vision classes, out of the incidental funds raised during the Week, was given a dollar with which to start a bank account."

Once shown how, most state and local groups continued this type of program as an annual public relations activity. While the depression, followed by the war years, interrupted the practice, it was later resumed and in some cities remains a permanent feature in the continuing effort to create public awareness of the problems and the potential of blind men, women and children.

But many states lacked any sort of organizational structure to carry on work for their blind citizens. Charles Hayes, whose responsibilities made him in effect the Foundation's first director of field services, traveled across the country to tackle this fundamental problem. From the 1923 annual report:

> One of the first undertakings of the Foundation was directly in response to an appeal made by the State of Rhode Island. There are over 800 Blind in the state, and up to that time they had no Association, no Commission, no Workshop—in fact no assistance of any kind or character, with the exception of two Home Teachers. They wrote us that they desired to establish an Association and had no other source to turn to.
>
> After an active campaign, conducted by the Foundation, in which the interest and support of the Governor and the Catholic Bishop of Rhode Island were enlisted, together with that of the Mayor of Providence and two hundred representative citizens, meetings were held in Brown University. An Association to serve the entire state was formed, with a Secretary and a splendid Board of Directors. This Association is now functioning exceedingly well. Honorable William S. Flynn, Governor of the State of Rhode Island, has addressed a personal letter to the Foundation thanking us for the assistance in this matter.

And in the same report:

> In October, 1923, the Foundation was requested to send a representative to Des Moines, for a conference with the Governor and other state officials, regarding the needs of the Blind in Iowa. As a result of this conference, a tentative plan was outlined, to be used as a program for the work of the State authorities.

This kind of basic spadework was to preoccupy the Foundation for years to come, and at many different stages of development. The making of a plan, tentative or otherwise, was only the first step. There had to be enabling legislation, followed by appropriation of public funds, followed by effective programming, followed by recruitment and training of personnel. The progression was by no means automatic; frustrated local groups were to call upon the Foundation over and over again to help reactivate programs that had stalled along the way.

Another of Hayes' responsibilities was taking over editorship of the quarterly *Outlook for the Blind.* One of the most taxing demands on his versatility came a year or so after the Foundation opened its doors, when he was called upon to act as major domo of what was called "the Helen Keller Party" as it toured the United States in the Foundation's first national fund-raising drive. Of this more will be said later, but it is a revealing clue to Hayes' unflappable nature that he could cope with the conflicting, sometimes explosive, pressures that arose in these tours and yet remain in the good graces of all concerned. Even the hard-to-please Anne Sullivan Macy reacted favorably to him. "He has a genius for harmonizing conflicting individualities," she wrote the Foundation's president after the first coast-to-coast campaign tour.

The same could hardly have been said of Hayes' colleague, Robert B. Irwin, a man of an entirely different stripe. It was not merely a question of Hayes' being sighted while Irwin was blind. The more significant contrasts lay in temperament. Where Hayes was easygoing and flexible, Irwin was doggedly persistent. Where Hayes' first interest was people, Irwin was more concerned with concepts. The common touch which was second nature to Charlie required a conscious, not always successful, effort on Irwin's part. Nor was modest self effacement Robert Irwin's long suit. His undeniable strengths lay in other directions.

Robert Benjamin Irwin, born in Rockford, Iowa, on June 2, 1883, was a three-year-old tot when his parents boarded the newly completed Northern Pacific Railroad to take up a homestead on the shores of Puget Sound's North Bay, in what was then the Washington Territory. The father, a pharmacist, opened a small drugstore which also served as the post office of the tiny settlement. To feed his growing family, which ultimately numbered three sons and nine daughters, the senior Irwin supplemented his income by working in the lumber camps that dotted the area's virgin forests.

One way and another, the family got by, but just barely. Although Robert Irwin was later to lead a comfortable, financially secure life, he never forgot the taste of poverty and never stopped fearing it. Colleagues often joked, both in his presence and behind his back, about his tight-fistedness when it came to tipping waiters or picking up bar checks. They charged it up to his Scottish ancestry, but it is quite likely that carefulness with money was an enduring heritage of his youth.

A robust, venturesome child, young Robert enjoyed exploring the scenic surroundings of his new home. With his father, the little boy went fishing, clam digging, rowing to points around the bay, gathering starfish and other sea specimens, climbing the cliffs to poke a curious finger into sea pigeons' nests. The alluring memories of towering fir trees, foaming surf, and snow-capped mountains drew him back to Puget Sound when he retired from professional life in 1950.

The boy was five years old when a feverish infection, which he later described as inflammatory rheumatism, affected his eyes. According to an account written by his wife in 1945:

Olympia, the nearest city where good doctors could be found, was two days away by rowboat, the only means of transportation. His parents were young and inexperienced, and did not consider the inflammation in their little boy's eyes especially alarming. When at last they took him in the big steamer to

San Francisco to see a specialist, the sight in one eye was gone and that in the other eye was so seriously affected that in another year it too had flickered out.

The child's blindness was total; he was never again to distinguish either light or form. Although an agile mind and a fearless spirit helped him quickly find his way again in the familiar surroundings of the homestead, his parents had to face the painful decision that if their eldest son was to get an education, it could not be at home.

The same year that the Irwin family moved west, the State School for Defective Youth (now the Washington State School for the Blind) was established in the city of Vancouver, just across the Columbia River from Portland, Oregon. Like many other institutions of its day, the school housed under a single roof all types of children who needed special help with education: the blind, the deaf, and the feeble-minded. It was this institution Robert Irwin entered at the age of seven, and left in 1901 as the school's first blind graduate. He was never to live at home again, for the following September he entered the University of Washington in Seattle. During his 11 years at the school, he saw his family only during summer vacations.

The effects on a young child of separation from his family was another experience Robert Irwin never forgot. Throughout his life he favored keeping blind children at home by establishing special classes for them in the local public schools.

Irwin was also convinced, based on his own experience, that blind people could manage perfectly well in ordinary business enterprises. To earn the capital that would keep him going through four years at the University of Washington, and the three years he spent in graduate work, he had turned his hand to a variety of money-making schemes. That first summer after graduation from the school for the blind, he took a young brother as a guide and canvassed the surrounding countryside, selling stereoscopic views to farmers and townsfolk. During succeeding vacations, according to the biographical sketch written by his wife and published in the University of Washington's alumni magazine, Robert

ran a cigar stand inside one of the office buildings in downtown Seattle, he leased a house and sublet parts of it to cover the cost of his own lodging, and each summer he continued his canvassing, once on a tandem bicycle with another young man as a guide. With kettles and pans hung on the handlebars, they toured Washington and Oregon, cooking their meals and sleeping in the open. . . ."

Irwin received his A.B. in 1906. Aided by a scholarship from the University Club of Seattle, he then went east to spend a year earning a master's degree in history from the Harvard Graduate School. By then his vocational aim had crystallized: he would work in the field of education of the blind. He continued at Harvard for the next two years, taking education courses and working on a thesis, "The Administration of Schools for the Blind."

The first public announcement of the advent of this newest recruit appeared in *Outlook for the Blind* in January 1909. Referring to the thesis in preparation, a news item said that the young graduate student was "supplementing the facts derived from the special literature upon the subject and the files of reports of the various schools with a series of questionnaires to superintendents. . . . He will [also] visit several of the institutions for the blind. With this exhaustive preparation he is fitting himself to take his place in the movement for improving the condition of the sightless."

A few months later the resourceful Charles Campbell, founder and editor of the *Outlook,* remembered Irwin when organizing a symposium on the recurrent issue of whether there should be a separate college for the blind or whether the blind should try to secure passage of federal legislation to provide scholarships in existing colleges. Irwin's opinion, published in the Summer 1909 issue, recited various practical objections to a college established exclusively for the blind. Such a college would have to be "virtually a university" because its curriculum would have to embrace not only liberal arts but law, osteopathy, theology, music, and other professional specialities; it would never be able to build a sufficiently large and up-to-date reference library in tactile print; and its diploma would not carry weight with the public for a long time. Furthermore, "every educator of the blind knows the deleterious effect of collecting the blind together in isolated groups. . . . A College for the Blind would deepen the ruts out of which its students must be got before they can hope to succeed in the world with the seeing."

With equal firmness Irwin came out against automatic scholarships for every blind person aspiring to higher education. Seemingly taking it for granted that his own achievements should serve as a universal yardstick, he assumed a rather dogmatic stance:

> All that is needed by a blind man who has fight and ability enough to succeed in competition with his sighted brothers is sufficient pecuniary aid to enable him to employ all the reading he needs. He can then attend with very little handicap, any college he chooses. Any handicap which still remains is that which is his lot as a blind man. This he must face throughout his life and the sooner he faces it the better it will be for him.

By the time he left Harvard in June of 1909, Robert Irwin had already lined up a job of the kind he wanted. The Cleveland Board of Education hired him to organize that city's first day school classes for blind children. During his 14-year tenure there, he blazed a number of new trails.

It took him only a few months to reach the conclusion that children with partial sight did not belong in the same classroom as those who were totally blind. He therefore proceeded to organize one of the nation's earliest sight-saving classes for children who could function in a regular public school with proper room arrangement, good lighting, and special equipment, particularly large-type books. He established an independent non-profit company to publish such books, having first methodically experimented with different type sizes and faces to determine the most legible. This firm, the Clear Type Publishing Company, remained in existence throughout his lifetime. There would come a day, he predicted, when commercial publishers would enter the field of large-type book production. Time proved him right.

Irwin had his first taste of legislative victory when he secured passage in the Ohio legislature of a law that liberally subsidized public school classes for blind and partially sighted children. Thanks to passage of this bill, he was able to expand his territory from Cleveland to other cities in Ohio, becoming the first statewide supervisor of education for visually handicapped children.

As his scope widened, so did his acquaintanceship with every element of work for the blind: the leaders, the institutions, the traditions, the public attitudes that blocked blind people from progressing toward parity with the sighted. He took advantage of every opportunity that came his way to flail at these barriers.

Was there a shameful scarcity of brailled books for the adult blind? A year after coming to Cleveland, Irwin interested a local philanthropic group in organizing the Howe Publishing Society to produce such books. In so doing, he incidentally acquired a technical knowledge of braille production processes that was to stand him in excellent stead in succeeding decades.

Were there other, subtler, more complicated factors that were holding back development of adequate reading materials in tactile form? In 1911, Irwin gained an insight into these when he was named to membership on the AAWB's Uniform Type Committee. This was at the point when "the battle of the dots" was raging full force. He did not do well with the committee. Twenty-five years later, in a tactfully worded reference to Irwin's initial experience with this thorny issue, Henry Latimer wrote that the new member's views "were, to say the least, unconventional; and when, a year later, limited funds made it necessary to reduce the size of the Type Committee, his name was found missing from the membership."

Irwin was renamed to the group in 1918, by which time it had been greatly enlarged and had been turned into a commission jointly sponsored by AAWB and AAIB. The ultimate irony, as Latimer put it, was that when the whole problem of uniform type was turned over to the American Foundation for the Blind in 1923, "it became Mr. Irwin's direct responsibility to guide this movement to its . . . conclusion."

The beginning of Irwin's work in education coincided with the growth of the new science of psychology. There was much interest in educational circles over the intelligence scale devised by the French psychologist Alfred Binet. Binet's work was considered particularly useful in establishing early identification of mental retardation.

In the United States, major experimentation with the Binet scale was under way at the Vineland, New Jersey, Training School for the Feeble Minded under the direction of psychologist Henry H. Goddard. Irwin's awareness of the educational problems presented by mental deficiency among blind children led him to take the initiative of spending the summer of 1914 at Vineland to work out, in collaboration with Dr. Goddard, an adaptation of the Binet tests that would make them suitable for use with blind children. This meant devising oral or tactual substitutes for the large number of test questions involving pictures or diagrams.

Irwin's adaptations were ultimately found to be imperfect in several essential respects, and it remained for other psychologists, notably Dr. Samuel P. Hayes, to refine and develop the work in succeeding years. But that summer at Vineland added one more dimension to Robert Irwin's range of knowledge and interests, and brought him once again into the national limelight as an innovator.

When Irwin came to the Foundation, his mental luggage included yet another piece of conviction that was to influence his thinking for years to come. In 1918 the American Red Cross Institute at Evergreen had commissioned him to make a survey of existing state pension laws for blind persons. The resulting monograph, "Blind Relief Laws and Their Administration," was a cogent, well-written document that described and analyzed such legislation in 13 states, examined the manner in which these laws were administered, and struck out boldly at the concept of pensions granted purely on the grounds of blindness and regardless of need. It offered a model statute designed to overcome the shortcomings of the existing laws.

Irwin was assuredly aware that many of these laws had come into being through pressures generated by organized groups of blind people. He must also have realized that his strong recommendations to do away with across-the-board pensions would not endear him to the beneficiaries of such giveaway programs. Nevertheless, his somewhat righteous sense of fairness to the taxpayer prevailed over his desire for solidarity with his fellow blind. Both he and the Foundation were ultimately to pay a price for this high-principled indifference to popularity. As it happens, Irwin later modified his stand against special privileges for the blind and in the late Thirties campaigned hard, albeit unsuccessfully, for a "handicap allowance" which was essentially a pension under another name. His change of viewpoint was sincere enough, but it came too late to bridge the uncomfortable gulf between the Foundation and the organized blind.

In his execution of the Red Cross monograph, Irwin had a co-author: Mary Blanchard, a social worker in the employ of the Cleveland Society for the Blind, whom he married in 1917. A capable woman of notable intelligence and charm, Irwin's wife, who was sighted, never resumed her own career after her husband came to the Foundation. She devoted the rest of her life to serving as companion, homemaker, aide, and helpmeet to the brilliant but demanding man she had married. She died on April 23, 1949, at the age of sixty-five.

A sturdily built man just above medium stature, Robert Irwin was blessed with rugged health and a copious fund of energy. He had fair skin, often flushed with high color, a longish straight nose, and a wide, well-shaped mouth. While the thick brown hair of his youth eventually turned gray, he retained most of it. People meeting him for the first time were made instantly aware of his blindness by the dull-glazed spectacles he affected in the once-common belief that they were less conspicuous than dark glasses. Usually composed and affable, Irwin was always dignified and sometimes rigidly formal. His sense of humor was not of the back-slapping variety but more apt to be of an ironic cast, especially when the joke was on him.

Endowed with excellent physical coordination, he moved about with relative ease, using an ordinary stout walking cane. For routine travel between home and office, he dispensed with a sighted companion, relying on trains, taxis, and other public conveyances. When dog guides were introduced in the United States in the late Twenties, Irwin dismissed them for his own use as too much bother. Actually, he may then have been a little old to undergo the necessary training; he was also too stubbornly proud of his independence to rely on so conspicuous a travel aid as a dog. When it came to longer journeys, of which he took many, he was usually accompanied. It was his awareness of the expense of carfare for two that led him to initiate one of the Foundation's first tangible accomplishments in the legislative field. This was the federal law, followed by agreements with interstate carriers, that provided blind travelers and their guides with the one-fare privilege they retain to this day.

Some of Robert Irwin's qualities—his driving perfectionism, his controlling and paternalistic attitudes toward subordinates, his competitive spirit, his occasionally ungovernable temper—surfaced only after he had gained secure stature as a nationally respected thinker, leader, and doer. But enough was known about both his abilities and his personality during the Foundation's formative days to evoke confidence in some quarters, uneasiness in others.

The residential school superintendents, in particular, regarded Irwin as a natural enemy, largely because he was so outspoken an advocate of the day school classes in public schools that seemed to threaten the future of the residential schools. A revealing last-ditch attempt to keep Irwin away from the seat of national power was made by two of these superintendents. On November 29, 1922, Olin Burritt of the Pennsylvania school wrote to Foundation president Migel that he and Edward Allen of Perkins had talked over "the best way in which the Foundation can utilize Mr. Irwin's services" and had arrived at the following plan: "Let us associate Mr. Irwin with the Foundation as the director of research work but let him remain in Cleveland."

Migel ignored this transparent maneuver and proceeded to bring Irwin to New York. Two strong men were now poised on the verge of a partnership neither would have occasion to regret.

4

The Second Career of Major Migel

The practice of philanthropy in America has brought to the fore some extraordinary personalities, but few so singular as the man who turned his unpaid labors for the blind into the second career of a long and colorful lifetime.

If one were compelled to assign a single explanation to Moses Charles Migel's unique role as champion and benefactor of the blind, it would have to be that his exacting sense of order was offended by needless chaos affecting an entire stratum of society. It was his steadfast belief that commonsense principles of organization, of the kind that are second nature to any businessman, should be able to straighten out an untidy state of affairs.

Leaders in work for the blind had never even heard the name Migel when he appeared, seemingly out of nowhere, and proceeded to assume a strategic role in a hopelessly stalemated situation that reflected precisely the kind of disorder he could not abide. This was the tactile type question, "the war of the dots."

Ever since the first schools for blind children were founded in the 1830s, there had coexisted in the United States a number of separate systems of raised writing designed to be read by the fingertips. As Charles W. Holmes summed it up soon after the turn of the century:

> The lamentable fact is that we have at present five distinct codes of embossed print. . . . In order to avail himself of the full range of literature (which at best is woefully limited) the blind reader must learn, and keep well up in, all these codes. How long would our seeing friends stand for such a state of affairs in ink type? Imagine for a moment the ridiculous situation that would arise, if the daily papers published in Boston had an entirely different system of characters from those used by New York publishers.

The implications of this "ridiculous situation" were anything but ridiculous.

The small sums available for books were being dissipated because the same titles
had to be produced in different types. Communication among blind people was
rendered nearly impossible because they could not read one another's letters.
Professional energies that could have been devoted to constructive efforts were
being burned up in passionate internecine struggles.

By 1911 more than a decade of concentrated effort on the part of leaders in work
for the blind had produced some improvement. Through a complex process of trial
and error, negotiation and compromise, the field of battle had been reduced to
New York Point and American braille.

At its biennial convention that year, the American Association of Workers for
the Blind concluded that the only way to decide the question of which of these
systems should be universally adopted was through an impartial research study that
would test the reading performance of an equal number of users of each system.
AAWB members raised a small sum with which its Uniform Type Committee
could begin conducting such a study. In the months that followed, twelve hundred
American readers were tested, without either system demonstrating a commanding lead. What proved really unsettling to the research team was the discovery that a third system—British braille—apparently gave better results than
either the American version of braille or New York Point. It looked as though the
entire process would have to start over again.

At this juncture M.C. Migel entered the picture. Up to that time, his interest in
blindness had been confined to spending each Monday evening reading aloud to
the residents of a New York home for blind men and women, the Society for the
Relief of the Destitute Blind. But he had become personally aware of the type
problem when, having brought a braille book from England as a gift for one of the
home's residents, he found to his astonishment that her fingers, trained to read
New York Point, could not read it. Now, he heard, there was a movement afoot
that might correct this senseless situation.

The brother of one of the home's residents was Walter G. Holmes, editor of the
Matilda Ziegler Magazine for the Blind, a periodical which, like most other embossed literature, was being produced in separate editions of American braille and
New York Point. Migel called on Holmes to find out more about the group that
was attempting to work out a single finger-reading system. "Would it be worth
while," he asked, "for me to give this Uniform Type Committee a thousand
dollars?" Holmes, to whom such a sum represented the larger part of a year's
salary, gave a guarded reply. "It depends," he said, "on how much a thousand
dollars means to you." "That's a minor point," said Migel. "Something really
ought to be done to straighten things out."

It was the beginning. By 1914, when the AAWB's Uniform Type Committee
had joined forces with a parallel committee of the American Association of Instructors of the Blind, the name of M.C. Migel appeared as treasurer of the
combined task force, renamed the Uniform Type Commission. From that point
onward, he became the commission's sole source of funds, supplying whatever it
needed for staff work, travel expenses, publication and distribution of its reports.

As will be seen in a later chapter, the question of a single dot code for the United
States was settled by 1917, but it was to take some 15 years of calendar time and
uncounted man-years of patience before the ultimate goal was reached of a uniform

system of raised type that could be read throughout the English-speaking world. Although patience was not his long suit, Migel stuck with the problem throughout. Had this been his sole accomplishment for blind people, it would have earned him an honored place in their gallery of greats. But a host of mightier feats were in the offing.

What manner of man was Moses Charles Migel? What prompted him to devote more than half his lifetime to the cause of blind men and women? It was many years before even those who worked most closely with him learned much about the man, his background, or his motivation. In 1941, when the AAWB was preparing to present Migel with its Shotwell Medal, the chairman of the award committee wrote Robert Irwin asking for background material about the man Irwin had been intimately associated with for 20 years. "Strangely enough," Irwin wrote in reply, "I can tell you very little about Mr. Migel's biography except that he was formerly a silk manufacturer but retired many years ago. . . . Mr. Migel is very shy about publicity."

Throughout his long lifetime—he died a few days before his ninety-second birthday—Migel knew far more about the blind than the blind knew about him. As a man who always lived in the present, he was so little given to reminiscence that even his children were unable to supply authenticated details of either his ancestry or his early years. Much of what they recalled was told them by Migel's mother, Hannah, who died in 1926.

Migel's parents began their married life in New York City during the Civil War, living in a house on Canal Street where their first child, Clara, was born in 1864. Soon thereafter, the young husband developed an asthmatic condition which necessitated a change of climate. The family traveled to Houston, Texas, where their second child, Moses Charles, was born November 3, 1866. The Texas climate having failed to bring about the desired remedy for Migel senior, the family moved south, by way of Panama, to Peru and then to Chile. Three other children, two sons and a daughter, were born during these wanderings. However, the father's health continued to deteriorate; he died soon after the family came back to New York and just before the birth of a sixth child, a daughter.

Left in modest circumstances, the widow moved across the East River. The census of 1880 showed Hannah Migel, widow, aged thirty, living at 278 McDonough Street in a middle-class district of what was then the independent city of Brooklyn. The census entry listed six children: Clara, fifteen; Moses, thirteen; Saul, eleven; Linda, five; Julius, two; Bella, one.

Moses Charles Migel, then, was orphaned in his early teens; as the eldest son he became the man of the family and apparently assumed the role of breadwinner as soon as he was out of school. After a series of jobs as office boy, clerk, and salesman for various firms, he somehow got into the silk business. The Brooklyn city directory for 1893, at which time he was twenty-seven years old and his brother twenty-five, listed Moses Migel, silks, and Saul H. Migel, silks, at 370 Grand Avenue, which was also given as the residence of Hannah Migel, widow. The directory for the following year showed the silk business to have been moved to 58 Greene Street, Manhattan; the Brooklyn residence remained unchanged until 1897.

By 1898 Migel and his mother (and probably the younger children) had moved their residence to West 88 Street in Manhattan. Two years later the business listing for Moses C. Migel, silk, showed not only a Greene Street address in downtown Manhattan but also one in an industrial section of Long Island City, the latter probably a factory or warehouse. In the course of time, there were also silk mills in Providence, Rhode Island, and elsewhere, employing three thousand people. The Migel mills specialized in spun silk, made out of short fibres. One of the outlets for this product was telephone wire insulation, for which the mills held a profitable contract. This and other lucrative products made of silk during the days before synthetics came on the market enabled the self-made young industrialist to gain so strong a start and so substantial a capital that when, at the age of forty, he became a married man, he was in a position to retire from managerial activities. He retained his financial interests, however, for he was still sufficiently involved in the silk industry a dozen years later to be able to render his country a signal service when the United States entered World War I.

The War Department was in need of silk—more than 25 million yards of it—for cartridge bags to contain the smokeless powder used in firing cannon. Silk had the advantage over cotton of leaving no residue after firing, so that ramrod cleaning of the barrel was eliminated and reloading could be done at once. Since the breeding of silkworms was centered in the Orient, Migel volunteered to form an import firm, the Allied Silk Trading Corporation, to bring in the needed fibres from China and Japan and to supervise the manufacture of the cartridge cloth by a combine of American mills. Without waiting for a formal contract, he tied up $500,000 in working capital to import 6,900,000 yards of silk. The price quoted the government was cost plus 7½ percent, a reasonable markup in view of the delays and uncertainties of payment. At war's end, these difficulties having proven less than anticipated, the Allied Silk Trading Corporation voluntarily reduced its profit margin to 3 percent and rebated $2 million to the federal treasury. A distinguished service certificate from the War Department was its principal reward.

Immediately after the Armistice, the American Red Cross asked Migel to take charge of preliminary adjustment services for American servicemen blinded in battle who were in various French hospitals awaiting return to the United States. By then he was not only nationally known for his association with the Uniform Type Commission but had acquired official status through appointment by New York Governor Charles S. Whitman as chairman of the New York State Commission for the Blind. He not only accepted the overseas assignment but assembled a group of eight trained nurses to accompany him abroad at his own expense. In Paris the group set up headquarters for the Red Cross Bureau of Reconstruction and Reeducation which, in addition to attending to the needs of blinded American soldiers and sailors, established an experimental farm school near Chenonceaux for a group of French *mutilés de la guerre,* supplied it with tractors and other agricultural machinery and staffed it with expert instructors who would train for a future livelihood in agriculture those disabled men who could no longer pursue their pre-war occupations.

The bureau also established a factory for the manufacture of artificial limbs for legless French veterans and, once it was in full operation, made a gift of it to the

French government. As disbursing agent for the American Red Cross, it distributed several million francs to various French relief organizations. For these services to France, Migel was subsequently made a Chevalier of the French Legion of Honor.

Migel's work for the war-blinded continued when he returned to the United States after nine months in France. He served on the five-member Committee of Direction of the Red Cross Institute for the Blind at Evergreen, an experience which added one more dimension to his understanding of the problems of the visually handicapped.

Where his colleagues in work for the blind were concerned, Migel's wartime activities yielded a handy by-product. Then, as now, Red Cross officials working with the armed forces were given assimilated military ranks. Migel's assignment in France carried the rank of major, and "Major" became the familiar form of address used by people who knew his aversion to the use of his given name. He had long since adopted the practice of using only his initials in business. Old friends gave him the nickname of "Migs"; his Chilean-born wife invariably addressed him as *Hijo* (son) or its fond diminutive *Hijito* (sonny). It became a favorite family anecdote that when Migel was overseas for the Red Cross and sent affectionate cables to his wife at their summer home in Monroe, New York, a rumor swept the small town that Mrs. Migel was carrying on an affair with someone named Hijito.

There could hardly have been a less likely candidate for naughty behavior. Elisa Parada, whom Migel married in 1906, grew up in the Victorian age and never really left it. Born in Santiago, Chile, in 1877, she was orphaned while young and spent her growing-up years at Santiago College, a Methodist boarding school for girls. For all her ninety years, she remained an old-fashioned, straitlaced lady who never cut her hair, never shortened her ankle-length skirts, never wore a sleeve that ended above the elbow, and objected on moral grounds to alcohol, tobacco, gambling, and swearing. Her husband, on the other hand, was a bon vivant. He was a master mixer of giant-sized old fashioneds, a confirmed cigar and cigarette smoker until he gave up tobacco for health reasons late in life; a man who played cards for high stakes, bet heavily on horses and even owned a few.

The glue that held the marriage together was Mrs. Migel's Spanish background. She was a submissive wife who took it for granted that her husband should be undisputed master of the house and that his outside life was no concern of hers. For a man who had been catered to by an indulgent mother until the age of forty, it was an ideal arrangement. The Major worshipped the petite, dark-haired beauty he called "my little Carmen" and told people "she's the one who'll get me into Heaven." Having thus taken care of the future, he felt free to do as he pleased in the here-and-now. He did, however, pay his wife the compliment of not flaunting his freedom in her presence. At the country home where they entertained extensively, the famous old-fashioneds were mixed and consumed in the pantry, out of sight of the lady of the house. The Major refrained from telling his wife about the nickel-a-point bridge games he played at the Lotos Club, and she refrained from asking.

One subject on which the Migels saw eye to eye was strict discipline for their three children. Even when they were quite small, daughter Parmenia and sons

John and Richard were expected to report to the breakfast table at eight o'clock sharp, washed, dressed, and combed. Lunch was promptly at one o'clock. The child who came a few minutes late to the table had to begin with whatever course was being served at the time; greater tardiness usually meant banishment from the dining room until the next meal.

Another thing the Migels had in common was a love of nature and a firm belief in the healthful effects of outdoor living. The spacious country estate called Greenbraes, located in the Ramapo Hills some forty miles from New York City, was their real home; their city apartment was little more than a *pied à terre,* for the restless Major was constantly on the go, spending most winters in Palm Beach, spring months in Arizona or New Mexico, and autumn months in Europe.

It was the Migels' belief in the benefits of country air that led them to undertake a personal charity which gave them much satisfaction. When a five-acre piece of property adjoining theirs became available in 1923, they bought it and turned it into a free vacation home for blind women. Called Rest Haven, the property could accommodate 35 guests at a time. Each year, between May and October, six successive groups of women who could not otherwise afford a country vacation were accommodated at Rest Haven for 18-day stays. The question of guides was ingeniously solved by including a few sighted women in each group. There was no charge for anyone, blind or sighted; even the round-trip transportation from New York City was supplied.

The Migels personally supervised the conversion and decoration of the house and grounds at Rest Haven into a comfortable resort adapted to the needs of blind persons. They and their children visited frequently, enjoying the pleasure of their guests, many of whom were women the Major had known during his weekly visits to the Society for the Relief of the Destitute Blind.

Until just before World War II, when it was closed down for a period, all of Rest Haven's expenses were defrayed by the Migels. In 1944 the Major deeded the entire property to the American Foundation for the Blind. Although the Foundation's executives and trustees knew that there were now other vacation facilities available to blind women, and were aware that this type of direct service activity for individuals was not really appropriate for a national organization, Rest Haven was kept going out of respect for the Migels and was not closed down until after the death of Mrs. Migel in 1967. The purchase, maintenance, and operation of Rest Haven over a 15-year period probably cost the Migels some $200,000. They never for a moment doubted it was worth it, even when it meant a little financial strain.

It was characteristic of the Major that when Rest Haven first opened, it was credited to "an anonymous friend of the blind." Migel had yet to learn that money could be more easily raised for a cause if donors were publicly identified, and that it was up to him to set the example.

Although the American Foundation for the Blind was the recipient of most of the gifts Migel made in his lifetime, he maintained other private charities in addition to Rest Haven, such as financing the college education of several deserving young men. His interest in the Society for the Relief of the Destitute Blind continued long after he stopped being a weekly reader for the residents. Periodically he would organize parties at the institution, bringing in groups of musicians or actors to provide entertainment. He was also a lifelong contributor to the National Society for the Prevention of Blindness, of which he had been one of the founders.

Mrs. Migel's main interest was in her alma mater. When she visited Chile in 1924 and found Santiago College in need of new buildings, the Migels made a gift of $150,000 to the school and Mrs. Migel became president of its board of trustees.

M.C. Migel was not the type of man to pass unnoticed in a crowd. He was a handsome figure whose erect posture and jaunty tread were outward symbols of a healthy self-regard. A bit of a Beau Brummell, he usually sported a flower in the lapel of his custom-tailored suit; he wore his hat tipped to a rakish angle. A full head of white hair was combed smoothly back to frame a clean-shaven, craggy face whose outstanding features were a pair of keen, somewhat hooded, brown eyes, a Roman nose and a full-lipped, sensuous mouth. Until he required an operation for cataract when he was nearly ninety, his sole physical impairment was a mild hearing loss, the result of a childhood bout with scarlet fever.

Toward women, the Major's manner was courtly but tinged with indulgent condescension. Intellectual brilliance or business competence on a woman's part never failed to amaze him. Grace S. Harper, who worked with him during his Red Cross stint in Paris, so impressed him by her ability to prepare a complicated budget that, on her return to the United States, he used his influence to have her appointed executive secretary of the New York State Commission for the Blind, of which he remained chairman until 1924. It was a post Miss Harper filled with distinction for 32 years until her retirement in 1951.

Ability to handle figures was an essential qualification for anyone who worked for Migel. There came a time when, after hiring a private secretary who was perfect in all other respects, he discovered she simply couldn't add. He discharged her and, determined not to make the same mistake twice, prepared a long column of figures with which to test the arithmetical ability of candidates for the job. Having added up the column himself and jotted down the sum, he interviewed each applicant, then handed her the sheet of figures and told her to go into the next room and add them up. To his dismay, one young woman after another failed the test.

When Amelia Landor's turn came, she listened to his instructions and said, "It's quite unnecessary for me to go into another room. I'll add up the figures right here and now." Which she proceeded to do. When she announced her sum, he compared it with his. "Sorry, my dear, it's the wrong answer."

"It's no such thing," came the tart reply. "If you got a different answer, sir, it's you who made a mistake." He took the figures, recalculated, and burst into laughter. Miss Landor was right, and so had been most of the other applicants he had rejected. But he hired Amelia Landor on the spot, not merely because she knew how to add but because she had the spunk to defend her work. She remained in charge of his private business office until the day he died.

Major Migel admired brains and mettle and he liked people who argued with him. What he didn't like was losing the argument, as those who worked with him at the Foundation were to find out. Because he was quick to anger, people who knew him well learned to recognize the warning signal: a sharp sucking-in of cheeks and tightly pursed lips preceded an outburst of temper. Had Robert Irwin been able to see, he might have evaded a few of the stormy encounters which were to punctuate the otherwise harmonious team effort that began when M.C. Migel took over active direction of the national strategy to serve the interests of blind people.

5

The Facts of Blindness

M.C. Migel and Robert Irwin, two of the three principals in the venturesome new undertaking, were now on stage. The third principal, Helen Keller, waited in the wings. Before the curtain rises on Act One, some program notes:

What, exactly, is blindness? In spite of efforts extending over many decades, this seemingly simple question has never found a simple answer.

The conditions commonly subsumed under the heading of blindness actually fall into three categories: total blindness, legal blindness, and functional blindness.

Total blindness was always easily understood. It was sightlessness—the absence of any light or image perception whatsoever.

Legal blindness was defined in a formula adopted in 1934 by the American Medical Association, subsequently incorporated in the Aid to the Blind title of the Social Security Act of 1935, and further embodied into law in federal and state statutes providing various special services and benefits for blind persons. Because it is the eligibility criterion for so many tangible benefits, from welfare assistance to income tax exemptions, legal blindness is sometimes referred to as economic blindness. The basic definition establishing it was this:

> Central visual acuity of 20/200 or less in the better eye with corrective glasses or central visual acuity of more than 20/200 if there is a visual field defect in which the peripheral field is contracted to such an extent that the widest diameter of the visual field subtends an angular distance no greater than 20 degrees in the better eye.

What this means in ordinary language is that a person is deemed legally blind (a) if, even with perfectly fitted eyeglasses, his better eye can see no more at a distance of 20 feet than a person with normal vision can see at a distance of 200 feet; and/or (b) if his central visual field is so restricted that he can only see objects within a 20-degree arc, in contrast to the visually normal person's ability to see objects in a much wider arc above, below, and on each side of the line of sight.

Measurements of visual acuity—the ability to discern detail—are made on the familiar Snellen Chart, whose printed letters are so sized and shaped that the ability to read a certain line from a distance of 20 feet denotes normal vision, designated as 20/20. The person who from that distance is unable to see more than the single large letter which is the chart's top line is said to have 20/200 vision. This is the entry point of legal blindness.

Totally blind persons, of course, fit within this definition of legal blindness. So do those who can distinguish between light and darkness but have to bring objects within an inch or two of their eyes in order to identify them. So do those who have "tunnel" or "gunbarrel" vision and can see objects straight ahead of them but not on either side. So do those persons who have only lateral vision.

All such persons—and in 1972 estimates of their number in the United States ranged from 441,000 to 1,700,000—have sufficiently severe visual impairment to function as legally blind, even though many included in the higher estimates are not officially classified as such.

According to a study made in 1972, an additional 4,700,000 Americans had lesser degrees of visual impairment which rendered them functionally blind, i.e., unable to read ordinary newspaper print even with perfectly fitted eyeglasses. "Partially sighted" is a term sometimes used to describe people with these lesser degrees of visual disability.

One reason for the great disparity in blindness estimates is that no agreement has ever been reached on a standard definition that would encompass all persons severely handicapped by visual loss. At least 16 different definitions are used in the United States, according to one authority. The official legal definition of blindness tends to be narrowly interpreted in some states, loosely interpreted in others. It is mandatory in some situations, such as eligibility for financial aid, but not in others, such as eligibility for vocational rehabilitation training. Where education of children is concerned, it has been gradually abandoned in favor of visual efficiency, which includes many factors other than the two specified in the legal definition.

Over the years, ophthalmologists have repeatedly criticized the weaknesses of the legal definition. Dr. Richard E. Hoover, chief of ophthalmology at the Greater Baltimore Medical Center, called it "inadequate, unrealistic, inequitable, prejudicial and restrictive," noting that the definition takes into account only two visual characteristics—distance acuity and central fields—while ignoring other factors that affect the ability to see, such as peripheral fields, muscle balance, and depth perception. The definition calls for separate measurements of each eye but ignores the performance of both eyes together. It does not allow for individual differences in ability to use residual vision, nor does it distinguish between the degree and type of vision required for vocational pursuits and that needed for ordinary activities of daily living.

Equally serious is the fact that there are no provisions to insure standardized measurement and reporting, even of the two characteristics specified in the definition. It is thus entirely possible for different ophthalmologists examining the same person to report different findings.

In the absence of agreement on what constitutes blindness, how has it been possible to make even an educated guess as to how many blind or visually impaired people there have been at any given time?

Among the early tasks assumed by the American Foundation for the Blind was devising, in cooperation with the National Society for the Prevention of Blindness, a standard report form for eye examinations that could serve as a basic tool. That form, a single sheet of paper, had some astonishing effects. As various schools for the blind were persuaded to try it out, professional examinations uncovered scores of children whose sight could be restored or substantially improved through surgery. Relaying this information to Helen Keller in 1933, Robert Irwin wrote: "Now we are confronted with a situation where there is no money to pay for these operations, and no local eye specialist who is willing to perform the operations without pay. Of course we will work it out somehow. . . ."

One way or another, it was indeed worked out. Many years later, Senator Jennings Randolph recalled that during this period, when he was district governor of the Lions Clubs in West Virginia, the Lions paid for the hospitalization of such children, while a local eye surgeon, Dr. Jay Blades, performed all of the operations free of charge. Comparable solutions were found in other states.

The jointly sponsored Committee on Statistics which developed the eye examination report form also worked out a scheme for standard classifications of causes of blindness, likewise in the interest of laying the groundwork for uniform statistics. The classification schedule, as later revised, was ultimately adopted internationally.

Once these statistical tools had been shaped, the committee, headed for three decades by the eminently qualified social statistician Ralph G. Hurlin, secretary of the Russell Sage Foundation, tackled the task of constructing a formula for estimating the nation's blind population. The formula it evolved, which has been the fundamental yardstick of blindness prevalence in the United States for many years, was the basis for the lowest figure in the range of 1972 estimates. At no time did it ever pretend to produce more than a reasonable guess. A brief description of the formula and its origin will illustrate why this is so.

Under the Hurlin formula, the extent of blindness in the nation is estimated through the use of a rate originally derived from one particular state in which a reliably complete register of blind persons was maintained. This basic rate is then weighted for each of the other states by three social factors: (1) the proportion of aged persons in the state's population (because the older people are, the more susceptible they are to severe visual loss); (2) the state's ethnic composition (because non-white groups tend to receive less eye care); (3) the state's infant mortality rate (because the same inadequate health programs which produce higher-than-average infant death rates tend to result in higher-than-average blindness).

The state whose blindness register provided the basic data to which these estimates were initially anchored was North Carolina. Why North Carolina? In 1937, when the Hurlin formula was first worked out, there were a number of states which maintained registers of their blind residents. Few of these registers were either up-to-date or complete, but the Tar Heel State's was relatively trustworthy because North Carolina had been the scene, just a few years earlier, of an exceptional effort to make a comprehensive census of its blind residents. Such a census was vital in persuading the state legislature to establish a commission for the blind, and a commission was urgently needed. North Carolina was then the only state that, apart from its 90-year-old school for blind children, did not have a single voluntary or public resource for blind adults.

In the circumstances, when George E. Lineberry, superintendent of the state school for the blind, asked for help in building the case for a state commission, his request was given top priority. Charles Hayes and the Foundation's staff devised and executed a meticulous plan for surveying the counties comprising the largest cities in the state. In each county they organized a committee whose membership included representation from every large or small organized body that could be found. Members of the field staff visited the selected counties, conducted public meetings to explain why the survey was being made, and armed the local committees with census forms to be filled out for every blind person located.

Invariably, the field team was met in each county with the assertion that only a handful of its residents were blind. Invariably, too, the facts proved otherwise. In one county, officials estimated the blind population to be 35; the very first sweep located 218. A second sweep, in which six of the major counties were subjected to a house-by-house check, utilizing a crew of workers employed under a Civil Works Administration program, uncovered many additional cases.

As a result of the year-long project, the legislature established a state commission and appropriated $25,000 for its first year's operation; three voluntary county associations and a statewide association for the blind were organized; a sheltered workshop was set up; home teachers were employed; a committee for the prevention of blindness was established; Lions Clubs were activated to lend their assistance.

From a national standpoint, the significance of the North Carolina census was that its findings demolished the 1-per-1,000 rule of thumb that had long been used for estimating the prevalence of blindness in the United States. Testifying before a Congressional committee some years later, Dr. Hurlin said that his 1937 estimates, based on the North Carolina census, proved the extent of blindness in the nation to be "from two to two-and-one-half times as great as was commonly supposed."

Additional pilot studies, made in other states, caused further modifications in the formula. For the 1940 census Dr. Hurlin arrived at a blindness rate of 1.75 per 1,000, yielding a national total for that year of 230,000. Ten years later, the formula yielded a higher rate, 1.98 per 1,000, giving a total of more than 308,000. For the 1960 census, the blindness rate was estimated to be 2.14 per 1,000, and the total 385,000. The 1972 estimate of 441,000 blind persons was calculated at the same rate, taking into account the nation's population growth during the preceding dozen years.

Since the decennial federal census presumably reached every household in the nation, could it not have been used to take a count of the blind members of those households? Such an effort had been made for an entire century, and it had failed. Beginning with the census of 1830, enumerators were instructed to ask about blindness, but there were so many deficiencies in the method (enumerators forgot to ask, families chose not to acknowledge) that the findings could not be taken seriously. For example, the census of 1920 yielded a national figure of 57,444 blind persons. This, it was shown immediately thereafter, was 20,000 less than the total reported in a special study, also made by the United States Census Bureau, for the very same year. Leaders in work for the blind challenged both estimates, believing the actual figure at that time to be in the neighborhood of 100,000. Following the 1930 census, which proved equally unsatisfactory in yielding a reliable figure, the Census Bureau decided to drop the blindness item from subsequent enumerations. It was never reinstated.

An amusing sidelight on the questionable validity of census figures was cited by Gabriel Farrell in *The Story of Blindness.* The census of 1880, he wrote,

> reported 48,929 blind persons. This was double the number enrolled in the report of ten years previous, which was 20,220. Workers for the blind were concerned that blindness might have doubled in a decade. A possible explanation for the doubling, however, was the fact that [the 1880 census] enumerators received a bonus of five cents for each case of blindness reported!

There is no equally transparent explanation for the fact that more contemporary efforts to arrive at a definitive figure have also produced amazingly wide discrepancies. Whereas the 1960 revision of the Hurlin formula gave a legal blindness rate of 2.14 per 1,000 of population, a national health survey made by the United States Public Health Service in 1957-58 put the prevalence rate of "severe visual impairment" at 5.17. A repeat national health survey two years later gave an even higher rate of 5.6, and in 1963–65 the same survey came up with a rate of 6.6 per 1,000, placing the number of Americans with severe visual impairments at 1,227,000.

In 1962 an effort was begun to pinpoint data on incidence (new cases) as well as prevalence (existing cases) of blindness. The system used was designated the Model Reporting Area for Blindness Statistics (MRA); it was initiated by the National Institute of Neurological Diseases and Blindness and transferred in 1969 to the just-created National Eye Institute. MRA started with 11 states which voluntarily agreed to update and maintain their blindness registers, using uniform definitions of blindness, uniform classification of causes, and agreed-upon procedures for registering persons certified as blind by ophthalmologists or optometrists. As of 1972 there were 16 participating states contributing their findings to the federal body.

The most frequently cited figure for incidence of new blindness during the Sixties was that 30,000 persons lost their sight each year in the United States. A much higher rate was projected in 1971 by the director of the National Eye Institute, who predicted that 50,000 persons would become blind within the year and 500,000 within the next decade.

In only one respect have all the surveys found general agreement. The crucial factor affecting both incidence and prevalence of blindness is the increasing longevity of the American population. More than 50 percent of the nation's visually impaired persons are over sixty. In 1967 a specialist in biometrics projected an "army of the aged blind" by 1985.

The realistic likelihood is that it will never be possible to obtain an exact count of the nation's blind population, particularly the geriatric blind. One reason for this is that an aging person whose blindness is caused by diabetes is more apt to be reported as a diabetic than as a blind person. Nor do public records supply a reliable index. In many states, needy blind persons receiving public welfare assistance who reach the age of sixty-five are automatically transferred from the Aid to the Blind roster to the Old Age Assistance category. There is also the factor of "the hidden blind"—isolates who desire no care and avoid contact with agencies serving blind persons.

Blindness would be easier to define and count if it were a condition stemming from a single cause. But there have been scores of causes, and while some were eliminated through prevention or cure or changing conditions, others appeared to take their place.

One of the most dramatic crusades against blindness was already well along the road to successful completion by the early Twenties. This was the fight against ophthalmia neonatorum—popularly called "babies' sore eyes"—an inflammation in the eyes of newborn infants usually caused by the presence of gonorrheal infection in the mother's birth canal.

The simple precaution of routinely putting drops of an effective prophylactic, silver nitrate, into the eyes of newborn infants halted the onslaught of this disease, which at one time was responsible for as much as 30 percent of all blindness in children. A 20-year campaign to introduce and enforce state laws mandating the use of such drops by doctors, nurses, or midwives brought about a steady decline, year by year, in this particular cause of blindness.

Extensive public education campaigns were launched to secure enactment of the needed laws. This was no easy feat: mention of venereal disease was taboo in polite society, and it took courage for editors to allow discussion, even in euphemistic terms, of the reason so many infants suffered loss of sight. Helen Keller, who authored articles on the subject in the *Ladies' Home Journal* in 1907, credited the magazine's editor, Edward Bok, with a key role in penetrating the barrier of public ignorance.

State and local agencies took aggressive stands. In 1910 the Massachusetts Charitable Eye and Ear Infirmary published a study of 116 cases of infants blinded by ophthalmia neonatorum:

> In practically every instance the cause of the child's disablement is failure on the part of the physician to recognize and give warning of the serious nature of the disease. . . . The general practitioner has yet much to learn of the disease, and the parents know nothing of it. Upon these two groups—the practitioners and the parents—the baby must depend for the gift of sight.

The report made another trenchant point: the venereal disease that produced ophthalmia neonatorum could also kill, and some of the infants treated in the Infirmary did not survive.

The formation, in 1908, of what later became the National Society for the Prevention of Blindness was a direct outgrowth of the need to carry on a nation-wide fight against "babies' sore eyes." Progress made in halting the disease was reflected in yearly statistics showing how many of the pupils newly admitted to schools and classes for the blind were its victims. In the 1907–08 school year, the percentage was 26.5; ten years later it had dropped to 15.2. With the passage of another decade, the percentage in 1927–28 went down to 9.1, from which point it slowly tapered off. That cases of ophthalmia neonatorum crop up even in modern times can only be ascribed to inexcusable carelessness.

The other venereal disease, syphilis, was at one time also responsible for a substantial share of blindness. In the United States, as in most other nations observing modern health standards, medical progress in the treatment of syphilis with antibiotics has brought about a noticeable improvement, but venereal disease remains responsible for considerable blindness in less developed areas of the world. The disparity among nations is even more marked in relation to trachoma, an infectious virus disease endemic in the Middle East and in some areas of Asia and Africa, but now rarely encountered in the United States due to stringent enforcement of immigration regulations which bar admission of persons with trachoma symptoms.

The advance of medicine has helped abate or eliminate the spread of several other disease entities—including tuberculosis, smallpox, typhoid, and scarlet fever—which formerly gave rise to blindness in American children and adults. Improved surgical techniques have also played a part in mitigating, and sometimes reversing, visual defects. Most notable among the successful surgical interventions are corneal transplants, the use of laser beams in treating detached retinas, and simplified cataract extractions.

Offsetting the progress made in reducing the incidence of blindness due to infectious disease are several new factors. Degenerative processes that accompany aging produce a high rate of blindness in the form of cataract, glaucoma, and retinal deterioration. Diabetes, which once killed its victims within a few short years, has been brought under control with insulin; diabetics live longer, but simultaneously have a longer exposure to the risk of blindness that can be a result of the disease. In the Sixties and Seventies, diabetes accounted for nearly 15 percent of all new cases of blindness. Almost exactly the same percentage was attributable to glaucoma, while just under 14 percent of new blindness derived from senile cataracts.

Where the very young are concerned, epidemics of blindness intermittently crop up, seemingly out of nowhere, and leave a lamentable legacy of visual impairment before the causes are discovered and proper preventive measures introduced. Such was the case with retrolental fibroplasia, which left some 12,000 children blind during the Forties and up into the early Fifties, when its astonishing cause was identified. And such was the case with the rubella (German measles) epidemic of the mid-Sixties. Not only blindness but many other grave impairments, including deafness, heart defects, and mental retardation, were discovered in newborn infants whose mothers had contracted rubella during the early months of pregnancy. Some 30,000 multihandicapped children were born during that epidemic; an estimated 5,000 to 6,000 of these numbered blindness among their impairments.

Epidemics of German measles tend to arise at approximately seven-year intervals. In the late Sixties and early Seventies, the medical and public health professions mounted a sweeping immunization campaign in what, as this is written, appears to have been a successful effort to protect pregnant women from exposure to the rubella virus before the arrival of the next epidemic cycle.

But there remain the constants. These include the hereditary or congenital eye defects, most common among them glaucoma and retinitis pigmentosa. Safety precautions manage to hold industrial accidents in check, but the traffic casualties of a nation on wheels, and the social casualties of a society increasingly wracked by violence and crime, tend to counterbalance them. And of course there is the most tragic accident of all: war.

To serve the nation's visually impaired men, women, and children there existed in the United States in 1972 several hundred voluntary and tax-supported bodies. Depending on how they were counted—whether units or branches of multi-service agencies were considered separate or subsumed under the parent organization—the total was put at slightly over 400 or just under 800. The gross expenditure of these organizations, in whichever way they were counted, was calculated to have been $469 million for the fiscal year 1967. According to the government-sponsored study which produced this estimate, about 57 percent of this sum ($268 million) was federal money, 29 percent ($131 million) came out of state tax funds, and the remaining 14 percent (just under $70 million) was spent by 274 voluntary organizations.

A functional breakdown of the $469 million total ascribed the expenditure of $270 million to income maintenance, $69 million to education, $48 million to vocational services, $10 million to residential care, $2 million to research, and more than $70 million to a great variety of technical, personal, and social services ranging from braille and recorded books to dog guides, mobility training, rehabilitation, social and psychological counseling, aids and appliances, recreation, camping, etc.

One way to measure the change in the lives of blind Americans during the past half century would be to compare these figures with the less than $31 million reported as the nation's total expenditures for services to blind persons in 1919.

One final program note. Only one legally blind person in ten is totally without sight. Modern practice is careful to make a semantic distinction among types of visual deficiency, reserving the term "blindness" for total or nearly total absence of sight and using "visual impairment" to denote the other degrees of visual loss which are severe enough to qualify as legal blindness. However, for most of the period covered by this history, "blindness" was the term used for all types of serious visual handicap. Considerations of historical accuracy require that it be so used in this book.

6

The Perfect Symbol

Had the organizers of the American Foundation for the Blind set about inventing a torchbearer for their cause, they could have done no better than to create a Helen Keller. This radiant woman embodied both tragedy and triumph. The message conveyed by her very existence was stunningly simple. If a Helen Keller, who was not only blind but deaf, could be lifted out of what she herself called "the double dungeon of darkness and silence," then there was surely reason to believe that others could be similarly freed.

In the modern era, electronic communications have made instant celebrity a commonplace occurrence. Fame was harder to achieve fifty or more years ago when the written word and the public platform were the sole means of transmitting information. But Helen Keller was already a figure of world renown in Victorian times. Every school child knew the story, as emotionally satisfying as any fairy tale, of how seven-year-old Helen, blind and deaf since the age of nineteen months, had been a half-savage little creature, raging with frustration over her inability to understand or make herself understood, until she was released by the magic key of language transmitted through her fingers. In school auditoriums the world over, children joyously reenacted the climactic scene in the pump house, in which the gush of water on one of Helen's hands, while the word w-a-t-e-r was being simultaneously finger-spelled into the other, brought about the blazing insight that unlocked the doors of her mind.

The story of Helen Keller's childhood was even better than a fairy tale, for it did not stop with a bland "and so they lived happily ever after" but went on to tell, in gratifying detail, how Helen, once she had grasped the idea of communication, learned to read and write braille, to write script and use the typewriter; how she even mastered the technique of oral speech; and how she succeeded, in spite of her heavy handicaps, in earning a college degree from Radcliffe. It also had a most reassuring feature. Helen's fairy godmother did not disappear after waving her magic wand, but became the little girl's lifelong teacher, companion, and guide.

Although the Helen Keller "miracle" was extensively (and often exaggeratedly) treated in the press from the time in 1887 that Anne Sullivan reported her first successes with her deaf-blind pupil, the major source for the thrilling real-life story was a book that Helen wrote in 1903 while she was still in college. *The Story of My Life* recounted the events that began with March 3, 1887, the day that "Teacher"—twenty-one years old, herself half-blind and not yet fully recovered from an eye operation—arrived at the Keller farm in Alabama from the Perkins Institution in Massachusetts. It continued through the painstaking years of education, telling of the friendship of a galaxy of greats that included Alexander Graham Bell, Oliver Wendell Holmes, and Mark Twain, and noting that a group of wealthy and devoted patrons had supplied the financial help that made everything possible.

For the general public, interest in the Helen Keller story ended there. She was a legend, and one did not think of legends as dealing with the ordinary concerns of life. From time to time, however, her name surfaced in specialized circles. A series of articles she wrote for the *Ladies' Home Journal* in 1907 pleaded for public support of the campaign against ophthalmia neonatorum. Through the influence of John Albert Macy, the writer and editor Anne Sullivan married in 1905, Helen became a Socialist and made occasional public appearances on behalf of anti-war and other liberal causes. She was a supporter of the movement for women's suffrage and wrote one or two articles on this subject.

Much of Helen's time was given over to maintaining a large correspondence, not only with the many persons who had befriended her as a child but also with parents of blind children who sought her advice, scholars who wanted to know more about the methods used in her education, organizations for the blind and organizations for the deaf that asked her to help them raise funds.

Soon after Helen's graduation from Radcliffe, she and her teacher bought an old farmhouse in Wrentham, Massachusetts, a suburb of Boston. When Anne Sullivan became a bride, John Macy joined their household. The marriage was a troubled one, however, and although it was apparently never legally terminated, John Macy took his departure in 1914, never to return. He died in 1932.

While still in college, Helen had written a charmingly modest essay, "My Future As I See It." She thought she might become a traveling emissary "from the teachers in this country to those of Europe . . . to carry a message of encouragement to those who, in the face of popular prejudice and indifference . . . are struggling to teach the blind and give them means of self-support. She also thought she herself might teach. And, of course, "Whether I teach or not, I shall write. . . . I may perhaps translate from the classics and from the modern languages." Settlement work, she noted, attracted her as a "way in which I may render service to others with my own hands." And she liked the idea of taking care of the sick and thought she might study massage.

Her predominant interest, however, was in assisting the deaf and the blind:

> I am not competent now to discuss their problems, but I shall find out what these problems are and study the methods of solving them. . . . I shall keep track of all the measures adopted in behalf of the deaf and the blind, and to the best of my ability support the most efficient.

Helen was twenty-three when she laid out these dreams and hopes in December 1903. Ten years later, none had materialized in any substantial way. Editors, it developed, were not interested in having her write on any subject other than herself—and that particular topic, she felt, had been exhausted. Translating jobs did not come her way. No one brought her a deaf-blind child to educate, nor could she have afforded to do the job if such a child had been produced. She was as far from self-support as she had ever been. Moreover, some of her former patrons had dropped out of the picture. A particular disappointment was that John Spaulding, "the sugar king of Boston," who had made her a generous annual allowance ever since her childhood, had died without providing for her in his will. Her teacher was subject to frequent and serious illnesses; the emotional and financial crisis precipitated by one such illness in 1913 led Helen to swallow her pride and accept the $5,000-a-year stipend from Andrew Carnegie she had proudly refused a few years earlier.

Money had always been a problem. The Keller family had no funds to speak of; indeed, Helen's father was unable to continue paying Anne Sullivan a salary soon after she and Helen left Alabama for the North. Helen and Anne managed, for the most part, by staying for long periods as house guests of wealthy friends and by accepting help from any and every promising source. Helen was later to write of this period that her teacher's "desire to have me educated and equipped to be a cupbearer of good to others was stronger than any fear of monetary difficulties. Nothing could resist the mingled dignity and audacity with which she pleaded my cause."

When Helen announced her determination to prepare for college, a group of her patrons set out to raise a fund to make this possible. In this effort, Mark Twain played a pivotal role. He himself had been rescued from deep financial difficulty through the help of the Standard Oil magnate H.H. Rogers, who, out of admiration for the writer's talent, had taken over management of the disastrous debts growing out of Twain's unlucky ventures into the publishing business. It seemed only natural to Twain, when he heard of Helen's dilemma, to seek help for her from the same source. From London, where he was spending a year trying to finish a book, Twain wrote to his patron's wife in November 1896:

> For & in behalf
>   of Helen Keller
>   Stone blind & deaf, &
>   formerly dumb.

Dear Mrs. Rogers,—Experience has convinced me that when one wishes to set a hard-worked man at something which he mightn't prefer to be bothered with, it is best to move upon him behind his wife. If she can't convince him it isn't worth while for other people to try.

Mr. Rogers will remember our visit with that astonishing girl at Laurence Hutton's house when she was fourteen years old. Last July, in Boston, when she was 16 she underwent the Harvard examination for admission to Radcliffe College. She passed without a single condition. She was allowed only the same amount of time that is granted to other applicants, & this was shortened in her case by the fact that the question-papers had to be *read* to her. Yet she scored an average of 90 as against an average of 78 on the part of the other applicants.

It won't *do* for America to allow this marvelous child to retire from her studies because of poverty. If she can go on with them she will make a fame that will endure in history for centuries. Along her special lines she is the most extraordinary product of all the ages. . . .

Mrs. Hutton's idea is to raise a permanent fund the interest upon which shall support Helen & her teacher & put them out of the fear of want. I shan't say a word against it, but she will find it a difficult and disheartening job, & meanwhile, what is to become of that miraculous girl?

No, for immediate and sound effectiveness, the thing is for you to plead with Mr. Rogers for this hampered wonder of your sex. . . .

Twain's scheme proposed that Rogers involve the Rockefellers and the "other Standard Oil chiefs" in underwriting the cost of Helen's college education. That it worked is clear from his next note to Mrs. Rogers:

It is superb! And I am beyond measure grateful to you both. I knew you would be interested in that wonderful girl, & that Mr. Rogers was already interested in her & touched by her; & I was sure that if nobody else helped her you two *would;* but you have gone far & away beyond the sum I expected. . . .

Helen and Anne would have been infinitely better off had they followed Mark Twain's example and asked H.H. Rogers or someone like him to take charge of their finances. But Teacher, in particular, had a stubborn myopia on this subject. In her biography of Anne Sullivan Macy which was published in 1933, Nella Braddy was to write that the friends who raised Helen's college fund "hoped that the possession of money of their own would teach the girls how to manage it, but this last was a vain hope. The mystery of finance remained forever a closed book to Annie Sullivan, and if the whole truth be told, to Helen also."

Helen herself was to write, in 1929: "My sense of pride mutinies against my confession; but we are the kind of people who come out of an enterprise poorer than we went into it." At another point in the same book, *Midstream:* "Financial difficulties have seemed nearly always an integral part of our lives, and from time to time many people have tried to help us extricate ourselves from them." That such help was acceptable only if unaccompanied by advice, she made clear in the resentful statement that "all through my life people who imagine themselves more competent than my teacher and I have wanted to organize my affairs." Those who were really appreciated, she wrote, were "the friends who have not tried to manage me."

Some of the wellsprings of this prickly attitude may be detected in Helen Keller's memoir, *Teacher,* published 20 years after Anne's death:

It required a powerful temperament for Teacher to protect me against interference and the zeal of strangers who wished to run my affairs. . . . From bitter experience she suspected that many people who offered to help us wanted in reality to use me for their own purposes.

It is doubtful whether the trustees of the American Foundation for the Blind were prepared for the "powerful temperament" they were to encounter in Anne Sullivan Macy when they decided to enlist Helen Keller's services. They did know that Helen could only be dealt with as part of a package that included her teacher and Polly Thomson, who had joined the Keller-Macy household in 1914. Each of the three had a distinct role to play. Helen, obviously, could not appear on a platform by herself. Her laboriously acquired speech was never perfected to a point where she could be readily understood by the unaccustomed ear. Nor was she capable of a sustained speaking effort. Her public appearances, therefore, followed a pattern. First Mrs. Macy would appear, alone. She would tell how the concept of communication had been conveyed to a child who could neither see, hear, nor speak, and would describe the methods used in educating a liberated young mind to a high degree of culture. Then Helen would walk on stage and, taking hold of her teacher's hand, give a brief talk. After each sentence she would pause while her teacher repeated it in her clear diction with its faint trace of Irish brogue.

If more than a few minutes of speaking were involved, Helen might begin orally and then finger-spell the rest of her message into Mrs. Macy's hand. They would then field questions from the audience, with Mrs. Macy transmitting what was said into Helen's hand and Helen responding, either vocally or manually. Polly Thomson usually stood by in the wings, ready to go on as an alternate for Mrs. Macy if the latter was too tired or too unwell to carry her half of the program.

It was a tested "act." They had tried it out during cross-country lecture tours in 1913 and 1915, and had perfected it a few years later when they were engaged by the Keith Orpheum Circuit for two coast-to-coast seasons in vaudeville. The principal trouble was that no matter how much money they earned, it all seemed to disappear. The three women were fond of clothes and justified the cost of their liberal wardrobes by citing the necessity of being well-dressed for a variety of public appearances. When they had a few dollars to spare, they spent the money joyously on gala vacation excursions, on improvements to the rambling house in Forest Hills, New York, to which they had moved in 1917, or—often enough—on gifts for friends.

It was primarily the chronic shortage of cash, and mounting concern that she might die and leave her aging life companion unprovided for, that made Helen eagerly accept the offer to appear in a movie based on her life story. She and Anne went to Hollywood full of zeal and happy expectation. The picture, a concoction of fact and fantasy called *Deliverance*, opened to kindly notices in 1919 but was a box-office failure. The only money Helen and Anne got out of it was a substantial advance, all of which was used up before they ever left Hollywood.

The vaudeville experience which followed was financially more rewarding, but after two full seasons this string, too, was just about played out. They had only one story to tell, and few audiences were interested in hearing it a second time. There was no way for them to create fresh material equal in impact to that initial drama.

From many viewpoints, therefore, Helen Keller and Anne Sullivan Macy were ready for new directions as 1924 began. At the same point, the American Foundation for the Blind, having survived its first year of operation, was ready for a major effort to achieve national recognition and support. It seemed a perfect conjunction of mutual need and opportunity.

No inspired stroke of genius was needed to conceive the plan that Helen Keller should join forces with the Foundation. Helen Keller was not only the perfect symbol, her name was a household word. She could be counted upon to attract large audiences to any public meeting at which an appeal would be made for support of a new movement to assist America's blind people.

The Foundation's first director-general, Joseph Nate, had made a tentative approach along these lines to Helen and her teacher, but nothing concrete had materialized. With Nate's departure, the responsibility for devising a way to finance the Foundation's work fell to M.C. Migel. In a letter to Charles F.F. Campbell, then director of the Detroit League for the Handicapped, the Foundation president set forth the organization's situation as of late November 1923 and the plan developed by the trustees for building a nationwide membership body.

A minimum budget of $42,500 had been adopted for 1924, he told Campbell, adding that the Foundation could easily use twice that sum for work already on hand:

> Our present idea is to have the Foundation underwritten for a period of three years by . . . possibly fifty men and women who might pledge themselves for three years to $1,000 per annum. I believe this might not be so extremely difficult, as several people whom I have approached have already pledged various large amounts, and we have possibly $24,000 per annum underwritten.
>
> With this accomplished the Foundation would be safe for a period of three years, and in the interim, we propose to secure at least five thousand members at Ten Dollars per annum. With the securing of the latter, we would be more or less safe for a long period. . . . Naturally, an endowment is the answer to the entire problem, and we feel that after three years, if our work is worth while, we can proceed on that. Our great problem at present is as to the securing of this large membership, and if we can devise the proper plan, this should not be insuperable.

Did Campbell have any practical suggestions on how this plan might be realized? What did he think of the possibility of large public gatherings? Campbell's reply, couched in characteristically enthusiastic terms, was prompt and specific:

> For years, I have felt very keenly that the most practical method of raising money is to avail oneself of the services of Miss Helen Keller and her teacher. . . . I am convinced that nothing would please them more than to do their part in a campaign to raise funds for the Foundation.

He proceeded to outline a detailed plan:

> A series of "drawing room" meetings could be arranged in the leading cities throughout the country to which a select group of wealthy people could be invited. These meetings should be made distinctly social events. . . . At each of these gatherings, a brief, clear-cut statement with regard to the needs of

the blind and the plans of the Foundation should be given. . . . After such an introduction, Mrs. Macy could give, in a very few minutes, an outline of the way in which Miss Keller received her education and then Miss Keller would make a personal appeal for the blind of the country.

A born romanticist, Campbell went on to remind Migel that Helen Keller had been dramatically effective as a fund-raiser while she was a small girl. In the late 1880s he pointed out, Michael Anagnos, then head of the Perkins Institution,

raised astonishing sums of money for the kindergarten for the blind in Massachusetts by letting Helen make the appeal. The scenes enacted by Henry Ward Beecher, when people of wealth came forward and threw money and jewelry at his feet when he made his appeals in behalf of the slaves, were repeated, to a certain extent, in the presence of Helen Keller when she made her plea for little blind children.

Campbell then tackled the crux of the matter:

One question will, inevitably, arise: namely, how should Miss Keller and Mrs. Macy be paid. At first thought it might be suggested that a fixed sum, plus a commission upon all over a certain amount raised, should be given, but it would be infinitely more effective if some of the present donors to the Foundation would underwrite the Helen Keller campaign so that it could be truthfully said that . . . she received no portion, whatever, of the money raised during her tour. . . . It goes without saying that Mrs. Macy and Miss Keller should receive a very handsome honorarium for this service. . . . The success of such a campaign is assured, provided (and this is of the utmost importance), a high-grade, capable individual is employed to plan the undertaking.

Campbell may very well have had himself in mind as the "high-grade, capable individual" to direct the campaign. Less than two months later, Robert Irwin wrote him:

You will be interested to know that as a result of your suggestion to Mr. Migel some time ago, the Foundation is arranging for a series of meetings in and around New York . . . at which Helen Keller will be the star performer. It is planned to follow much the same program as you outlined in your letter.

We are very anxious to make these first meetings a thorough-going success. Mr. Migel feels that after Helen Keller speaks he would like to have the champion spellbinder of the work for the blind make the appeal for funds. Accordingly he has asked me to write you, asking if you would be able to come on for three or four days for this purpose. As this is but an experiment and the Foundation cannot get too deeply involved, we are hoping that you will be able to come and put this thing over simply for your expenses, plus the gratitude of everybody concerned.

The "champion spellbinder" agreed to help out with three initial meetings in Westchester, but the plan promptly ran into a muddled conflict of dates. While Irwin was scheduling events in Westchester, a member of Charles Hayes' staff was setting up a series of meetings in New Jersey for the identical period.

The New Jersey work was in the hands of an energetic woman named Ida Hirst-Gifford, whom Hayes had employed the preceding year to assist him in field service. During World War I, Mrs. Gifford had gained national prominence through the successful placement and supervision of 50 blind employees as armature winders in the New Jersey factory of the Crocker-Wheeler Electric Manufacturing Company. She had many important connections throughout the state and used these to organize three meetings in March and two more in early April.

Since an undeclared contest seemed to have arisen between him and Mrs. Gifford, Campbell withdrew after the first two Westchester meetings. Mrs. Gifford, whose accomplishments included musicianship, not only organized fund-raising meetings but occasionally filled in as a piano accompanist for the musical interludes that were part of every program. She developed a harmonious relationship with the Helen Keller party and remained a member of their entourage in subsequent campaigns. In the intervals between these drives, she undertook other promotional and field service assignments for the Foundation. In later years, she served as administrator of Rest Haven. She retired in 1947 and died the following year at the age of sixty-eight.

The trustees were pleased and excited over the first fruits of the Helen Keller experiment. On April 18, Migel sent a graceful note to Campbell in Detroit:

> . . . we have been working for some little time with the assistance of Helen Keller and Mrs. Macy, and thus far have held seven meetings, addressed about 10,000 people, and have had subscribed to our Foundation approximately $8,000—a most wonderful record. . . . Both Mrs. Macy and Helen Keller have been indefatigable, most willing and disinterested. They really feel that they wish to help the cause.
>
> As you were practically instrumental and took the initiative in recommending that we proceed with them, I know you will be highly pleased, and it is because of this that I am writing you.

All the meetings followed a more or less standard procedure. Each featured a performance by one or more blind artists: Edwin Grasse, who played both the violin and the piano; Abram Haitowitsch, violinist; William Fuhrmeister, baritone; or Guy Envin, the French soldier-poet, who gave dramatic recitations. Then there was a brief talk by someone representing the Foundation—most often Charles Hayes—describing its purposes and goals. This was followed by the climactic appearance of Helen and her teacher. After Helen's appeal for support of the Foundation, there was another musical interlude while ushers moved through the aisles, distributing membership blanks and collecting cash donations.

If M.C. Migel and Mrs. Gifford and ten thousand members of the public were impressed by Helen Keller's impact, so was Anne Sullivan Macy. No sooner had the first series of meetings been concluded in the spring of 1924, than Mrs. Macy declared she and Helen were convinced there was no need to wait three years before beginning to build an endowment fund. They thought it could be done at once, with an objective of $2 million. The magnitude of the goal appealed to their imaginations; they were confident it could be reached. Swayed by their confidence, the Major allowed himself to be diverted from his original timetable. If

$2 million could be raised, he reasoned, the income from such a nest egg would surely make it unnecessary for the Foundation ever again to turn to the public for funds. It was an immensely appealing prospect for a man who found asking others for money distasteful.

Should she and Helen embark on a $2 million endowment campaign, Mrs. Macy informed the Foundation, they would require much more substantial compensation than the previous honorarium of $50 per meeting plus expenses. The need to make such a change had already been recognized by the executive committee, which at its meeting of June 4, 1924, authorized the president "to make arrangements with Miss Helen Keller and Mrs. Macy at the rate of $750 per month and expenses, for a period of six months, to address meetings to increase the funds of the Foundation."

Mrs. Macy did not regard this as satisfactory. She wanted $2,000 a month for the six-month campaign period, out of which Helen and her two companions would pay their own traveling expenses. For this, Helen would agree to make four public appearances a week, three with Mrs. Macy and one with Polly Thomson. What appeared unreasonable to the Foundation in this counter-offer was the stipulation that the monthly fee was to be no less during periods when the campaign was conducted in the New York area, where traveling expenses were minimal, than when the party was booked in distant cities. Robert Irwin and Charles Hayes were sent to Forest Hills to negotiate this point. They got nowhere.

There followed what was to be the first of many brushes between Anne Sullivan Macy's "powerful temperament" and M.C. Migel's equally forceful personality. The Major bridled at being presented with an ultimatum. He was offended that Anne had called in her lawyer, William Ashley, to handle the negotiations instead of dealing face to face with the trustees. There might be only one Helen Keller, but there were other ways to raise money. The Foundation had, in fact, been approached by several well-regarded fund-raising firms. As a matter of prudent business management, the Major felt the alternatives should at least be weighed.

On her side, Mrs. Macy felt she could afford to be single-minded in her demands; she, too, had been approached by commercial firms with various promotional schemes that seemed financially promising. Her principal responsibility, as she saw it, was to protect Helen's interests. All other considerations were secondary.

For Migel, however, the question had implications that transcended personalities. Publicly contributed money was a sacred trust; in his view it would be unconscionable if too large a percentage of the funds given for service to blind people were to be dissipated in expenses. Characteristically, his first thought was to solve the problem by reaching into his own pocket. He offered to underwrite personally the $2,000 monthly salary, so that this sum would not be charged against the money raised. This arrangement, he felt, would protect the Foundation from accusations of extravagance.

Some of these points had already been conveyed to Mrs. Macy when Migel proposed, in early August, that a conference be held at which the matter could be settled. He had yet to find out how rigid Teacher could be when thwarted. On August 6, she sent two stiffly worded wires. The one to Migel said:

I SHALL NOT BE AT CONFERENCE TOMORROW. IF YOU THINK OTHER AGENCIES
CAN RAISE THE TWO MILLION DOLLARS WITHOUT HELEN KELLER, WE SHALL BE
MOST WILLING TO WITHDRAW.

To William Ashley, she wired:

MR. MIGEL HAS ASKED ME TO BE PRESENT AT YOUR CONFERENCE TOMORROW.
THINK I HAD BETTER NOT. UNDERSTAND HE BELIEVES FUND CAN BE RAISED
WITHOUT HELEN KELLER. HOPE THIS IS TRUE. WE SHOULD BE GLAD TO BE
RELEASED. IF WE MUST CONTINUE, WOULD PREFER TO HAVE OUR SALARY COME
OUT OF EXPENSES INCIDENTAL TO RAISING MONEY THAN TO BE UNDERWRITTEN
BY MIGEL.

One can only speculate about the outcome of so defiant a challenge had Anne
Sullivan Macy been a man. What salvaged the situation, on this and subsequent
occasions, was Migel's attitude toward women. It would have gone against his
grain to take on a woman in open battle. Moreover, Helen Keller and Anne
Sullivan Macy were no ordinary women. The Major had already developed a
genuine affection for Helen that was to grow and deepen until the day he died. He
had sincere respect and admiration for Anne's accomplishments; moreover he felt
great compassion for her deteriorating health. He and she were the same age, but
he was hale and hearty while she was not only fast approaching total blindness but
was also plagued with numerous other ailments, including a form of septicemia that
manifested itself in painful carbuncles.

Migel did not at that time know about the horrifying childhood years Anne had
spent in the Tewksbury poorhouse until, at the age of fourteen, she clawed her
way out and gained admission to the Perkins Institution for the Blind. It was not
until Nella Braddy's biography of her appeared in 1933 that the world learned of
the trials she had undergone before she ever heard of Helen Keller. What the
Major did recognize (and it touched him deeply) was the unique nature of the tie
that bound Helen and her teacher into a kind of Siamese twinship. Closer than
mother and daughter, closer than sisters, closer than husband and wife, these two
women all but shared a single heartbeat. Although Helen had an independent mind
and spirit and personality, she was helpless without someone who could be her eyes
and ears and voice. Anne had chosen to be that someone and had subordinated her
own life so that Helen's might be as rich and full as possible. Such gallant
selflessness could not help but move a man who was a sentimentalist at heart.

There can hardly be any other explanation for the well-nigh angelic patience
that the normally quick-tempered Migel displayed toward Helen's teacher on the
many occasions when she proved difficult. In the present instance, he agreed to her
terms, continuing to insist only on the proviso that he would privately underwrite
the salary.

The plan for the endowment campaign was announced in the Fall 1924 issue of
Outlook for the Blind:

In order to insure the perpetuity of the national work for the benefit of the
blind, it has been deemed imperative that an endowment fund be established,
sufficient to maintain the minimum activities of this organization.

As the American Foundation for the Blind embodies a dream which has long been cherished by Miss Helen Keller, she and Mrs. Macy have consented to devote their time and energies to assisting with the endowment fund campaign.

The campaign is under the direction of a committee of men and women of nation-wide reputation, of which Dr. Henry van Dyke is chairman. Efforts will be made in every large city of this country to enlist friends and obtain contributions toward the endowment fund. This will be done principally through the medium of mass meetings which will be addressed by Miss Keller, Mrs. Macy and others.

The Foundation wishes to impress upon its friends the fact that such a national campaign depends for its success upon the active cooperation of workers for the blind in every community.

A representative of the Foundation will call upon workers for the blind in each community, several weeks in advance of Miss Keller's visit in order to perfect arrangements for the meetings.

The Foundation will in all cases be guided by the judgment of those in charge of local organizations, in order that the best interests of all may be served.

Omission of the $2 million campaign goal figure and the careful wording of the closing paragraphs were designed to avoid alienating local agencies. Rumors, some accurate and others exaggerated, were already flying thick and fast. In some cities, agency heads openly expressed resentment over the prospect that the Foundation drive might divert large sums of money from local services. In other cities, the objections centered around reports that Helen Keller would be paid a lavish salary. In still others, a highly moral tone was assumed: Was not the Foundation callously exploiting the infirmities of a handicapped person?

Echoes of disaffection were not slow in reaching New York. Robert Irwin, attending a committee meeting in Ohio, heard that Cincinnati was up in arms. In early December, Charles Hayes informed Migel that the Chicago Council of Social Agencies had voted to disapprove any Foundation campaign in that city. "This vote," he wrote, "was based on the facts that they did not endorse any national organization asking for an endowment and that they did not have sufficient knowledge of the activities of the Foundation." The "big objector," Hayes went on, was Edith Swift, executive director of the Chicago Lighthouse, who was the daughter of a former mayor of Chicago and influential in the city's business community. Hayes continued:

> She will not endorse the Helen Keller meetings. She claims that they are purely sentimental and that such meetings would be damaging not only to the work for the blind in Chicago, but to the Foundation. . . . The more I see of the Chicago situation, [the more] I am convinced it would be extremely unwise to launch our campaign at present.

Chicago, Hayes concluded, "has an injured air, and the best way to cure it is to leave it alone now and come back later." Hayes was right in his diagnosis, wrong in his prognosis. Chicago never did permit Helen Keller to campaign there. Neither did St. Louis and several other major cities.

Understandably upset over these negative reactions, Migel suggested that Irwin spend a week or two with the campaign party as an observer. Irwin attended three meetings in Ohio, talked to a lot of people, and sent a preliminary report of his findings to Migel on January 13, 1925. He found a good deal to criticize:

> We are going too fast to any more than skim off the cream. There is a lack of coordination among the different parts of the machine. After the advance man sells the proposition to the community leaders, there is not sufficient follow-up work to enable the committees to function intelligently, they are left in the dark on too many points. . . .

What concerned him most was how to avoid the irritations being stirred up by the fund-raising firm which had been employed to handle advance arrangements, press coverage, follow-up mailings, and other details. He urged strongly that this outfit be dismissed and that the Foundation build its own campaign organization instead.

The trustees agreed. On February 4, 1925, the executive committee acted to cancel the contract with the outside firm and voted that the campaign be continued until June 1 "under the direct management of the Foundation."

The decision to push on with the drive, despite all the vexations, was spurred by the brilliant success of the campaign effort in Detroit, where more than $40,000 was raised. Much of the credit for this gratifying result was due to Charles Campbell, who had almost single-handedly planned and directed the Detroit strategy. With his usual generosity of spirit, Campbell proceeded to detail, for the Foundation's future guidance, every step he had followed in organizing his community for liberal giving and to call attention to a pitfall: "Unfortunately, a good many thoughtful givers look somewhat askance upon national agencies." He also offered an important insight into the fast-changing economic patterns of the newly industrialized Middle West: ". . . few people outside of Detroit realize that this city has doubled its population within the last ten years. This means that the great majority of the men here who are rich are young and still chiefly occupied with making, and not giving, money. . . . Most of them still have to learn to give."

To everyone's disappointment, there were to be no other banner triumphs even remotely comparable to Detroit during the balance of the 1925 campaign. As the group moved westward, crowds came to hear Helen Keller in every city they visited, but the amounts contributed were often little more than token sums. High hopes had been pinned on Los Angeles, and particularly on the money to be garnered from the motion picture colony, but results proved as illusory as the images projected on the silver screen.

The 139 speeches made by Helen Keller in 53 cities over a period of nearly seven months in this first endowment campaign represented only part of her effort. She also wrote endless thank-you letters, addressed special appeals to potential "big givers," and suffered through innumerable receptions, luncheons, and other social functions. These were an ordeal for her. "I know that nearly everybody has heard of me, and that people want to see me, just as we all want to see places and persons and objects we have heard about," she later wrote. Still,

I do not know a more disturbing sensation than that of being ceremoniously ushered into the presence of a company of strangers, who are also celebrities, especially if you have physical limitations which make you different. As a rule, when I am introduced to such people, they are excessively conscious of my limitations. When they try to talk to me, and find that their words have to be spelled into my hand, their tongues cleave to the roofs of their mouths and they become speechless. And I am quite as uncomfortable as they are.

In one of the rare flashes of humor to appear in her published writings (as opposed to her private correspondence, which often sparkled with wit), she ended the foregoing passage with this:

Even now, where people are gathered, I say little, beyond explaining patiently that I am not Annette Kellerman [the champion exhibition swimmer credited with popularizing the one-piece bathing suit for women during the Twenties], that I do not play the piano, and have not learned to sing. I assure them that I know day is not night and that it is no more necessary to have raised letters on the keys of my typewriter than for them to have the keys of their pianos lettered. I have become quite expert in simulating interest in absurdities that are told me about other blind people. Putting on my Job-like expression, I tell them blind people are like other people in the dark, that fire burns them, and cold chills them, and they like food when they are hungry, and drink when they are thirsty, that some of them like one lump of sugar in their tea, and others more.

Helen felt differently about platform appearances which did not involve social chit-chat. She derived understandable pleasure from the warmth with which audiences responded to her. But she could never bring herself to enjoy fund-raising. The very need for philanthropy conflicted with her Socialist beliefs. As she once wrote: "in our present civilization most philanthropic and educational institutions are supported by public donations and gifts from wealthy citizens. This is a wretched way, but we have not yet learned a better one. . . . "

Needless to say, her campaign speeches did not reflect such views. Basically all alike, their major themes may be sampled in excerpts from the address she made in June 1925 to the International Convention of Lions Clubs:

Try to imagine how you would feel if you were suddenly stricken blind today. Picture yourself stumbling and groping at noonday as in the night, your work, your independence gone. In that dark world wouldn't you be glad if a friend took you by the hand and said, "Come with me and I will teach you how to do some of the things you used to do when you could see"? That is just the kind of friend the American Foundation is going to be to all the blind in this country if seeing people will give it the support it must have.

You have heard how through a little word dropped from the fingers of another a ray of light from another soul touched the darkness of my mind and I found myself, found the world, found God. It is because my teacher learned about me and broke through the dark, silent imprisonment which held me that I am able to work for myself and for others. It is the caring we want more than money. The gift without the sympathy and interest of the giver is empty. If you care, if we can make the people of this great country care, the blind will indeed triumph over blindness.

. . . I appeal to you, you who have your sight, your hearing, you who are strong and brave and kind. Will you not constitute yourselves Knights of the Blind in this crusade against darkness?

Where the Lions Clubs were concerned, this was an irresistible appeal. This nationwide organization, founded in 1917 to promote civic welfare, had already taken on the cause of the blind as one of its major projects; after Helen's talk the sponsorship became permanent. Over the years, local Lions Clubs initiated and supported educational weeks for the blind; raised funds for the brailling and sound-recording of books; supplied blind persons with canes, radios, typewriters, and other useful appliances; arranged entertainments, outings, and camping programs; paid tuition fees for blind students; organized and supported eye clinics and other medical services for the blind; contributed funds to local agencies and fulfilled in innumerable other ways the crusading role that Helen Keller had urged them to adopt.

As this first nationwide drive drew to a close, the fund-raising party recognized with deep chagrin that Helen's appeals had failed to stimulate an equally gratifying response when it came to actual cash results. Seven months of campaigning had produced $130,000 in cash and $40,000 in pledges. The Foundation's executive committee, which received this news at its September 1925 meeting, also learned that the expenses involved in raising this sum were embarrassingly high, even allowing for the fact that $14,000 in salary for the Keller-Macy-Thomson trio was not being charged against campaign results. The Foundation, it appeared, could expect at best to net about $100,000 from this endowment effort; this sum, when invested, would produce an annual income of no more than $5,000.

M.C. Migel, though deeply disappointed, was not one to carp. Shortly before the final campaign meeting, which was held in San Francisco on June 15, he wrote a kindly and tactful letter to Mrs. Macy on the west coast proposing that they confer during the summer to "map out a programme whereby Helen and you and Miss Thomson would continue with us for a long period, should you care to do so, and under an arrangement that naturally would be satisfactory and fair to both sides."

The reply that came from Mrs. Macy so perfectly typifies this complex woman's tenacity of purpose, as well as her ability to be simultaneously blunt and gracious, that it deserves to be quoted at length if not in full. It was dated June 25, 1925.

I won't harass you by going too deeply into the history of our unsuccessful efforts to secure the Endowment Fund, all the more that we have failed so obviously; but I must plead for my delay in acknowledging your letter of May 12th. Its genuine kindness went straight to my heart, and I cannot thank you enough for writing in such a splendidly generous spirit. . . .

I need not tell you, Mr. Migel, that I—that we all—deplore our failure to come nearer to the goal of our expectations in the matter of raising the Fund, though I now understand that those expectations were naively childish. The idea of raising two million dollars in six months for a new and scarcely heard of organization mocks at common sense.

I have often tried to project myself in imagination into your mind to get your reaction on the situation, with indifferent success. I have never been a capitalist; so I find it difficult to sense what a capitalist's state of mind is when a pet investment yields a negligible dividend. Humanly speaking, you must have felt keenly disappointed sometimes, and asked yourself if such large expenditure was justified by the meager contributions we were sending in; and perhaps you have thought that we might have done better. But as the days passed, I am sure you have felt in the depths of your generous nature that we have all done our very best. Right here I wish to say, we have been much impressed by your attitude of patient waiting for results that have not been forthcoming. Not once have you complained, or shown us by any sign that you were dissatisfied with our procedure. . . .

You may recollect that when we first discussed methods of raising money, I thought we should get it from the people in small donations, and, you, on the other hand, thought we should try to get large gifts from the rich. Now I am convinced that we must get a large part of the Fund from the common people before we can hope for big donations. . . .

The last few meetings, when we asked the people for a pledge of twenty-five cents a month for a year, the response was spontaneous, and quite satisfactory. . . . When the people once get this idea, the Fund will grow rapidly, and then wealthy givers will see that our work has a just claim to be taken seriously.

Less than six months later, the same woman who expressed such heartfelt gratitude for Migel's "splendidly generous spirit" was firing a volley of angry accusations at him:

[Y]our treatment of Helen Keller and me does not confirm the high opinion I had formed of you. Your words and your deeds do not harmonize. While expressing a profound appreciation of our endeavors to raise the Endowment Fund for the Foundation, you bargain with us like a railroad magnate employing stokers or road menders. When talking business, you apparently have little sense of the nature of the work we are doing for the Foundation, or of anything except securing our labor as cheaply as possible.

Several factors were responsible for this about-face. Helen and her two companions had vacationed lightheartedly on the Pacific coast for several months following the end of the campaign tour. They returned to Forest Hills in October to discover that their bank balance was alarmingly low and their house needed major repairs. The only solution they could see was to negotiate a larger salary for the 1926 campaign effort. They apparently felt such desperate financial pressure that they found it hard to recognize that the Foundation, too, faced some very real dilemmas.

For one thing, there was genuine disagreement on the part of the trustees with Mrs. Macy's theory that an endowment fund could and should be built out of small donations from "the common people." This approach might be valid, but it would take far too long and cost far too much. Migel and his associates still thought the fund would have to be raised through pace-setting large gifts from the wealthy. The trustees fully recognized the educational and other merits of building a mass body of supporters, but it would be more advantageous, they felt, for money from this source to be in the form of memberships. Endowment giving was a one-time affair; memberships, on the other hand, were annually renewable, and renewals could be solicited by mail at far less cost than the initial gift.

Of even greater importance to those operating the Foundation's steadily expanding service program was that membership fees could be used for current operations, whereas only the income from endowment gifts could be thus employed. The Foundation's operations were already moving fast in many directions, and funds to finance continued momentum were urgently needed.

An overriding consideration was that the elected officers and trustees of the Foundation could not blink at a basic problem of ethics—what price fund-raising? The cost of the first campaign had been distressingly high, even allowing for the public education benefits that had accrued. The trustees could not, in good conscience, justify any fund-raising program in which fifty cents out of every contributed dollar was used up in expenses. Nor could they risk any further undermining of their relationships with local agencies for the blind, many of which were openly expressing resentment over so ambitious a capital funds drive. A membership campaign would make much less of a stir and encounter far less opposition.

All these factors were weighed before the executive committee voted in late September 1925 to renew the Keller-Macy contract for the first five months of 1926 on the same $2,000-a-month basis as the previous year. But the proposed contract contained an important protective proviso: ". . . if, in the judgment of the American Foundation for the Blind, the expenses of the Helen Keller Tour seem excessive, as compared with income from mass meetings, this agreement is to be modified."

In a less tempestuous mood, Anne Sullivan Macy might have seen the merit of this position. But she was in no emotional state to be judicious. She felt frustrated at every point. She and Helen regarded themselves as morally committed to completing the endowment fund; in their view, appealing for $5 and $10 memberships would be a comedown compared with the lofty goal of a $2 million endowment. Mrs. Macy was offended at the rejection of her firm conviction that, despite the disappointing results of the previous year, such a fund could still be built through mass support. She wanted to see penny banks distributed to the nation's school children and was annoyed that no one seemed to take this suggestion seriously. Most immediate of all, she was distressed at her inability to secure a sufficiently high level of compensation to alleviate the household's financial stress.

Nevertheless, she signed the contract for 1926 after a few compromises had been worked out. The campaign would be concentrated in a smaller territory so that travel expenses would be lower. Any gifts of more than $100 obtained through the mass meetings or through direct solicitation by Helen would be placed in the endowment fund; in addition, at least 10 percent of the total money received through memberships and renewals would be credited to the endowment fund.

With this face-saving agreement, the 1926 campaign was launched and, despite its stormy beginnings, proved to be a resounding success. With Charles Hayes and Ida Hirst-Gifford doing the organizing and the legwork, the campaign party barnstormed through nine northeastern states, addressing 120,000 persons at 110 meetings in 70 cities during a five-month period. The money raised amounted to $134,000, almost all of it in small sums, at a cost of less than 30 percent of the gross.

The campaign schedule was grueling. There were two, sometimes three, meetings in a single day. They might address a noontime audience of 900 in a church in Gouverneur, New York, and that same evening face 700 people gathered in a school auditorium in nearby Ogdensburg. Some of the meetings were financial disappointments; others exceeded expectations. By this time, the campaign party had developed experience and sophistication in fund-raising. They had learned, for example, that the events that attracted the largest and most eminent audiences were not necessarily those that raised the most money.

The showpiece of this 1926 campaign was its opening gun—a mass meeting in the nation's capital under impressive sponsorship. The list of patrons was headed by Mrs. Calvin Coolidge (the President himself had agreed to become honorary president of the Foundation and was so listed), Vice-President and Mrs. Dawes, Chief Justice and Mrs. Taft, several other Supreme Court justices, virtually every member of the Cabinet, a dozen senators and congressmen, and thirty-odd foreign ambassadors, ministers, and other members of the diplomatic corps.

Three thousand people gathered in the Washington Auditorium to hear an opening address by Dr. Henry van Dyke, the clergyman-educator who was chairman of the Helen Keller National Committee. The meeting was chaired by Dr. Gilbert Grosvenor, son-in-law of Alexander Graham Bell. Edwin Grasse, the versatile blind musician who participated in this tour as he had in the previous one, provided several musical interludes. At one point he played the overture to *Lohengrin* on the organ; later, he switched to the violin to play several Fritz Kreisler solos; at a third juncture he performed the "Meditation" from Massenet's *Thaïs* with Ida Hirst-Gifford accompanying him on the piano. The climax, as always, was the joint performance by Helen Keller and her teacher, following which members of Washington's Junior League, acting as "Helen Keller's Aides," moved through the audience collecting cash and membership pledges.

Although the $8,400 raised that evening was not especially impressive in relation to the potential of so large and wealthy an audience, the publicity value of the illustrious patronage had its impact on the meetings that followed. In Rochester, New York, where Helen's old friend, Mrs. Edmund B. Lyon, sponsored a reception for 150 selected leaders, just over $7,000 was garnered over the teacups. This was followed by two mass meetings, attended by 3,700 people in all, at which an additional $4,300 was raised.

In Newark a series of mass meetings, plus a private tea, brought in some $6,500. In Worcester, Massachusetts, one of the Foundation's trustees, Mabel Knowles Gage, brought together a group of 75 friends at a private reception and raised more than $5,000; an additional $2,900 was gathered in smaller amounts from two public meetings whose audiences totalled 2,100. There were just enough of these gratifying high points to keep up the spirits of the weary campaign group.

Following the contretemps with Mrs. Macy that preceded the 1926 campaign agreement, Migel withdrew from active contact with the Keller household. As it happened, he spent much of 1926 abroad and it fell to Robert Irwin to help stage-manage the Foundation's relations with Helen and her teacher. Irwin not only wrote them encouraging notes while they were on the road but arranged for several of the trustees to do likewise.

The executive committee also went formally on record, at its meeting of June 10, 1926, by adopting a resolution to convey to the Helen Keller party "a wholehearted vote of gratitude" for their accomplishments. The three campaigners appeared in person at this session and Helen accepted the resolution with a graceful speech.

However, she said, "we must all realize there is still a long way—a very long way—to go. . . . Frankly, there are very pressing reasons that make us pause before going on with this task. The fact is we cannot afford it, but my teacher will explain this to you."

What her teacher had to say was all too familiar. According to the minutes of the meeting: "Mrs. Macy felt that the party could not continue with the campaign work under the present financial arrangement, nor did she think favorably of the suggestion that the party, instead of campaigning, devote their energies to soliciting large sums from private individuals."

It was the same old impasse and the meeting ended without reaching a decision. In mid-July Irwin wrote the Foundation's treasurer, Herbert H. White, suggesting a possible way out which, he reported, Mrs. Macy had indicated she would consider favorably. This was a proposal

> that Miss Keller be placed on the staff of the Foundation at $5,000 a year, in addition to the amount paid when on the road. Miss Keller would, for this amount, allow us the use of her name in connection with all of our financial and other publicity, and would prepare special articles and special letters for us upon various topics.

At about the same time, White received a long and discontented letter from Helen Keller, written from her sister's home in Montgomery, Alabama, where she and her companions were vacationing. It was in response to one which he, in his capacity as treasurer, had sent a few weeks earlier, enclosing a check for $1,000 as a bonus for special gifts. Helen's letter re-echoed some familiar themes:

> I have not written to you before because I needed to consider very carefully the advisability of accepting the check. My first impulse was to accept it; for I felt that Mrs. Macy and I had earned it. . . . Besides, we needed the money badly. . . . As we told the Executive Board, every cent of our salary went for expenses. . . . [I]t is utterly impossible for three women to live as we must live on such a meagre salary. . . . two thousand dollars a month for five months would not be extravagant compensation to pay me alone. . . .
>
> Frankly, the attitude of the Foundation towards Mrs. Macy and me has always been that of an employer, governed solely by practical considerations. It has assumed that we were for sale, and has negotiated to buy us as cheaply as possible. . . . But we are not for sale at a bargain any more. We are capable of earning our living with much less effort and strain. . . . Under the

circumstances, we feel quite disinclined to work for the Foundation next year. I doubt even if a more equitable arrangement would induce us to continue.

Why was it Helen Keller, and not Anne Sullivan Macy, who signed this querulous communication? Probably for the same reason that the letter transmitting the check had been signed by the Foundation's treasurer and not its president. The latter undoubtedly felt he had had enough of Mrs. Macy for a while, and she felt the same way toward him and his associates. So pervasive was the tension that it found a childishly petty outlet for annoyance. The resolution of thanks at the June meeting had voiced its appreciation to Helen Keller, Anne Sullivan Macy, and Polly Thomson. "When the Executive Board wished to express its appreciation of Mrs. Macy's and my services to the cause of the blind, it included Miss Thomson on equal terms with us in its vote of thanks," Helen's letter to White noted indignantly. "If the Board wished to honor Mr. Migel for his contributions to the Foundation, would it inscribe the name of his secretary on parchment in a similar manner?"

The upshot of all this was the return of the check "because Mrs. Macy and I feel that it would in some subtle way hamper us, and curtail our freedom of decision when the time comes to discuss plans for the future."

Caught in a crossfire that he recognized was aimed at another target, Herbert White responded with a gallant attempt to smooth ruffled feathers. White was at this time a man in his late sixties. The son of a family that had lived in New England since Colonial times, he had begun his working career at age fifteen, starting as a bank clerk and later moving into the employ of the Connecticut Mutual Life Insurance Company, of which he became treasurer in 1906. His interest in work for the blind had been constant since 1893, when he helped found the Connecticut Institute for the Blind. He was a dedicated, patriotic, and civic-minded person whose approach to life was described, when he died in 1934, as one of "unquestioning faith that ultimately there would be found a right and best way to accomplish necessary ends."

White's temperate response to Helen assured her that there was no thought of "bargain and sale" in the Foundation's dealings.

It is my recollection that the costs of campaign and terms were arranged on what at the time was agreed to be fair and satisfactory to all. If the estimates have been found incorrect it is because of our inability to forecast clearly unforeseen contingencies. . . . It seems to me, therefore, that misunderstanding has arisen and should be cleared up.

The returned check "is still at your disposal," he concluded. "It was sent you in good faith and it would seem to me that without loss in self-respect or without complicating the situation, which I hope may be set right, you may safely use it."

It was a troubled situation. One of the people in whom Mrs. Macy confided about it was Charles Campbell, who wrote her after reviewing the correspondence with the Foundation she had forwarded for his information. He found her feeling toward Migel unfortunate and hoped she would continue her affiliation with the Foundation. Neither White's conciliatory approach nor Campbell's impartial advice affected the immediate outcome. When the executive committee met in September, it adopted the suggestion of an extra $5,000 a year in salary for Helen. The offer was turned down. However, the letter in which Helen explained the reason for her refusal was far more moderate in tone than the one she had written in mid-summer.

The Foundation's offer had been conveyed in a letter signed by Olin H. Burritt as secretary, and it was to Burritt that Helen replied on October 22. She had made up her mind to bring her autobiography up to date, and although "the money difficulty remains the same" and "we may have to augment our income by lecturing once in a while," she was determined that "this question must not interfere with my decision; for the book must be done Now or Never. I think I can do it this winter if there are not too many interruptions. Next October, God willing, I would be ready to take to the road."

The Foundation had no choice but to accept this decision. It did act to insure some continuity by arranging to pay Helen a substantial honorarium for the preparation of some written material that could be used in mail appeals; beyond that, it could only wait until the book was finished. Four months later, Burritt sent a follow-up note asking Helen whether her availability in October could be counted upon. Her reply contained dismaying news:

> The truth is, my autobiography is not progressing as fast as I at first thought it would. . . . Mrs. Macy has gone through the material with the assistance of one of Doubleday and Page's staff; but that is the merest beginning. The material must be gone over many times, and read to me besides. We were getting along nicely until Mrs. Macy's eyes gave out the middle of January. . . .
>
> When Dr. Berens * says Mrs. Macy's eyes are better, my spirits soar, and I think the book will be nearly finished by June. When he says she must not read a word for several days, my hopes fail. . . .

As things worked out, Helen was not free that October, nor the following one, nor the one after that. It was 1932 before she was in a position to go back on the road for the Foundation and by then the country was so deep in economic depression that the results were a pittance. Her teacher's condition was such that there were long periods when she could not use her eyes at all. The principal saving grace in the situation was the presence of the person Helen had referred to as "one of Doubleday and Page's staff." This was Nella Braddy Henney, who not only played an essential role in the composition of Helen's book *Midstream* but in the process gained the confidence of Anne Sullivan Macy to such a degree that the latter allowed her to write her biography. Mrs. Henney became a cherished intimate of all three members of the household; the friendships she forged with Anne, Polly, and Helen lasted until each of them died.

(Indeed, where Anne was concerned, the friendship extended beyond the grave, for Mrs. Henney served as a consultant to William Gibson when he

---

* Dr. Conrad Berens was an eminent eye surgeon who was head of the Eye Clinic of the New York Lighthouse and prominent in the work of the National Society for the Prevention of Blindness. He was not only Mrs. Macy's physician but a close friend of the Keller household.

dramatized the story of Helen Keller and her teacher in *The Miracle Worker,* first as a "Playhouse 90" production on the Columbia Broadcasting System television network in 1957, then as a full-length Broadway play, and finally as the 1962 motion picture that brought Academy Awards to Anne Bancroft and Patty Duke for their respective roles as Anne Sullivan and Helen Keller.)

It was the news of Mrs. Macy's disabling illness that brought M.C. Migel back into the life of the Helen Keller household. He might have resolved never again to negotiate business arrangements with Helen and her teacher, but sickness and suffering were something else again. Now that their financial relationships with the Foundation had been settled by other officers, the Major felt free to call at Forest Hills as a friend. He went to see Helen and Mrs. Macy during Christmas week of 1926 and offered his personal financial help. He would place a fund at their disposal, he said, and they were not to hesitate to draw upon it whenever they wished. They could have a check at once if they needed it. This they refused, but the following April Anne wrote asking whether he would finance a chauffeured trip to New England that would enable them to revisit Wrentham and other scenes of the past that Helen was trying to recapture in *Midstream.* He agreed at once, and she replied she would ascertain the cost and let him know. On May 18 she wrote saying that "five hundred dollars will take care of it handsomely." Her letter continued:

> But I am going to make a further request. Once having screwed my courage to the point of asking you for money, I find I am quite shameless in availing myself of your generosity. Frankly, our finances are very low. Thus far we have succeeded in paying our bills; but next month will bring doctors' bills which I shall not be able to manage. May I have a thousand dollars in addition to the five hundred, please? If you will be so good, you will relieve me of considerable anxiety, and make it easier for all of us.

Migel wrote back on May 20, enclosing a check, but alas, the Major and Mrs. Macy were destined to stumble into one unfortunate misunderstanding after another. Migel's check had been drawn on the President's Fund he had established at the Foundation. This fund consisted of his own money, to be used under his direction for non-budgetary expenditures. A check drawn on it was as much a personal gift from Migel as one drawn on his private checking account. But Anne did not know this, and she was mortified that anyone at the Foundation should be privy to a confidential transaction.

"I regret deeply that I ever swerved from my resolve not to ask you for money," she wrote him when he returned from abroad. "I had a very strong intuition that such a request would create a humiliating situation, which it has." She enclosed her own check in repayment of $1,500. Even though she ended her letter with a dignified statement ("Many times I have thanked you for your kindly intentions. I must still believe that you mean well."), it was to be a long time before the two got back on cordial terms.

Two years later Anne underwent an unsuccessful operation on her right eye. This was a period of such intense anxiety for Helen that Migel's heart went out to her, and he ventured once again to offer financial help. In June 1929 he wrote suggesting that Helen, her teacher, and Polly take a vacation; he enclosed a check (his personal voucher this time) for $1,000 to pay for a cruise on the St. Lawrence River. His note went on: "Also, please send me a memorandum, giving me a rough idea of your hospital bills, and I shall defray same for you."

There was an ecstatic reply from Helen saying that the vacation would be doubly appreciated because Mrs. Macy would have to have a cataract operation on her other eye in September. There was also a postscript:

> It is most dear of you to ask about our hospital bills; but we shall not send them. You may have heard of a golden windfall that dropped into our unexpectant hands in the shape of a bequest from our lifelong friend, Mrs. William Thaw. It will take care of the hospital bills and quite a budget of other obligations.

In October the Major received a long, friendly letter from Anne herself, telling him how much improved she was in health and spirits after the cruise and spending the balance of the summer in the Adirondacks. "It's time to say how much I thank you for all your goodness to me," she ended. Three months later, however, she sent him a bitter letter of grievance. It differed from her previous outbursts only in that she now drew a distinction between Migel's personal relations with Helen and herself and what she described as the Foundation's "niggardly treatment of Helen." The Foundation, she said, "has not the slightest conception of the labor" entailed in Helen's work for the blind.

> Helen is a slow, painstaking worker. She makes many mistakes she does not know of until the letter is brought to me, then she must write it all over herself, as we have no stenographer. . . . Sometimes a letter has to be re-written five or six times before it is ready to mail.
>
> I am sure also that the trustees do not know how much time we three give each day to Foundation business—opening and reading letters, telephoning, autographing books and photographs, wrapping and addressing and mailing them . . . and taking them to the post-office—there is no one to do this mechanical labor. . . . Over seven hundred books have been autographed here in the past three months! It is necessary for either Miss Thomson or me to stand over Helen, keeping the line straight while she writes the inscription with painful slowness. All this standing and trying to see the words between her fingers is a terrible strain on my eyes.

Anne might have stopped right there; she had made her case. But she was in a mood to lash out and went on for five pages with passionate criticism of the Foundation's work and of its staff, even threatening to send an open letter to the press "showing up the treatment one blind person has received from the Foundation." The letter also voiced some hyperbolic claims: "It is Helen who has interested the public in the Foundation—put it on the map, so to speak. . . . Without Helen's name the Foundation could not exist, unless you personally financed it."

The clue to this extraordinary communication was contained in another letter to Migel, written the same day, from Helen herself. As always, she knew exactly what Mrs. Macy had written because she, Helen, had typed the letter. (She was always the household typist. Polly Thomson, who was called her secretary, could neither type nor take shorthand; even her handwriting, bold and dashing, was nearly illegible.)

"There is no disguising the fact that things are going very badly with my teacher these days," Helen wrote.

> She has not been able to read even the headlines of a newspaper for more than a week. She is very nervous, and naturally discouraged. . . . Please, dear Mr. Migel, try to be patient with our complaints and difficulties . . . these days we are living at high tension, and all around us is uncertainty and the dark. And what are friends for, if not to worry them a little?

Migel's reply to Helen reflected the forbearance he had learned to exercise toward the Forest Hills menage: "As to being impatient with you, my dear, that I shall never be—you know how I feel toward you all, although occasionally Teacher does try one a little."

His reply to Anne took the form of prompt action. At the next executive committee meeting a new financial arrangement was executed, giving Helen a salary of $6,000 a year plus a $1,200 allowance for clerical help. For this, Helen would write appeal letters to wealthy individuals and form letters for use with the Foundation's now large mailing list of members and contributors. She would testify on behalf of the Foundation at legislative hearings when indicated and would take on such other special assignments as would benefit from the use of her undeniable influence.

This new setup satisfied everyone. Helen wrote Migel a long and charmingly contrite reply to the letter notifying her of it. She cited Victor Hugo's parable about the man who tried to prevent a bee from dashing itself to death against a window pane. Attempting to capture the confused insect so as to free it through an open window, the man was stung for his pains.

> Now it seems to me we have behaved very much like the bee. You have always been our friend; but we have conducted ourselves in the manner of the stupid, suspicious drone. . . . Our narrow views and individual preoccupations have obscured the inner vision, so that we could not see your effort to befriend us, and plunged ahead into rash things. Like the bee, we have dashed ourselves against obstacles that didn't exist!

Now, she went on, "we are . . . feeling a little stunned and foolish, but grateful to you for having saved us from the consequences of our rashness. We hope we may prove ourselves worthy of your magnanimity."

It was almost the end of the cross-purposes and misunderstandings that had intermittently punctuated the relationship of Helen Keller and her household with the Foundation and its president. There were to be future differences of opinion and occasional angry explosions, sometimes from Anne in the five years of life that remained to her, sometimes from Helen herself. But neither Helen nor her teacher ever again questioned the genuine devotion of their friend, M.C. Migel, and he never ceased to give evidence, in ways large and small, of his unending concern for their welfare.

He sent them liberal checks and imaginative gifts at Christmas, at Easter, on Helen's birthday, and on numerous other occasions. When *Midstream* was published, he not only bought dozens of copies to give as gifts to his friends but underwrote the purchase of 2,500 copies of a low-cost edition to be sold by blind vendors at a profit to themselves. When Nella Braddy's biography of Anne Sullivan Macy appeared, Migel was again a large-scale buyer. He also arranged for the Foundation to send thousands of letters to agencies for the blind, praising the book and promoting its sale.

Nothing was too much trouble. When Anne was convalescing from her final eye operation, she was disturbed by street traffic. A park was being built in Forest Hills, and the heavily loaded construction trucks rumbling by in a continuous stream were literally shaking their house's foundations. Migel wrote to Robert Moses, then chairman of the State Council on Parks, explaining the situation and making a forthright request: "I am wondering if you would be good enough to order the rerouting of these trucks for a month or two, until Mrs. Macy recovers." Commissioner Moses cooperated; a member of his staff wrote Migel that as much of the hauling as possible would be diverted to a parallel street.

The most significant change in relationship took place at the end of 1932, when Anne finally yielded to Migel's urging that the management of Helen's financial affairs be put in charge of a three-man committee of trustees: himself; the banker Harvey D. Gibson, who was president of the Manufacturers Trust Company and a trustee of the Foundation; and the industrialist William Ziegler, Jr., also a member of the Foundation board.

It was not an easy decision for this proud woman to make. But Anne was by then nearly seventy years old; the sight of one eye was gone, only 10 percent vision remained in the other and this, too, was ultimately to be lost. She could no longer be at Helen's side in public appearances; that role had now become Polly Thomson's. Her sole remaining obligation toward Helen was to insure her against want. With a mixture of reluctance and relief, she transferred that obligation to the man she had finally learned to respect and trust. When death came to Anne Sullivan Macy on October 20, 1936, it found her serene in the knowledge that her affairs, and Helen's, were in order at last.

There remained Helen, never a docile soul, who had inevitably absorbed much of her teacher's determination to stick with whatever course she set out upon, no matter what. For Helen, the period that began during the mid-Thirties was one of steadily broadening horizons as she gradually modified her fixed ideas. One of the first to go was the notion that the endowment fund could only be completed through innumerable small donations. Although she had vehemently protested, "I am not gifted with the magic of charming large donations out of the coffers of the rich," she was extraordinarily successful at it.

The next barrier to crumble—although this took repeated assaults—was her insistence that her public and private appeals be made solely for the purpose of completing the endowment fund and not for current program needs. Curiously, she fought hardest of all against involvement in the drive to launch the Talking Book, one of the landmark achievements in services to blind people.

It was only when Helen finally conceded that the raising of that magic $2 million was not to be the only star in her crown of accomplishments that the second and more constructive phase of her work for the blind really began. Once she had shaken loose of the endowment obsession, she was free to pursue a more diversified program of service, using her talent with words, her winning personality, and the magic of her name in all the areas where they could make an impact: testimony before legislatures, personal appearances, national and international tours, letters and visits to men in high places. In this many-sided role she remained on the staff of the American Foundation for the Blind (and later also on that of the Foundation's sister agency, the American Foundation for Overseas Blind) for the rest of her life.

For the rest of her life, too, she remained under the solicitous stewardship of the personal trustees who served as her financial counselors and ultimately as the executors of her estate. The three original trustees predeceased her; they were replaced, one by one, by other men affiliated with the Foundation, which maintained a guardian account for her and ultimately became her residuary legatee. At the time of Helen Keller's death on June 1, 1968, her trustees were Jansen Noyes, Jr., then president (later chairman of the board) of the Foundation; Richard H. Migel, younger son of the Major and then treasurer (later vice-chairman of the board) of the Foundation; and James S. Adams, a banker and a Foundation trustee (later retired).

At no point did Helen's trustees see their responsibility as limited to shielding her from fear of privation. They took over management of all her affairs. They stood by her during the prolonged final illness of Polly Thomson, who died in 1960 at the age of seventy-five. Under their supervision, the Foundation's executive director (first Robert B. Irwin and, after 1949, M. Robert Barnett) saw to it that her household was staffed and run smoothly, that her house and grounds were kept in repair, that she had adequate clerical help for her work and proper nursing care during her last years. The trustees and the Foundation executives went beyond their official obligations. They behaved as friends, and because they took a personal interest, Helen Keller lived out her days in the comfort and dignity that her beloved teacher had spent a lifetime struggling to insure.

To do justice to the rich and varied texture of the latter half of Helen Keller's life would require the full biography that will surely be written one day. Many of the major milestones of those final forty years will emerge in the context of succeeding chapters. However, even as sketchy an outline as space in this volume affords must include mention of one other friendship that grew out of her work for the Foundation.

Gustavus A. Pfeiffer, the farmer's son who started life as half-owner of a drug store in Parksburg, Iowa, and ended as head of what became the billion-dollar pharmaceutical and cosmetics firm, Warner-Lambert, Inc., first encountered Helen in 1929 when he received one of her fund-raising appeals in the mail. It was a form letter, but he did not treat it as such. "Your letter goes right to the heart and opens the purse," he wrote her, enclosing a $500 check. Her personal note of acknowledgment produced a series of other, increasingly generous, contributions. These were sizable enough to prompt M.C. Migel to seek the acquaintance of this new benefactor of the blind, and the two struck up a warm friendship. Pfeiffer was impressed by what the Major told him of the Foundation's accomplishments and of its goals for the future; in due course, he agreed to serve on the board of trustees.

Pfeiffer was a devoutly religious man and when he met Helen in person he was struck by her spirituality and her intimate knowledge of the Bible. He wanted her to meet his nephew, Robert, who was a professor of Semitic languages and history at Harvard University and a man who had done intensive research on Biblical literature. A bond of mutual interest and affection developed and "Uncle Gus," Robert Pfeiffer, and other members of the family became close friends of Helen's household. When, following her teacher's death, Helen mentioned that she would like to leave Forest Hills and live in the country, "Uncle Gus" and his wife invited her to occupy one of the houses they had built for the use of artists and writers near their country estate in Westport, Connecticut.

Helen was charmed with the idea of Westport and said so, whereupon Pfeiffer decided that none of the existing houses in the colony was quite suitable for her. Instead he donated four acres of land to the Foundation for a residence to be built tailored to her particular needs. Helen's trustees saw to the disposition of the Forest Hills house and arranged for the financing of the new structure; "Uncle Gus" contributed not only the land but much of the cost of building and furnishing. His thoughtfulness extended to ordering a miniature model of the ten-room colonial-style building, so that Helen's fingers could familiarize her with the layout of her new home before she even moved in.

When the house, which was named Arcan Ridge, was almost totally destroyed by fire while Helen was abroad in 1946, Pfeiffer promptly cabled to reassure her that he would have it rebuilt. It was at Arcan Ridge, in its original and rebuilt versions, that Helen spent the last thirty years of her life, secure in the knowledge that she could safely devote all of her energies to the welfare of others, and it was from Arcan Ridge that in June 1968 her ashes went to their final resting place in St. Joseph's Chapel of the Washington Cathedral.

7

"Action Is Our Watchword"

To Helen Keller and her campaign entourage criss-crossing the country, the American Foundation for the Blind during the Twenties must have seemed a bottomless purse, its wide-open clasp hungry for every coin that could be cajoled out of the citizenry. An utterly different image was held, however, by those whose efforts were directed at translating organizational goals into working realities. To trustees and staff, the new organization was more like a bushel of fertile seeds, each bursting with the promise of a rich harvest of benefit for blind men, women and children. The potential was prodigious, the problem one of priorities. But the selection of those priorities was not always within their control. Prudent planning might dictate one course of action, outside pressures might precipitate another, while the emergence of unexpected opportunity might cause both to be postponed in the interests of *carpe diem*.

Nevertheless, an astonishing number of basic programs took root during the early years. Before the Twenties were over:

• Solid inroads had been made in the field of education through research on teaching methods and curricula, the initiation of teacher training programs, and sponsorship of an experimental school for the primary grades. There had also been an important breakthrough: the establishment, in Mississippi, of that state's first class for blind black children.

• The groundwork had been laid for production and dissemination of a larger, cheaper, more efficiently produced, and more widely distributed supply of literature for blind adults.

• An active field service had been established to assist local agencies in strengthening their programs, in obtaining needed legislation and appropriations, and in creating statewide commissions and associations to spearhead expansion and improvement of services for blind residents.

• A start had been made in opening up vocational opportunities through surveys and studies of occupations in which blind people were functioning successfully. A consulting group of vocational specialists had been convened to determine the most effective methods of training and placement.

• An engineering laboratory had been established to test, adapt, and improve mechanical devices that could be helpful to blind individuals and the organizations serving them, and a system initiated for distribution of aids and appliances specially adapted to the needs of blind persons.

• Publication of *Outlook for the Blind* had been taken over and its circulation greatly expanded. A second periodical had been started for educators of blind children and a program begun of publishing original books, monographs, and other literature dealing with aspects of blindness and work for the blind.

• Most exhilarating of all, the new organization had ventured into legislative waters and found the experience salutary and the results rewarding.

"Action is our watchword; action will bring results," the Foundation proclaimed in a ringing statement of purpose issued soon after it opened its doors. Even before it had a staff or an office, a satisfying opportunity arose to lend credibility to this watchword.

In the fall of 1922, M.C. Migel, accompanied by a committee of blinded World War I veterans, called at the White House to impress upon President Warren G. Harding the shocking paucity of books for the adult blind. Some 450 blinded American soldiers and sailors, the delegation pointed out, were now dependent on finger-reading. They had laboriously learned the system known as Revised Braille Grade 1½, but there were only about 300 titles available for adults in Grade 1½. As Migel later wrote President Harding in a summary of their discussion: "There is no endowment for printing books for the adult blind. When we consider that blind individuals are even more dependent upon reading . . . to profitably fill in otherwise idle and lonely hours, than are the seeing, the imperative necessity arises of satisfying their requirements by increasing the supply of embossed literature."

The federal government's subsidy to the American Printing House for the Blind (then at the rate of $50,000 a year) was restricted to the production of textbooks, and it was insufficient even for this purpose, allowing less than $7 per capita for blind school children. What the delegation asked for was an appropriation of $50,000 a year for three years for books for blinded veterans. The original idea was that this would cover the cost of producing 300 copies each of eight new titles a year, to become the personal possessions of braille-reading veterans. Later thinking revised this plan in favor of producing a greater number of titles in smaller quantities, using libraries for the blind and veterans' homes and hospitals as loan depositories.

"The cost of printing and embossing books for the blind is very considerable," the Major's letter to Harding pointed out. "Heavy paper must be used for proper embossing, and the cost of making the brass plates is very large" when prorated to the limited number of finished books made from the plates. He cited some examples comparing the cost of inkprint editions of popular books with the braille versions of the same titles. Even without taking the cost of plate-making into account, the comparisons were startling:

Pilgrim's Progress—85¢ in ink, $21.15 in braille
Robinson Crusoe—85¢ in ink, $20.80 in braille
A Tale of Two Cities—85¢ in ink, $16.45 in braille
Huckleberry Finn—$1.75 in ink, $31.10 in braille
Vanity Fair—85¢ in ink, $55.95 in braille

To clinch the comparison, the Major enclosed a photograph showing the relative sizes and weights of the inkprint and braille editions of *David Copperfield*. The former measured 4½ × 7 inches and weighed a little over one pound. The latter required six volumes, 9 × 12 inches, each weighing 4 pounds, or 32 pounds in all; 30 inches of shelf space were needed for the six volumes.

It was a thoroughly successful intervention. The Veterans Bureau, to which Harding referred the matter, not only endorsed the delegation's request but went even further. "I recommend that $100,000 be added to the item 'Vocational Rehabilitation' in the appropriation for the United States Veterans Bureau for the fiscal year ending June 30, 1924, for the purchase of embossed literature in Revised Braille for the use of blinded ex-servicemen," the bureau's director wrote to the chairman of the Senate Appropriations Committee on January 11, 1923. Congress approved the appropriation and Migel wrote exultantly to Olin Burritt: "If the Foundation did not do another stroke for a whole year, I think this one thing would have justified its existence."

Asked by the Veterans Bureau to submit a proposed list of titles to be produced under this appropriation, Robert Irwin formed a committee of librarians and other specialists in literature to draw up the list while simultaneously canvassing the various braille printing houses to see how much of this work they could handle in the limited time before the appropriation lapsed. It soon became apparent that under no circumstances were the existing printing houses capable of producing $100,000 worth of new braille books within the time limit.

There was talk for a while of setting up a new non-profit corporation to manufacture the books, but this idea was dropped as being neither politic nor feasible. Ultimately, the American Printing House for the Blind, which had originally signified it could handle no more than $30,000 worth of the work, undertook to produce double that amount. It was given a contract and printed 68 titles, in editions of 15 copies each, at a cost of about $60,000. At least part of the disappointment at the loss of the balance of the appropriation was allayed when the Veterans Bureau was induced to allot a new grant of $15,000 for the production of 20 additional titles the following year.

What was thought to be significant about this venture was not so much the direct benefits to blinded veterans as the fact that the expensive brass plates, once made, could be used to produce additional copies of the same book for the much larger group of blind civilians. Early in 1927, Irwin essayed a delicate probe to ascertain whether the Veterans Bureau might finance additional books. The answer was negative. The bureau, wrote its director, Frank T. Hines, "is in no position to justify the need for additional Braille literature for blind ex-service men at this time considering . . . the limited number of blind veterans who have availed themselves of the loan of these books in the past."

The turndown came as no surprise to Irwin, who had accurately sized up the situation some time earlier. He had written to a colleague in mid-1925:

> The truth is, our Veteran readers are not anything to brag about. In the first place they are inexperienced in Braille; in the second place they have had the new Government books only a few months, and in some cases only a few weeks; and in the third place many of them probably use their compensation to pay for readers.
>
> The important thing is, [the veteran] must be made a habitual reader and unless he is given a considerable selection of books in which he is interested, he will never acquire the habit. Few sighted people would acquire the habit of reading if they had no more books available than did the blind.

If the Veterans Bureau was no longer a source for the printing of braille books, the only remaining recourse was to seek voluntary gifts for this purpose. The year 1927, as it happened, was one when Helen Keller was not on the road for the Foundation, so the dependable Ida Hirst-Gifford was available to initiate a campaign to secure underwriting of braille book production from organized groups and philanthropic individuals. It was a slow process; in three years she secured cash and pledges of close to $25,000 for the production of 70 titles requiring 131 volumes. These were printed in editions of 11 copies each, one for each of the nation's leading libraries for the blind.

Some of the books were produced as memorials. Mrs. Andrew Carnegie, one of the earliest subscribers, gave $1,140 for the brailling of her husband's autobiography in six volumes. Rodman Wanamaker paid for the brailling of two books in memory of his father, the founder of the John Wanamaker department store chain. Now and again, an author generously financed the brailling of his own work. One such was former New York State Governor Alfred E. Smith, who contributed the cost of brailling his autobiography, *Up to Now*.

By far the largest number of books were underwritten by Lions Clubs and Junior League groups. These were mostly popular new novels, ranging from John Galsworthy's *The Forsyte Saga* to Willa Cather's *O Pioneers* to Warwick Deeping's *Sorrell and Son* and Zane Grey's *The Thundering Herd*. There was a refreshing absence of the kind of "inspirational" literature that had traditionally constituted the bulk of brailled works, presumably on the theory that blind people were either more spiritual than others or more in need of uplift. For once, blind people were reading the same best sellers as their sighted friends.

Gratifying as this campaign may have been, it by no means represented a satisfactory solution to the overall problem of literature for blind adults. But as will be seen in the next chapter, the Foundation was simultaneously moving in several other directions in an effort to introduce a degree of order into what it described as "the more or less chaotic condition of library work for the blind in the United States."

When Migel informed President Harding in 1922 that reading was the principal way in which blind individuals could "fill in otherwise idle and lonely hours," he—along with most others—was oblivious of the towering potential of that brand-new invention known as radio. In less than two years, the ability of this new form of communication to open up undreamed-of worlds of information and diversion became vividly apparent. For the blind, radio represented a special boon. Once they turned the dial and adjusted the earphones or the loudspeaker, they were at full parity with the sighted.

The idea of mounting a campaign to furnish radios to blind people was the brainchild of a burgeoning industry and of several enterprising newspapers which saw promotional possibilities in supporting a drive with such unmistakable human interest. But neither the American Radio Association nor the cooperating newspapers were in a position to select recipients for the sets to be purchased with the funds they raised. To take care of the sifting of applications and actual distribution, they turned to a natural outlet, the new national organization established for assistance to blind people.

A Foundation report in 1925 noted that it "was asked to act as trustee of this money, and to see to it that the receiving sets were distributed where they would do the greatest amount of good." This it agreed to do "with some misgivings." Announcement of the campaign, which began in November of 1924, stipulated that the Foundation would depend on local agencies "for allotment to proper persons, also for assisting in installation" of the sets, which in those early days involved assembly of the receiving apparatus, the tubes and the loudspeakers, all of which came as separate units.

Radios were given free to those blind persons certified by local agencies as being unable to defray any part of the cost; they were available for purchase by others at discounts of 40 percent or more. By the end of 1925, the $62,000 raised in the newspaper campaign made possible the distribution of 2,550 sets. This was an impressive number, but it could not begin to satisfy the demand. What was to be done with the waiting list of those whose requests were still unmet?

The Foundation turned for help to the radio manufacturers. In 1926 and 1927, Powel Crosley, Jr., president of the Crosley Radio Corporation, Cincinnati, came to the rescue by donating 1,000 receiving sets, while the Radio Corporation of America donated the tubes. The funds to defray the costs of processing, shipping, and record-keeping had to be found elsewhere. In January 1928 the Foundation's financial secretary reported to the executive committee that Crosley "had been prevailed upon to donate 500 additional radios, and the Radio Corporation, 1,000 tubes, bringing the cost of equipment and distribution down to $2,500, of which Mr. Migel has generously consented to bear $2,000."

The following year, Powel Crosley was replaced by A. Atwater Kent of Philadelphia, who supplied 250 fully equipped radios at nominal cost in response to a letter from Helen Keller. In succeeding years, radios were contributed by other benefactors. One of the most consistent was Robert W. Jameson, who was president of United Cigar Stores when he made his initial gift of 100 radios in 1931. In the course of the next ten years, he donated another 800 sets. By the time wartime conditions halted civilian radio production, the Foundation had distributed free radios to 6,200 blind people. Jameson resumed his devotion to this particular form of philanthropy after the war; from 1949 until he died four years later, he contributed an additional $7,500 for radio purchases.

During his later years, Jameson was chairman of the executive committee of the McCrory Stores Corporation. A few months before his death, some of his business associates decided to honor his seventy-seventh birthday by establishing a revolving fund to make interest-free loans to blind persons wishing to start a business, complete an education, or pursue other productive ends. The Jameson Loan Fund, which was later augmented by a $10,000 bequest from Jameson himself, remained in operation until the Foundation made a policy decision in the early Sixties to discontinue direct assistance programs for individuals. The fund's principal was subsequently used for professional fellowships.

Reactivated in 1947, the radio campaign remained in force until 1964, by which time the total number of radios given to blind men and women was close to 25,000. It, too, was dropped as a result of the new policy of discontinuing services for individuals that could now be furnished through local voluntary or tax-supported sources.

The situation had been quite different, of course, when the bedrock national welfare programs and social insurances were not yet in existence and, even in those few states which provided pensions or other financial help to the blind, the level was pathetically low. Thus, when Robert Jameson's friend, John D. Burger, president of the Reiss-Premier Pipe Company, made it a practice to contribute a thousand or more smoking pipes annually, the Foundation gladly distributed them to blind men through local agencies. By the time he died in 1943, Burger had donated 24,000 briars. The warm expressions of pleasure and appreciation from the recipients prompted his widow to continue her husband's practice for another 15 years. The Burgers sought no public recognition of these benefactions; the pipes were distributed as gifts of an anonymous friend.

The radio campaign was the Foundation's first direct service for blind individuals. It was soon followed by another, growing out of the Foundation's pivotal role in securing and administering the one-fare law, a badly needed economic boon for blind people who were unable to travel without a sighted companion and had to pay fares for two persons.

For some years, certain railroads had made rate concessions to blind travelers and their guides under a "charity" classification, which was the only loophole open under the existing Interstate Commerce Act. The Foundation set about getting an amendment to the Act that would stipulate blindness as a separate classification without the demeaning aspect of "charity." The amendment, Public Law 69-655, went through in February 1927. The problem now was getting the railroads to agree to its provisions.

The first road to go along by allowing a blind person and his guide to travel for a single fare was the Baltimore & Ohio. Other lines proved more difficult to persuade. A report to the executive committee in January 1928 noted that the Foundation's president had been in personal touch with 30 railroad officials in an effort to secure favorable action. The power of decision, he discovered, rested with the six trunk line associations into which the nation's railroads were divided. A year later, the Eastern Trunk Line Association agreed to a plan under which the Foundation would assume responsibility for certifying that persons given this one-fare concession were entitled to it. This was the crucial breakthrough; the other trunk line associations followed in swift order, and four years after the initiation of the one-fare service the Foundation was able to report, "more than $21,000 has been saved to blind travelers in this country by tickets bought through the Foundation alone."

A new dimension was added to this transportation service once dog guides had been introduced in the United States. A news item in the December 1931 *Outlook* reported:

> The Pennsylvania Railroad has recently announced that it will permit blind persons to travel in the regular day coaches accompanied by their guide dogs without any extra charge. The passenger traveling with such a dog must present an identification certificate issued by the American Foundation for the Blind, which will certify the dog as having been trained by a recognized training agency.

In due course, this action was formalized through a further amendment to the Interstate Commerce Act. The transportation effort did not stop with railroads. In succeeding years, several interstate and interurban bus lines were persuaded to extend travel concession privileges to blind riders; transatlantic steamship companies made a partial concession by allowing a blind person and his guide to travel for one and one-half fares. However, efforts to induce the airlines to adopt similar practices proved unavailing. Bills introduced into Congress to gain this privilege were successfully resisted by the Air Transport Association on the grounds that airlines provided enough by way of personal service to passengers to obviate the need for sighted escorts.

The original arrangements for validation of one-fare applications involved a great deal of clerical detail and also meant that the applicant had to anticipate his trip well in advance in order to secure the necessary letter of authorization from the Foundation. In 1938 a more efficient system went into effect: the Foundation issued annual coupon books which enabled holders to buy their tickets from local ticket agents on presentation of a voucher. This system remained basically unchanged in 1972, when qualified blind persons were first issued laminated photo identification cards and began paying a nominal annual fee of two dollars to cover as many coupon books as they required during the year.

Also initiated during the Twenties was the distribution of watches and other timepieces adapted for use by blind persons. This service, which had originally been handled by the *Matilda Ziegler Magazine for the Blind* as an accommodation for its readers, was taken over by the Foundation in 1926 at the magazine's suggestion. The arrangement, initially with the Waltham Watch Company, which enabled blind people to obtain reliable timepieces at low cost became the nucleus of the Foundation's Aids and Appliances Division, whose mail-order and over-the-counter sales in 1972 embraced 300 items including 30 different styles of brailled pocket and wrist watches, seven styles of clocks and a dozen types of timers.

Over and above the tuition and living costs common to all students, blind aspirants to higher education needed readers. As early as 1907 a brilliant young

graduate of the California School for the Blind, Newel Perry, who was taking
postgraduate work at Columbia University, persuaded the State of New York to
institute annual stipends that would defray the cost of reader service for blind
college students. The amount was modest, initially only $300 a year, but it was a
start. Other states followed, but it was not until the federal Vocational Rehabilitation Act was amended some decades later that the practice became universal.

Because scholarships were a popular philanthropic tradition, some of the earliest
monies contributed to the Foundation were earmarked for this purpose. A Committee on Scholarship Awards was established in 1924 and announced a few
months later that for the academic year beginning September 1925 four scholarships of $250 each would be granted "for professional, vocational or definitely
pre-vocational study of any sort, at any approved school, college or university . . .
to capable and worthy blind students" who showed "satisfactory certification of
exceptional merit covering character, ability and promise." A fifth scholarship was
added almost immediately through a gift from the New York banker, Felix M.
Warburg; the following year, several additional benefactors made it possible to
expand the program to 9 students. By 1928, the number had been further enlarged
to 15.

Three men and two women were the first scholarship recipients. Two, a man
and a woman, enrolled in schools of osteopathy, then considered one of the most
promising fields of work for blind persons. The other two men studied philosophy
at Harvard and journalism at Johns Hopkins respectively, while the second woman
enrolled at a music conservatory. All five did well enough in their studies for their
grants to be renewed in succeeding years. In 1929, when the *Outlook* published an
article about blind people who were successfully functioning as teachers of the
sighted, the Scholarship Committee was gratified to read a tribute by the head of a
school in the Appalachian Mountains to the excellent performance as a music
teacher of the young woman who had been one of the first five scholarship
grantees.

The scholarship program never reached large proportions, although the
cumulative amounts added up to a respectable total. In 1951, when the program
was 25 years old, the Foundation calculated that its grants had benefited 220
individuals at a total cost of $101,000. When, a dozen years later, the scholarship
program was discontinued, the overall number of recipients exceeded 300 and the
dollar figure came to $600,000. The latter embraced not only the regular academic
and vocational scholarships but also a fellowship program begun in 1951 and the
practice, begun much earlier, of granting special summer study stipends for blind
or sighted students taking special courses in work for the blind, and for qualified
teachers of the deaf preparing to specialize in the education of deaf-blind children.
Grant amounts went up gradually over the years; they were upped to $300 in
1944, to $500 in 1956, and to $800 in 1958 when eligibility was restricted to
persons doing graduate work. The fellowship stipends, which ranged up to $2,000
a year, went to graduate students preparing for professional careers in agencies
serving blind persons. Scholarship awards were discontinued by the Foundation in
1963 because of the flood of federal money available for higher education in the
Sixties, but fellowships, research grants, special summer study stipends, and a

limited number of undergraduate scholarships for deaf-blind students continued to be awarded for some years thereafter.

The end of the scholarship program also saw the end of the annual award of the Captain Charles W. Brown Memorial Medal to the recipient whose work was deemed to be most outstanding during the academic year. The man in whose memory the medal was given, one of the first supporters of the Foundation's scholarships, was a colorful personality who had begun life as a sea captain but later turned to land-based occupations and eventually became president of the Pittsburgh Plate Glass Company. When Captain Brown died in 1928 at the age of seventy, M.C. Migel donated a gold medal for scholastic achievement in his honor. A review of 20 medal recipients, which appeared in the October 1954 issue of *New Outlook for the Blind,* noted that almost all had been successful in their chosen vocations: law, social work, teaching, osteopathy, writing, and business occupations. The 1948–49 medallist, incidentally, was Kenneth Jernigan, then a graduate student in education at George Peabody College for Teachers. In 1972 Jernigan was director of the Iowa Commission for the Blind and also president of the National Federation of the Blind, in which capacity he will be encountered in a later chapter.

Another educational effort which had its beginning in the fertile early years was the initiation of summer study programs for teachers of the blind. Robert Irwin gave the first—for home teachers of blind adults—in 1924. It was an improvised, homespun effort, but it set a significant precedent for continuing use of Foundation staff in undergraduate, graduate and in-service educational programs.

This first course was a cooperative effort of the Foundation and a committee representing the New York Institute for the Education of the Blind, the Brooklyn Bureau of Charities, and the New Jersey Commission for the Blind. The teamwork was along practical lines: "The Foundation furnished the director of the course and the classroom. The cooperating committee provided the secretary of the course and the industrial instructor and met the various other incidental expenses. The New York Public Library very kindly loaned . . . the necessary books."

With a substantial array of projects under way, and an even larger body of work clamoring to be begun, the Foundation quickly outgrew its original small quarters on Union Square. A search for larger offices was in progress in late 1924 when Robert M. Catts, owner of the Grand Central Palace Building on East 46th Street, offered a two-year rent-free lease on office space there. The gift was accepted with gratitude, and the move took place in the summer of 1925. Two years later, the allotted quarters had also grown too crowded and it was necessary to rent additional space on another floor.

As early as 1928 the Major began to speak of the desirability of erecting a permanent headquarters building for the Foundation, and a committee was appointed to look into the matter. A few months later, however, second thoughts prevailed and it was decided that it would be prudent to defer this kind of capital expenditure until the endowment fund had been completed.

There were high hopes, at this time, that the $2 million goal might be met.

Expectations had been given an invigorating boost by John D. Rockefeller, Jr.'s agreement in late 1926, to contribute $50,000 outright. He said he would consider an additional gift once the endowment total, which then stood at $300,000, reached the half-million-dollar mark. Spurred by this powerful incentive, the Foundation's trustees signed up for a total of $160,000, led by a $50,000 contribution from Felix M. Warburg, a similar amount from the Major, and $10,000 from William Ziegler, Jr. To raise the remaining $40,000, a letter appeal written and signed by Helen Keller was sent broadside, explaining the circumstances and beseeching a swift and generous response from friends of the blind. It came. In June 1928 the *Outlook* boxed a full-page statement under the jubilant headline, "The First Fulfilment," announcing the attainment of the half-million dollar figure. Rockefeller promptly made good on his offer of an additional gift; he sent a second (and unconditional) check for $50,000 to propel the fund toward its next milestone, a full million. With the advent of the depression years, this goal proved elusive. It was largely through bequests rather than contributions that the million-dollar mark was finally reached in April of 1934, and it took an additional 14 years before the original target of $2 million was achieved.

The endowment gifts were not the first Rockefeller money to come to the Foundation. Beginning in 1924, badly needed budgetary funds had been contributed by the Laura Spelman Rockefeller Memorial: $15,000 toward the 1924 budget, $12,500 for 1925, and $10,000 for 1926, each grant contingent on the Foundation's raising successively higher multiples from outside sources. It was the availability of this seed money, among other factors, that prompted the decision to aim the 1925 and 1926 campaigns at raising operating income through memberships.

As that income grew, annual budgets moved upward in a steep line. Expenditures went from $45,000 in 1925 to $63,000 in 1926 to $100,000 in 1927 to $116,000 in 1928 to $126,000 in 1929. Budgetary controls were strict, especially during the period when the Foundation's president was simultaneously functioning as administrator. Migel examined each month's figures with an eye that overlooked nothing. In November of 1925, for example, he addressed a stern letter to the two department heads, Hayes and Irwin, noting that in the previous month several minor expenditures had been made and several small salary increases granted without specific authorization from the executive committee. This would not do. It would be desirable, the Major stipulated,

> to establish the following rule, which must be rigidly adhered to, i.e.
>
> That no expenditures of any kind or character be made, excepting for trifling petty cash items, without the same being submitted to the Executive Committee previous to arranging for said expenditures—
>
> That no advance in salaries be granted by anyone, excepting under the above condition—
>
> That no additions to the force of any kind or character be made excepting under the above condition.

Irwin raised an immediate protest. "I do not see how we could function under a plan by which all purchases were approved in advance by our Executive Committee, which meets but four times a year," he wrote Migel the following day. He proposed an alternative: that the annual budget be divided into 12 monthly parts, and that he and Hayes be permitted to operate within these monthly allotments, shifting items within them if need be, and turning to the executive committee for permission only in exceptional instances.

Bright as he was, Robert Irwin had not yet learned that the fiscal area was one in which there was little hope of winning an argument with M.C. Migel. At its next meeting, the executive committee solemnly proceeded to discuss salary increases ranging from $2 a week for the switchboard operator to $5 a week for the bookkeeper. (All were approved.) To spare itself the awkwardness of dealing with such trivia at each meeting, the committee then voted that all staff salaries should be reviewed at a stipulated time each year. Presumably this was done through a subcommittee, if at all; subsequent minutes recorded no further discussions of clerical salaries, although wage adjustments for major staff members did come up for consideration from time to time.

Once the Foundation was operating at a six-figure level, with a steadily expanding staff and an increasingly complex service program, it was time to reconsider the question of centralizing administrative control in the hands of an executive director. The issue was first precipitated in mid-1927, when Migel suggested to the trustees that they begin seeking a new president. He conveyed the message through Irwin, who reported to Henry Latimer: "He says that he will continue as a trustee for a while, and will help some financially, but he thinks that the Foundation is now on its feet, and he wishes to withdraw. Have you any suggestions?"

Latimer did have a suggestion, and it was succinct: persuade the Major to stay on another year and then keep him as a member of the executive committee. Irwin agreed with the former, but was dubious about the latter because of Migel's dominating personality: "It makes little difference where he is on the executive committee, he would still be the leader."

Latimer made a personal effort to cajole the Major into continuing and Migel yielded to this and to similar entreaties from other trustees on the proviso that less of his time would be demanded in the future.

The trustees, having agreed that the time had come for the Foundation to have a full-time executive director, appointed a subcommittee to seek the proper man. Apparently little action was taken on this, and in May of 1928 Latimer, who was a member of the subcommittee, sought to expedite a decision. He addressed a lengthy communication to the executive committee in which he defined the qualities he considered essential in an executive director: knowledge and experience in work for the blind, ability to delegate responsibility and coordinate staff, experience in handling budgets and in formulating fund-raising plans, an analytic turn of mind, acceptable levels of scholarship, tact, generosity, and approachability. After setting forth these criteria, he went on:

> In my opinion Mr. Robert B. Irwin possesses the foregoing qualifications . . . plus an intimate acquaintance with the aims and operations of the Foundation, a wide acquaintance among men of affairs, and likewise an acquaintance

among workers for the Blind both here and abroad, which will stand the
Foundation in good stead.

Anticipating some of the objections that might be raised against his nominee,
Latimer continued:

> In the event that Mr. Irwin's physical blindness is offered as an obstacle to
> the proper exercise of the duties of this office, I submit that such an objection,
> in light of his manifest ability and success, is wholly unworthy of consider-
> ation by those who, like ourselves, are constantly teaching, preaching and
> professing to believe in the capabilities of blind people.
>
> Should it be objected that Mr. Irwin is not a financial man, I again submit
> that he is as much such a man as is presently needed by the Foundation, and
> as is presently available.

The records give no hint of what may have gone on behind closed doors while
this proposal was considered, nor is there any indication that the Foundation
engaged in a talent search such as that conducted before the hiring of its first
director-general, but the fact is that a full year went by before Robert Irwin was
named executive director of the American Foundation for the Blind. Oddly, the
appointment, which took effect in June of 1929, was never officially announced in
the Foundation's periodical; the first hint readers of the *Outlook* had of Irwin's
elevation came through a passing reference to "Robert B. Irwin, executive director," in a report of the annual meeting published in the September 1929 issue.

If Irwin, who liked public recognition as much as any man, was bothered by this
lack of fanfare, he did not betray it. He was, in any event, far too busy struggling
with a variety of urgent projects. Predominant among them was one that had
occupied much of his time and thought for a half-dozen years: how to increase the
supply, decrease the cost, improve the production, and enlarge the distribution of
literature for the blind.

8

The Language of the Fingers

Like so many of the inventions that have been blessings to mankind, it came about accidentally. Opening up the world of written language to the blind was the furthest thing from the mind of the man who devised the basic concept that made it possible. He was Charles Barbier, an officer in Napoleon's army, and he was after a method of sending coded military messages that could be employed under cover of darkness. He called it *écriture nocturne*—night writing—a system of raised dots the fingers could interpret without the need for a betraying light.

The military value of Barbier's system was that these dots were not tracings of the ordinary alphabet. They were arranged into a secret code, based on a twelve-dot unit or "cell"—two dots wide by six dots high. Each dot or combination of dots within this cell arrangement stood for a letter or a phonetic sound.

Theoretically, Barbier's system was a breakthrough; in practice, it failed to work. It was too complex, too clumsy, too spread out. It did not take into account the limited area the human fingertip could span with a single touch.

In 1808, when *écriture nocturne* was presented to the French Academy of Sciences, it was rightly acclaimed as a brilliant invention. In succeeding years, Barbier experimented with variations of his system, employing different numbers of dots and different cipher codes. These were duly submitted to the Academy, and their published reports were widely circulated. Eventually, one such report found its way to the National Institution for the Blind in Paris where the twelve-dot system was tested and rejected as impracticable. But—and it is a large but—it was there that a thoughtful and creative member of the student body perceived that dot writing did have possibilities. The student was Louis Braille, who was only eleven years old and newly enrolled at the school when Barbier's invention was tried out there in 1820. Nine years later, Braille achieved his own breakthrough by finding a way to overcome the two fundamental flaws in Barbier's system. First he cut the number of dots in half so that a fingertip could encompass the entire cell unit of six dots in one impression. He then devised a new code, alphabetic rather than phonetic, employing combinations of these six dots.

The genius of Louis Braille's system was its simplicity. He arranged his dot cell into two parallel columns, three dots high. Starting with the letter *a*, he used the single dot in the cell's upper left-hand corner. For the next letter, *b*, he added the dot directly underneath. To denote the letter *c* he used the *a* dot and its corresponding dot in the upper right-hand corner. For identification purposes in teaching the system, he numbered his dots:

$$
\begin{array}{ccc}
1 & \bullet \quad \bullet & 4 \\
2 & \bullet \quad \bullet & 5 \\
3 & \bullet \quad \bullet & 6 \\
\end{array}
$$

The first ten letters of the alphabet, from *a* through *j*, employed only the dots in the upper two rows of the cell. Braille then made the next ten letters by adding the bottom left-hand corner dot, #3, to each of his first ten letters. Now he needed five more combinations (the French alphabet, which at that time omitted the letter *w*, had only 25 letters). For this purpose he used the lower right-hand dot, #6, adding it to his previous combinations. The accompanying diagram illustrates these principles.

Because Braille's code was arbitrary, his symbols were capable of standing for anything that followed an accepted sequence: not only the letters of the alphabet but numerals, musical notes, chemical tables, etc. All the reader had to know was which code was being used. For the numerals 1 through 9, for example, Braille's code used the same symbols as the first nine letters of the alphabet. The tenth letter stood for zero. When numbers appeared in the context of a reading passage, a coded signal alerted the reader to the fact that the next cell represented a numeral and not a letter. This coded signal, called the numerical indicator, is identified as # in Line 6 of the diagram.

Since six dots could be arranged into 63 different patterns and the alphabet required less than half of these, there was room within Braille's code for this numerical signal and a good many others to represent diphthongs, conjunctions such as *with* or *and* or *for*, common letter combinations such as *ch* or *th*, and other useful adjuncts to written language.

The braille code shown in the diagram is the modern version, but in most essential respects it is unchanged from the alphabetic code Louis Braille published in 1834. Five years earlier he had worked out and published his code to music notation; this, too, has remained basically unchanged.

Louis Braille was not the first to realize that fingers were to the blind what eyes were to the sighted, but he was the first to work out a practical method of employing the fingers to do the work of the eyes. Official recognition of his genius came only after his death, but within his lifetime he had the satisfaction of knowing that his students at the school for the blind in Paris could learn and use and profit from the key he had fashioned.

Born January 4, 1809, in the village of Coupvray, not far from Paris, Louis was the son of a harness maker. While playing with one of his father's tools, a sharp knife, the three-year-old child accidentally slit one of his eyes. The resulting

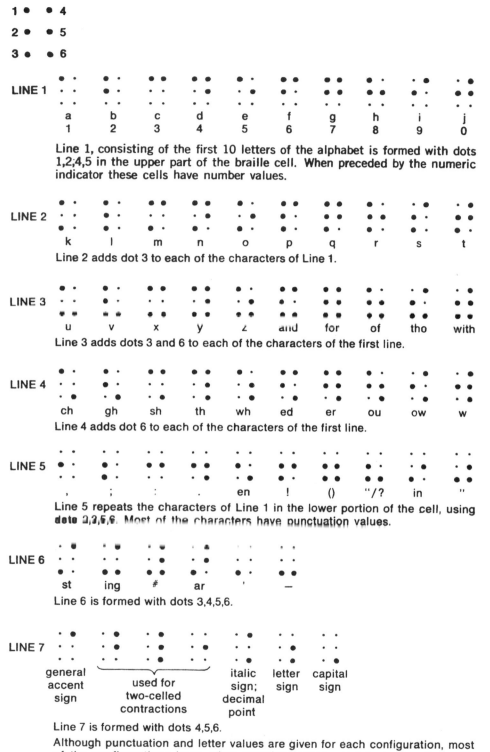

1 ● ● 4

2 ● ● 5

3 ● ● 6

LINE 1

a	b	c	d	e	f	g	h	i	j
1	2	3	4	5	6	7	8	9	0

Line 1, consisting of the first 10 letters of the alphabet is formed with dots 1,2;4,5 in the upper part of the braille cell. When preceded by the numeric indicator these cells have number values.

LINE 2

k   l   m   n   o   p   q   r   s   t

Line 2 adds dot 3 to each of the characters of Line 1.

LINE 3

u   v   x   y   z   and   for   of   tho   with

Line 3 adds dots 3 and 6 to each of the characters of the first line.

LINE 4

ch   gh   sh   th   wh   ed   er   ou   ow   w

Line 4 adds dot 6 to each of the characters of the first line.

LINE 5

,   ;   :   .   en   !   ()   "/?   in   "

Line 5 repeats the characters of Line 1 in the lower portion of the cell, using dots 2,3,5,6. Most of the characters have punctuation values.

LINE 6

st   ing   #   ar   '   —

Line 6 is formed with dots 3,4,5,6.

LINE 7

general accent sign | used for two-celled contractions | italic sign; decimal point | letter sign | capital sign

Line 7 is formed with dots 4,5,6.

Although punctuation and letter values are given for each configuration, most of the configurations have other meanings when used in conjunction with different braille characters.

infection also destroyed the vision of the other eye; a bright little boy was now totally blind.

For some years Louis attended the village school with his brothers and sisters, but in 1819 his father brought him to Paris and the National Institution for the Blind. Here he remained, first as a student and then as an instructor, and it was here that he adapted the Barbier system to the needs of blind persons everywhere. His health was frail, however; whether due to tuberculosis or some other respiratory ailment, he coughed so incessantly that it became increasingly difficult for him to lecture. Eventually, he had to give up and return to Coupvray. There he died on January 16, 1852, two weeks after his forty-third birthday. He was buried in the family plot in the village cemetery until, on the centennial of his death, his body was exhumed and ceremoniously transferred to the Pantheon in Paris. In deference to Coupvray, which had erected a monument to Braille in its main square, the skeleton of his right hand—"the hand with the reading fingers"—was left to repose forever in its native earth.

A major virtue of Barbier's system, which Louis Braille recognized and retained, was that it could be written as well as read without benefit of sight. Barbier had invented a writing frame, consisting of a board and a stylus, which Braille adapted. The governing principle of this device remains in effect today in the form of the modern braille slate. This consists of two metal or plastic plates, hinged together at one end and open at the other to permit a sheet of paper to be inserted between them. The upper plate is pierced by little windows, each the exact size of a braille cell. Directly under each window, on the lower plate, are six shallow pits arranged in the braille cell pattern: two pits wide by three pits high. Embossing takes place when the stylus is placed in a window and is pressed downward against the paper in order to form each braille character, dot by dot, against the corresponding pit of the lower plate.

To read what has been embossed, the paper must be turned over so that the dots protrude upward. Turning the paper transposes left and right, as in a mirror image. Therefore, writing by means of a braille slate is done backwards, from right to left instead of vice versa, so that the letters, when the paper is turned, will read in the customary left-to-right order. Confusing as it may sound, this practice soon becomes quite automatic for the blind user of braille.

It was the fact that blind people could write it as well as read it that gave braille a commanding advantage over other early methods of embossed writing. These were tried, in varied forms, for many years both before and after the braille code made its appearance.

Most of the other efforts to produce tangible type—letters cut out of wooden blocks or cardboard, letters carved in relief on wood or incised into wood or wax—suffered from a common error of logic. They simulated the linear alphabet of the sighted and thus, as the blind French philosopher Pierre Villey put it, made the mistake of "talking to the fingers the language of the eye." Specifically designed for tactile use, the braille code could not be easily read by the eye. This was one reason why, despite its instant appeal to blind students, braille encountered considerable initial resistance from sighted teachers. Obviously, it was easier for such teachers to supervise and correct a student's work if they could follow visually what the student was writing tactually. There may well have been another reason too; braille could be taught by blind teachers, and this constituted a threat to the job security of the sighted.

In the English language, various forms of tangible type in linear form were developed in England and Scotland during the nineteenth century. Only one of these survived. Moon type, named after its originator, Dr. William Moon, consisted of stripped-down and simplified versions of roman capital letters. The letter *A,* for example, appeared without its crossbar; the letter *D,* without its front vertical line. Moon type was first produced in England in 1847 and was introduced in the United States in 1880. As will be seen in a later chapter, it proved particularly useful as a reading method for persons blinded late in life who felt unequal to mastering braille.

Early American efforts at production of literature for finger-readers were also in linear type. The most enduring of these was Boston Line Type, an angular modification of roman letters in both upper and lower case. It was devised by Dr. Samuel Gridley Howe, founder of the Perkins School for the Blind in Massachusetts. The first book printed in Boston Line Type was *Acts of the Apostles,* which Perkins produced in 1835. This was soon followed by editions of the New Testament and the Old Testament.

Of greater importance than the Scriptures in the education of children were the textbooks that were printed for the students at Perkins and adopted by many of the other schools for the blind that were then rapidly emerging in other parts of the United States. Boston Line Type, which thus became the predominant print medium for the blind in the United States for four or five decades, served for secular literature as well.

Among the books printed in this form was *The Old Curiosity Shop;* it makes an intriguing footnote to history that the $1,700 cost of this embossed edition was defrayed by Charles Dickens himself. Dickens had visited the Perkins school in 1842, during his first trip to the United States, and had been so impressed by what he saw there that he devoted 14 pages of *American Notes* to a description of the school, and particularly to an account of Dr. Howe's pioneering accomplishment in educating a deaf-blind girl, Laura Bridgman. Some forty years later, it was this passage that kindled in Helen Keller's mother the hope that her own little deaf-blind daughter might also be given a chance in life. With the help of Alexander Graham Bell, the Kellers approached the then director of Perkins, Michael Anagnos, to ask whether the school could furnish a teacher familiar with the methods that had brought enlightenment to Laura Bridgman. Anagnos, who was Howe's son-in-law, chose one of the brightest of his recent graduates, young Anne Sullivan. Thus was forged the chain of coincidence that brought together the twosome, Helen and her teacher, whom Mark Twain called the Miracle and the Miracle Worker.

By the time Anne Sullivan became a student at Perkins in the early 1880s, the dot system was already in use in most American schools for the blind. Soon after braille's official adoption in Paris in 1854, Dr. Simon Pollak, one of the founders of the Missouri School for the Blind, was traveling in Europe. He learned about braille and brought the new code back with him. Some of the school's faculty offered the usual objections of the sighted to this alien style of finger-reading, but the students seized upon it with delight. It was said that they used braille to pass surreptitious notes—sometimes love letters—to one another, knowing that the messages, if intercepted, could not be read by their teachers. The school's music teacher was the first to yield; soon thereafter the rest of the faculty followed and instruction in literary braille was begun.

As the dot system gradually began to prevail over linear types in Missouri and elsewhere, various educators of the blind started trying to improve the braille code. These well-intentioned efforts led to unfortunate results, for it was the simultaneous existence of differing code systems that ultimately precipitated the "war of the dots" that raged over so many decades.

To a lesser degree, somewhat the same sort of chaos arose in England, but the British resolved their differences with greater speed and firmness. By 1905, British braille had been systematized and a uniform code adopted and divided into two levels. Grade 1 was basic braille, in which each word was spelled out, letter by letter. Grade 2 introduced 197 space-saving contractions or abbreviations for frequently used words. In the United States, it took an additional dozen years and a great deal more controversy before agreement was reached on the uniform type system known as Revised Braille Grade 1½. This was essentially the same as British braille, except that it rested partway between the two British grades, employing only 44 of the Grade 2 contractions. This half-step, which was officially adopted by American schools and agencies for the blind in 1917, left enough of a gap between the two English-language systems to hinder free exchange of literature across the Atlantic Ocean.

To close that gap and establish a uniform braille code was one of Robert Irwin's objectives during the early years of the American Foundation for the Blind. His confidence was bolstered by a favorable omen. In the mid-Twenties, negotiations were begun aimed at achieving international agreement on a universal braille code of musical notation. This was an important need. Music was a major vocational outlet for blind people, and one in which gifted blind singers, pianists, organists, and violinists the world over achieved professional renown. The study of music traditionally occupied a prominent place in the curriculum of every school for blind children. Many of the graduates earned their living as performers, music teachers, or piano tuners. Music scores for the sighted used an internationally recognized set of symbols; why should this not be so for the blind? But several styles of music notation in braille had been evolved, and until there was agreement on a single style, a blind musician in London could not readily make use of a braille score produced in Philadelphia or Vienna or Rome.

A five-nation conference held in Paris in the spring of 1929 reached agreement on an international music code for the blind; thirteen other nations had agreed in advance to accept the conference decisions. "The world is at last in accordance in the usage of braille musical symbols," the *Outlook for the Blind* reported joyfully in its account of the conference. "We may congratulate ourselves on sharing in the final triumph of the braille system."

The man who represented the United States in this triumph was Louis W.

Rodenberg, who was in charge of braille printing at the Illinois School for the Blind (now the Illinois Braille and Sight Saving School). The Illinois institution, a pioneer in the development of mechanical aids for braille production, had long been a leader in the printing of musical scores. Rodenberg, who became associated with the school in 1912, had worked out a key to braille music notation which brought him a national reputation when it was published in 1917. In 1924 the Foundation commissioned him to expand his earlier work into an encyclopedia of braille music notation; it was issued the following year.

Rodenberg had evolved a particular style, known as "bar over bar," for the arrangement of braille music. He had also experimented with various ways to publish songs that would enable blind singers to learn words and music simultaneously. The year after the Paris conference he achieved a long-cherished dream when he began editing the American edition of *Musical Review for the Blind*, the country's first professional music journal in braille. His pioneering achievements in brailled music were honored in 1943 when he was awarded the Foundation's Migel Medal. Rodenberg retired from the Illinois school in 1963 and died three years later at the age of seventy-four. He lived long enough to see established in the Library of Congress a comprehensive collection of brailled musical scores, texts, and instructional materials to be made available for nationwide use under a federal bill enacted in 1962.

It may seem odd that Robert Irwin, who regarded books for the blind as a top priority, encouraged progress on a music code before tackling the knottier question of achieving uniformity of braille literature in the English-speaking world. He had his reasons. For one thing, he was working on improving the mechanical aspects of braille production so as to reduce costs. For another, as he was to point out in his posthumously published reminiscences, *As I Saw It*, both the American readers of braille and the printing houses that produced it were thoroughly tired of changes. The printers had had to scrap thousands upon thousands of costly printing plates in earlier versions of braille after Grade 1½ was adopted; they were understandably reluctant to undergo the same wasteful expense should Grade 1½ have to be modified or abandoned by virtue of an agreement with the British. As for blind readers, wrote Irwin:

> Many still living had first learned [Boston] linetype, then New York Point, then American braille, then Revised braille grade 1½. The rank and file of finger readers had a good deal of sympathy with a speaker at one of the national conventions who in a burst of oratory said, "If anyone invents a new system of printing for the blind, shoot him on the spot."

The right psychological moment for change drew nearer as plans were developed for the convening of a world conference of the blind in New York in 1931. In an atmosphere of international cooperation, and with the way already paved by the agreement on braille music, the climate might prove opportune for a final accommodation with Great Britain. To win over those still reluctant, Irwin added a dollars-and-cents inducement by having a staff assistant, Ruth E. Wilcox, conduct a statistical "contraction study" to determine the relative amounts of space (and thus, of expense) required by the British and American grades. The study demonstrated that Grade 2 occupied from 12 to 14 percent less space than Grade 1½. For example, the six-letter word *nation* in Grade 2, using an *n* followed by the two-cell contraction for *ation,* needed only three braille characters, whereas the same word written in Grade 1½ contained all six letters and therefore required six braille cells.

On his way to a meeting in Vienna in the summer of 1929, Irwin stopped off in London and found the British more receptive than in the past. He wrote Migel about his discussions: "I really believe that, if we put sufficient drive behind this thing, we can bring about almost complete uniformity." His optimism was justified when Sir Ian Fraser (later Lord Fraser of Lonsdale), chairman of St. Dunstan's Executive Council and an acknowledged leader of the British blind, told the opening session of the World Conference on Work for the Blind in 1931: "It is my belief that a little common sense and a little give and take on both sides of the Atlantic may bring about a uniform type. . . ."

The give and take duly took place; in September 1932 the *Outlook* triumphantly headlined an article: "Uniform Braille for the English-Speaking World Achieved." The compromise version, named Standard English braille, was immediately adopted for all adult literature. For some years, schoolbooks for beginning readers retained the easier Grade 1½, but this was gradually abandoned and all books came to be produced in Standard English braille.

This does not mean, however, that the braille codes remain static. Because braille communicates a living language, it needs ongoing surveillance and periodic updating to reflect the new words, concepts and processes of a scientific and technological age. To insure consistency of treatment by braille printing houses, a group known as the American Braille Commission was organized soon after the agreement with the British. This was superseded in 1950 by a larger group, the Joint Uniform Braille Committee of the AAIB and AAWB, which gave way, eight years later, to a more permanent jointly sponsored body, the Braille Authority.

In 1968 a National Advisory Council to the Braille Authority was formed. It consisted of educators and service program leaders, the objective being to establish closer liaison between the producers and the users of braille materials. The Braille Authority and its advisory body concern themselves with such problems as improved methods of embossing maps, diagrams, charts and tabular material, the development of advanced computer symbol transcriptions and of notation systems for higher mathematics, the introduction of a music code specifically adapted for the percussion and plucked instruments popularized by rock and country music, and comparable changes designed to enable braille readers to be part of the modern world.

When the Foundation asserted in a 1924 report that "no more valuable contribution could be made just now than to discover ways of reducing the cost" of braille literature, it did not have in mind merely economies that could be effected through greater use of contractions. American methods of printing literature for finger-readers were inefficient and far behind European methods. To understand the steps initiated to remedy these flaws, it is necessary to go back in time to review the progress made in dot-writing after the development of the braille slate.

A sheet of embossed dots produced by means of a braille slate is just that: a single sheet. To obtain more than one copy requires duplicating machinery of some sort. Early efforts to accomplish this were adaptations of standard inkprint production methods. Movable type set up the dot pattern in high relief. This was then locked into a frame, placed in a flat press, and applied to heavy paper with sufficient pressure to make dents in the paper without piercing it. Sometimes the movable type was cast into metal bars before being put on the press. Another method was to punch dots in a metal plate by means of a heavy stylus and a hammer. The hand-punched plate then served as a stereotype whose dots could be transferred to paper with the use of a flat or rotary printing press. Since all of these methods involved hand composition, they were necessarily slow. There was yet another time factor: once the heavy braille sheets were embossed, they had to be varnished and dried to preserve the raised dots.

When the first commercial typewriter was successfully marketed toward the end of the nineteenth century, its operating principle offered a way of achieving much greater speed in brailling. In 1890 Frank H. Hall was appointed superintendent of the Illinois Institution for the Education of the Blind. The forty-nine-year-old Hall, who had had twenty-five years of teaching and supervisory experience in public schools, was appalled to discover what primitive educational tools were available to his blind students. It occurred to him that the typewriter principle could be made applicable to the production of dot-writing. Only six keys would be needed, one for each dot in the braille cell. With fingers on the keyboard, a blind person could strike the combination of keys needed to produce a braille character embossed on the paper in the machine's roller. It would be a little like playing a chord on the piano. The carriage would then move the paper along to where the next braille cell would be made, while word separation could be achieved with a space bar.

With the help of G.A. Sieber, a skilled machinist, Hall completed his work on the braille version of the typewriter in less than two years. Exhibited at the 1892 convention of the American Association of Instructors of the Blind, his invention was received with acclaim. Those who saw Hall's daughter give a demonstration on the machine at a speed of 100 words a minute "were almost dumbfounded with surprise and delight," according to one eyewitness.

Hall's machine, called a braillewriter, was a significant factor in giving braille a commanding edge over its principal competitor, New York Point. The latter was also a dot system. It had been devised in 1868 by William B. Wait, superintendent of the New York Institution for the Blind (later named the New York Institute for the Education of the Blind), as an improvement over Louis Braille's code and, because of certain desirable features, it was popular with many educators.

New York Point differed from braille in two essential respects. Whereas Louis Braille had developed his code in what appeared to him to be a logical sequence, starting with a single dot for *a* and gradually increasing the number of dots as the end of the alphabet neared, Wait thought it more scientific to take into account the frequency of occurrence of the various letters. The letter *t*, for example, occurs much more often in the English language than the letter *k*. In braille only two dots are needed to make *k*, which is the 11th letter of the alphabet, whereas *t*, the 20th letter, requires four dots. Wait changed all that by assigning the fewest dots to the most frequently used letters.

The other difference was that whereas braille had as its unvarying base a cell two dots wide by three dots high, the New York Point cell was only two dots high, but the width of its base could be one, two, three or four dots, depending on the number needed to denote a particular letter.

That New York Point was a good and sensible system was undeniable. Why, then, did it fail to win out over braille? Over-promotion may have been one important factor. Wait was a brilliant man but so hard-driving and zealous that he antagonized many in influential quarters. Opposition spurred him on to ever more militant measures, which ultimately cost him the loyalty of even those who shared his high opinion of New York Point. It became a vicious, inflammatory spiral. To review the detailed records of the "war of the dots" is to uncover the stuff of melodrama, a sorry tale that victimized the very people the battling adversaries were trying to help.

Frank Hall was a conscientious educator. Once given charge of a school for blind children, he lost no time in making a thorough study of the relative merits of braille and New York Point. There was a powerful practical argument to sway him in favor of the latter; in 1890, virtually all the schoolbooks for blind children produced under federal subsidy by the American Printing House for the Blind were in New York Point. Hall's school had access to free books if its students were instructed in Wait's system. Textbooks in a form of braille developed at the Perkins school in Boston and known as American braille were being produced by the Howe Memorial Press, a Perkins affiliate, but these were not federally subsidized and had to be paid for. The Illinois institution, like most other schools for the blind, had a small printing shop of its own and produced much of its educational material in that way.

What, then, decided Frank Hall in favor of a machine that would write braille rather than New York Point?

> At first I thought of making [a machine] to write New York Point, but when I took into consideration that the letters of that system were not of uniform length, [while] each braille character occupied precisely the same amount of [horizontal] space as any other character, I determined to attempt the easier task. . . . When they made the first typewriter ever made, the first thing they had to do was to make the letters of uniform length. The *i* in the Remington occupies exactly the same space as the *m*. . . . It seemed to me that was the only proper system on which to attempt to make a machine to write for the blind.

It did not take long before Wait developed a comparable writing machine called the Kleidograph to handle New York Point. But the Hall braillewriter had the inside track and its existence had already precipitated a significant change in the production of educational materials for blind children. As additional school superintendents saw the potential of the braillewriter, they switched from New York

Point and successfully demanded that the American Printing House use part of its federal grant to manufacture textbooks in braille as well as in New York Point.

Once there existed a machine that could punch braille dots on paper, the logical next step was to make it strong enough to punch through metal and produce a stereotype from which copies could be duplicated. A year later this had been accomplished. Hall also devised a method of motorizing the machine. "The work is done by the electric motor," he explained, "and all the fingers have to do is to select the keys and they do it almost as fast as you can play a piano."

Hall made these remarks during one of the crucial battles in the war of the dots. This was the series of hearings held in 1909 by the New York City Board of Education to decide whether braille or New York Point should be the medium of instruction in the day school classes for blind children the city was about to institute. The defeat of New York Point in the city of its birth was a crushing blow to the aging William Wait. He died in 1916, and was thus spared the pain of seeing his brainchild receive the coup de grâce the following year, when agreement was reached to print all future literature for the blind in braille Grade 1½.

By that time, Hall was also gone. He had left the Illinois school in 1903 and worked in the field of agricultural education until his death in 1911. He never patented his machines, refusing any personal profit from their invention. His attitude was squarely in the tradition, unbroken to this day, that equipment for the use of blind persons was to be sold at cost.

Because of the diversion of energies resulting from the battle over types, little progress was made in American braille production methods during the thirty years following the invention of Hall's braillewriter and stereotyper. One of the earliest steps taken by the Foundation was to call a conference of the leading braille printers and some of their major customers for a pooling of ideas on how to make braille books better, cheaper, and less bulky. Their principal recommendations were that the size of braille books be standardized, and that books be printed on both sides of the page.

Two-sided book printing, which had long been standard practice in Europe, had never successfully evolved in the United States. To study European methods, a three-man committee consisting of Robert Irwin, L.E. Bramlette (superintendent of the American Printing House for the Blind), and Frank C. Bryan (manager of the Howe Memorial Press) visited braille printing plants in Great Britain, France, Germany, and Austria during the summer of 1924. The committee concluded that it would take six months to a year to adapt American production methods to the more efficient and economical systems used abroad, and they recommended that some experimentation be undertaken before any of the expensive European equipment was imported.

The committee's time estimate proved optimistic; it was to take a lot longer than a year, a great deal of costly engineering, and a wholly unanticipated series of setbacks before two-sided book printing became standard practice in the United States.

The process involved in printing braille on both sides of the same sheet was called interpointing. It required a precise placement of plates and paper, so that the dots embossed on one side would fall between the lines of the dots embossed on the other so that fingers reading one side of the sheet would not be confused by the dots on the reverse side.

That interpointing was possible with American equipment had already been shown. The *Ziegler Magazine* shop had adapted its Hall stereotyper to produce two-sided printing some years earlier. Results were far from perfect, but the magazine's readers were so happy to get twice as much reading matter in the same number of pages that they got used to the imperfections. However, while relatively crude work might get by in something as ephemeral as a monthly magazine, a much higher quality of production was needed in books designed to be circulated and read by many over a period of years.

The dominant producer of printed matter for blind readers was then, as it had been for many decades, the American Printing House for the Blind in Louisville, Kentucky. This unique organization, originally an offspring of the Kentucky School for the Blind, was founded in 1858 by action of the Kentucky Legislature. It became an official printer of schoolbooks for the United States in 1879, when Congress passed "An Act to Promote the Education of the Blind."

Under this act, a perpetual trust fund of $250,000 was set up, to be invested in United States interest-bearing bonds, the income from which, at 4 percent, would go to the Printing House on condition that the $10,000 annual yield be spent on the manufacture of books and tangible apparatus to be distributed, free of charge, to tax-supported residential schools for the blind. Distribution was to be on a pro rata basis, in proportion to the schools' enrollment of pupils. A further provision was that the superintendents of these schools were to serve as ex-officio trustees of the Printing House. (In 1961, five years after the act had been amended to make Printing House services available to visually handicapped children attending regular public day schools as well as those enrolled in special schools and classes for the blind, a further amendment enlarged the ex-officio trusteeship category to include representatives of state education departments.)

In 1906 the bond feature was eliminated in favor of a direct federal grant of $10,000 to be made annually in perpetuity. In 1919, an additional annual grant of $40,000 was voted, reflecting the nation's population growth and consequent increase in the number of children attending schools and classes for the blind. As the latter continued to grow, so did the Printing House grant. It was upped to $75,000 in 1927, to $125,000 ten years later, to $260,000 in 1951, then to $410,000 in 1956. In 1962, the ceiling on appropriations was lifted, and the Printing House was charged with seeking each year's budget on the basis of proven needs. Its scope of service was enlarged in 1970 when parochial and private schools were permitted to participate along with the tax-supported residential and day schools in free receipt of educational materials for their blind pupils.

In the fiscal year ending June 30, 1972, the federal grant to the Printing House amounted to $1,590,000. This sum, known as the quota fund, supplied 21,846 pupils in schools and classes for the blind with educational materials in the form of books in braille, large type, or sound recording, as well as maps, globes, slates, music scores and equipment, and a wide range of other educational aids and apparatus.

The overall operations of the American Printing House now encompass far more than the materials produced under the federal grant. To supplement their quota allotments, schools purchase additional supplies and equipment that are sold on a non-profit basis. The Printing House also handles contracts from government bureaus, voluntary and business organizations for the manufacture of various kinds of books, periodicals and tangible aids for the blind. Outside of its federal grant, therefore, the Printing House functions as a non-profit organization, part of whose funds come through contributions from the public. With a full-time staff of 550 and an overall business volume which in 1972 exceeded $7,500,000, it remains the world's largest publishing house for the blind.

In the early Twenties, virtually all the other braille printeries in the United States were offshoots of schools for the blind. There were a dozen or so all told, only two of which—the Howe Memorial Press in Boston and the Clovernook Printing House for the Blind in Cincinnati—were large enough to handle more than local work. (The endowed *Matilda Ziegler Magazine for the Blind* was bigger than either, but it was in a class by itself.) Like the American Printing House, all these smaller braille presses were long established and settled in their ways.

At the point where the Foundation decided to take forthright action to modernize braille publishing practices, a fresh wind began to blow in from the west in the person of J. Robert Atkinson of Los Angeles. Atkinson, who had founded the independent Universal Braille Press in 1919, was a blind man endowed with an abundance of ability, ambition, and aggression. Over the next two decades he was to administer several salutary shocks to sting the established printing houses out of lethargic complacency. His actions were also to give rise to bitter personal rivalries, passionate partisanships, and unruly public controversies that proved deeply disturbing to blind people throughout the nation.

A publicity release issued by Atkinson's organization in 1944 began: "J. Robert Atkinson lost his sight in an accident in 1912 when working as a cowboy in Montana." Atkinson almost never bothered to contradict the impression that this accident had taken place out on the open range. Even the obituary put out by his organization when he died in 1964 stated, "Bob Atkinson was blinded by backfire from a revolver while working on his brother's cattle range in Montana." In actual fact, however, according to an authorized biography published toward the end of Atkinson's life, the accident took place in a Los Angeles hotel room.

Atkinson's tendency to evade inconvenient truths was one of the traits that made him a storm center in work for the blind. On the other side of the ledger was his admirable degree of grit. Following the accident that cost him his sight, he refused to be overwhelmed by blindness and proceeded to teach himself all forms of finger-reading. Simultaneously, he developed an interest in Christian Science and obtained permission from that church's headquarters in Boston to hand-transcribe the works of Mary Baker Eddy into braille for his private use. This undertaking had two results. He began to think about braille production, and once he had established himself in business as a braille printer, the Christian Science Church became one of his principal customers.

In 1919 Atkinson set up the Universal Braille Press in the garage of his home in

Los Angeles. With the financial help of a philanthropic couple whose interest he had attracted, he began in business by printing the King James version of the Bible in the newly approved Grade 1½ braille. This was a five-year project, in the course of which he began experimenting with improvements in braille printing methods.

The initial bylaws of the American Foundation for the Blind stipulated, as one of the ten categories of special interest groups to be given places on the board of trustees, "technical heads of embossing plants and departments." At the Vinton convention, where these bylaws were adopted, Atkinson, though not present and a newcomer to the field, was named to represent the embossers category. He attended the first meeting of the Foundation trustees, which was held in New York in November 1921. On his return to California he submitted a bill for his travel expenses, with the explanation that the trip from the West Coast was too costly to be met out of his personal funds. He had to travel with his wife as a sighted escort, which meant two fares at that time. While this voucher was honored, the board was not in a financial position to go along with Atkinson's formal proposal that the expenses of trustees attending future meetings be routinely met. At the expiration of Atkinson's three-year term, the embossing plant delegates elected another representative to serve on the Foundation board.

In 1924 Atkinson announced the development of an improved braille stereo-typer and wrote an article to which the *Outlook for the Blind,* in its first issue under Foundation auspices, gave considerable prominence. The Foundation had just sent three men abroad in search of improved printing methods. Naturally it was interested in examining the machine which Atkinson's article called "superior to any model on the market." In December 1924 the executive committee authorized a three-man committee to visit Los Angeles for the purpose of seeing the Atkinson stereotyper and its performance. Atkinson demurred on the grounds that the equipment was undergoing further refinement. But he did agree to bring the stereotyper to New York for a meeting of braille printers the following September, and the Foundation acceded to his request that it meet his travel costs.

At that meeting, two other stereotypers capable of being adapted to two-sided printing were also exhibited—one by Frank Bryan of the Howe Press in Boston, and the other by Joseph Brusca of the *Ziegler Magazine* plant in New York. In the course of the two-day session demonstrations were given and the machines carefully inspected. All three had merit, but none met the desired standard.

While encouraging further work on the three models (a $3,000 fund was raised to help meet the expense of mechanical modifications), the printers attending the conference reached the same conclusion as the delegation which had visited the European printing plants the previous year: a mechanical shop was needed in which experimentation could be carried out and new equipment and processes thoroughly tested for performance, ease of operation, reliability, and durability. They urged that the Foundation establish such a shop.

Inasmuch as the end product would be better, cheaper, and less bulky books for the blind, a logical source of financing was the Carnegie Corporation, whose major interest was library work. The Foundation turned to the American Library Association with a request that it use its influence to secure a Carnegie grant of $10,000 annually. This plan succeeded; in May of 1926 the Carnegie Corporation voted the Foundation $10,000 for 1927 on a matching basis.

In January of 1927 the Foundation's mechanical shop, forerunner of its engineering division, was born. It began with the utmost modesty in space rented in the *Ziegler Magazine* plant. Julius Hurliman, a Swiss mechanical engineer with extensive experience in the printing field, was put in charge. He and a helper constituted the entire staff. Hurliman was "an original fellow, a hard worker, and deeply interested in the humanitarian as well as the mechanical aspects of his job," according to Irwin, who made this statement in a letter to Dr. Frederick B. Keppel, president of the Carnegie Corporation, reporting the shop's progress six months after its opening. Two-sided printing was already under way in Atkinson's plant, he wrote, but the process was not yet reliable enough. However:

> If our shop can have support sufficient to continue its operation we will within two or three years revolutionize the method of printing for the blind in this country. Four Braille publishing plants have already advised us that they will adopt two side printing just as soon as we can recommend satisfactory machines.

In this account of early experimental efforts, the American Printing House for the Blind has been conspicuously absent. Even though its superintendent, E.E. Bramlette, was a Foundation trustee and had been drawn into every step of the effort to improve braille production, the Printing House had assumed an attitude of studied indifference toward interpointing. In an attempt to elicit some action, Foundation president Migel wrote to the Printing House's president, John W. Barr, in June 1926, asking that the question of two-sided printing be put before the latter's trustees. The reply was a flat rebuff. The Printing House, Barr wrote, had concluded that

> interpointing, while it saves about one-third of the paper, space and binding, costs about one-half more labor. This extra cost of labor much more than offsets the saving in material. [Furthermore, interpoint printing] could not apply to Primary and Intermediate text books for the schools and is of very doubtful use in the high school texts. Therefore, while interpointing may save space for the librarian and adult readers, it will undoubtedly be of little or no use to the schools for the blind.

There was only one weapon left that might prevail over intransigence, and the Foundation proceeded to use it. Its braille memorial fund campaign was under way and monies were being collected from various organizations to underwrite the brailling of adult books. Irwin directed the bulk of this business to the Universal Braille Press, and they agreed to produce the books in interpoint. With experience, prices came steadily downward, thus demolishing the Printing House's argument of higher labor costs. Although his equipment needed improvement, Atkinson's work was of high quality and he was eager to have the business. "The work we have received from the Foundation has undoubtedly helped us wonderfully and perhaps enabled us to survive," he wrote.

After a year or so of watching order after order go to California, the American Printing House for the Blind was aroused to the point of complaining publicly about the Foundation's failure to assign it the lion's share of the contract work. Its argument was that if all braille printing were concentrated in a single shop, there would be more efficient use of plant and lower costs that would benefit all blind readers, children and adults alike. Irwin thought just the opposite: "A little friendly competition is good for any large organization, little as the management may enjoy it."

In one way, the spur of competition had the desired effect. Reversing its stand, the Printing House decided that interpointing was practicable after all and began bidding aggressively on contracts for two-sided printing. In another way, however the effects were regrettable. With the support of a number of school superintendents, Bramlette mounted a vigorous campaign to swing public opinion in favor of centralizing all braille printing in Louisville. Atkinson, whose temper had a low flash point, reacted with understandable sharpness. In mid-1928 he wrote Bramlette accusing him of seeking a monopoly and alleging that the Printing House quoted prices below cost when bidding competitively but at the same time charged unreasonably high prices on non-competitive contracts.

Atkinson circulated copies of this letter far and wide. But he, too, was reluctant to face increased competition. He wrote Migel: "I do not think it wise for [the smaller braille plants] to become too ambitious, nor do I think it wise for other plants to be created." Here he was intimating an idea he was later to proclaim publicly: the Universal Braille Press in the West and the American Printing House for the Blind in the East should divide the country between them.

It is worth noting that at this stage Atkinson clearly regarded the Foundation as his ally. Bramlette thought so, too, and was sufficiently exercised over what he regarded as favoritism toward Atkinson to bring the matter up before the Foundation's executive committee. Yet not many months later Atkinson was to appear before a Congressional committee to denounce the "entangling alliance" between the Foundation and the Printing House, and although there was not in fact any such alliance, the Foundation was to speak up forcefully in defense of the Printing House against some of Atkinson's accusations. Then, only a year or two thereafter, the Printing House was to strive mightily to defeat a Foundation proposal which it regarded as threatening to its interests. Such was, is, and probably always will be the price of nonpartisanship.

Before any of this transpired, the Foundation itself was swept into the field of competitive fire. Rumors were rampant that its experimental shop was designed to become a braille publishing house. So widespread was this impression that it was deemed advisable, in early 1928, to address a circular letter to all organizations and professional leaders in work for the blind, specifically denying any such intention and reiterating that it was purely a "mechanical research laboratory."

The fact that the Foundation shop did produce a limited amount of embossed literature was due partly to the conditions of the Carnegie grant. Carnegie support, which was continued for 1928, was predicated on the Foundation's working with the American Library Association in "a reading course project for the blind, including experimentation in Braille printing." The literature produced consisted of a number of reading course pamphlets plus braille editions of a Foundation professional journal, the *Teachers Forum*. At a later point, the shop also printed the first braille editions of the *Outlook for the Blind*.

That the shop did indeed function as a mechanical research laboratory was soon demonstrated. The Cooper Engineering Company of Chicago announced its intention to discontinue manufacture of the Hall stereotyper, the Hall braille-writer, and other equipment for the blind it had been producing ever since the days of Frank H. Hall. For the Cooper firm, whose principal business was the manufacture of such heavy industrial equipment as oil well machinery and gas main couplings, the production of mechanical appliances for blind users constituted a small, unprofitable sideline. The Foundation agreed to buy the Cooper jigs, dies, and other production equipment; while it did not intend to become a manufacturer of appliances any more than it intended to become a braille publishing house, it felt sure that its shop could effect some greatly needed improvements, particularly in the braillewriter.

The end product of the Foundation's efforts to modernize braille production was that two-sided printing became standard practice. As for the Foundation's experimental printing shop, which remained in existence until the beginning of 1932, it chalked up three major accomplishments: the development of a functional stereotyper, the development of a new braillewriter, and the successful adaptation of a European method for duplicating hand-transcribed braille manuscripts.

Once the shop had perfected a stereotyper capable of consistently precise performance in producing interpoint work, the machine was submitted to the American Printing House for the Blind for testing under actual production conditions. Two other stereotypers, one of them Atkinson's, were simultaneously subjected to the same use test. The Printing House agreed to adopt, and to manufacture in its own facilities, whichever model it found to be best. The test results favored the Foundation's machine, so a contract was duly signed in February 1932 under which the Printing House would manufacture the stereotyper in the future while the Foundation would market it. In all, 16 of these machines were produced; 13 were sold in the United States for installation in four printing houses, four schools for the blind, and two large local service agencies. The remaining three were bought by braille printing houses in Canada, South America, and England.

(In the years following these pioneering efforts many of the advances achieved in general printing were adapted for use in braille publishing. Probably the most dramatic of these was an automated process, put into limited production at the American Printing House for the Blind in the Sixties. It employs a key punch computer program to translate inkprint text into braille characters which, by means of magnetic tape, then embossed directly onto metal stereograph plates. The key punch operator does not have to know braille; the coding is done by the computer. As of 1972, however, most braille manufacturing continues to use trained stereotypists who operate braillewriting machines to translate inkprint copy onto the metal plates. The reason is cost.)

Development of a greatly improved portable braillewriter was completed in the experimental shop at the beginning of 1932. The new machine was more precisely engineered, easier to maintain, more efficient in operation, and considerably quieter than the Hall braillewriter. When it came to commercial production, however, a serious dilemma arose. Because of a necessarily limited market, the unit cost of a braillewriter was far higher than blind people could afford to pay; no production run would be large enough to amortize the cost of tooling. Production plans were deferred for some months while the Foundation shopped for the lowest possible price. In 1933 a deal was worked out with the L.C. Smith & Corona Typewriter Company under which the Foundation agreed to pay $19,000 for the production dies and tools and to advance $12,500 in capital to finance the manufacture of each lot of 500 braillewriters. Marketing was handled by the Foundation, which sold the machines at manufacturing cost. The first machines of the initial lot of 500 came off the assembly line late that year. They were an instantaneous success.

The Howe Memorial Press in Boston, which had been manufacturing its own braillewriters since 1921, decided to discontinue them following the introduction of the Foundation's model. In announcing this decision at the 1933 convention of the American Association of Workers for the Blind, Howe's manager, Frank Bryan, was generous in his praise. The Foundation's braillewriter, he said, "has everything one could want for brailling and is a real boon to the cause." By the time World War II requirements restricted the supply of aluminum for civilian use, 1,500 Foundation braillewriters had been distributed. In the midst of the war the *Outlook* published an emergency appeal for people to sell back machines no longer in use, but the yield was small. For the most part, blind civilians had to make do with whatever they had. However, in early 1945 a special dispensation was secured from the war production authorities for manufacture of braillewriters for blinded servicemen, and 900 Foundation machines were produced for this purpose that year and the next.

Well before wartime restrictions halted production of this braillewriter, efforts were under way to seek further convenience for blind users in the form of a smaller, lighter machine that might fit into a person's pocket or briefcase. Toward the end of 1938 a young engineer named Raymond Lavender constructed a crude model of a miniature machine weighing less than three pounds. It had serious deficiencies, but was regarded as sufficiently promising to warrant further investigation. In the course of the next two years, the Foundation advanced several thousand dollars in grants to the inventor in exchange for title to the finished product. The results were unsatisfactory, and the project was dropped in late 1941 when Lavender, who had accepted wartime employment with a large industrial firm, became unavailable for further experimentation.

Robert Irwin, who never gave up easily, applied to the Carnegie Corporation for a grant to go on with the development of a lightweight, compact machine. An urgent need existed. The Foundation braillewriter weighed 16 pounds, even though it was largely made of aluminum. "Now that aluminum is well nigh impossible to obtain, it will be necessary to cast the machine of iron, which will make it so heavy as to be no longer portable," Irwin wrote on October 8, 1941, in requesting $6,000 to perfect a writer that could be carried about conveniently, and an additional grant of $15,000 to begin manufacture of such a model when designed. The Carnegie people agreed to the development grant and left the way open for a later application to finance the tooling up. By this time, however, the United States was fully at war and neither skilled labor nor raw materials could be had for non-essential enterprises.

In 1945 the Foundation contracted with the Armour Research Foundation of the Illinois Institute of Technology to complete development of a lightweight writer. The Armour people started with the Lavender machine but soon abandoned it. Several new designs were tried out during the following two years, but not one measured up. In the end, failure had to be acknowledged.

At this point there was a turnaround that spoke well of the growing spirit of unity and cooperation in work for the blind. During the war years an engineer associated with the Howe Memorial Press of the Perkins School had developed a nine-pound braillewriter designed on entirely new principles. In 1947 a working model of this device, called the Perkins Brailler, so impressed the Foundation that it voted to endorse the new machine and terminate efforts to produce a new model of its own. The Foundation went even further by persuading the Carnegie Corporation to allocate to the Perkins Brailler the $15,000 tooling grant half-promised to the Foundation six years earlier. This would be matched by a similar sum to be raised by Perkins.

By the end of October 1949, M. Robert Barnett, who had then just succeeded Irwin as executive director of the Foundation, was able to report to the Carnegie Corporation that the first Perkins Braillers would come off the assembly line in the spring. As an earnest of the Foundation's confidence, he noted, it had placed an order for 500 machines for resale, thus providing Perkins with an assured market for their initial production run.

Over the years the Perkins Brailler has proved its excellence; it has become the most popular machine of its kind, with sales far outrunning two other American-made braillewriting machines. One of these is the New Hall Braillewriter, which the American Printing House redesigned after the war; the other, surprisingly enough, is the Lavender Writer. Raymond Lavender reappeared in the world of work for the blind in 1950, by which time he had redesigned his small machine and elicited interest from several major braille houses. In the course of the next decade, the Lavender writer was finally perfected; in 1962 it began to be manufactured and marketed by the American Printing House for the Blind. It was the lowest-priced of the three American machines, but weighed only a half-pound less than the Perkins Brailler. A truly pocket-sized braillewriter was still awaiting invention in 1972.

The third aspect of braille production in which the Foundation experimental shop achieved useful progress was the Garin process.

Maurice Garin was a French engineer who invented a method of duplicating hand-transcribed braille. It consisted of filling the pitted side of a page of braille manuscript with a mixture of plaster and glue. This fixed in place the raised dots on the other side and hardened the paper sufficiently to serve as a printing plate from which 50 or more copies could be struck.

A process of this sort was of great importance in France and other European countries, where hand-transcribing had long been a major resource of library collections for the blind. In the United States, however, hand-copying did not begin in earnest until World War I, when blinded servicemen required literature in the newly adopted braille Grade 1½. Mrs. Gertrude T. Rider, head of the

Reading Room for the Blind in the Library of Congress, was put in charge of the library at Evergreen, where she trained volunteers to braille stories, news reports, and anything else the trainees asked for by way of reading material. By 1920, Evergreen reported that its braille library held 500 press-made and an equal number of hand-copied volumes. By the time it closed its doors in 1925, it possessed 1,500 volumes; these were transferred to the Library of Congress, where Mrs. Rider and her staff continued to circulate them by mail to the discharged men as well as to other blind readers.

Hand-copied books, however, were hardly a total answer to the needs of several hundred blinded men, so at the same time that Mrs. Rider was organizing a volunteer corps of hand copiers, she invoked the help of the Committee on War Services of the American Library Association in securing funds for press-brailling. As the American Foundation for the Blind was to do, the Library Association asked authors, publishers, clubs, and individuals to finance the cost of embossing books in the new typeface. Many authors responded generously by paying for the brailling of their own works. Booth Tarkington gave $300 for the embossing of *Penrod;* Mary Roberts Rinehart sent a check for $500 to make the plates for her newest book, *Love Stories.* Civic organizations and philanthropic individuals financed not only fiction but books on practical aspects of making a living for blind men.

The Library Association's interest was not limited to the war-blinded. At the same time that the newly press-brailled volumes in braille Grade 1½ swelled the Evergreen collection, copies went to the principal libraries which circulated books for the civilian blind.

It was in promoting the hand-copying of books by volunteers, however, that Mrs. Rider made her greatest contribution. Starting with a woman who turned up at Evergreen, she discovered that motivated people could be trained in a few weeks of concentrated study to produce readable braille. Through the Red Cross she had access to a nationwide network of women, eager to serve, who needed only to be told what to do and how to do it. By 1921, when the national board of the American Red Cross officially adopted braille transcribing as part of its volunteer service, there were already 25 chapters in 13 states and the District of Columbia enthusiastically pounding away at braillewriters. The volunteers contributed not only time and effort but, in most instances, bought their own braillewriting machines and supplies of braille paper.

As head of the Reading Room for the Blind in the Library of Congress, Mrs. Rider was in a position to combine the library's facilities with Red Cross manpower to develop correspondence courses in braille transcribing for the guidance of the volunteers. Handbooks for proofreading were also published, and a certifying system was established. A volunteer braillist won her certificate to make permanent transcriptions by submitting 50 pages of accurate and neatly transcribed work. In the early days, all volunteer transcriptions were sent to Washington, where the pages were corrected, shellacked, numbered, collated, and bound into volumes before presentation to a library. Much of the work, particularly the proofreading and correcting, was done by blind people paid out of Red Cross funds. The collating and other processing tasks were handled for the most part by volunteers from the District of Columbia chapter of the Red Cross.

So much care and thought went into this entire movement that someone even found an ingenious use for the test sheets submitted by would-be braillists. These were sent to blind people who had tuberculosis or other communicable diseases which barred them from participating in the regular circulating book system.

The principal drawback of hand-transcribing was that hundreds of hours of volunteer labor produced but a single copy of a book. The Garin duplicating process had become known in the United States shortly after the end of the war, but due to the differences between American and European brailling methods, the process needed modification before it could be used.

When the Foundation sent its team of technical experts abroad in 1924 to investigate braille production methods, one of the team's purposes was to look into the Garin process. Robert Irwin got in touch with the inventor in Paris and commissioned him to work out adaptations of his equipment to fit American requirements. One adaptation involved page size, since American transcribers used a different number of characters per line and lines per page. The other problem to be solved was somewhat more intricate. European hand-transcribers preparing material to be duplicated worked with a slate and stylus, whereas American volunteer copyists were accustomed to working on braillewriting machines. However, there was one style of braillewriter, a British model, that could be modified to accommodate the Garin equipment, and Irwin arranged to have it sent from London to Paris, so that Garin might work out the necessary mechanical adjustments. This was eventually accomplished.

Because it was tricky to handle and produced uneven results at best, and because it did not lend itself to two-sided printing, the Garin process was only partially successful in duplicating books. Its real usefulness proved to be as the braille equivalent of the mimeograph for making multiple copies of school examination papers, circular letters and other short-lived materials. It had the further advantage of being inexpensive. Ultimately the development of plastics following World War II made possible a vacuum-forming process which allowed hand-transcribed materials to be mechanically duplicated.

By the time Gertrude Rider retired from professional life at the end of 1925, she had certified 900 volunteer braille transcribers in 149 Red Cross chapters and other women's groups from Maine to California. She had also seen a change in the distribution system that greatly stimulated the continuing interest of the volunteers once the appeal of blinded soldiers had abated. Hand-transcribed manuscripts were no longer solely collected and distributed through the Library of Congress in Washington; groups working in large cities which housed major libraries for the blind had the option of working for and with these local institutions. Volunteers not only brailled for their local libraries but helped out in the processing, collating and binding of the finished volumes.

Succeeding Mrs. Rider at the Library of Congress was Adelia M. Hoyt, a blind woman who had been her assistant since 1913. Under Miss Hoyt's direction the braille transcribing service was maintained at a high level and after 1932 was safely shepherded through the transition from Grade 1½ to Standard English braille.

Two years after Miss Hoyt's retirement in 1938, she was awarded the Foundation's Migel Medal in recognition of her achievements. A few years later, a Foundation medal was presented to a layman whose leadership in hand-copying of books for the blind antedated even Mrs. Rider's. This was Harold T. Clark, a Cleveland lawyer, who, before World War I, had organized a volunteer corps of braillists under the banner of the Cleveland Society for the Blind and kept it going until the service was officially adopted by the Red Cross.

One of the first coordinating services undertaken by the Foundation immediately after its establishment was the compilation and maintenance of a card catalog called the Embosser's List. It served as a clearing house of braille books published anywhere in the United States. To prevent duplication of titles, all braille printers registered their books with the Foundation and refrained from beginning work on a new title until they had ascertained, by means of the catalog, that it had not already been brailled elsewhere. Each issue of the *Outlook* printed a list of newly press-brailled books so that librarians, schools, and agencies serving blind adults might know what was available, and where.

Where hand-transcribed books were concerned, so long as all of these were processed by the Library of Congress, an automatic clearing house was in effect. Once volunteer transcribing was decentralized, however, the need arose to prevent duplication of titles in hand-copied as well as press-brailled books. Initiative toward this end was taken by the American Library Association's Committee on Work for the Blind under the chairmanship of Lucille A. Goldthwaite, librarian for the blind of the New York Public Library. Lists of the hand-copied books in the possession of various local libraries were compiled by Miss Goldthwaite and published regularly in the *Outlook* beginning with the March 1927 issue.

The *Outlook* stopped printing these lists at the end of 1931, by which time Miss Goldthwaite had begun, under the joint sponsorship of the New York Public Library and the American Braille Press in Paris, a monthly braille magazine, the *Braille Book Review,* which carried lists of all new press-brailled and hand-copied volumes along with descriptive annotations, reviews, and other book news of interest to finger-readers. Budgetary stringency caused the American Braille Press to withdraw from the partnership in 1934, and the New York Public Library used a small bequest to carry the full cost for some months until the Library of Congress took over a share of the financial responsibility.

Inasmuch as the *Review* was issued in braille, its contents were not conveniently available to sighted persons who had a professional interest in them. In 1940 the Foundation began to publish a mimeographed version for distribution to libraries, schools, day classes, and agencies for the blind. Miss Goldthwaite, who won a Foundation medal in 1946 for her leadership in creating this useful adjunct to reading for the blind, continued to edit both editions of the *Braille Book Review* until mid-1951. The last nine years of her editorship were under the auspices of the Foundation, whose staff she joined following her retirement from the New York Public Library in 1942.

The *Review* went from mimeograph to inkprint in 1953, at which time the Library of Congress assumed the total cost of publication. As of 1972 it was continuing as a bi-monthly, with the editing and distribution of the inkprint edition handled by the Foundation's Publications Division in cooperation with the Library of Congress. The latter likewise financed production of the *Review*'s braille edition, which also incorporated announcements of books issued in sound-recorded form. The publication was sent free of charge to the 11,000 braille readers registered with regional libraries for the blind.

What was it about brailling that so swiftly attracted the willing eyes and fingers of thousands of volunteers? Part of the answer could be seen in any list of hand-transcribed books. Beyond their sense of service and the fact that the program was begun before press-brailled books were available through federal appropriations—and before the days of recorded books and large-type printing—the women who sat down at their braillewriters forty and fifty years ago had the pleasant task of dealing with contemporary best sellers. A 1927 list of hand-copied books included titles by Michael Arlen, Willa Cather, Rafael Sabatini, P.G. Wodehouse and other popular authors.

The spirit of the early volunteers was perhaps most eloquently expressed in a letter from one of them who wrote, "I should like nothing better on my tombstone than 'She Brailled a Book.' " The appetite for brailling seemed self renewing. In the Forties a New York agency for the blind reported that a seventy-three-year-old volunteer had transcribed 337 volumes of textbook material, fiction, poetry, and plays—35,302 pages in all—in 13 years, and a New Jersey woman was cited for transcribing 316 children's books in an eight-year period.

World War II brought about an administrative change in volunteer brailling. Preoccupied with other wartime responsibilities, the American Red Cross discontinued its sponsorship of the transcribing service and the Library of Congress picked up the national certification program. As had been the case in the years 1914 to 1918, war evoked a new surge of interest in service for the blinded. A nationwide organization of volunteer braillists took shape in 1945. The National Braille Association, which by 1972 had some 2,500 members, conducted workshops for the improvement of transcribing methods, maintained a program for recognizing length of service, made awards for outstanding accomplishment, and met regularly with organizations engaged in all types of work for the blind.

The appreciable extent to which hand-copied books continue to swell the range of literature available to finger-readers can be seen in almost any contemporary issue of the *Braille Book Review*. Of the 775 new braille titles put into circulation during 1970, nearly 600 were hand-copied. In addition to the national program of the Library of Congress, major hand-transcribing programs offering nationwide circulation are currently conducted by three large public libraries—New York, Philadelphia, and Chicago—and three voluntary organizations in New York City—the Jewish Braille Institute, the Jewish Guild for the Blind, and the Xavier Society for the Blind. The denominational auspices of these agencies are not reflected in their book transcriptions, which are mostly of a general and nonsectarian nature.

One of the most significant by-products of the volunteer braillist movement has been the overflow of interest into other aspects of service for blind people. Local agencies—often the instruction and training centers for volunteer braillists—have benefited from their contact with a corps of dedicated, deeply committed members of the community who constitute a unique and precious bridge between blind people and the sighted world.

The work of volunteer braillists in the Seventies includes a substantial volume of technical and reference books and periodicals which are indispensable to blind students pursuing an education, to professional workers whose careers require keeping up with the technical literature in their particular fields, to scholars who need special reference material. While the development of other channels of communication has lessened the blind person's overall dependence on finger-reading, nothing has yet replaced Louis Braille's six-dot cell as a basic medium for serious study.

9

Books for the Blind

It was all very well to improve the quality and reduce the cost of braille literature through two-sided printing, efficient production equipment, and expansion of volunteer hand-copying, but none of these measures, beneficial as they were, solved the basic problem of a sufficiency of books and adequate channels for their distribution.

Very few blind people were affluent enough to own personal book collections of any size. For all but a few, cost and bulk dictated dependence on public library facilities. Around the turn of the century, when free public libraries were growing fast, collections for the blind were started in about 75 of them. Before long, however, the blind people in these communities had read everything on the local shelves and began writing to libraries in other cities in search of fresh material. This threatened to become too expensive a procedure for libraries and borrowers alike until the federal government, in 1904, amended the postal law to extend free mailing privileges to books loaned to blind readers. It was, incidentally, Canada and not the United States which took the leadership here; free mailing began in Canada in 1898.

The mailing privilege alleviated the problem but did not solve it. Libraries budgeting funds for purchases had to weigh the fact that a single copy of a finger-reading book cost fifteen or twenty times as much as an inkprint copy of the same book. They needed to decide whether this book for blind readers should be ordered in braille or in New York Point or in Moon type or in all three. They had to allot shelf space to the thick, oversized volumes. They had to have staff to service mail requests, which entailed more than simply taking a book off the shelf and shipping it out. Readers, knowing how little was available, did not always specify the books they wanted. Librarians had to keep records of which books the borrower had already received, and form some judgment as to each reader's tastes.

Library growth in the United States had been a haphazard process. Most libraries were freestanding institutions, spontaneously established and supported by states or municipalities or philanthropic organizations for the benefit of local residents. It was a real question whether such institutions were empowered, or could afford, to serve readers from faraway places. In the spirit of fellowship that exists among book lovers everywhere, a few did so unhesitatingly. Many schools for the blind also circulated their book collections, in some instances only to their own graduates, in others, to blind people anywhere. But in a good many cities, library collections of books in raised print gradually fell into disuse. In *As I Saw It,* Robert Irwin described what happened:

> The library departments for the blind at first attracted much public atten-
> tion. When, in time, they seemed neglected by sightless readers, who soon
> had read the entire collection, the library authorities gradually lost interest in
> these departments. Books which had first been displayed conspicuously in
> the front room of the library found their way gradually to a back room, then
> to the attic, and then to the furnace. New readers might drop into the library
> to borrow a book but could find no one readily available who even knew
> where the books were. . . . As a final irony, blind people were pronounced
> uninterested in library service.

Those libraries that did maintain a service were plagued by the differing forms of type in books for the blind. When, in 1917, braille Grade 1½ was adopted as the uniform type for all future instruction, it held out promise of relief in the future but, for the moment, merely meant one more type style. The libraries could not, and did not, scrap their collections in the earlier types, for these were still in demand by readers, not all of whom could be induced to master the new style of braille. Indeed, according to Lucille Goldthwaite, a considerable number of readers, "disgruntled by the loss of their favorite medium of reading . . . dropped from the [borrowers'] lists forever, constituting a sort of 'lost battalion' in the battle of the types."

There was great unevenness in the size of state and local library collections, in their circulation policies and in the services they rendered to borrowers, and even greater irregularity in their geographic positioning. Most of the active collections of books for finger-readers were clustered in the northeastern quarter of the country, with all but three or four east of the Mississippi and north of the Ohio River.

This chaotic picture, distressing to blind people and librarians alike, led the American Association of Workers for the Blind at its 1927 convention to adopt a resolution asking the Foundation to join forces with the American Library Association in studying library conditions "with a view to developing a comprehensive plan for serving the blind readers of the country." In 1928 an extensive survey was begun.

All libraries for the blind in the United States and Canada were sent questionnaires designed to ascertain who their readers were: age, sex, occupation, kinds of reading matter borrowed. In order to discover the extent to which the same individuals used several libraries, the names and addresses of all readers were requested. The questionnaires also inquired into the methods used by the libraries in servicing reader requests.

The 34 American and 2 Canadian libraries that cooperated in this survey embraced all the important centers of reading matter for the blind. Analysis of the returns yielded statistical proof of the pattern that leaders of work for the blind had long suspected. No more than about 10,000 separate individuals used library services. Most southern and southwestern states had no reading resources for the blind; to the extent that readers in those areas obtained books at all, it was through long-distance mail service, the major burden of which fell on a few large collections.

Not only was there a serious deficiency of touch literature, but much of what the libraries did have bore little relation to what the borrowers wanted to read. As Robert Irwin explained when he addressed the meeting of the American Library Association in May of 1929:

> Most of the printing concerns for the blind in the United States are sup-
> ported by agencies primarily interested in the education of the blind
> child. . . . As a result nearly all of the books published in this country are
> selected with their educational aspect in mind . . . selected because they form
> a part of the literature which blind people *should* read. . . . If our public
> libraries for the seeing were restricted to only the titles to be found in our
> braille libraries, many of our librarians would be looking for other jobs.

One can only guess at the reason why the Foundation's executive director, in that same speech, said: "We probably cannot count upon the government to assist in any large way in the publication of books for adults . . . the production of braille books for the mature readers must be left to philanthropy."

What was notable about this assertion was the fact that at this very point in time the Foundation had already begun conversations with the Library of Congress to probe avenues of action by means of which the federal government would, in fact, finance the publication of books for blind adults. It may be that Irwin was being canny in not wishing to raise premature hopes among his hearers. He himself may not have been overly sanguine about the outcome of the exploratory talks. Likelier still, he probably did not wish to dangle before the librarians any temptation to defer budgeting and buying books for the blind on the grounds that such books might soon be made available at federal expense.

However sound his motives may have been, it did not take long for events to make Robert Irwin wish he had been more open. A public declaration of what he had in mind in May of 1929 might have spared the Foundation, and Irwin personally, a good deal of unpleasantness in the next two years.

The findings of the library survey had made it abundantly clear that meeting the needs of blind readers would require both large amounts of money and a more equitable distribution pattern of reading resources. These were the twin objectives of the bill introduced into Congress on January 23, 1930, by Representative Ruth Baker Pratt of New York.

H.R. 9042, "a bill to provide books for the adult blind," was drafted by Irwin in consultation with library authorities in the autumn of 1929. It was taken to

Washington by M.C. Migel, who discussed it with one of his intimate friends, Senator Reed Smoot of Utah. The latter agreed to sponsor the bill in the Senate but advised that it should first be introduced in the House of Representatives. The Foundation president then took the proposed legislation to Mrs. Pratt, a member of the House Committee on the Library. The Republican congresswoman from New York City, then serving her first term in the House, endorsed the idea so promptly and enthusiastically that the Foundation people were taken by surprise. Irwin later said he had not expected such speedy action, and would in fact have preferred enough of a delay for the bill to be reviewed by leaders in work for the blind before it was dropped into the legislative hopper.

The bill introduced by Mrs. Pratt was a briefly worded measure calling for a federal appropriation of $75,000 a year to be made to the Library of Congress "for the purchase and publication of books for the blind, such books to be loaned to blind residents of the United States."

It contained only one other provision:

> In order to facilitate the prompt and economic circulation of books among the blind people of the United States, the Librarian of Congress may arrange with such local public libraries as he may judge appropriate to serve as local or regional centers for the circulation of such books, under such conditions and regulations as he may prescribe. In the lending of such books preference shall at all times be given to the needs of blind persons who have been honorably discharged from the United States military or naval service. [The last sentence was later dropped.]

Mrs. Pratt's bill was referred to the House Committee on the Library for consideration. On its face, it was hardly the kind of legislation to provoke a year-long controversy. But such proved to be the case, for on the very same day Congressman Joe Crail of California introduced a competitive measure, H.R. 9052, "a bill authorizing an annual appropriation to the Braille Institute of America (Incorporated), for the purpose of manufacturing and furnishing embossed books and periodicals for the blind and designating the conditions upon which the same may be used, and for other purposes." In addition to the direct appropriation of $100,000 a year to the Braille Institute of America, the major feature of H.R. 9052 was that books manufactured under the grant were to be distributed to libraries according to a pro rata formula based on their total number of blind borrowers.

The Braille Institute of America was a newly organized non-profit corporation located in Los Angeles. It had been created by J. Robert Atkinson in 1929 to provide a structure that would be better suited than his privately owned Universal Braille Press for competing with the non-profit American Printing House for the Blind. Under a quota system, the latter had been receiving federal funds for schoolbooks since 1879; the Crail bill was aimed at securing for the Braille Institute comparable grants for books for blind adults.

Atkinson had announced the forthcoming creation of the Braille Institute at the AAWB convention in June 1929: "We have what we believe is a very feasible plan for raising an annual appropriation of one hundred thousand dollars a year." What that "very feasible plan" was, he refrained from saying. No doubt he had a federal appropriation in mind but, for reasons of his own, Atkinson was being just as cagy in addressing his fellow workers for the blind as Robert Irwin had been a month earlier in his talk to the librarians.

Unfortunately the Pratt and Crail bills were referred to different committees of the House of Representatives. The Committee on the Library was a small, five-member group with comparatively few measures to consider. The Pratt bill was thus scheduled for a relatively early hearing. The Crail bill had to wait two months longer before the broadly based Education Committee could hold a hearing on it. Complicating matters even further, Representative Lister Hill of Alabama introduced a third bill, calling for an appropriation of $100,000 to be expended under the direction of the American Library Association, although that organization's executive committee had already voted to endorse the Pratt bill. The Hill proposal was the brainchild of a few individual blind men who maintained that the Library of Congress was not sufficiently knowledgeable about blind people to be entrusted with selecting books for them. The Hill bill was also referred to the House Committee on Education.

The hearing on the Pratt bill before the Committee on the Library took place on March 27, 1930. The lead-off witness was M.C. Migel. The principal point in his brief, extemporaneous statement was that although the American Foundation for the Blind considered the Pratt bill to be the soundest of the three proposals, "all we want is books for the blind," and the particular bill which could produce that result was a secondary consideration.

The Major was followed by Robert Irwin, who made a formal presentation illustrated by several exhibits. One was a map showing the existing locations of libraries for the blind and identifying the 15 libraries whose volume was sufficient to employ one or more full-time staff members to handle processing of books for the blind. Also pinpointed were five locations in the under-served areas of the country where, in Irwin's opinion, regional library centers for the blind might logically be established.

Another exhibit was an inkprint edition of the Bible and the 22 oversized volumes that constituted its braille equivalent. Irwin's point was that the bulk and expense of producing braille books restricted their potential buyers to libraries, and that so limited a market offered no incentive to commercial publishers.

Representative Robert Luce of Massachusetts, the committee's chairman, asked Irwin: "Would you contemplate that the library [of Congress] itself would establish a printing plant, or that it would be better for it to contract with existing printing plants for the actual production of the books?"

The reply should have been reassuring to Atkinson and his supporters, were they in a mood to listen. Irwin said there were at least three very good printing plants, located respectively in Boston, Louisville, and Los Angeles, and that the Librarian of Congress "would save himself a lot of grief if he did not attempt to establish a new printing house but made contracts with these different printers. Let these organizations bid on them and give it to the man who could give him the best quality for the least amount of money."

Irwin was followed in the witness chair by several persons who spoke briefly in support of the Pratt bill: Charles F.F. Campbell, executive director of the Detroit

League for the Handicapped; H. Randolph Latimer, executive director of the
Pennsylvania Association for the Blind; Carl H. Milam, executive secretary of
the American Library Association; and Adelia M. Hoyt, head of the service for
the blind of the Library of Congress.

The committee chairman then called on Helen Keller. Although she had
testified before many state legislatures, this was her first appearance before a
committee of Congress. Her impact, as always, was memorable. In a short,
unabashedly emotional speech, she declared:

> Books are the eyes of the blind. They reveal to us the glories of the
> light-filled world, they keep us in touch with what people are thinking and
> doing, they help us to forget our limitations. With our hands plunged into an
> interesting book, we feel independent and happy.
>
> Have you ever tried to imagine what it would be like not to see? Close
> your eyes for a moment. This room, the faces you have been looking
> at—where are they? Go to the window keeping your eyes shut. Everything
> out there is a blank—the street, the sky, the sun itself. Try to find your way
> back to your seat. Can you picture yourself sitting in that chair, day in and
> day out, always in the dark and only the dark gazing back at you? What you
> would not give to be able to read again! Wouldn't you give anything in the
> world for something to make you forget your misfortune for one hour? This
> bill affords you an opportunity to bestow this consolation upon thousands of
> blind men and women in the United States.
>
> When you closed your eyes just now you were assuming the sable livery
> of the blind, knowing all the time how quickly you could fling it aside. You
> felt no heavier burden than a grateful sigh that your blindness was a mum-
> mery. We who face the reality know we cannot escape the shadow while life
> lasts. I ask you to show your gratitude to God for your sight by voting for this
> bill.

When Congressman Crail appeared before the committee, he said that the
Library of Congress was not the proper agency to handle books for the blind
because it was not under the management of blind people, whereas the Braille
Institute of America was the creation of a blind man. The California congressman
seemed undeterred by the fact that he had just finished listening to testimony given
for the Library of Congress by Adelia Hoyt, herself a blind woman. He then
introduced, as part of his statement, a letter he had brought with him from the
Braille Institute of America.

The letter made some stern accusations. It claimed that the Pratt bill was the
product of "an entangling alliance" between the American Foundation for the
Blind and the American Printing House for the Blind. In language reminiscent of
his 1928 broadside, Atkinson asserted that the Printing House had had "a complete
monopoly on embossed printing" until his firm entered the field, and that this
monopoly came about through the Printing House's having been given a federal
subsidy for books for blind children. This arrangement, he said, "jeopardizes
initiative, restricts trade and impedes progress in the field of printing for the blind."
In the very next paragraph, however, the letter said that the Printing House

contract with the federal government constituted a precedent that could apply equally well to a contract subsidizing the Braille Institute to print books for blind adults. This agile use of both sides of every argument was a hallmark of Atkinson's forensic style. It had been seen in the past and was to become even more evident in the months to follow.

The librarian of the Cincinnati Library for the Blind, J.H. Ralls, testified next. He said he had drafted the Hill bill, which he was now willing to drop provided the legislation specified that the appropriation be spent exclusively for the publication of new books and that the Library of Congress be required to work in conjunction with the American Library Association's Committee for the Blind in making book selections. Since the Hill bill was subsequently withdrawn, Ralls' testimony would not be worth mentioning were it not for the fact that he said he had suggested to Robert Irwin the previous evening that a conference be held among the various factions, and that Irwin had refused to consider compromise because of "a certain tendency toward obstinacy." Atkinson was to make much of this statement later.

The final witness was Thomas P. Gore, a blind Oklahoman who had formerly served in the Senate. Gore put in a bid for the institution of which he was president, the National Library for the Blind. This was a quasi-public institution, organized in 1910 during a brief period when the Librarian of Congress took the position that the collection of books in its Reading Room for the Blind more properly belonged in a local public library. Although this viewpoint was soon reversed and the collection was brought back to the Library of Congress, the National Library for the Blind remained in existence, serving blind residents of the District of Columbia and maintaining a mail service for borrowers in other states. The burden of the ex-Senator's testimony was that it would be more efficient and economical if his institution were designated as the sole repository of books for the blind for national circulation, instead of allocating this function to a number of regional depositories.

On April 9, 1930, the Pratt bill was reported out by the Committee on the Library with the appropriation request upped to $100,000. On May 9, a companion bill introduced by Reed Smoot was favorably reported by the Senate Committee on Education and Labor; it was passed by the Senate without debate three days later. Mrs. Pratt then moved to have her bill called up on the House's unanimous consent calendar for passage, but her motion was automatically defeated when objection was raised by Congressman Crail on the grounds that the House Committee on Education had scheduled a hearing on his opposing measure for May 28.

The House Committee on Education was chaired by Representative Daniel A. Reed of New York. It had 20 other members, 6 of whom attended the hearing. Except for the chairman, who had some familiarity with the work of the New York City Lighthouse, none of the members apparently knew much about work for the blind. In the course of the day they received a concentrated but bewildering education.

The hearing opened with a statement by Congressman Crail in which he set forth and elaborated the same charges he had presented to the Committee on the Library. Congressman John C. Schafer of Wisconsin interrupted with a question:

"Is there anything to prevent this Braille Institute from submitting to competitive bidding with the Louisville or any other institutions, should Congress enact the so-called Pratt bill?" Crail's answer: "No; there is not anything directly in the bill, but there is in practical effect, yes." He did not explain what he meant by "practical effect" other than to reiterate that the Printing House's federal appropriation for schoolbooks gave it a competitive advantage because "its overhead, equipment and salaries are being paid by the Government of the United States."

The chairman then called on John W. Barr, president of the American Printing House for the Blind, who had asked to be heard in order "to make an accurate statement of the past history" of his organization and to "correct the impression that it is a private institution." Following his account of how the Printing House had come into being, how it operated, and how it expended and accounted for its federal appropriation for schoolbooks, Barr was subjected to a good deal of confused cross-examination by members of the committee, who found it difficult to grasp the dual nature of the Printing House structure. It was in the course of some digressive, rapid-fire questioning that Crail asked: "Is it not true that your last annual report says that you made a profit of $30,000 on a contract which you had with the United States Veterans Bureau, and that you used that $30,000 for putting a third story on the building of your factory?"

Barr, who had earlier indicated he had a train to catch, gave a hurried and inadequate answer: "We did make a profit, but it was under competitive bidding and that all inured ultimately to the benefit of making at a lower cost the books which we distributed to these various States for the student blind of those States."

The Printing House president had not been prepared for a question which bore so little relation to the issue before the committee and even less relation to reality. The "last" annual report referred to was for 1926; there was, in fact, no $30,000 figure in it; the sum could only have been hypothesized by putting together a number of unrelated figures. But Barr either did not remember the details or was unable to take the time to go into them. This was regrettable, for even though its existence was eventually disproved, the charge of a $30,000 profit was to be repeated many times in the course of the day and in the months ahead.

Crail was quick to capitalize on what Barr had said.

> I am very glad we have had this chance to cross examine Mr. Barr because it has developed that $30,000 profit in that one line was made possible because of the fact that they used government money in equipment, printing presses, type, paper, pay roll, to compete with other people in the same business.

By this time Congressman Schafer had begun to wonder if all this smoke might not betray the presence of fire. He raised the question of whether Congress ought not to repeal the Printing House's long-standing schoolbook appropriation and place all printing for the blind, children and adults alike, under the direct jurisdiction of a governmental agency such as the Library of Congress. Since this was the very last thing the California group wanted to see happen, Crail hastened to demur:

> We do not come here to split or destroy the Louisville institution. They have done good work within their appropriation, but our people have set up an

exactly identical institution as theirs for the adult blind. Now, if this committee . . . thinks that the whole policy of the government has been wrong and that there should not be any private institution entrusted with this work, and will put every institution on a par, it would be agreeable to us, but if the policy of the government is to maintain the Louisville institution subsidized, we would like to have the bill come through as it is.

Then he moved to attack on another front:

There is one other point I would bring to the attention of the committee, and that is that the Librarian of Congress has declared that he was no proper person to carry on work for the blind, and in a report which he made to Congress some years ago he stated that he wanted to get out of the Library of Congress this work of distributing books to the blind, as it was no part of his duties or functions, and, that being so, evidently he is not the person who should be intrusted with this great responsibility.

What Crail did not tell the committee (perhaps he himself had not been accurately briefed) was that the statement referred to had been made 20 years earlier, in 1910, and that it had dealt not with nationwide distribution of books but with the use then made by blind residents of the District of Columbia of the reading room on the Library's premises. (It was this action, later revoked, that had led to the establishment of Senator Gore's institution.)

Crail then introduced a new letter from the Braille Institute of America, 10,000 words in length, expounding the arguments in favor of having a federal appropriation allocated to itself. There were some extravagant claims:

That the Universal Braille Press has contributed more toward facilitating the production of Braille printing in America in 10 years than has any other institution in this country over a period of 50 years; and that to it belongs the credit for introducing in America and perfecting the method of printing Braille books on both sides of the paper . . .

And there were some extraordinary gratuitous disparagements of the Foundation, without whose help, as Atkinson had freely acknowledged in the past, he might have had to close the doors of his business:

Its knowledge on this subject [of printing books for the blind] is acquired through its bureau of research, which bureau obtains its information secondhand through the experience of executive heads in charge of printing plants for the blind. Mr. Atkinson has been very generous in supplying this bureau with technical data growing out of his varied experience. We think it unethical, to say the least, for a junior organization with no first-hand experience in the publishing business to criticize or belittle the work of a senior organization which has demonstrated its resourcefulness, and whose benevolence is felt in a wide field of benefaction.

Although every member of the Committee on Education had received a copy of this massive missive in advance of the hearing, J. Robert Atkinson, who was then called upon to testify, repeated most of its substance in his statement.

"Fully 90 percent of the blind readers of the United States are behind this bill," he then went on to say, offering as proof a number of petitions in support of the Crail bill his organization had circulated throughout the country. He echoed Crail's allegation that the Pratt bill had "originated overnight, as it were" as a copy-cat measure. He accused his opponents of strong-arm methods to intimidate blind readers and librarians.

Atkinson's testimony also dwelt at length on his personal life history and his efforts to overcome the handicap of blindness. Through his brailling of the works of Mary Baker Eddy, he said, "I really became the pioneer in the field of hand-transcribing." At the same time he claimed, "the Universal Braille Press is today the most modernly equipped printing plant for the blind in the world" and "we also have the distinction of publishing the first, and as yet the only secular braille magazine in the United States, whose postal entry permits the printing of advertisements." The qualifying clause in the latter statement allowed him to ignore the existence of the *Matilda Ziegler Magazine for the Blind,* continuously published since 1907 and with a circulation at least fifty times greater than that of Atkinson's *Braille Mirror.*

When the committee reconvened following a luncheon recess, Atkinson, who was due to resume his testimony, was late in returning. The chairman therefore called on the next scheduled witness, Robert Irwin, who made a brief statement describing the findings of the library survey and recapitulating the reasons for the Foundation's belief that the Pratt bill offered the most viable solution to the problem of securing and distributing books for blind adults. "Leaving aside the question of working out a comprehensive library system," said Irwin, "it resolves itself down to a question of whether or not it is good public policy to have the purchase of books handled by a government agency or by a private agency. . . . Some of us who have given quite a bit of study to the subject feel rather strongly that it should be handled by a government agency."

He also challenged the assertion that 90 percent of blind people were for the Crail bill and called the committee's attention to the desirability of a "more businesslike relationship" between Atkinson's two corporations. But while he did try to put some of Atkinson's boasts into perspective, Irwin gave him a generous measure of credit for what he had accomplished in braille printing, particularly in interpointing, which he "took to . . . more quickly and with more enthusiasm than any of the other braille publishers."

In concluding his statement he voiced the hope that the issues raised concerning the American Printing House's contract for the printing of children's books would not result in holding up action on books for blind adults. He urged the committee to do what it could to "expedite some bill which will correct the present situation."

One of the questions asked by committee members following Irwin's statement came from Congressman Paul J. Kvale of Minnesota. Kvale had received a letter from a blind constituent complaining about the "extremely narrow" moralistic viewpoint of the superintendents of schools for the blind in relation to literature. The letter said, "They are self-constituted bulwarks of our morals. Nothing but what they conceive to be the cleanest literature, no matter how insipid, can come under our fingers. . . . at one time it was seriously contemplated giving us an expurgated edition of the Bible."

What, the Congressman asked, was Irwin's opinion as to who should be entrusted with selection of books for blind adults? The response satisfied Kvale.

I do not believe books for the adult blind should be selected by educators who were thinking of the needs of their children. . . . My suggestion has always been the Librarian of Congress should appoint a committee consisting of three librarians and two laymen to select those books.

Congressman Crail then tried to assail Irwin's credibility as an impartial witness in a machine-gun interrogation that was soon halted by the chairman's sharp reminder to Crail that "this is not a criminal proceeding."

Atkinson then resumed his testimony, focusing now on a direct attack on the American Printing House. He alleged that the Printing House had engaged in a form of commercial espionage by sending an ostensible job-seeker to Atkinson's plant for the purpose of spying out its equipment and production methods. He accused the Printing House of price juggling and other unfair methods of competition, of extravagance, of careless management, of indifference to the welfare of blind people. He insisted that the Pratt bill was designed to favor the Printing House because of the "coalition" and "interlocking" interests of the Printing House trustees and the American Foundation for the Blind, choosing to ignore the fact that neither was mentioned in the Pratt bill, which specified only that appropriations were to be allocated to the Library of Congress.

In the course of a long and tedious afternoon, testimony was taken from two blind men who supported the Crail bill on the grounds that blind people had to be given a greater voice in the selection of books for their use as well as in all other work conducted on their behalf. Finally George S. Wilson, superintendent of the Indiana School for the Blind, made an attempt to clarify once and for all the nature and operations of the American Printing House for the Blind, of which he had been a trustee for the 33 years he had headed a school for the blind. His explanations were cogent, but they came too late to be of help. By 5:45 P.M. the committee was thoroughly befuddled over how the Printing House could administer a government-subsidized grant for schoolbooks and simultaneously operate as a nonprofit publisher of other books for the blind. Members of the committee were not only confused but concerned. Some grave accusations had been leveled at the Printing House and these, they felt, could not in good conscience be passed by without intensive scrutiny.

Just about the only thing that was clear to the House Committee on Education at the end of an exhausting day was that blind men could be strong individualists, imbued with as much ambitious drive as anyone else, and that they could be hard fighters in pursuing their ends. If the committee had ever held any vague notion of "the blind" as a homogeneous group of resigned and helpless people, that notion had been dispelled.

The 152-page printed record of the May 28 hearing contained a number of supplemental statements filed in ensuing weeks. Among them was one from Irwin, which observed that the Foundation

has for the past two years secured competitive bids from the American Printing House for the Blind and the Universal Braille Press and our records have shown that when the same quality of material and workmanship was required, the Universal Braille Press has underbid the American Printing House quite as often as the reverse has been the case.

The main thrust of Irwin's statement, however, was that "the adult blind people of America have waited all too long for their books." In urging the Committee on Education to recommend immediate passage of the Pratt bill, he pointed out that this need not stop an investigation into the total operations of the Printing House: "If the American Printing House subsidy is a mistake, it will require legislation, and the Pratt Bill can be amended at the same time if necessary."

A communication from John Barr, the Printing House president, was also among the supplemental statements. Accompanying it was a letter from public accountants who audited the Louisville organization's books. Both documents explained how the Printing House accounts were kept and convincingly disproved the allegation that there had been a $30,000 profit on the Veterans Bureau contract. Much the same ground was covered in a statement filed by Representative Maurice H. Thatcher of Kentucky.

None of this availed in getting the 71st Congress to act before adjournment. A final effort by Mrs. Pratt to get her bill through on the unanimous consent calendar was defeated when Congressman Schafer objected on the grounds that no action should be taken until the Committee on Education had had an opportunity to consider all of the controversial issues raised at the May 28 hearing.

During the months before Congress reconvened, the communication wires in work for the blind hummed ceaselessly. A newsletter, the *Braille Trumpeter*, was launched as the official organ of the Braille Institute of America. In its first issue it rehearsed and embroidered all of Atkinson's charges and urged readers to write members of Congress expressing their support for the Crail bill and their opposition to the "circumventive and secondary" Pratt measure. The latter's sponsors were scornfully dismissed as "a negligible group." The Crail bill, proclaimed the *Braille Trumpeter*, was sure to receive "an overwhelming majority of votes in both houses."

The proponents of the Pratt bill were not idle during the Congressional recess, but they refrained from broadsides and concentrated instead on lining up support from the nation's legislators. The Crail bill died in committee, and in December 1930 the Pratt and Smoot bills were reintroduced in the House and Senate respectively. The Senate bill passed without debate in January. The House measure would come up for action on the last day of February.

M.C. Migel, who had never taken his eye off the main target—to get books for the blind as soon as possible and in whatever way had a chance of legislative passage—sought to reach an accommodation with the California group, fearing that continued in-fighting would kill all chances for any bill. On January 9, 1931, he had a conference with Congressman Crail in Washington. That same evening, without informing or consulting Robert Irwin, who was in New York, the Major sent Atkinson a telegram. According to a typewritten draft in the Foundation's files, dated and annotated in what appears to be the Major's handwriting, that telegram read:

TO ATKINSON

HAVE HAD CONFERENCE WITH CONGRESSMAN CRAIL WHO WILL WIRE YOU. IN MY OPINION UNLESS OPPOSITION IS WITHDRAWN, THERE IS VERY LITTLE CHANCE OF SECURING ANY LEGISLATION WHATSOEVER. THE BLIND OF THE UNITED STATES SUFFERING THEREBY. LIBRARY OF CONGRESS ASSURES ME THEY HAVE ABSOLUTELY NO LEANING OR COMMITMENT TOWARDS LOUISVILLE PLANT OR ANY OTHER AND I AM PERSONALLY AND ABSOLUTELY CONFIDENT THAT YOU WILL SECURE YOUR SHARE OR MORE OF ALL PRINTING. FOR THE SAKE OF ALL THE BLIND OF THE COUNTRY, IN WHICH WE ARE BOTH WHOLE-HEARTEDLY INTERESTED, I SUGGEST YOU WITHDRAW OPPOSITION.

Whether this is the wire that was actually sent cannot be ascertained. In later years Atkinson claimed that Migel had wired guaranteeing him half of the Library of Congress business if he would withdraw, but he never produced the document to substantiate his claim. In any event, Migel's attempt at intervention failed. It was to be a fight to the finish.

When the Pratt bill came up on the floor of the House on Saturday, February 28, Congressman Crail let fly. This bill, he said, "would be vicious in its operation" unless amended. Although he did not specify what sort of amendment he had in mind and never actually introduced one, it appeared from a remark made by Congressman Kvale during the ensuing debate that an amendment would be offered to limit the percentage of the total work under the appropriation that could go to any one printing house.

Crail's speech to the House recited once again the charges that the Pratt bill would unduly favor the American Printing House for the Blind, that it would "absolutely shut out" the best-equipped printing house in the world, etc., etc. Once again he raised the spectre of the "$30,000 profit" and even though Congressman Thatcher promptly rose to point out that this had been factually disproven, Crail refused to give ground.

Unexpectedly, it was Representative Schafer who finally dispelled this particular myth. The Wisconsin congressman said:

I did most of the cross-examining during that hearing, and my cross-examination was based on the gentleman's [Crail's] statement indicating a $30,000 profit on the Veterans Bureau contract.... I have been unable to find anywhere in that or any other record the report of this Louisville concern where they indicated they made $30,000 on the Veterans Bureau contract. The cross-examination was very rapid, and it may have been that the words were put into the witness' mouth and he did not deny them, but he also did not affirm them.... I will very frankly state that I was led off the trail, as was the Committee on Education, with a statement which I have not been able to substantiate.

Not even this direct challenge fazed the headstrong California congressman. He went on with his argument and it began to look as though the floor of Congress was fated to witness a complete playback of the events of May 28, 1930, until Representative Frederick Lehlbach of New Jersey, another member of the Commit-

tee on Education, observed dryly: "If we, after the hearings, had desired to report
out the bill sponsored by the gentleman from California, we were perfectly able to
do so; but we concluded not to do so, because the committee is for the Pratt bill."

The final blow to Crail's and Atkinson's aspirations came when Education
Committee chairman Reed put himself on record as favoring the Pratt bill
"because no service would be rendered to the blind by entering into any controversy at this time as to just what we should do." A few minutes later the House
passed the bill. The Pratt-Smoot Act, Public Law 71-787, was signed by President
Hoover on the following Tuesday, March 3, 1931.

Ironically, later the same year, when the Library of Congress was letting its first
contracts for braille printing under the federal appropriation, Atkinson wrote
Migel that he had been awarded contracts for 6 out of the first 16 books, "which is
as much if not more than we really could expect. . . . we feel well satisfied."

But that contented state of mind was not to last very long and, as will be seen in
the next chapter, Atkinson soon found a new issue over which to launch a public
quarrel. Where braille printing was concerned, the Braille Institute of America
gradually fell behind the competition. Once the Printing House had upgraded its
production equipment, Atkinson found himself losing most bids for Library of
Congress work and once again raised the cry of "monopoly." At least these
subsequent laments were merely intramural; the U.S. Congress was never again to
provide a public stage for so virulent a squabble among blind people and those
striving to serve them.

The Pratt-Smoot Act underwent a series of amendments in succeeding years,
and library service for blind readers came to achieve proportions undreamed of in
1931. The original number of 19 regional distributing libraries was steadily
expanded; in 1972 there were 51. For that fiscal year Congress approved a total of
$8,572,000 for this program, which embraced not only books in braille but in
recorded form. It served blind children as well as adults and extended to music
scores and instructional texts on music. In addition to blind people, the bill
embraced physically handicapped individuals who were unable to read or handle
normal printed material, and it reached out to the libraries of state institutions such
as residential schools and hospitals for the disabled.

Library of Congress statistics for fiscal 1972 showed nearly 300,000 readers
enrolled in the books for the blind program. Only about 18,000 of these, however,
were finger-readers; the overwhelming majority received their literature through
the medium of the ear. Probably no more than 10 percent of the nation's legally
blind persons are still active readers of braille. Most of those who do depend on
finger-reading were born blind or were blinded at an early age. For them, a
knowledge of braille remains fundamental to securing an education. *Understanding
Braille,* one of the Foundation's most widely distributed public information book-
lets, explains why:

> Without the opportunity of actual reading experience, blind persons never
> would be able to conceptualize spelling, the sentence, the paragraph, the use
> of punctuation marks, methods of numeric computations, the arrangement of
> information into charts and tables, the use of footnotes, the use of the
> dictionary, and other aspects of written information that are so familiar to the

literate sighted. The benefits inherent in direct visual or tactual reading experiences cannot be replaced by listening to the printed word through someone else's voice.

If, in the Seventies, all visually handicapped people, young and old, have ready access to a respectable volume of literature in whatever form or forms appeal to them, it should not be forgotten that the 40-year flowering of modern library service for the blind grew from the single seed of the Pratt-Smoot Act of 1931. In retrospect, the punishing struggle entailed in planting that seed was clearly worth it.

10

The Talking Book

In the ordinary course of events, blind people lag behind their sighted fellows in reaping the benefits of technological progress. There was, however, one shining exception. For fourteen years before their seeing neighbors caught up, blind people were using the long-playing phonograph record popularly known as the LP. They had another name for it. It was called the Talking Book.

Of all the devices that blazed paths of progress for blind people in the twentieth century, the Talking Book was in a class by itself. With a single spin of a turntable, it opened the world of reading to the three out of four blind adults who had never mastered finger-reading well enough, if at all, to use it as a satisfactory means of communication. That the Foundation's development of the Talking Book in 1934 followed so closely on the heels of the braille breakthrough it had itself engineered is, as one observer put it at the time, "a coincidence not without irony." From the start, the Talking Book was destined to overtake braille, speedily and permanently, as the broadest channel of literature and information for blind people of all ages.

The basic idea was not new. When Thomas Edison applied for a patent for his Tin-Foil Phonograph in 1877, one of the ten potential uses he listed for his invention was "phonograph books, which will speak to blind people without effort on their part." Interestingly, this item was second in his list of ten; "reproduction of music" was fourth.

Why, then, did it take more than fifty years before Edison's idea found practical application? It was primarily a matter of technology. Edison's invention used revolving cylinders coated with tinfoil, wax, hard rubber, or similar substances. Just before the turn of the century, the flat platter replaced the cylinder, and shellac became the major ingredient used in molding such platters. For many years thereafter, the standard phonograph record was played on a spring-wound or electrically driven turntable revolving at 78 revolutions per minute. At this speed the two popular record sizes—10 and 12 inches in diameter—had playing times of three and five minutes respectively. These early 78 rpm shellac records reproduced music with reasonable fidelity, but they also had significant drawbacks. They were expensive. They were heavy—the average 12-inch record weighed more than half a pound. They were fragile—a dropped record meant a broken record.

During the Twenties, the advent of radio brought about some radical changes in recording techniques. Programs and commercials recorded in New York studios had to be shipped to radio stations all over the country to be put on the air in accordance with local schedules. The breakable shellac records could not withstand the vicissitudes of postal handling. Moreover, a half-hour program would have required the playing of at least six large platters with irritating gaps in continuity between changes. To overcome these obstacles radio engineers developed what were called electrical transcriptions that could play continuously for 30 minutes. These were 16-inch discs, made out of aluminum or a semi-flexible cellulose acetate compound, and designed to be played on oversized turntables revolving at the slower speed of 33⅓ rpm.

This, the reader will recognize, is how modern long-playing records perform, but it was not until 1948 that both the LP and the instrument to play it were perfected to reproduce music well enough for the commercial market. In the Twenties there were still too many unsolved technical problems. In the Thirties, when some of these problems had been overcome, economic conditions militated against successful promotion of luxury goods, and during most of the Forties wartime shortages of materials and labor had the same effect.

An extra spur to the science of recording during the late Twenties was the newest entertainment miracle—the talking motion picture. To provide the sound tracks for early talkies, major film and recording companies invested lavishly in research and development. It was in the engineering laboratories of these studios that the basic experiments were conducted which, after examination of the many alternate methods and materials capable of reproducing sound, opted in favor of a constant turntable speed of 33⅓ rpm using flexible, relatively unbreakable records manufactured out of acetate mixes.

One person who followed all of these technical developments with keen interest was Robert Irwin. In 1924 he was visited by John W. Dyer, a young man whose father, Frank L. Dyer, had just applied for several patents covering variations on existing recording methods: turntable speeds slower than 78 rpm, grooves narrower than the prevailing standard and spaced more closely together than the customary 90 to 100 lines per inch. The senior Dyer was a mechanical engineer turned lawyer who had been patent attorney, then general counsel, for the Edison companies. At the time of his son's visit to the Foundation he was in independent practice as an engineering consultant.

Irwin was immediately intrigued by the potentials of the Dyer patents. He wrote a friend in April 1924 that there was "a scheme simmering in which I am tremendously interested. . . . for making phonograph records which will contain 15,000 words on a side of a 12-inch disk," which could be manufactured cheaply and played on an inexpensive playback machine. "If we do not die too young, you and I may both live to see some revolutionary changes in books for the blind," he wrote another friend a few months later.

The prospect that records could be used to read books to blind people had strong appeal for Irwin. He once confided: "I have always dreamed of books on phonograph records ever since my first hearing of a squeaky Edison cylinder. I was never a rapid braille reader. . . . When I was a boy . . . and had earned a few pennies to spend, I used to save up those pennies to hire a rapid finger reader to read stuff to me that I wanted to hear."

Irwin knew nothing about the phonograph business in 1924, but he acquired a liberal technical and commercial education in succeeding years. Among other things, he eventually learned that the Dyer patents, which were granted in 1927, did not stand up in court. Dyer had counted on having the major record companies buy the rights to his patents; when they refused and went ahead with their own development of slow-speed, close-grooved records, he sued for patent infringement. His suits lost, on the grounds that his patents did not introduce original principles but merely differences in degree of existing processes. Although aware of these lawsuits while they were in progress, the Foundation deemed it prudent to go along with Dyer, inasmuch as he had agreed from the first to forgo royalties or any other financial gain from any use made of his patents on behalf of blind people. By way of non-monetary compensation, however, he asked that his contributions be publicly acknowledged.

In an agreement formalized by an exchange of letters in early 1932, a major stipulation was that all Talking Books produced by the Foundation would acknowledge that the use of royalty-free patents had been given in memory of Dyer's late wife. This pledge was honored even after Dyer's lawsuits lost.Between 1934 and 1948, by which time the patents had expired and Dyer himself was dead, each Talking Book label carried the legend, "Isabelle Archer Dyer Memorial Record."

The other legal hurdle that had to be cleared before the Talking Book could become a reality concerned copyrights. If Talking Books were to command a wide audience among blind readers, they would have to include new and current books as well as literary classics in the public domain. In principle, authors and publishers who had long permitted their copyrighted books to be reproduced in braille were equally well disposed to making their work available to blind readers in this new form, but they raised some understandable objections. "If such discs were used for public halls, or especially for broadcasting purposes, they would fall into the realm of public performance and therefore would be decidedly in competition with books in print," *Publishers Weekly* for April 21, 1934, pointed out.

How to protect the interests of the copyright owners was the subject of a year-long series of negotiations conducted by the Foundation, first with the Author's League and then with the National Association of Book Publishers. The formula ultimately agreed upon was that a token fee of $25 per book would be paid to protect the copyright principle; that every Talking Book record would be labeled "solely for the use of the blind" and would acknowledge permission of the copyright owner; and that Talking Books would never be sold to sighted people, never be used in public meetings or broadcast on radio. These agreements, originally for a one-year trial period, were subsequently renewed. With minor changes, the same conditions continued to prevail in 1972.

It was no part of the Foundation's original thinking that it could or should itself become a producer of recorded books. With extensive research going forward in the laboratories of the major recording studios, the logical course was to ask for their help in devising a method to make such books available to blind readers at low cost. As early as 1927 approaches were made to both the Western Electric Company and the Edison Laboratories. Charles Edison, son of the inventor, seemed responsive, but his staff saw no commercial possibilities in the idea and the only tangible result was an experimental recording played for the Foundation's board at its meeting three years later.

Another year passed and it became increasingly clear that, in the absence of profit potential, none of the commercial manufacturers had any interest in producing low-cost recorded books. The Foundation made one last try. In February of 1932 Migel went to see David Sarnoff, president of the Radio Corporation of America, with a plan he subsequently confirmed in writing. The Foundation would provide the narrators to record the books and would handle distribution of the finished product if RCA would manufacture the records and sell them at cost.

Sarnoff, like Charles Edison before him, gave the plan his general blessing, but discussions with his manufacturing chiefs quickly revealed that, even on a non-profit basis, the use of a large plant's facilities for the tiny production runs the Foundation had in mind would entail prohibitive costs.

There remained only one option: do-it-yourself. The following month the Foundation made a formal approach to the Carnegie Corporation. Carnegie grants in 1927 and 1928 had been instrumental in effecting major reductions in the cost of braille books, Irwin reminded Dr. Frederick A. Keppel, the Carnegie president. There was now in prospect a new method of publishing books that would yield even more dramatic benefits to blind readers:

> I have in my office a record capable of playing 25 minutes on each side, and containing approximately 4500 words [per side.] Every word is perfectly clear and pleasant to the ear; surface sound has been almost entirely eliminated; and what is most gratifying, the cost of production has been reduced to the point where phonograph record books can be produced as cheaply as braille books were a few years ago.

Recorded books, he noted in a follow-up communication, "could be loaned scores —if not hundreds—of times before they were worn out. What is perhaps of most importance—nearly every blind person, after two or three lessons, could learn to operate the phonograph, and thus read to his heart's content."

In requesting an initial grant of $15,000 for experimental work, Irwin admitted candidly that this would be just the beginning. An additional $35,000 to $40,000 would be needed for equipment to begin production. The Foundation had a long-range plan in view; it would launch a campaign to supply blind people with inexpensive phonographs to play Talking Book records and would try to have part of the annual $100,000 federal appropriation for books for the adult blind used for books in recorded form.

Nowhere is the boldness of Robert Irwin's imagination better illustrated than in the unqualified statement he made to Keppel: "I believe that the libraries for the blind of the future will be stocked with phonograph records instead of braille books, and that these records will be loaned through the mails just as braille books are today."

Irwin's daring was all the more remarkable in view of the economic and psychological climate of the time. Nineteen thirty-two was one of the bleakest years of the depression. The Foundation itself was in financial straits. Its operating budget, which had reached $126,000 in 1929, had been cut and cut again. The figure for fiscal 1932 was under $100,000 and would shrink to $87,500 the following year. Not only had contributions fallen off but the yield from invested funds was also reduced. Corporate and municipal bonds were in default, dividends on stocks were cut or omitted, and the real estate holdings and mortgages which had been fruitful investments in the Twenties were not producing their customary income. Fortunately, the investment policy had been thoroughly conservative and in the long run relatively few capital losses were sustained. But stringent measures were required to avoid yearly operating deficits. In 1933 staff members were asked to accept salary cuts of 14 to 18 percent as well as mandatory two- to four-week summer vacations without pay. In some instances they did not even take the vacations, but contributed their unpaid services.

Paradoxically, the very fact of the depression helped the Talking Book become a reality. At precisely the right moment an industrial layoff brought precisely the right man into the Foundation orbit. He was a talented young electrical engineer named Jackson Oscar Kleber, whose experience included employment in the recording laboratories of both the Radio Corporation of America and Electrical Research Products, a subsidiary of the Bell Telephone Laboratories. Kleber was not only up on all of the latest developments in sound-recording technology but, through former colleagues, had access to news of what was going on in all of the major laboratories. With Kleber on staff, Irwin wrote Dr. Keppel in a final follow-up on May 23, 1932, "we start our investigations right where the RCA Victor and Bell Telephone Labs have left off."

At its meeting the next day, the Carnegie Corporation board voted a $10,000 grant. To raise the balance of the required amount, the Foundation applied to John D. Rockefeller, Jr.'s General Education Board, but was turned down. The last arrow in its quiver, however, hit the target. Mrs. William H. Moore was a wealthy and generous woman who in 1930 had contributed $20,000 to the endowment fund. Asked to give the $5,000 that would make up the difference between the Carnegie grant and the $15,000 needed for initial experimentation, Mrs. Moore not only assented but made a similar gift the following year and, when the Foundation was constructing its own building in 1934, gave $15,000 more to meet the cost of equipping the Talking Book studios.

J.O. Kleber got to work at once. A restless, quick-witted individual, he was the prototype of the "basement inventor"—the kind of man who constantly toyed with ideas for mechanical and electrical gadgets and who approached every problem with the delighted anticipation of a child working at a puzzle. "The doggondest collector of odds and ends I ever knew," is the way one colleague described him. "Anything that looked as if it might be useful in some Rube Goldberg experiment would be pried loose from a junk pile and carted off to his house. . . . things like electric motors, pumps, old amplifiers and speakers, and probably anything else that had wires going to and from it."

Given this type of mind, Kleber was not in the least fazed by the staggering array of technical questions before him. What type of compound would produce records flexible enough to be shipped by mail, durable enough to stand up under circulating library use, thin enough to occupy minimum shelf space? What kind of needle could play such records without damaging them? Could a sturdy record player be developed out of standard parts at a cost low enough for the average blind person to afford? What would be the most economical method of manufacturing Talking Books in editions as small as 100 copies? Which of several methods of recording should be used in making the masters? How close together could the grooves on the records be cut without loss of clarity or durability? (The greater the number of grooves, the greater the amount of text on a platter.) What would be the best reading speed for the narrators whose voices were to be recorded? What vocal qualities would be desirable in such narrators?

Kleber's confidence and enthusiasm were shared by Irwin, who was sufficiently sanguine over the prospects of the Talking Book to make a public announcement of the new project at the 1932 convention of the American Association of Instructors of the Blind, dramatizing his remarks with the playing of test recordings.

By November of that year, when the Foundation applied successfully to the Carnegie Corporation for a second $10,000 grant, it had nearly finished equipping a makeshift studio for production of master recordings, was completing arrangements for the masters to be processed and pressed at relatively low cost, had developed two designs of inexpensive electric playback machines, and was working on a spring-driven model for use in rural homes not equipped with electricity.

Some months earlier, steps had been taken to clear the way for an essential element in the overall strategy: having recorded books made eligible for purchase and distribution by the Library of Congress on the same basis as braille books. The Pratt-Smoot Act of 1931 had authorized annual appropriations simply for "books for the adult blind." When Senator Smoot and Congresswoman Pratt filed an amendment to include books in recorded form, objections were promptly raised by the braille publishing houses. Senator Jesse H. Metcalf of Rhode Island, who headed the Committee on Education and Labor which had jurisdiction over the bill in the upper house, solicited the views of the Librarian of Congress, Herbert Putnam. The Librarian's response was on the cool side:

> Since the purpose of the original bill was to increase the literature available to the Blind, an amendment which simply enlarges the form in which such literature may be provided seems in principle consistent.
>
> The particular form just now suggested—a phonograph record—is not yet perfected. Its success depends upon apparatus inexpensive as compared with

the existing phonographs, and which may therefore be brought within the means of the blind themselves.

Assuming the records to be produced, the availability of them to any blind person will depend upon his possession of the phonograph itself. Until some assurance of that possession generally (either through purchase by the blind themselves or by free distribution through some fund not yet in sight), the prospect of the employment of such records seems remote.

When the Senator forwarded a copy of this letter to the Foundation with a request for comments, Migel replied that in order to have blind people supplied with talking machines, there would have to be funds for recorded books. He went on to state: "When it has been made perfectly clear that the blind book appropriation may be used for the purchase of phonograph record books, our Foundation proposes to launch a nation-wide movement to interest local communities in supplying their blind citizens with talking machines." Moreover, "there is nothing mandatory in S 5189. It simply authorizes the Librarian of Congress at his discretion to publish books for the blind on phonograph records."

That the braille publishers were not mollified became apparent when the Senate Committee on Labor and Education held a hearing on S 5189. In a letter dated February 23, 1933, Irwin wrote his friend Calvin Glover in Cincinnati:

> Dear Cal:
>
> Well, I got on to Washington in time to appear before the Senate Committee and tell them about the Talking Book. When I arrived in town I called up Senator Metcalf's secretary to ask if they needed to have me appear before the Committee. He said he had just received a flock of telegrams from various superintendents [of schools for the blind] protesting against the bill, which would make it possible to divert some of the Pratt-Smoot law to Talking Books. . . . I called Senator Metcalf's attention to the fact that all of these people were either owners or trustees of braille publishing concerns, whereupon they read the telegrams with much greater interest.

In *As I Saw It* Irwin added a revealing detail to this sequence of events. When, in the course of the hearing, one senator asked whether anyone would be apt to object to the bill, the chairman, relaying the information Irwin had given, said there had been no opposition except from braille publishers. "Perhaps fortunately," Irwin's book observed slyly, "the members of the committee did not realize that these were non-profit organizations." Needless to say, he did not volunteer to enlighten them.

By holding his tongue during the committee hearing, Irwin may have outflanked the opposition, but he did not underestimate it. The battle two years earlier to secure passage of the original Pratt-Smoot Act had shown him how greatly lawmakers could be influenced by letters from their constituents, and he ended his letter to Glover by asking for a lot of written support.

When, immediately following committee approval, the bill to amend the Pratt-Smoot Act came up on the Senate's unanimous consent calendar, several senators who had received the same telegrams as those sent to the committee asked for deferral. The same thing happened two days later. On March 3, the last day of the 72nd Congress, when the bill was brought up once again, Senator Robert M. LaFollette, Jr. of Wisconsin rose to oppose it. The arguments he raised were that "in the first place there are many persons who are not equipped with proper reproducing machinery to use these records; and in the second place, the funds now provided for the publication of books in braille type are too limited and more money instead of less should be provided [for braille books]."

Objections to the bill, LaFollette said, had come to him, not from a braille publisher but from the superintendent of the Wisconsin school for the blind, "who is absolutely disinterested." That phrase was just as disingenuous as had been Irwin's silence at the committee meeting. The Wisconsin superintendent was J.T. Hooper, who, like all other heads of schools for the blind, was an ex-officio trustee of the American Printing House for the Blind. Furthermore, the superintendent's daughter, Marjorie Hooper, was on the staff of the Printing House.

With Congress slated to adjourn that afternoon, LaFollette then proposed an amendment that would limit to $10,000 the amount to be spent on recorded books out of the $100,000 appropriation available for books for the blind. Senator Frederic C. Walcott of Connecticut pointed out that since the bill had already been passed by the House, any change would force it into conference, for which there was no time left before adjournment. He made a counter-offer. If LaFollette would withdraw the proposed change, "we can declare ourselves here in favor of instructing Doctor Putnam not to exceed in his appropriation for this experiment $10,000 during the first year." The bill was then given a third reading and passed as Public Law 72-439. It was signed by President Herbert Hoover the following morning (March 4, 1933), his last day in office.

The first hurdle had been cleared. A $10,000 limitation on Talking Book expenditures for the 1933–34 fiscal year was not as serious as it sounded. Library of Congress officials had made it clear they would not allocate a single dollar for Talking Books until a sufficient number of playback machines were in the hands of blind readers, and this would take time. Just how many constituted "a sufficient number" was an unanswered question.

There were other questions, too, that demanded immediate answers. What was the best and fastest way to get playback machines into the possession of those who would benefit from them? Only a small number of blind persons would be in a position to buy their own, even at the modest price of $25 or $30. The majority would have to receive Talking Book machines as gifts.

There were three possible ways to finance such gifts. The Foundation could mount a national campaign to raise the money and then distribute the machines to qualified blind individuals, much as it had done with radios. It could forgo a public campaign and turn, instead, to a small number of philanthropic individuals and foundations to underwrite the cost of one or two thousand machines.

The Foundation opted for the third alternative; it would assign field agents to help each state's local agencies for the blind raise funds to supply machines to the people of their own communities. This might be a slower, and perhaps costlier, procedure than either of the others, but it was better statesmanship because it would protect the Foundation from any accusation of taking funds out of local communities for national purposes. Whatever funds the Foundation might be able to raise for its own account could then be used for development and perfection of the Talking Book product, on which much remained to be done.

To spearhead the publicity that would be needed to launch a state-by-state campaign, the obvious choice was Helen Keller. Helen, who was spending the year in Scotland with Anne Sullivan Macy and Polly Thomson, cabled the Foundation in September 1933 to ask whether she would be needed for campaign purposes that winter. Migel wired, then followed up by letter, to say yes. Knowing Helen's determination to reserve her fund-raising efforts for completion of the endowment fund, he wrote that this could be the primary objective but that the Talking Book project was also a possibility.

On receipt of Migel's cable, but before she could receive his letter, Helen cabled back a flat rejection:

> IF EXECUTIVE COMMITTEE DECIDES CONTINUING ENDOWMENT CAMPAIGN WILL
> RETURN AT ONCE. TALKING BOOKS A LUXURY THE BLIND CAN GO WITHOUT FOR
> THE PRESENT. WITH TEN MILLION PEOPLE OUT OF WORK AM UNWILLING TO
> SOLICIT MONEY FOR PHONOGRAPHS. AFFECTIONATELY KELLER.

Once Migel's letter reached her, she sent a long, apologetic note saying that a sudden deterioration in her and her companions' health would rule out the possibility of their campaigning for any purpose that winter. "The only thought which sustains me in my upset state of mind," she wrote, "is that under the economic difficulties which continue in America we should not be likely to raise much money this year; and from all reports Dr. Nagle is doing well."

(The Dr. Nagle to whom she referred was J. Stewart Nagle, a former clergyman whom the Foundation employed as a fund-raiser from time to time. It was he who had initially enlisted the support of Mrs. Moore and who persuaded her to make her gifts to the Talking Book program. A man of earnest, jovial personality who was generally well liked. Nagle for some reason irritated Helen and her associates. Anne Sullivan Macy mockingly referred to him as "Jolly Boy," at one point going so far as to exact a promise from Irwin that Nagle would be kept away from the Keller household. It can only be surmised that any successful fund-raiser weakened Anne's oft-stated conviction that Helen Keller alone could attract substantial support for the Foundation.)

Helen's resistance to participation in the Talking Book campaign surprised and dismayed the Foundation trustees. Some attributed her attitude to her own deafness, which might cause her to underestimate the importance of the spoken word. Others thought it to be a reflection of her lifelong Socialist convictions, which understandably put bread ahead of "luxuries." Whatever the reason, she later proved open to persuasion, and although she never went out to raise funds for the Talking Book program, she did make a number of vital contributions to publicizing it.

The opening gun of the Talking Book machine campaign was an article, in the *Outlook* for October 1933, describing the instrument—referred to as the Talking Book "reproducer"—developed in the Foundation's studio:

This machine is approximately fifteen inches square by eleven inches deep, weighs thirty pounds, and, at present prices of material and labor, can be built in quantities at a cost of approximately thirty dollars each. . . . The instrument has various controls which make possible a variation in speed, tone and volume of the reproduced sound, thus giving the reader an opportunity to alter the sound to suit his personal requirements. The case may be closed and the entire instrument carried as a suitcase. . . . [A] spring-driven model can be constructed in quantities at a cost of approximately twenty dollars each.

The accompanying photograph showed an unidentified man (it was Kleber), back to the camera, holding a slim stack of records in front of the opened machine. Propped up on the table for visual comparison were three bulky braille volumes containing the same number of words as the records.

By the following spring, committees organized in 17 states had accepted quotas toward a national goal of 5,000 machines in the hands of blind readers within the next 12 months. Their campaigns looked sufficiently promising for the Foundation's executive committee to authorize the immediate manufacture of 600 Talking Book machines. The Library of Congress, which had decided to begin ordering sound-recorded books once 300 machines had been sold, was now willing to spend the $10,000 set aside in its 1933–34 budget and to commit some funds out of the following fiscal year's appropriation.

What should those first titles be? With the passage of the Pratt-Smoot Act in 1931, Dr. Herman H.B. Meyer, who headed the Legislative Reference Service of the Library of Congress, had been given the additional assignment of directing what was called "Project, Books for the Blind." Dr. Meyer, a scholarly man nearing retirement age, shared the views of Herbert Putnam that books published under Library of Congress auspices should be of "an informing nature" and more or less permanent character, i.e., literary classics. On the other hand, Robert Irwin knew—and scores of letters from blind people confirmed—that overemphasis on the classics could easily kill the fledgling program. The first group of titles, he wrote Meyer, should "include books which the rank and file of seeing people would rush to the library to borrow."

They compromised. As noted in the 1934 annual report of the Librarian of Congress, the Library's first order was for the following titles:

The Four Gospels
The Psalms
Selected Patriotic Documents:
    Declaration of Independence and Constitution of the United States
    Washington's Farewell Address and Washington's Valley Forge Letter
      to the Continental Congress.
    Lincoln's Gettysburg Address, Lincoln's First and Second Inaugural
      Addresses.
Collection of Poems
Shakespeare:
    As You Like It, Merchant of Venice, Hamlet, Sonnets.

Fiction:
  Carroll: *As the Earth Turns*
  Delafield: *The Diary of a Provincial Lady*
  Jarrett: *Night Over Fitch's Pond*
  Kipling: *The Brushwood Boy*
  Masefield: *The Bird of Dawning*
  Wodehouse: *Very Good, Jeeves*

Even the order in which these titles was listed was a sensitive matter for the Library. Dr. Meyer sent specific instructions on this point: "when you list [the titles] for which the Library of Congress stands sponsor, be sure to print the Gospels and Psalms, the Patriotic Documents, the Collection of Poems, the Shakespeare Plays, *first*. Where you put the rest doesn't matter."

The initial Library of Congress orders were for 100 sets of each title, distributed according to a circulation formula to the same 24 regional libraries for the blind as those receiving books in raised print. A bill drafted by the Foundation to amend the postal law to extend to Talking Books the same free mailing privileges as braille books was enacted in May 1934.

An immediate dilemma in getting the Talking Book program under way was how to finance the required capital expenditures. Funds had to be laid out for the parts used in manufacturing the hundreds of playback machines for which contingent orders were on hand. Production of the initial batch of records ordered by the Library of Congress meant advancing money for supplies and labor. It was estimated that a revolving fund of $50,000 would be needed to handle these outlays, in addition to $15,000 for continuing research and development. Application was made to the Carnegie Corporation for a $65,000 grant, but this time the cash register rang only faintly, to the tune of $15,000. Appeals to other philanthropic bodies were even less successful. The Foundation, it appeared, would have to borrow from its own endowment fund, with consequent loss of income to its other work. The situation was temporarily alleviated with the providential arrival of a legacy, against which some of the operating funds were borrowed (at the prevailing annual interest rate of 2 percent) until, a year later, an altogether different solution emerged.

Money was not the only headache. The Talking Book program had barely begun rolling when a new controversy was originated by "Fighting Bob" Atkinson of the Braille Institute of America. Although he, along with his fellow braille publishers, had inveighed strongly in 1933 against allowing the Talking Book to come under the Pratt-Smoot Act, he had evidently decided to climb aboard the winning vehicle. Less than three months after passage of the amendment that brought Talking Books within the Pratt-Smoot purview, Atkinson put the Foundation on notice that he had been negotiating "for some time" with a Los Angeles engineer who had patented a "revolutionary" invention for sound recording, called the Readophone. According to Atkinson, the Readophone could outperform the Talking Book in every way: length of recording, price, sound quality, etc. The Foundation responded to this intriguing bit of news by urging Atkinson to bring his machine and some specimen recordings to the AAWB convention, scheduled for later that month in Richmond, Virginia. Atkinson declined, but during the next few months kept up a barrage of publicity to promote the Readophone. It began to look as though a new "war of the dots" was in the offing.

Ever the mediator, Migel urged Atkinson to send the Readophone to New York for examination. If Atkinson or his engineer thought it best to accompany the machine for demonstration purposes, Migel wrote on March 21, 1934, the Foundation would pay half the traveling expense. Atkinson demurred on the grounds that he could not afford the other half. The Foundation then proposed to send its own engineer to Los Angeles, but this suggestion was rejected because, Atkinson wrote, "there are those who are ever eager to copy the work of others and against these we must protect ourselves." His counterproposal was that both he and his engineer would bring the machine to New York, provided the Foundation met all expenses. The Foundation agreed, and May 28, 1934, was set as the demonstration date. There followed a series of almost daily letters from Atkinson, concerned with financial and other details. He estimated his travel cost at $300 and asked for an advance, then revised the figure to $700, and finally announced that he had decided to have his wife accompany him in addition to the engineer. His travel bill, which ultimately came to over $900, was paid by Migel out of his own funds.

Far more irritating than the petty bargaining was the fact that Atkinson repeatedly deferred the demonstration date as he made use of his free trip to arrange stopovers for Readophone demonstrations in Cleveland, Chicago, Boston, and Washington. The delay was serious because—just in case the Readophone should turn out to be everything its sponsor claimed for it—the Foundation had suspended its own Talking Book production.

Inasmuch as the Readophone employed a different recording principle than that used in the Talking Book, an impartial committee of experts was assembled to evaluate the two machines. This unpaid "jury" consisted of six sound-recording engineers: two from the staff of RCA Victor, one employed by the Electrical Research Products affiliate of Bell Laboratories, and three associated with independent recording studios.

The demonstration finally took place on June 12, and immediately thereafter the technical group filed a unanimous report rejecting the Readophone. Their major point was that its "revolutionary" principle—known as the constant linear method of recording—had been in existence for many years and had been tried repeatedly but that no commercial manufacturer, despite heavy investment in engineering research, had succeeded in perfecting it to yield consistently good performance. The report concluded by recommending that the Foundation should continue to "adhere to the system of constant turntable speed as is utilized in commercial machines. . . ."

Although the Foundation now felt confident about resuming its production of Talking Book machines and recordings, it was not in Atkinson's nature to take a defeat lying down. He went ahead with his scheduled demonstrations and urged the groups of blind people who attended to write the Library of Congress, asking it to sponsor recorded books that could be played on the Readophone. Because of the difference in recording techniques, Talking Books could not be used on Readophone machines, and vice versa.

Even before his trip to New York, Atkinson had notified Library officials of the development of the Readophone and they had given him the same response they had given the Foundation. The Library would not begin to purchase any type of recorded books until at least 300 machines for playing them were in the hands of blind readers. Moving on to Washington after the New York demonstration, Atkinson demonstrated his machine to Dr. Meyer. He also took the precaution of providing himself with an alternative. He wrote Migel that "when I told him [Meyer] that we could easily equip to make talking book records for the machine developed by the Foundation, he said he would give us a chance to bid on such records."

The latter possibility never materialized. Neither did production of the Readophone. The principal effect of the entire affair was arousal of uneasy suspicions in thousands of blind people. It was the Library of Congress that finally put an end to this troublesome situation. When nearly a year had passed and, despite the hullaballoo, only a handful of Readophones had been ordered, Dr. Meyer wrote Atkinson on February 21, 1935, that the Library would not buy any records that could not be played on the Foundation machine. It refused "to be precipitated into a fight between rival reproducing machines for the use of the blind, a fight similar to the struggle over embossed types of several decades ago."

The Readophone affair undoubtedly contributed to thwarting the Foundation's goal of placing 5,000 Talking Book machines in the hands of blind readers within 12 months. Something was needed to move the program back into high gear and the person to supply the motive power was Helen Keller, who had now returned to the United States. Helen was not free to go out campaigning because her teacher was again gravely ill, and she was steadfast in her refusal to raise money for the Talking Book program. But she agreed to use her influence in its behalf. The Foundation had a promise from the Columbia Broadcasting System to devote a network broadcast to promotion of the Talking Book, and in November of 1934 Helen wrote letters to outstanding radio personalities soliciting their participation.

Alexander Woollcott—wit, critic, essayist, storyteller, anthologist, and public personality—had an enormous listenership for his weekly "Town Crier of the Air" broadcasts. Effervescent, impulsive, sentimental, he was an early and ardent advocate of the dog guide movement and had met Helen and her teacher at a fund-raising dinner for the Seeing Eye. He promptly added them to his eclectic circle of friends. When he learned of Anne's hospitalization he sent roses every day to brighten her sickroom; he also dropped in to read to her at every opportunity. It was said that when she died, two years later, the last words she tapped into Helen's hand were, "You must send for Alexander. I want him to read to me."

Helen's letter to Woollcott about the broadcast, written with typical poetic grace and imagery, brought his assent. Also saying yes were Edwin C. Hill, the eminent news commentator, and the noted Irish tenor John McCormack.

Will Rogers went even further. Two days before Christmas he published in his widely syndicated newspaper column most of the letter he had received from "the world's most remarkable woman." Rogers had never met Helen Keller; theirs was a pen-pal friendship which had begun in 1929 when, as part of the endowment fund drive, copies of Helen's book *Midstream* were sent to numerous celebrities. Rogers had been among the few who did not acknowledge the book or its accompanying note. Helen then wrote an impishly coquettish letter asking him, as "the magician of words," to devote a column to an appeal for public support of the Foundation.

Rogers had responded by sending a check for $500. "Here's my little dab," he wrote, "it's not much on the way to two million but I just don't want Rockefeller to be the only one in the R's." He had promised to write something about the campaign for funds if he could think up a way to approach the subject, but this never materialized. His publication of the letter Helen wrote him four years later may have been his way of making good on that overdue promise.

The network broadcast and other major publicity efforts were a help; so was the growing list of Talking Books which the Library of Congress now began to order. By January of 1935 the number of titles had reached 35, with 20 more promised before the end of the 1934–35 fiscal year. The American Bible Society and the New York Bible Society, which had joined in financing the first recordings of the Gospels and the Psalms, said they would sponsor recordings of the full texts of the Old and New Testaments.

In reporting these developments to the Carnegie Corporation, Robert Irwin also mentioned the need for research to develop an inexpensive method of disc recording which "would render practicable the transcription of Talking Books by volunteer workers somewhat similar to the work carried on by volunteer hand braille transcribers at present." It was to take more than a dozen years before this idea became a reality, but its place in the grand design was clearly visualized when the Talking Book was in its infancy.

Midway through the 1934–35 fiscal year it became apparent that $100,000 a year could not be stretched by the Library of Congress to cover the needs of blind readers in both braille and sound-recorded form. Talking Books had received nearly a third of the year's appropriation. To allocate any more in order to satisfy the clamor from readers for recorded books would be to inflict serious damage on the publishing program for finger-readers, and no one wanted to see that happen. It was time to raise the ceiling on the federal appropriation. An amendment to the Pratt-Smoot Act authorizing an increase to $175,000 was introduced early in 1935 and passed without difficulty in May.

That there was no organized opposition this time around was due to the stipulation in the amendment that the Library of Congress could expend up to $100,000 for braille books and up to $75,000 for literature in recorded form. With their original allocation restored, the braille publishers had no reason to complain, although some thought it would be better if the two appropriations were divorced. A.C. Ellis, who in 1930 had succeeded the late Edgar E. Bramlette as superintendent of the American Printing House for the Blind, was one of these. He sent Irwin several firmly phrased letters urging separation, but eventually yielded to the latter's conviction that the bill would be more acceptable to the Library administrators if they were left free to decide how the appropriation should be allocated. In the course of this correspondence, Irwin ventured the shrewd guess "that you will [some day] wish to push the publication of Talking Books yourself . . ." and offered him assistance at the proper time. Ellis admitted "there is some probability that the Printing House will some day develop a phonographic book department." He took Irwin up on the offer of assistance and asked for information about costs and other factors entailed in equipping a recording studio. Kleber prepared detailed estimates and subsequently went to Louisville to discuss them with Ellis and his staff.

As to the bill raising the appropriation for books for the blind, one point made in the brief discussion which took place on the floor of the House before unanimous passage was voted is worth noting. In presenting the Library Committee's affirmative recommendation, Congressman Kent Keller observed that "the machines for using these records are not to cost the Government a penny. They are provided for the blind people of the country by liberal-minded people who are interested in them."

This was true enough at the time, but it was due to undergo complete reversal within a matter of months. It was with that reversal that the Talking Book finally came into its own.

There is no clue in the files of the American Foundation for the Blind as to just who conceived the idea of having Talking Book machines manufactured as one of the work relief projects initiated under the New Deal. The first document bearing on this, a letter written to Franklin D. Roosevelt on April 17, 1935, discloses a fully thought-out plan. After explaining the Talking Book and what it meant to blind persons, it stated:

> Through private channels our Foundation has been able thus far to place in the hands of the blind thirteen hundred Talking Book machines—sold at actual cost of manufacture. There should be at least ten thousand machines in the hands of the blind, but, unfortunately, the blind as a whole are not people whose means would enable them to procure these machines.
>
> We, therefore, respectfully submit to you the request that either through the Public Works Administration, or through any other means within your power to grant, a sufficient sum be appropriated for the production of, say, five thousand Talking Book machines.
>
> The manufacture and assembling . . . would give employment to several hundred people directly and indirectly in the production of tubes, motors, cases, radio sets, earphones, etc. So that, in addition to the benefit conferred upon the blind, the employment of a large number of people would be a considerable aid to industrial recovery.
>
> These machines can and should remain the property of the Federal Government, and might be distributed through the Library of Congress or loaned to the various State Commissions for the Blind to be loaned without charge to the blind.

Signed by M.C. Migel, the letter ended with a request that he and Helen Keller be allowed to discuss the proposal with the President. At the conclusion of that meeting a few weeks later, F.D.R. picked up the telephone and instructed Frank C. Walker of the National Emergency Council to expedite the project. He also communicated his personal interest to Harry L. Hopkins, administrator of the Works Progress Administration, and to Frances Perkins, Secretary of Labor.

Helen had never been face to face with Franklin D. Roosevelt before this meeting, but they had exchanged letters. Their correspondence had a curious beginning. In 1929 one of Helen's fund-raising letters had gone to Roosevelt, then governor of New York State, inviting him to become a member of the Foundation. He declined, but forgot to sign his note. Impulsively, Helen sent the letter back to Albany with a handwritten message on the back. In her square printed script, she painstakingly lettered:

Please, dear Mr. Roosevelt sign your full name. Something tells me you are going to be the next President of the "Land of the Free and the home of the

brave" and this seems a good time to get your autograph. It may interest you to know I have never asked for any ones autograph before.   With all good wishes

I am, Cordially yours
Helen Keller

Roosevelt returned the letter to her, signed, and thus began a relationship of mutual regard which Helen nourished by sending him occasional admiring notes when he made public pronouncements that particularly pleased her. At a political dinner in Washington attended by the President early in 1935, Will Rogers, serving as toastmaster, casually mentioned his forthcoming broadcast on behalf of the Talking Book, whereupon F.D.R. jotted on a card passed to Rogers, "Anything Helen Keller is for, I am for." Rogers quoted this in the course of his broadcast appeal.

Such incidents may have helped pave the way for Roosevelt's sympathetic response to the Foundation's request. Also helpful was the fact that a member of the Foundation board, Mary V. Hun of Albany, New York, was a close family friend and long-time political associate of Roosevelt; during his governorship she served as chairman of the New York State Commission for the Blind. Finally, there was the fact that just a few months earlier, Franklin D. Roosevelt had become honorary president of the American Foundation for the Blind.

It was commonly believed, during the Roosevelt era, that a strong element in his generous attitude toward work for the handicapped was the fellow feeling that grew out of his own physical disability. Whatever the reason or reasons, F.D.R.'s personal endorsement of the plan to have Talking Book machines manufactured as a work relief project was probably the only thing that saved it from strangulation by red tape.

Technically, the plan did not actually qualify as a work relief project. The Works Progress Administration had been established to give jobs to the unemployed, and its administrative policy stipulated that 75 cents out of every dollar should be spent for direct labor. The manufacture of Talking Book machines, however, was primarily an assembly job using commercially available turntables, motors, speakers, amplifiers, etc. These were purchased from a dozen different sources; the labor component, which involved assembling and fastening, represented less than 40 percent of the total cost of the finished product.

Threading through the bureaucratic layers to gain permission for this deviation from the WPA formula was no easy task. Another challenge was obtaining the agreement of the Library of Congress to take title to the Talking Book machines once they were manufactured. The Library was not keen on the idea; involvement with ownership and distribution for record players was an unprecedented, seemingly alien, function for a scholarly institution. The Foundation offered to do everything in its power to ease things.

"If you wish us to do so," Migel wrote in a letter to Librarian of Congress Herbert Putnam,

> the Foundation will arrange with the State Commissions for the Blind in each State to be responsible for the machines allotted to that State—the different Commissions to determine which blind people may receive machines on an indefinite loan under such conditions as you may wish to prescribe. If you desire, the Foundation will undertake to arrange for the Commission or any other agency in each state to check up on the machines periodically and to give instruction in their use. In short, the Foundation will relieve the Library of Congress so far as you may desire of all details connected with the distribution of these machines. . . .

It was on this basis that the Library was persuaded to "sponsor the orphan child," as Irwin put it in a chatty letter to Helen Keller at the end of August. Supervising the manufacture of 5,000 machines at a cost of $210,000 would be "a nice messy job." Still: "What a job it would be to raise this money from private sources!"

On September 19, 1935, President Roosevelt signed the executive order to the Treasury transferring $211,500 to the Library of Congress for the construction of Talking Book machines. The Library then appointed the American Foundation for the Blind as its agent to supervise the project; Robert Irwin was sworn in as a dollar-a-year Assistant of the Library of Congress for this purpose.

By December a loft had been rented at 475 Tenth Avenue in Manhattan and some of the men who had been assembling Talking Book machines in the basement of the Foundation building moved over to set up production lines in the new premises. Project NEC No. 11,620 was on its way.

WPA projects as a whole were the subject of innumerable jokes in those days; the satiric term "boondoggling" came into the language to describe the activities of little or no practical value to which some WPA workers were assigned. The Talking Book machine project, however, was one of the glorious exceptions. Although its white-collar workers were totally inexperienced in assembly operations, the enthusiasm and skill of the supervisory crew brought them rapidly into line. Among both workers and supervisors (the latter earned $20 for a 40-hour week, the former $16.40) were several unknowingly beginning lifetime careers in work for the blind. Arthur Helms, who became production manager of the Foundation's Talking Book Division, began in the WPA shop. So did Charles G. Ritter, who later sparked the growth of the Foundation's aids and appliances service.

In charge of the shop as project manager was "the other Kleber"—Chester C. Kleber, known as "C.C." to distinguish him from his cousin, "J.O." J.O. continued at the Foundation, concentrating on design research and supervising production of Talking Book records. C.C. was no inventor; he was an administrator and sales executive, whose skills fitted him admirably both for the managership of the WPA project and for the post he ultimately occupied as general manager of the National Industries for the Blind.

Despite its numerous problems (the inexperience of the workers, a constant turnover as men gradually found their way back to white-collar employment, supplies arriving late or in unacceptable condition, repeated bureaucratic interference from overlapping government units charged with control of WPA expenditures), the Talking Book project went so well that it was renewed time and again over a seven-year period. By the time it was finally discontinued in 1942, it had produced 23,000 Talking Book machines at an overall expenditure of $1,181,000. The contract renewals were by no means automatic; there were several cliffhanging episodes when the threat of imminent termination was averted only by direct appeal to Franklin D. Roosevelt. Increasingly, however, the project made additional friends in influential quarters. New York Congressman Matthew J. Merritt, who inspected the project six months after it opened, was so impressed that he inserted an account of his observations in the *Congressional Record:*

My first impressions . . . were those of simplicity, energy, and good management. There are 300 men working on one large floor, which is divided into the necessary sections to cover all phases of manufacture, from preliminary inspection of parts to shipping. It is impossible to doubt that every one of these men derives his inspiration from the sign which hangs at one end of the room. It reads "Every man working here is doing his part to make the blind of the country happier." There is adequate evidence of this in the cheerfulness and energy which these W.P.A. men apply to their work.

Quite early in the game, a logical question arose. If the assembly process could be sufficiently streamlined to fit the fumbling fingers of former clerks, could it not be adapted for blind workers as well? A few unemployed blind men were tried experimentally, aided by special jigs and guides devised for their use in the various operations. This proved so successful that additional blind and disabled people were hired; at one point, when there were 197 WPA men working in the factory, 89 were visually handicapped and 33 others were either deaf or had cardiac limitations.

Blind people everywhere were ecstatic over the WPA-manufactured machines. As for the state and local agencies for the blind handling distribution, their reactions reflected both gratification and distress. Typical was this letter from a home teacher of the blind in Jefferson City, Missouri:

> I have 16 counties with over 800 blind people and 13 WPA Talking Book machines to use in the territory. . . . I am certain I could use four or five times as many machines as I can get, so what shall I do? My plan is to loan a machine for two or three months to a person, then pick it up and let someone else use it for a while.

This teacher ended her letter with an urgent plea for spring-driven machines as well as the electrified ones. So many similar requests were received from rural districts that provision was made for the WPA project to produce several thousand players that could be hand-cranked.

Throughout the life of the WPA project, and for some years thereafter, the Foundation continued to produce its own Talking Book machines for sale to people who wanted permanent possession of their instruments and were unwilling to wait for one on loan from the Library of Congress. There were various improvements introduced as the years went on. All told, about 5,000 such machines were produced and sold from 1934, when the first ones were put on the market, until 1951, when the Foundation stopped production.

By the beginning of 1937, when 10,000 WPA machines had already been distributed and 5,000 more were in process of manufacture, it was obvious that the 1935 appropriation ceiling of $75,000 for recorded books was wholly inadequate to serve a readership whose number had increased tenfold in two years and was slated to go on growing. A new amendment to the Pratt-Smoot Act was therefore introduced, raising the Talking Book ceiling to $175,000. It passed Congress without difficulty and was signed into law on April 23, 1937. Three years later, by which time the number of Talking Book machines in circulation was up to 20,000, the authorized figure was raised to $250,000. It was next increased in 1942, when the WPA project had ended and for the first time the Library of Congress had to use some of its own appropriation for repair and replacement of the older machines. A further increase in 1944 permitted the expenditure of up to $400,000 for both records and machines. The amount allowed for the machines was relatively small because both labor and parts were in short supply during the war years. Not until the war ended could a substantial sum be spent for new machines. The Talking Book appropriation for the following fiscal year was accordingly more than doubled ($925,000). In this same year, 1946, the ceiling for brailled literature for adults, which had remained constant at $100,000 since 1935, was also doubled.

These levels of expenditure were maintained for a decade. In 1957, when the call for additional funds was sounded once again, Congress decided not to go on patchworking the Pratt-Smoot Act with an endless series of amendments but to lift the legislative ceiling altogether and require the Library of Congress to apply for each year's appropriation on the basis of justified need. Since then appropriations have moved steadily upward. The million-dollar figure, which appeared gargantuan in 1947, was only one-ninth of the sum approved for 1972–73.

Not all the changes dealing with books for the blind concerned rising budgets. There were four which affected the basic nature of the program. The first went into effect in 1939. A phrase was inserted into the law specifying that in the purchase of Talking Books the Librarian of Congress "shall give preference to non-profit-making institutions or agencies whose activities are primarily concerned with the blind." This was to protect the program from lowering of standards through commercialization. A second change, enacted in 1952, removed the word "adult" from the law. A third, ten years later, broadened the program to include musical scores and instructional texts on music in braille and sound-recorded form. This enabled the Library of Congress, by consolidating the holdings of various regional libraries and acquiring additional materials from all parts of the world, to create its national circulating and reference collection for blind musicians and students.

It was the fourth fundamental change, which took place in 1966, that was largely responsible for the quantum jump in Talking Book production, circulation, and expenditures. Public Law 89-522 expanded the eligibility for Talking Book service to all physically handicapped individuals unable to read or handle normal printed material. Readers of Talking Books could now include not only persons suffering from physical limitations caused by such diseases as multiple sclerosis, cerebral palsy, diplegia, Parkinsonism, etc., but also thousands of visually handicapped adults and children who had not previously been eligible because they did not qualify under the legal definition of blindness.

Although blind children were not eligible until 1952 for Talking Books produced under Library of Congress auspices, they began to benefit from recorded reading in 1936, when the American Printing House for the Blind obtained a ruling that permitted expansion of its schoolbook program for blind children on the same grounds that the 1933 Pratt-Smoot amendment expanded book publishing for blind adults: books were books, whether in raised print or recorded form. The Printing House built a complete recording studio and pressing plant and began, the following year, to manufacture, for distribution to schools under their quota allotments, such Talking Books as *Silas Marner, Treasure Island,* and *Gulliver's Travels.* At the same time it obtained a substantial increase in its annual federal appropriation.

Once the Printing House was equipped to produce recorded books for its school constituency, it was in a position to ask for a share of the Library of Congress' orders for recorded books for blind adults. As a matter of sound public policy, the Library welcomed the availability of an additional supplier. So did the Foundation. Having arranged for thousands of new playback machines to reach blind readers through the WPA project, and having secured legislation to more than double the appropriation for Talking Books, the Foundation was unable to produce enough records to meet the stepped-up demands.

Nor did it wish to. Robert Irwin had been sincere when he wrote that there was no desire for a monopoly on Talking Books. The Foundation saw its role as one of continuing research and innovation in all areas which affected blind people. To become primarily a recording studio would be to diverge from its main path. Besides, there were serious financial considerations to be taken into account. Even with part of the Talking Book production diverted to the Printing House, there was an immediate need to invest more capital in plant and facilities. Up to this point, manufacture of Talking Books had been a two-part operation, with the master recordings made in the Foundation studio and the remaining steps—electroplating of the masters and pressing of the finished platters—contracted out to the RCA-Victor plant in Camden, New Jersey. With the prospect that in 1937–38 the Foundation would be called upon to execute more than $100,000 worth of orders for the Library of Congress, prudent management called for investing in additional studio equipment and setting up a small plating and pressing unit. This, Irwin argued in persuading the Foundation board to agree to the new capital expenditures, "would make us more independent of the Victor Company, should they suddenly cease to be as friendly as they are now."

It was a foresighted move. Within a few years, the Victor Company, while friendly as ever, was too busy with high-priority war work to pay much attention to Talking Books. By then the Foundation had learned enough about record manufacturing to be able to handle every step of the process. Initially, this was on a limited scale; only after the war was there sufficient space and equipment to accommodate manufacture of the entire volume of Talking Book orders. In 1950, when a four-story wing had been added to the Foundation's premises, all subcontracting of record pressing came to an end.

The circumstances of the Printing House were different. Located on spacious, state-granted land on the outskirts of Louisville, the Printing House was equipped for all phases of production almost from the beginning. Once it was geared to full-scale operation, it became a full partner in the production of Talking Books. The Library of Congress adopted a conscious policy of dividing its business fifty-fifty between the Foundation and the Printing House, each of which repeatedly enlarged plant and facilities to accommodate the steadily rising volume.

Almost as soon as the Talking Book became a reality, Edward Van Cleve of the New York Institute for the Education of the Blind ordered a few sets of Talking

Books to try out in the school's upper classes. The selections were mostly short stories or classic poetry of the kind familiar to generations of high school English students: Byron's *The Prisoner of Chillon*, Gray's *Elegy Written in a Country Churchyard*, etc. In mid-1936 a teacher in Van Cleve's school reported on the ways in which he made use of such recordings and concluded that the Talking Book was "an ally rather than a rival to braille."

This was a point that worried some educators. If blind children learned to depend on recorded books, what motivation would they have to master the difficult and tedious process of finger-reading? The question was valid enough to warrant a serious study that would examine the respective roles of braille and recorded books in the education of blind children. To finance such a study, the Foundation turned once again to the Carnegie Corporation, which responded with a $10,000 grant in late 1938. A few months later, the Foundation was once again fortunate enough to find the right man at the right time.

Berthold Lowenfeld, who had been head teacher at one of Europe's most eminent schools for the blind, the Blindeninstitut in Vienna, had just arrived in the United States as a refugee from Nazi-occupied Austria. A Ph.D. in psychology from the University of Vienna, Lowenfeld not only knew English but had spent the year 1930–31 in the United States as a Rockefeller research fellow studying teaching methods in American schools for the blind. With his long years of teaching experience, scholarly background, and intimate knowledge of blind children abetted by an exceptional degree of personal charm, Lowenfeld was ideally equipped to work with the school superintendents in exploring the educational role of recorded books. Under his direction the Talking Book Education Project, which lasted from 1939 to 1945, enlisted the cooperation of 14 leading schools for the blind in testing the ways in which the child's fingers and ears could work together to enrich his knowledge of the world he could not see.

The project approached its goals in several stages. The first step was to survey the literary classics already available in Talking Book form and select those which could fit into educational curricula at various grade levels. "Learning by Listening," an annotated catalog of such recordings, was distributed to schools and classes for the blind. To facilitate immediate use of the records, Foundation engineers designed a heavy-duty model of the Talking Book machine for production by the WPA project; more than 500 of these were distributed to schools and classes for blind children.

To test the relative educational values of braille and Talking Books, a number of special recordings were made. These presented standard reading material for third and fourth grade children in three different recorded forms: straight reading, reading with dramatization, reading illustrated with sound effects. A comparable selection of stories was presented in braille. Responses by children and teachers in the schools cooperating in the tests were unequivocal: material that seemed dry and uninteresting in braille captured the children's attention when presented in recorded form with sound effects and dramatizations.

To demonstrate the techniques by which imaginatively recorded books could be incorporated into the educational curriculum, a number of study units were put into recorded form. Social studies were enlivened by dramatizations of crucial events: *Across the Isthmus* (the story of the Panama Canal), *Wires Round the World* (the story of the telegraph), *Haste Post Haste* (the story of the postal service). Nature study recordings reproduced bird calls to illustrate a verbal text describing different species of birds, their habits and habitats.

Another objective of the education project was to demonstrate the Talking Book as an enrichment factor in the teaching process. "The speed of the average braille reader is comparatively slow, and this factor necessarily limits the quantity of reading material which may be absorbed by the blind child," Lowenfeld pointed out. The blind child could come closer to parity with the sighted child if, instead of tracing a story with his fingers at 60 words per minute, he could hear it read aloud at the standard Talking Book reading speed of 160 to 180 words per minute.

Practically no children's books other than texts existed in recorded form when the education project began. After examining the range of children's literature and consulting with library experts, Lowenfeld drew up a list of books which the American Printing House for the Blind was then persuaded to produce for distribution through the schools. In the course of the project, 115 such titles were issued in "illustrated" form with dramatized segments and sound effects inserted into the narration.

Once the basic principles had been established, the Talking Book Education Project gained the support of the W.K. Kellogg Foundation to extend its special techniques to additional study units. In music, for example, seven junior biographies of great composers were recorded. In place of the piano scores used in the inkprint editions of these books to illustrate the composers' work, the Talking Book editions played recorded excerpts from the compositions. Further enrichment was provided by "musical end papers"—beginning and ending each Talking Book in this series with selections characteristic of the composer's work. Thus the biography of Josef Haydn opened with a section of the *Toy Symphony* and closed with the final chorus of *The Creation*.

A report to the Kellogg Foundation describing this and similarly imaginative approaches to the educational needs of blind children also cited the results of tests conducted to identify the respective roles of finger-reading and ear-reading: "comprehension of narrative material is as good by listening to the Talking Book as it is by reading braille . . . but material which is mainly informative—as in textbooks of physics or chemistry—is better comprehended if read in braille." The comprehension test for narrative material had consisted of an elaborate experiment, in which a 700-page American history book was simultaneously published in braille and in Talking Book form (the former needed 10 volumes, the latter, 54 double-faced discs). So persuasive were the results that a permanent place was assured for recorded books in the education of blind children.

Lowenfeld, who was named director of educational research soon after he joined the Foundation staff, remained until 1949, when he resigned to become superintendent of the California School for the Blind. Although retired from this post since 1964, he continues to exert an active influence in the field of education as consultant, author and editor. Both his professional standing and his personal popularity were publicly recognized when he was honored by the Shotwell Award of the American Association of Workers for the Blind in 1965 and, three years later, by the Foundation's own Migel Medal.

11

The Beloved Voices

A major factor in the Talking Book's instant popularity was care in selecting the voices it reproduced. The winning formula was in the decision that actors could do a better job in bringing a book to life than such other public speakers as teachers (too pedantic), ministers (too preachy) or radio commercial announcers (too much "hard sell"). In the Thirties, heyday of soap opera, there were actors galore who were comfortable with a microphone, experienced in conveying characterization by voice alone and—the economy being what it was—glad to have a supplementary source of earnings even at the modest fees offered for Talking Book work. These were $5 a finished "page" (one side of a 15- or 20-minute record). Unlike the erasable magnetic tape later used in making master recordings, early masters were made on wax that could not be corrected. A mistake meant doing the whole side over again.

"This thing of recording a book is a tricky job," Robert Irwin observed in writing to a friend in January 1933. "It is quite a strain on a man to read for 20 minutes without mispronouncing a single word or placing the emphasis in the wrong place."

It was indeed a strain, especially in the first studio, a primitive eight-foot cubicle totally enclosed and sealed off from noise (and, simultaneously, from air). Alexander Woollcott, one of the first of the authors who recorded their own works on Talking Books, found the confinement so nervewracking that he had to have someone sit beside him as he read *While Rome Burns*. (Once the Foundation moved into its own building, its recording booths were professionally built and ventilated.)

Ethel Everett, who began recording Talking Books in 1935, was present on the occasion, in 1938, when the entire Talking Book management shared a state of alarm. Eleanor Roosevelt had agreed to record the first chapter of her book, *This Is*

My Story, with Miss Everett doing the rest. There were reporters, photographers
and newsreel cameramen on hand. When the appointed hour came and Mrs.
Roosevelt had not arrived, an embarrassing fiasco loomed. A hasty phone call was
made to the White House. Mrs. Roosevelt was not in Washington, she was in her
New York apartment, then located on Washington Square. A call there was
answered by an astonished Eleanor; the appointment had been wrongly entered in
her date book for the following day. Told of the circumstances, she dropped what
she was doing and, ten minutes later, the F.B.I. men stationed on the Foundation's
roof were relieved to see her striding along 16th Street. Apologetic but unflus-
tered, she posed for the necessary pictures and then went on to perform her role in
what might be considered a tiny footnote to history: the first Talking Book
recording to be made by a resident of the White House. In later years, the same
footnote might add, Talking Books were introduced by ex-Presidents Herbert
Hoover *(The Ordeal of Woodrow Wilson)* and Harry S. Truman *(Years of
Decision)*.

That they could hear the voices of famous personages may not have made a great
difference to the blind people who hungrily awaited each new Talking Book, but it
carried prestige in other quarters. One of the reasons the Library of Congress gave
for its reluctance to award the recording contracts to commercial firms was that
only a non-profit organization could attract the unpaid services of eminent
personalities.

The range of eminence was wide. In the first decade, Talking Book subscribers
heard such voices as those of the deep-sea explorer William Beebe *(Half Mile
Down)*, the poet Stephen Vincent Benét *(John Brown's Body)*, the novelist Edna
Ferber *(A Peculiar Treasure)*, the English authors W. Somerset Maugham *(Of
Human Bondage)* and Jan Struther *(Mrs. Miniver)*, the German novelist Thomas
Mann *(Buddenbrooks)*. In later years the list grew to include the foreign corre-
spondent William Shirer *(Berlin Diary)*, the political leader Wendell Willkie
(One World), the sportswriters John Kieran *(Nature Notes)* and Red Barber
(Rhubarb in the Catbird Seat), the literary critic Clifton Fadiman *(Reading I've
Liked)*, the playwright and historian Robert E. Sherwood *(Roosevelt and Hopkins)*,
the philosopher Bertrand Russell *(Freedom vs. Organization)* as well as such
popular novelists and writers as Christopher Morley, Glenway Westcott, Eric
Knight, Cornelia Otis Skinner, Emily Kimbrough, Bel Kaufman, Leo Rosten, Piri
Thomas, Archibald MacLeish, Ogden Nash, Nat Hentoff.

Equally impressive were the stars of stage, screen, radio, and television who lent
their talents to recording literature for blind readers. Some served as occasional
narrators: Eva LeGallienne, Otis Skinner, Walter Hampden, Dame Sybil
Thorndike, Alfred Drake, Jose Ferrer, Blanche Yurka, Zachary Scott, Jessica
Tandy, Tom Ewell, Donald Madden, Brian Aherne, Patricia Collinge, Ossie
Davis, Ruby Dee, Mildred Dunnock, Kevin McCarthy, Roddy McDowall,
Sheppard Strudwick, Peggy Wood. Some recorded their own autobiographies:
Joan Crawford, Ilka Chase, Victor Borge, Ruth Gordon, Pearl Bailey. Still others
acted roles in the recorded plays the Talking Book studios ambitiously undertook
in the early years. "Ambitiously" is perhaps too mild a term, given the circum-
stances. The only member of the Foundation studio staff with any theatrical

experience was William Barbour, who had played a few bit roles on Broadway. Barbour, a boyhood friend of J.O. Kleber, was in charge of the artistic end of the studio. His principal assistant, who served as the recording monitor, was a pretty blind girl named Jane Muhlfeld who later became Mrs. Barbour.

Their system for choosing Talking Book narrators was to have the candidate make a 15-minute test recording of a short story or group of poems. On such occasions the microphone was wired to two outlets. One was in the control room where Kleber could simultaneously regulate the recording apparatus and listen to the reading. The other was in a separate room where the recording was heard by Barbour, Miss Muhlfeld and—in almost every case—by Robert Irwin as well. The candidate's suitability was determined by vote, the only flaw in this democratic procedure being that veto power was reserved to Irwin.

The extraordinary thing was how well this amateurish casting system worked. The monitors were not easy to please. A report issued a decade after the Talking Book program began said: "we have auditioned literally hundreds of professional actors [and] have found less than ten readers who combine the qualities of educational background, voice, accuracy and stamina essential for this work." That the selection system was not perfect was revealed some fifteen years after the event when a staff member, looking through the audition records of early Talking Book candidates, came across a card with this notation: "Damn nice fellow. Pretty good reader. Might try out when we get some books." The name on the card: Gregory Peck.

The names and voices featured on Foundation-produced Talking Books in later years were well known to fans of television, radio, films, and the stage: Leon Janney, Arnold Moss, Guy Sorel, Kermit Murdock, Staats Cotsworth, George Rose, Norman Rose, Harold Scott, Eugenia Rawls. A comparable group recorded Talking Books for the Printing House. These professionals "give to the works they present a sparkle and vivacity which must be heard to be believed," their ultimate boss, the head of the Library of Congress' Division for the Blind and Physically Handicapped, testified.

What was their motivation? While the 1972 fee of $30 per recorded hour was far more respectable than the original pittance, it was still considerably less than what these same performers commanded for other professional assignments. Alexander Scourby spoke for them all when he told an audience at an American Library Association convention that no work he ever did gave him greater gratification. The Talking Book, he said, was the one activity he would never give up "as long as I can speak and as long as I am acceptable to the Foundation and to the people who get the books [and] as long as I can stand on my feet and get to the studio."

John Knight, who narrated the very first Talking Book, left his tribute to the program in the form of a bequest to the Library of Congress. The funds left by the actor, who died in 1964, were used in 1971 to construct a new tape recording studio at the headquarters of the Library's Division for the Blind and Physically Handicapped.

The most treasured rewards of all for those who recorded Talking Books were the letters they received from listeners. A Baltimore minister wrote to Scourby:

Fifteen years ago I lost my sight in a hunting accident and prior to that time had read *Les Miserables.*

Then I thought it was a great book, but yesterday I finished on my Talking Book the first two sections which are read by you, and words fail me in attempting to express to you my appreciation for what you have done in the rendition of this story.

You have given the characters personality. I do not know when I have been so stirred. It is one thing to read a book to the blind, another to make them actually feel the pulse and reality of events that move before them.

This you have successfully done, and your effort will greatly help my future preaching. On Sunday morning I am preaching on the suffering of Christ and am quite certain that Jean Valjean will appear somewhere.

The recipients of such fan letters usually acknowledged them; sometimes this led to a prolonged correspondence. A girl student at the Texas School for the Blind wound up a two-year exchange of letters with Buckley Kozlow by inviting him to attend her wedding. Ethel Everett was the recipient, over the years, of so many poems written to and for her by a blind lawyer that she collected them in an album.

Listener responses were often augmented by letters from the authors of recorded books. The Talking Book version of Dean Acheson's memoirs, *Present at the Creation,* brought to Alan Hewitt, who recorded it, this note from the former United States Secretary of State:

Having heard myself on recordings, though with considerable difficulty in recognizing the voice as my own, I am not sure whether the comment of a friend of mine about your recording of *Present at the Creation* is or is not complimentary to you; but I thought you might be interested. He says that your voice and inflection were so similar to mine that he and his wife were sure I was in the house with them.

The Library of Congress received its share of grateful mail from blind readers and, on occasion, quoted from such letters in its annual reports. "It is the first time I have celebrated Christmas in October," one Talking Book subscriber wrote on receipt of some welcome new records. An even more concrete expression of appreciation came when a blind man bequeathed his modest home to the Library for use in furthering its work for the blind. The property of Nymphus Corridon Hanks of Heber City, Utah, added a little over $5,000 to the Library's trust funds.

Now and again, listeners had criticisms to offer. Some found women's voices · hard to take. Others objected to British accents. A letter from the regional library for the blind in Utah had this to say:

Many of our patrons, especially in Wyoming, hate British accents with a passion. One, who returned his books the day they arrived, enclosed a curt note saying he had shingles and was constitutionally unable to encompass British readers and shingles at the same time.

With new Talking Book titles being issued in the Seventies at the rate of 700 and 800 a year, such prejudices could be indulged. It was different in the early days, when only 40 or 50 new titles came out each year. Then the arrival of a new Talking Book was an occasion for pure rejoicing. Particularly well received were the full-cast recorded plays which, as *The New York Times* noted in December 1937, gave blind readers "an advantage over their seeing neighbors if they live in the many communities to which the spoken drama no longer comes."

Like many another a little theater group, the Foundation's studio got into play productions with Shakespeare. The small acting company assembled under a professional director, H. Lyle Winter, then moved into contemporary drama, beginning in 1935 with R.C. Sherriff's anti-war play, *Journey's End*, and going on, in succeeding years, to Maxwell Anderson's *Mary of Scotland*, Eugene O'Neill's *Anna Christie*, A.A. Milne's *Mr. Pim Passes By*, John Galsworthy's *The Silver Box*, and other stage hits of the time.

The original theatrical group included some actors who had already achieved recognition on the stage and others who were on their way. In addition to Alexander Scourby and Ethel Everett, there were such regulars as Wesley Addy, Lloyd Bridges, and Peggy Converse and such guest stars as Bert Lytell, Mady Christians, Grace Menken, Whitford Kane, Selena Royle. The regional libraries for the blind had a hard time keeping up with the demand for these recorded dramas. "Whereas the printed play has never caused much of a stir in either libraries or book shops, the spoken play on the Talking Book discs is always in circulation," the *Outlook* reported in 1942. During the fifteen-year span between the launching of the Talking Book and the advent of commercial LPs, only blind people could sit in their homes and be mentally transported to the theater by means of a slowly revolving disc.

Not even the most glorious of voices would have endeared the Talking Book to its listeners if the material transmitted by those voices had been boring. The early years saw a more or less constant tug of war between the Foundation and the Library of Congress, the former plumping for up-to-the-minute popular literature, the latter holding to the belief that it could properly sponsor only established classics or books of high literary value that gave promise of turning into classics. In the course of time, the Library gradually relaxed its literary purism, influenced in part by repeated urgings from the regional librarians, who knew at first hand what blind readers wanted, and by letters from the readers themselves. What ultimately tipped the scale, however, was the emergence of a new generation of Library leadership.

There is possibly some significance in the fact that the idea of serving blind readers did not originate with a Librarian of Congress, but with his wife. Soon after John Russell Young was sworn into the post in 1897, he proposed, at his wife's behest, "that some special accommodation should be made for the blind." It would not involve much extra effort. "Under the operations of the copyright law, we must have on our shelves a large number of publications especially printed for the blind. These might be kept together and attendants deputed to give them special care."

Examination of the Library's stock revealed a collection of about a hundred titles in raised letters; these were soon augmented by an equal number from various schools for the blind, and on November 4, 1897, the Reading Room for the Blind was opened in a corner of the basement of the Library of Congress. Some seventy blind persons living nearby were invited to make use of the new facility. To attract them, Mrs. Young organized a reading hour when volunteers, "ladies and gentlemen of Washington," took turns reading aloud from books not available in tactile print.

This was the origin of what was later called the Regional Library for the Blind in the Library of Congress and is today the National Collections for the Blind and Physically Handicapped. Operated under the overall Division for the Blind and Physically Handicapped, it functions in a dual capacity: first, like the other regional libraries, as a service for blind readers in its assigned area, and second, as a back-up national repository on which other regional libraries may draw as needed.

In 1899 Young was succeeded as Librarian of Congress by Herbert Putnam, who was to occupy the office for 40 years and then serve for an additional 16 years in the specially created position of Librarian Emeritus. It was Putnam who in 1910 questioned whether a service for local residents properly belonged in a federal library and ordered the transfer of the Reading Room's contents to the public library of the District of Columbia. The action was reversed two years later, but it was during that period that an apparent vacuum was filled by the creation of the National Library for the Blind. This was the organization of which Senator Thomas P. Gore of Oklahoma was president for many years; it remained in existence until 1946, when its contents and assets were merged into the Library of Congress.

Herbert Putnam was still the Librarian of Congress when the Pratt-Smoot Act was passed in 1931 and his institution found itself the custodian of $100,000 a year designated for books for the blind. He was in office in 1933 when the Talking Book was added to the program, and in 1935 when the Library was asked to take title to the Talking Book machines that would be manufactured under the WPA project. He retired at the end of 1939, by which time the books for the blind program had swelled to $275,000 a year and the Library held ownership of 21,000 Talking Book machines.

Despite the sizable responsibility entailed in administering large and steadily growing sums, direction of what Putnam regarded as a "project" was never more than a part-time side job for Library officials under his administration. The main responsibility of Herman H.B. Meyer, the first staff member to be put in charge, was as director of the Library's Legislative Reference Service. On retirement he was succeeded by Martin A. Roberts, who simultaneously continued his regular function as chief assistant librarian. When Roberts died in 1940 the program was transferred to a series of Library officials, each carrying it for a short period, until an administrative reorganization in 1946 gave books for the blind divisional status and a full-time director. The first was Xenophon P. Smith, a former Army librarian, who resigned two years later and was succeeded by George A. Schwegemann, Jr., a career employee who had been for many years in charge of the Library's Union Catalog Division and returned to that post in 1951. His successor was Donald G. Patterson, who remained until his retirement in 1957, at which point Robert S. Bray began the 15-year tenure which ended with his retirement in December 1972. During those 15 years Bray shepherded the program's steady growth from the slightly over $1 million appropriation the year he began to more than eight times that sum for fiscal 1972–73.

Viewed at long range, it is evident that the major shift in the Library's attitude toward service for blind readers took place with the retirement of Herbert Putnam and the naming as Librarian of Congress of a series of younger men: Archibald MacLeish (1939–1944), Luther H. Evans (1945–1953), and L. Quincy Mumford, who succeeded Evans and was still in office in 1972.

The transition from reluctant acceptance to enthusiastic affirmation could be traced in successive annual reports issued by the Library. During MacLeish's tenure there began to appear such prideful statements as "the Library of Congress is the world's largest publisher of books for the blind" and "the largest single publishing enterprise was its procurement of books for the adult blind." By 1959 the annual report, signed by Mumford, declared: "One of the most important human services the Library renders is that of providing books for the blind." Perhaps the ultimate testimonial to the program's solid status was the presentation to Bray of the Library's 1969 Distinguished Service Award in recognition of his "far-reaching vision and his brilliant and creative leadership of a continually evolving national program."

At the same time that the Library's attitude toward books for blind readers was changing from a cool handshake to a warm embrace, long years of continuous partnership with organizations whose steady focus was on the needs and welfare of blind persons brought about a growing degree of empathy in the Library staff. Not all of this was an unconscious process. In 1945 Robert Irwin suggested that the staff member in charge of reader service for the blind would gain insight by attending a six-week orientation course the Foundation was giving for social workers. Both the AAWB and the AAIB encouraged Library officials to participate in their conventions.

As the Library's sense of identification with blind people grew, so did its understanding of their needs and desires. All of this contributed to an ever more open viewpoint as to what books and periodicals would be desirable in Talking Book or braille form. It was a long but straight road that led from the Library's bluestocking attitude in the Thirties to its circulation of *Portnoy's Complaint* in 1970.

In making its selections the Library began, after a while, to seek formal guidance from both readers and librarians. A readers' advisory group, composed of 15 blind and 10 sighted persons, was organized in 1947, along with a separate group made up of librarians; these were subsequently amalgamated into a single advisory committee. When the 1952 amendment extended Talking Book service to children, the Library turned to the Children's Services Division of the American Library Association for assistance in choosing titles. In 1954, following a nationwide conference of regional librarians and others, the Library issued a formal policy statement on book selection which said: "A primary aim is to build up a balanced collection that will satisfy a wide diversity of reader interest. . . . with due allowance being made for the preferences of the preponderance of the readers for fiction and other popularly presented works." By 1970, the focus on popular titles enabled the Library to say: "It is highly significant that 90 percent of all books on the bestseller lists are issued on Talking Book records, on magnetic tape or in braille."

The selection policy became even more flexible after passage of the 1966 law which brought physically handicapped persons into the ranks of Talking Book readers. The composite reader profile which had guided book selections in the past could no longer serve. Many of the newly added readers were not persons of settled tastes or much experience in life. Typical of the new reader, the Library's 1968 annual report stated, "is a child with cerebral palsy, unable to handle a print book or magazine or to place a record on the turntable or to read braille." Such a child was also apt to be retarded in reading and communication skills: "his mind needs stimulation to introduce him to a world about which he knows amazingly little." Specialized material, recorded at a slower than normal reading rate, was devised to serve this kind of audience. Because the new readers also included thousands of Spanish-speaking persons, the small-scale program for foreign language recording had to be expanded.

That there was a need for many kinds of specialized material in recorded form had been recognized at a much earlier point. During World War II, Archibald MacLeish formed an advisory committee to develop plans for using Talking Books as an adjunct to the rehabilitation of blinded servicemen. One idea that emerged was to emphasize vocational opportunities open to blind persons. The Library suggested that the Foundation "prepare a general recording of talks by successful blind persons in [various vocational fields] and go on from there with more detailed material in each suitable profession."

Over the years Talking Books spanned a wide range of specialized needs. They supplied blind housewives with a variety of cookbooks, told scientifically minded readers about the nation's space exploration program, gave advice on financial planning and personal money management, dealt with particular health problems such as diabetes, put into vocal form the federal income tax guides for individuals and for small businesses. Blind or handicapped lawyers were supplied with weekly taped versions of Supreme Court decisions. Students of instrumental music were offered a series of instructional packages consisting of the same composition in taped, brailled, large-type, and regular printed score form.

Particular as well as general interests were served by a wide variety of magazines. In 1972 there were available for borrowing through regional libraries 24 periodicals on Talking Books and 12 others on tape. The majority of these could also be ordered as paid personal subscriptions by those unwilling to wait for magazines to reach them through the library circulation system. The magazines on Talking Books ranged from *American Heritage* to *Ellery Queen's Mystery Magazine*, from *Jack & Jill* to *Harvest Years*, from *Farm Journal* to *Newsweek*, from *Sports Illustrated* to *Good Housekeeping*. Those on tape were equally varied; they included *Foreign Affairs*, the *Personnel and Guidance Journal*, *High Fidelity*, and other periodicals geared to special interests.

The prospect of producing magazines in recorded form was the subject of correspondence between the Foundation and the Library of Congress as early as 1935. A Foundation plan to record the *Reader's Digest*, which had long been available in braille, fell through because of the cost factor. Four years later, the Printing House, which had initiated a braille edition with the help of contributions solicited through the Reader's Digest Association's Fund for the Blind, was able to secure a private gift with which to launch a Talking Book edition of the magazine. Both the braille and Talking Book editions were supported by funds raised through the Reader's Digest Association.

Cost factors were a constant concern. From the very beginning those in charge of spending the Congressional appropriations allotted for books for the blind were faced with painful choices: Should there be more titles in fewer copies, or fewer titles in more copies? In the early years, when relatively few Talking Book machines were in existence, the emphasis was on as many titles as possible, issued in editions of 100 copies. A distribution formula was worked out for the 25 regional libraries then in operation; each received from one to ten copies of each new title, the number based on population area served. The only exceptions to this formula were the two government-operated leper colonies. The blind people living in the leprosaria at Carville, Lousiana, and on the Hawaiian island of Molokai received Talking Book machines and records on permanent loan.

By 1936 the number of regional libraries had been increased to 28 and the Talking Book editions went up to 125. Although it took more than twenty years before there was a further expansion in the number of distribution centers, the Talking Book editions had to be increased, year by year, as the WPA-manufactured machines were distributed. At the windup of the WPA project in 1942 there were 25,000 blind people in possession of machines that could play Talking Books. If only 125 copies of a book were produced and all 25,000 readers happened to want it, the last in line might have to wait twenty years before his or her turn came. The Library's decision at that point was inescapable; editions had to be enlarged even if it meant fewer titles. The dilemma was resolved by increased appropriations; in 1972, when the number of titles exceeded 700, the average edition ran from 500 to 1,000, depending on the estimated popularity of the particular title.

A major help in satisfying the need for a wide variety of titles was the steady growth of volunteer-produced recordings. Although, as has been noted, the possibility of books recorded by volunteers was foreseen by Robert Irwin as early as 1935, it was not until 1947 that organized programs got under way. Just as the volunteer braillist movement was spurred by the needs of the men blinded in World War I, the desire to be helpful to the blinded veterans of World War II who were attending college under the G.I. Bill of Rights gave birth to spontaneous movements in many parts of the country to meet educational needs through volunteer recording.

A contemporary description by the librarian for the blind in the New York Public Library set forth the modest origin of what was to become an impressive nationwide program. It appeared in the *Outlook* for December 1947:

We were receiving requests from war-blinded veterans who hoped to continue their college work, for material which we had been almost wholly unable to supply. . . . Even if it had been available in braille, which it was not, they were not familiar enough with braille to be able to use it. Textbooks in history, sociology, psychology, all were required for these students; could we as librarians turn a helpless cold shoulder? There *must* be a way out, and there was.

The way out was an office dictating machine known as a SoundScriber; it used inexpensive small plastic discs on which 12 or 15 minutes of recorded material could be embossed. Such records were neither very durable nor of high reproduction fidelity, and they required special playback equipment—but they were a start.

Until sound recordings came into the picture, the average blind college student who did not know braille had to depend totally on live readers. Talking Books could supply him with literature of a general and recreational nature, but this was seldom what his professors required by way of course study material. Students who knew braille could get some help through hand-transcribed texts, but such students were seldom in a position to give enough advance notice of their needs for the required books to arrive in time. Under the provisions of the Vocational Rehabilitation Act of 1943, blind college students could receive funds with which to pay for reader services. However there was a ceiling—in some states as low as $20 per month—on such expenditures. Even more troublesome was the process of finding a paid reader, usually a fellow student, whose schedule could be dovetailed into that of the blind student.

Recorded texts solved almost all of these problems. As a midwestern counselor of blind students put it, a playback machine "never gets irritated when asked to repeat, never tries to explain a point, elaborate, refute the text, talk about next Saturday's football game, suggest a Coke or go to sleep."

The first volunteer-recorded books were so gratefully received that the movement spurted forward. All over the country so many groups were organized, under the aegis of libraries, state commissions, or voluntary agencies for the blind, that within a year or two a condition of near chaos developed. The volunteer groups were working independently, using different equipment, different techniques, different standards, and often unknowingly recording the same texts.

In an effort to achieve some form of coordination, a National Committee on Special Recording was organized toward the end of 1950. Consisting largely of New York people, this committee drew up a proposed program that would centralize title clearances, coordinate copyright applications, institute uniformity in circulation practices, and establish minimum standards for recording methods by volunteers. In January 1951 the committee asked the Foundation for a $15,000 grant to put its proposed program into effect. The Foundation thought the purpose would be better served if, instead of making an outright grant, it undertook to provide the committee with most of the services called for. M. Robert Barnett, then beginning his second year as the Foundation's executive director, met with the group to discuss the implications of the counterproposal. If they wanted to go ahead on their own, the Foundation would bow out of the picture.

Even before submitting its application to the Foundation, the committee had explored the possibility of the Library of Congress' taking leadership in the volunteer recording field. The initial response was one of distinct disinterest. However, a change in Library personnel was then taking place, and the committee felt more sanguine about ultimate sponsorship under federal auspices. With this in view, they decided to seek a demonstration grant from the Ford Foundation's Fund for Adult Education to get the program started "pending the time when the Library of Congress will take over." During the demonstration period they would depend on the Foundation to assist in technical and policy questions and to make certain production facilities available, principally the use of its new "instantaneous recording studio," then being installed. This consisted of a bank of 10 linked machines that could turn out simultaneous copies of a single embossed master. A special feature was that records embossed by this process could be played not only on SoundScriber equipment but also on any regulation Talking Book machine or commercial playback machine with a light pickup arm.

When the Fund for Adult Education agreed to make a three-year grant of $75,000, a schism in the membership of the committee brought about fundamental changes in its structure, leadership, and planned course. The original concept of serving as a national coordinating body for existing volunteer groups was dropped. A new body, incorporated under the name National Committee for Recording for the Blind, announced its purpose would be to establish new volunteer recording units throughout the United States, using as a prototype the unit functioning in a branch of the New York Public Library. Within a year, the first committee had been swept out of existence by a new group, controlled by a dynamic set of influential society women. Their head, Mrs. Ranald H. Macdonald, Jr., announced that they were no longer interested in having the Library of Congress take over the project but would turn to the public for operating funds.

Such was the origin of the organization now known as Recording for the Blind, Inc., which grew from a single volunteer unit operating out of a small library in New York City in 1951 to a publicly supported national group which raised $1,600,000 in 1972 to finance 23 recording studios in 14 states. The scope of the program expanded as well. From the original service for visually handicapped college students, the work branched out to recording material for visually handicapped high school and elementary school children as well as more general literature in the overall field of adult education.

Until 1957 the Foundation continued to provide Recording for the Blind with duplicating services for its embossed records; when the latter had acquired sufficient financial backing to handle this process for itself, the Foundation made it a gift of the duplicating and labelling equipment that had been used in producing RFB discs. Two years later, Barnett, who served as one of RFB's official advisors from its inception, resigned the post. With that, the Foundation's quasi-parental role came to an end.

Thanks to a vigorous public relations program, Recording for the Blind commanded much of the national spotlight as a source of specialized and supplementary literature for blind readers, but at no time did it have a monopoly on this field of service. Both before and after its organization there were volunteer groups working independently in numerous cities and states to provide the same sort of recorded literature for students and others with specialized interests.

Several national conferences were held under the auspices of the Library of Congress during the Fifties to promote uniformity of methods and procedures among these diverse groups. In 1960, by which time virtually all volunteer recording services had switched from embossed discs to magnetic tape, the Library undertook responsibility for national coordination and circulation of volunteer-produced tapes. Its long-established service for certification and coordination of the work of volunteer braillists was extended to embrace the tape volunteers and a program was launched to create an orderly national system, with the Library maintaining a central collection of master tapes and financing the duplication of selected titles for distribution through the regional libraries.

The thousands of volunteers enlisted in the Library's program either owned their tape recorders or had access to community-owned taping equipment. Prospective volunteers had to pass a voice test by submitting a sample tape, just as would-be braillists had to submit an acceptable sample of finished work in order to receive certification. Those who passed the voice tests were then assigned books to record and were supplied with the required blank tape.

Under the umbrella of the Library of Congress a great variety of people and groups taped books. They ranged from businessmen and housewives who worked out of their homes, to organized groups who raised funds to set up a tape studio in a central location, to prisoners serving sentences in penal institutions.

In Massachusetts the prison program, begun in the late Fifties, operated under the supervision of a voluntary agency, the National Braille Press in Boston. In Iowa, which started about the same time, the work was supervised by that state's commission for the blind. In 1969 a similar program was started in Maryland. These efforts were hugely successful, not only in what they produced for blind readers but as rehabilitative therapy for the inmates, all of whom did the recording in their free time and not as part of their prison work assignments. A remarkable range of subject matter, from higher mathematics to the Koran, was recorded by the prisoners.

Less confined volunteers demonstrated considerable ingenuity in fulfilling their assignments. Those who recorded in their own homes devised signals to ward against interruptions during taping sessions, a red balloon attached to a door knob or a single rose placed in a window serving to convey the same message as the warning light used in commercial studios: "Do not enter—recording in progress!" When a group of volunteers established a recording studio in the offices of Atlanta's Community Services for the Blind, they saved the cost of a plate glass window between the recording booth and the control room by using a glass table top.

In 1962 the Foundation produced a useful adjunct for all of these groups in the form of a down-to-earth handbook, "Tape Recording Books for the Blind." Written by Arthur Helms of the Talking Book studios, the handbook went into such specifics as how to select suitable voices, optimum reading speed, reading habits to be encouraged and those to be avoided, how to deal with foreign words and phrases, how to handle footnotes, illustrations, and tables of contents. In 1965 the Library of Congress began to provide a source of technical assistance by adding to its staff a recording consultant to help volunteer groups design and set up tape studios.

Talking Book readers also benefited from a different form of volunteer service provided from 1960 on by the Telephone Pioneers of America, an organization of 350,000 current and retired telephone company employees banded together for volunteer service. Members of Telephone Pioneers chapters across the country repaired and adjusted Talking Book machines and tape recorders—in some communities, even delivered and demonstrated the equipment to new users. They also conducted several other types of projects including tape recording, hand-brailling and construction of three-dimensional objects with which to illustrate braille books for children.

The service provided by the Pioneers helped solve a long-standing problem. The perennial question of repair had arisen almost as soon as quantities of Talking Book machines began coming off the production lines of the WPA project. The Library of Congress took title to them only on condition that the agencies which handled their distribution would keep the machines in working order. The problem for the agencies was not only in meeting the cost but in finding satisfactory sources of service. Two measures were taken by the Foundation to relieve the situation. One was securing passage of a bill that permitted Talking Book machines to be mailed for repair at the rate of one cent per pound. The other was broadening the WPA contract so that machines could be repaired as well as manufactured by the project's workers. With the closing of the WPA project in mid-1942, the Library of Congress turned to the Foundation to handle servicing of the WPA machines. This the Foundation was equipped to do; it merely expanded the shop which had always repaired its own Talking Book reproducers. The arrangement continued in effect until late 1946, when the Foundation asked to withdraw. The Library then awarded the repair contract to a commercial firm; in later years a non-profit agency, the Pennsylvania Association for the Blind, also bid successfully on both repair service and construction of new Talking Book machines in its sheltered workshop for blind workers. Later still, the Library adopted a decentralized plan under which machines were repaired by local service branches of a commercial manufacturer of record players. With the advent of the Telephone Pioneers volunteer service, it became possible to keep repair problems within reasonable bounds.

The repair question was serious because at the point where the early Talking Book machines might have been considered due for replacement there was no such possibility. When the first machines were ten years old, a normal lifetime for this type of appliance, the United States was deep in war, with manufacture of non-essential civilian goods suspended for the duration. An attempt made by the Foundation in 1942 to secure government permission for continued manufacture of Talking Book machines was only partially successful; a slow trickle of production was permitted to go on until the Foundation's stockpile of raw materials was exhausted. The one effort that did succeed was getting a priority rating on 30 million steel needles, so that blind people could at least continue to use the machines they had; on the models then in existence, a new needle had to be used every time a record was played.

During the war years, the "state of the art" in recording was at a standstill so far as civilian goods were concerned. It was known, however, that great technical strides were being achieved for military purposes. An effort to harness this new knowledge was made in 1945, when the Library of Congress convened a high-level conference on the future of the Talking Book. Those invited included members of the executive and engineering staffs of the Foundation and the Printing House, representatives of commercial recording firms, and a group of experts from several departments of the federal government, among them George W. Corner, M.D., chairman of the Committee on Sensory Devices of the wartime Office of Scientific Research and Development. In view of the extensive use made of Talking Books in hospitals for the war-blinded, it was thought that this committee, which was already working on advanced technological mobility and reading aids for the blind, might be willing to take on the additional task of modernizing Talking Book design. To the Library's disappointment, the committee refused on the grounds that the necessary improvements were within the competence of the phonograph industry.

Soon thereafter the Foundation completed development of a new model of its own Talking Book reproducer, but declined to submit it when the Library of Congress called for bids on a postwar model in 1946. The contract went to a commercial concern. It was the first time anything to do with the Talking Book program had passed out of the hands of non-profit organizations, a fact that caused Robert Irwin to worry—unnecessarily, as it turned out—about the possibility that Talking Book machines might be sold to sighted people not entitled to their use. What he might really have worried about was something he did not anticipate; the Foundation was never again to produce Talking Book machines for the Library of Congress.

The end was foreshadowed only a few months later. In 1947 the Foundation announced development of an entirely new model of Talking Book machine, the Sonograph. It was lightweight, inexpensive, and capable of playing not only pressed records but also the embossed discs that volunteer groups were just then beginning to record for blind students. When the Library of Congress called for bids on 2,500 new Talking Book machines for the 1948–49 fiscal year, Irwin was confident that the Sonograph—far lower in price than any of the dozen or so models submitted by commercial concerns—would be awarded the contract. It was with shocked dismay that the Foundation learned that, instead of being hailed as a design breakthrough, the Sonograph had been rejected by Library officials as having gone too far in the direction of economy and compactness.

Robert Irwin fired off an indignant protest to Luther Evans, Librarian of Congress. His letter brought a soothing but noncommittal reply from Evans, affirming that "the history of cooperation between your organization and the Library of Congress has been unusual" and voicing "great confidence that this will continue to be the case."

Irwin's protest may have been the reason that the Library thereupon decided to reject all bids and to seek the help of the National Bureau of Standards in rewriting the specifications before asking for new bids. The result of this action was twofold. When bidding was reopened on the new specifications, production of the Talking Book machines was awarded to a commercial firm, and the Library contracted with the National Bureau of Standards to provide it with a continuing program of research and development on records and machines.

These developments also had dual consequences. One was that the Foundation never again sought to manufacture Talking Book machines for the Library of Congress; for the next two or three years, it sold its Sonographs to blind persons wishing to buy their own equipment, and thereafter permanently phased out its manufacture of record-playing machines. The second was that the association with the National Bureau of Standards proved to be a mistake. The Library concluded, after four years, that the bureau's research and development services were "inadequate and uneconomical" and turned back for technical guidance to the organization that had given birth to the Talking Book: the American Foundation for the Blind. A research and development contract was negotiated with the Foundation in 1952 and was renewed for a number of years. Concomitantly, the Foundation maintained an independent research program financed out of its own funds as part of its continuing commitment to seek ways of improving all forms of service to blind persons.

The ongoing consultative relationship between the Foundation and the Library of Congress was instrumental in effecting twenty years of major improvements in Talking Book technology: the change from 12-inch discs to lighter-weight 10-inchers, the achievement of ever longer playing times as turntable speeds were halved from 33 1/3 rpm to 16 2/3 and then halved once again to 8 1/3 rpm; the additional increase in playing time as methods were worked out to groove records ever more closely, from the original 150 lines per inch to a pitch of 330; the introduction of sound sheets; the exploration, evaluation, and field-testing of tape recording techniques in open reel and cassette form. Similar attention was given to the design of Talking Book machines, in pursuit of better and more versatile performance, lighter weight, easier operation, and sturdier construction.

Not everything worked out. During the Fifties many months were spent in investigating European recording techniques on tape, film, and wire, only to arrive at the conclusion that these were not adaptable to the Talking Book. In 1956 the Foundation awarded a subcontract to Dr. Peter Goldmark, then head of the Columbia Broadcasting System Laboratories, to develop an 8 rpm record in 7-inch size, grooved so closely (550 lines to the inch) that it could play continuously for two hours. Testing of a prototype of this record and an analysis of the cost factors involved in its production led to the decision that so radical a change from the then prevailing system of 33 1/3 rpm records was premature.

Two years later Dr. Goldmark, serving as a consultant to Recording for the Blind, announced a design for a flyweight record player for his 8 rpm record. More or less simultaneously, the Foundation demonstrated its own version of an 8 rpm record. It differed from the Goldmark version in that it was compatible with the 50,000 Talking Book machines then in existence, whereas the Goldmark design required the use of a totally new reproducer, which would have meant replacing several million dollars' worth of equipment. Neither design was adopted at the time; instead, the intervening step was taken of recording at 16 2/3 rpm. This cautious approach was dictated by the rapid advances then taking place in tape technology, which seemed to suggest that an altogether different future direction was in the offing for recorded books.

During the years in which these and other experimental ventures were going forward in its engineering laboratories, some fundamental changes were also taking place in the Foundation's policies.

From the beginning, the Foundation's relationship to the Talking Book operated on two levels—one concerned with innovation, the other with manufacture. In the early days, the two were hardly separable; each technical innovation was promptly translated into manufacturing changes in the Talking Book records or in the machines for playing them. Evidently it did not occur to the Talking Book pioneers that a line might logically be drawn between experimentation with new ideas on the one hand and manufacture of Talking Books on contract for the Library of Congress on the other. The former admittedly entailed financial risks; the latter was supposed to be a breakeven proposition, yielding no profit to the Foundation but not resulting in operating losses either.

The absence of a clear distinction between these two levels of work was one of the first problems to confront M. Robert Barnett when he became the Foundation's executive director in the fall of 1949. It was also evident that the strategies employed under the former administration to minimize production losses had been ineffectual because wrongly conceived.

The major mistake had been reluctance to invest the capital needed to make the Talking Book plant self-sufficient in manufacturing all the work assigned to it by the Library of Congress. In 1947, Irwin had made an effort to raise $25,000 for these purposes from the Carnegie Corporation, but when the application was turned down, he did not bring sufficient pressure on his trustees to spend the needed money out of the Foundation's own funds. Under Barnett, the executive committee voted the necessary expenditures, and early in 1950 the Foundation proceeded to equip additional soundproof studios; to switch over from making master recordings on wax to the more up-to-date method of making them on tape; to procure and install enough additional plating and pressing equipment so that for the first time it would be in a position to manufacture all of its own Talking Books, from start to finish, on its own premises.

Another basic change was to separate the manufacturing and research functions by relieving J.O. Kleber of managerial responsibility for production. Kleber soon resigned and became director of research for another Foundation-fostered enterprise, National Industries for the Blind, where he remained until his death in 1958. Some of Kleber's functions were taken over by Manuel Powers, who supervised record production and also worked on design improvements for Talking Book machines. Powers, a chemist and electronics engineer, was a perfectionist who during his 14 years with the Foundation spent innumerable nights and weekends in pursuit of his goals. He, too, died in 1958.

By midyear of 1951, Barnett was able to inform the Library of Congress that the Foundation's Talking Book department was now equipped and staffed for three times as much production as the previous year. This was true; what was also true was that a careful cost analysis showed the Talking Book department to be costing the Foundation a great deal of money. In January of 1952 the executive committee debated quite seriously whether the Foundation was justified in going forward with the manufacture of Talking Books at all. On the basis of a detailed study made by Jansen Noyes, Jr. (then treasurer), a series of measures was recommended to cut down the operating losses. Confident that these economies would turn the tide, the executive committee went on record to state its conviction that the Talking Book was "of invaluable service to the blind of the nation." Because that belief has remained unshaken, the Foundation has continued over the years to invest large sums in building and maintaining an extensive, thoroughly modern plant.

Kleber was replaced as general manager of the Talking Book department by John W. Breuel, who later became director of the overall Manufacturing and Sales department. This department included four divisions: Talking Book, Tape Duplicating, Engineering, and Aids and Appliances. The department's structure, with the engineering division bridging all technical operations, was the logical outcome of a series of reorganizations begun early in Barnett's administration to tie technical research more closely to program goals. As part of the reorganization, the Foundation appointed several advisory committees. One of these, the Advisory Committee on Technical Research and Development, formulated the second major policy change affecting the Talking Book.

The committee was a high-powered group; members at the time were Karl M Dallenbach, chairman, Department of Psychology, University of Texas; Sherman M. Fairchild, president, Fairchild Recording Equipment Corporation, William C. Geer, Geer Laboratory, Ithaca, N.Y.; Peter C. Goldmark, president, CBS Laboratories; Jansen Noyes, Jr., Foundation treasurer; Edward J. Poitras, director of engineering, Fenwal, Inc., Ashland, Mass.; Jerome B. Wiesner, director of the research laboratory of electronics, Massachusetts Institute of Technology. There were also two associate members: Thornton C. Fry, assistant to the president, Bell Telephone Laboratories, and Edwin H. Land, president, Polaroid Corporation.

At the beginning of 1958 the committee recommended, after considerable discussion, that the Foundation "immediately and substantially reduce active research of its own on both tape and records" while continuing to encourage and assist research by others. The fundamental reason for this was that commercial research in magnetic tape and other types of recording was in progress that would inevitably outpace any efforts the Foundation could afford. Reduced activity in Talking Book research, furthermore, would free the Foundation to "take stock of its capacity for research and development in other areas of technology" affecting blind persons.

An initial objective of the Talking Book program was to make the cost of recorded books comparable with the cost of braille books. Once this goal had been achieved and surpassed, the aim became to bring the cost down to the price of the same book in a standard inkprint edition. This target was reached and overtaken (due in some measure to the rise in prices of inkprint books), and beating the cost of the paperback became the new aim. The 30-minute-per-side Talking Book record which cost $1 in the Fifties gave way to the 45-minute-per-side platter which cost 50 cents in the Sixties and 40 cents in the early Seventies. The Library of Congress' 1972 decision that, beginning the first of the following year, all new Talking Books would be recorded at 8 rpm (90 minutes per side) was expected to make it possible for the average 12-hour book to be produced for $3 or less. Nor would this necessarily be the end of the line. A 4 rpm record was experimentally produced by Foundation engineers as far back as 1966; it was a 12-inch disc which played for more than 10 hours.

A major factor in bringing down costs was the increasing use of automated equipment. The Foundation, which in 1972 was pressing 10,000 records a day, installed six new automatic presses that would increase the annual production to 3 million a year; its trustees voted that year to appropriate $340,000 for additional automated equipment and plant modernization.

A possibility for the future was that Talking Books might eventually be produced as flexible sound sheets, whose manufacturing costs would be lowest of all. The overall savings would be greater still: sound sheets would not be circulated but sent to the reader to keep or discard at will, thereby eliminating the handling and maintenance costs entailed in a circulation system. Another possibility was that the Talking Book of tomorrow would be a multi-track cassette at such slow speed (15/16 ips) that a two-track tape would produce 3 hours of reading and a four-track would double this. Marathon eight-track cassettes, which provided up to 13 hours of reading, replaced disc recording in the British Talking Book service in the early Sixties. In the United States the cassettes produced for the Library of Congress in 1972 were being recorded at 1 7/8 ips on dual-track tape, but experiments were going forward on slower speeds and additional tracks.

It is an accepted premise in research that not every avenue of inquiry will lead to useful discovery. Work on the Talking Book was no exception. One of the investigations which had yet to prove itself concerned methods of achieving speech compression.

If you, the reader of the inkprint edition of this book, read at average speed, you are encompassing about 300 words a minute. If you are a naturally fast reader, or have learned speed reading, you may be covering the pages at two or three times that rate. If, as a blind person, you are reading with your fingertips and are proficient in braille, your speed may be 100 words per minute. If you are listening to a recorded version, you are hearing the text read at about 175 words per minute, which is the optimum rate at which words can be spoken with accuracy and pleasing diction.

More than twenty years have been devoted to efforts to devise some form of "speed hearing" for blind listeners. There is a simple mechanical way to increase the delivery rate of recorded information: speeding up the turntable. Blind students were among the first to try this when three-speed turntables became commercially available shortly after World War II. By playing a 33 1/3 rpm Talking Book at 45 rpm, they increased the word rate from 175 words per minute to about 250. This simultaneously brought about a rise in pitch, but it was within tolerable limits. Tape could also be speeded up. When, however, attempts were made to play discs or tape at much more than 50 percent over the recorded speed, the sounds were those of an agitated Donald Duck.

Would comprehension suffer from increased speed? Tests conducted with blind school children by the psychologist Emerson Foulke of the University of Louisville demonstrated that the youngsters could absorb increases of up to 50 percent in word rate without significant reduction in their grasp of the recorded material.

Speech compression was one of the investigative areas proposed by the Foundation as early as 1953 under its research contract with the Library of Congress. It was not assigned a high priority. However, work on various electrical, mechanical, and electronic approaches was undertaken in a number of commercial and university laboratories during the Fifties and Sixties. The factor of economics defeated them all.

Speech compression, a process of squeezing sounds closer together, could be achieved in several different ways. One was by reducing or eliminating pauses between words—the aural equivalent of shortening or omitting the spaces between words in print. Another was by dropping out relatively non-essential words such as articles, pronouns, conjunctives. A third was by automatically eliminating minute bits of sound at fractional intervals, comparable to taking a series of tiny tucks in a length of material. A fourth was by condensing sounds electronically.

This last-named approach underlay what was called a harmonic speech compressor, an apparatus built by Foundation engineers toward the end of the Sixties. It was based on a complicated theoretical method developed by engineers at the Bell Telephone Laboratories for cutting sound frequency bands in half. The Bell engineers tested their theory by simulating the results on a computer but did not actually construct the apparatus. Foundation engineers were given the right to build an actual speech compressor and their construction of a prototype, completed in 1968, bore out the promises of the computer simulation. The speed of sound was doubled, to 320-340 words per minute, without pitch distortion.

Whether this intricate electronic device would ever move from the laboratory into actual application was still an open question in 1972, when it was being tested, along with other speech compression devices, at the University of Louisville.

Another possible approach to "speed hearing" was introduced toward the end of 1971. A commercial firm, the Cambridge Research and Development Group of Westport, Connecticut, had developed an electronic device called Variable Speech Control (VSC). VSC was an inexpensive solid-state module, smaller than a sugar cube, which, when built into a phonograph or tape recorder, enabled the user to control the rate of speech playback from ultra-slow to ultra-fast without alteration in tone or pitch. The developers awarded royalty-free licenses to produce and market machines incorporating the VSC to the Foundation and the Printing House.

As an interim measure, the newer models of Talking Book machines were equipped with an optional accessory, an attachment for variable motor speed which enabled the user to adjust the turntable rate to whatever degree of speed was both comfortable and comprehensible.

The 24 libraries that helped launch Talking Books in 1934 were those chosen to distribute braille books under the Pratt-Smoot Act of 1931. Regarded as regional depositories, each serving a designated area comprising one or more states, they functioned under various kinds of sponsorship. Some were units of state libraries, others were divisions of municipal public libraries, and still others were operated by state commissions, schools, or voluntary agencies for the blind. Federal funds for books for the blind were reserved wholly for supplying these libraries with reading materials and with the machines to play those in recorded form. Responsibility for housing, equipping, and staffing the libraries for reader service remained with their respective parent bodies.

As the federal expenditures grew, the libraries for the blind found themselves under steadily increasing pressure. At the outset of the program, they had 12,000 enrolled readers; by 1945, the number was 25,000; by 1950, it was 40,000; by 1960, it was 63,000; and five years after that, the active readership reached six figures. A great burst followed passage of Public Law 89-522, which opened the Talking Book program to the physically handicapped, with the result that, by 1972, Library of Congress officials cited the readership as 300,000 and climbing.

The growth pattern in the number of distributing libraries did not parallel this climb in readership. In 1936, two years after the introduction of the Talking Book, there were 28 regional libraries, but the next increase did not come until 1959, when two new units were opened; five years later, there were two more. The spurt in distribution began with the passage of the Library Services and Construction Act of 1966 which authorized, among other things, $25 million over a five-year period in grants to the states to provide or improve library service to the physically handicapped. Another provision of the same act authorized $50 million over a five-year period to improve library services in state institutions, including residential schools for the handicapped. Coupled with passage that same year of Public Law 89-522, there finally emerged the stimulus that saw the number of regional libraries shoot up to 51 in 1972. The ultimate goal of at least one distributing library in each of the American states, territories, and possessions now seemed within reach.

It might well have been achieved earlier. Soon after M. Robert Barnett became executive director of the Foundation, he met with Library of Congress officials to sound out their attitude toward federal subsidies to help meet the cost of distributing books for the blind. What the Foundation had in mind at the time—this was the summer of 1950—was introducing a bill in Congress that would simultaneously increase the number of regional libraries, which had been static for 14 years, and help relieve the shortages of staff and space that were choking the existing depositories.

At this meeting, the major problems facing the libraries were itemized: readership growing at a steep rate, annual circulation of close to a million volumes of braille and recorded books, the continuous issuance of new titles, the physical work burdens involved in distribution of the postwar Talking Book machines, the need to scrap and replace thousands of worn-out records and machines that had seen constant use for up to fifteen years. No systematic practice of obsoletion existed for Talking Books; out-of-date scientific tomes, for example, continued to be circulated in the absence of authority to withdraw them. Hard usage at the hands of one reader after another had resulted in numbers of broken sets; any set of Talking Books whose continuity was shattered because of a single missing or scratched record had to be withheld from circulation until it could be made complete. The libraries were unequipped to cope with all these mechanical problems and still give their subscribers the kind of personalized service needed by blind readers.

Library of Congress officials, while acknowledging the gravity of these difficulties, were not amenable to the idea of outright federal subsidy. Their position was that the distribution and servicing of the federally provided reading materials for the blind were properly the responsibility of the individual states. While less opposed to an alternative proposal for a matching federal-state system of support, they were unready to commit themselves. In the circumstances, any thought of introducing the contemplated bill was dropped, since the wholehearted backing of the Library of Congress would be essential to its chances of passage.

What did materialize from this discussion was a decision to convene a broadly representative national meeting of regional librarians and other interested parties. The first National Conference on Library Service for the Blind was held in November 1951. Of the 16 resolutions it adopted, only one even touched on financial questions, and that one merely proposed a study "looking to the amelioration of the burden now assumed by various distributing agencies and libraries." Most of the other resolutions called for strengthened service and leadership from the Library of Congress on such specific items as cataloging, retirement of surplus or unserviceable books and machines, and more effective communication links with and among the distributing libraries.

Many of these services were quickly instituted. The following year the Library of Congress began issuing printed catalog cards for Talking Book and braille volumes, cards similar to the centralized cataloging service it had long provided for books in inkprint. A system for periodic obsoletion of Talking Book records was soon begun. To provide additional service on a national scale, the staff of the Division for the Blind was steadily enlarged; the 18 authorized positions it had in 1950 went to 28 by 1960, 72 by 1970, and 92 by 1972.

While all of these measures helped to alleviate some of the pressures on the regional libraries, a nationwide survey conducted by the Foundation five years after the first national conference concluded that most of the depositories of books for the blind were still inadequately financed, housed, and staffed. A $20,000 grant from the Matilda Ziegler Foundation helped to finance this survey. The recommendations of the survey team, which consisted of 11 eminent librarians aided by an equally distinguished advisory committee, were substantially along the same lines as before. It was not, however, until passage of the twin library laws in 1966 that the libraries for the blind were in a position to effect any really substantial improvements. Not only were new ones opened, but in the older libraries staffs were expanded, new or enlarged quarters were secured, and services were augmented to encompass the new class of physically handicapped readers brought within the Talking Book orbit.

Robert S. Bray often talked about his first view of a regional library for the blind. Bray, who joined the Library staff in 1940 and had worked in several of the Library's divisions, was chief of the Technical Information Division in 1957 when the retirement of Donald G. Patterson created a vacancy in the Division for the

Blind. Bray happened to be attending a convention in a midwestern city when he received a telephone call notifying him that he had been chosen to succeed Patterson. As he subsequently related:

> There was a free afternoon, so I decided to learn something about what I was in for. I knew there was a regional library for the blind in that particular city, and so, without identifying myself, I went over to see what it was like. I was ushered into a low-ceilinged basement room that looked as though it might collapse at any moment. Everywhere my eyes turned, they encountered shelves heaped with black boxes. It was so crowded you could hardly walk—a regular rabbit warren. This had formerly been a furnace room; the old furnace was still there, in fact, and so were some of the old ashes.

Such desolate environments are now a thing of the past. Most libraries for the blind eventually acquired bright and spacious quarters. Some contained such features as soundproof reading rooms or carrels for quiet browsing. More important still, since most readers continued to be served by mail, they acquired adequate space and facilities for receiving and shipping the hundreds of sound-recorded and braille books that moved in and out each day, and clerical staffs to maintain the individual reader records and book catalogs. At least one regional library installed a 24-hour telephone tape system so that readers could phone in their book requests at any hour. Many equipped tape recording studios for use by volunteers, as well as duplicating machines to make multiple copies of the volunteer-recorded tapes.

A growing practice among regional libraries was to place deposit collections of Talking Books and tapes in such institutions as hospitals, rehabilitation centers, and convalescent and retirement homes, as well as in local schools and public library branches. This satellite system numbered 60 subregional centers in 1972; it was not only a convenience for the bed-bound and those with limited mobility but helped to produce greater awareness of the service among the handicapped people who were eligible to receive it.

One feature noted by Library of Congress officials in 1972 was the intensive usage being made by Talking Book readers, who were averaging more than 40 books a year. Readers are kept regularly informed of the new books available to them. All who are registered with the regional libraries receive, free of charge, the bi-monthly magazine *Talking Book Topics,* which contains annotated descriptions of new releases on records and tape. Every two years *Talking Book Topics* prints separate catalogs of the adult and children's books released during the period; cumulative catalogs of the total collection are also issued from time to time.

Each issue of *Topics* contains a detachable order form that the reader can use to request books from his regional library. So that blind people would not have to wait until a sighted member of the family could read them the publication's contents, the practice began in 1968 of binding into each issue a sound sheet giving the new book descriptions in recorded form.

Talking Book Topics originated in 1935 as a two-page mimeographed quarterly prepared by Alice Smith and Jane Muhlfeld, two blind members of the Foundation's staff, to inform the fewer than five hundred persons then in possession of

Talking Book machines of the hundred or so books thus far recorded. A year later, when the number of machine users had reached four thousand, *Topics* graduated from mimeograph to print.

The sound sheet also had an early antecedent. In 1939 the Foundation began to produce a recorded edition of *Talking Book Topics,* for which it charged a nominal subscription fee of $1 a year. As a matter of historical record, this was the very first periodical to be issued in sound-recorded form. It was discontinued in 1959 when the Foundation, which had been subsidizing its production, had to do some budgetary belt-tightening.

Financing of the inkprint edition of *Talking Book Topics,* originally edited and published at Foundation expense, was subsequently taken over by the Library of Congress. It became a joint endeavor, with the Foundation serving as editor and publisher and the Library meeting the costs of publication. *Topics* became a bi-monthly in 1953; in 1964 it changed format to a larger type and page size and expanded its editorial coverage. A sans serif typeface and additional space between lines were introduced a year or so later for the convenience of partially sighted readers. With a 1972 press run of some 200,000 copies, it constituted an essential link between producers and users of sound-recorded books.

To be eligible for Talking Book service, an applicant is required to submit professional certification of his inability to read ordinary print or to handle books. This requirement supersedes the pre-1966 regulation that stipulated legal blindness. Only once had an exception been made to the earlier eligibility rule. In 1955, when Dwight D. Eisenhower was stricken with a heart attack while vacationing in Denver, his doctors refused to allow him even the exertion of holding a book in his hands. The Talking Book was an obvious answer. The regional library in Denver did what it could while the Foundation immediately set about obtaining permission from the publishers of six light novels—westerns, mysteries, and adventure stories—to exempt the President of the United States from the "solely for the use of the blind" restriction. The books and a playback machine were air-expressed to Denver. A gracious note from Mrs. Eisenhower ("We are touched that you found it possible to make the President an exception to the qualifications necessary to receive the books; I know they will help pass many of the long hours of his convalescence.") closed the file on this footnote to history.

12

*A Share in the
General Welfare*

Do blind people constitute a special class entitled to special social protection?

For centuries past, the answer to this question seemed self-evident. Of course! The fact that in recent decades a good many responsible voices have challenged this assumption, or at least the extent to which it has been allowed to govern public programs, has created one of the unresolved contradictions in work for the blind.

At the one extreme have been those who, holding blindness to be a mere inconvenience, were sincerely convinced that if blind people were ever to become full-fledged members of society, they would have to desist from asking or accepting special favors. At the other extreme have been those who, with equal sincerity, adhered to the traditional view that blindness was so disabling a handicap that only if it were equalized through compensatory laws and regulations could blind people hope to approach parity with the sighted.

The traditionalist viewpoint was all but unanimous during the depression years, when the United States Government, struggling to cope with disastrous economic collapse, abandoned the tenet that America's system of free enterprise and local self-government could build a sufficient base of economic security under all its people.

The instrument chosen to deal with this changed view was the Social Security Act, a landmark in American history. The United States Constitution had laid upon the national government the responsibility to *promote* the general welfare. In 1935 the national government went a crucial step further; it moved into partnership with the states to *provide* the general welfare.

Conceived in crisis, patched together in haste, the Social Security Act was an imperfect instrument. How imperfect may be judged from the fact that nearly every Congress has amended it.

Matters might have been greatly simplified if the Act had been less of an omnibus measure, or if at least its major facets had been separated. One facet—what is now commonly referred to as Social Security—was a social insurance system which provided that working adults and their employers would contribute matched sums to a federally operated trust fund out of which monthly cash benefits would be paid to workers when they reached retirement age. (A subsequent amendment extended this protection to the families of insured workers.) A related form of insurance protection was unemployment compensation, fortified by a public employment system.

The other facet was public assistance, totally different in nature and purpose from social insurance. The Act's welfare provisions were designed to assist the states in meeting the subsistence needs of people who were uninsurable because they were incapable of working to support themselves: too old, too young, too incapacitated. These categories of uninsurables were specified in separate titles of the Social Security Act, and the provisions for federal-state cooperation in aiding them came to be known as categorical assistance.

As originally drafted and introduced into Congress in January 1935, the Wagner-Lewis bill, then called the Economic Security Act, contained not a single reference to blindness.

"A few days ago we were studying the Wagner-Lewis Economic Security Bill," Robert Irwin wrote to M.C. Migel on February 13, 1935, "and quite to my surprise I found it contains one section which provides that the Federal Government will match dollar for dollar money appropriated in the various States for carrying on work with crippled children." Why, Irwin went on, should not similar help be extended to the blind? The state agencies for the blind were in deep trouble; appropriations, never sufficient in the first place, had been cut or eliminated altogether. "If we could show [the states] that the Government would match any appropriation they made, I think we would be able to get things going."

With this in mind, Irwin had drafted an amendment to add a new clause to the bill, patterning it after the crippled children's section. It proposed that $1,500,000 in federal money be set aside annually to match state money expended for work with the adult blind. Such funds were not to be used for direct relief grants, but to support the constructive activities of the state agencies for the blind in casefinding, vocational training and placement, home care, and other rehabilitative services.

The proposed amendment contained two other features. The crippled children's section provided "facilities for diagnosis and care, hospitalization and after-care." Irwin wanted the definition of crippled children to be broadened so as to specify that it included children with seriously impaired vision. Another section of the bill, Title I, the old age insurance plan, called for benefits to be paid to workers at age sixty-five. Irwin wanted such benefits to be paid to blind workers at age fifty.

Hearings on the Senate version of the bill were already being held by the Senate Finance Committee when these ideas came to Irwin. In order to get them on record before the hearings ended, he ventured to testify even before notifying the Foundation president. He had been accompanied, he informed Migel in this same letter, by L.L. Watts of Virginia, president of the American Association of Workers for the Blind; S. Mervyn Sinclair of Pennsylvania, president of the Association of State Executives; and Lewis H. Carris of New York, executive director of the National Society for the Prevention of Blindness.

"We had a brief hearing yesterday," he reported, "but I do not think we will get anywhere unless we can get Wagner or some other member of the Finance Committee sufficiently interested to sponsor the matter vigorously when the Committee goes into executive session." Would Migel be willing to write his good friend, Robert F. Wagner, about it?

Migel, who was in Palm Beach, dashed off a characteristic response: "It is useless to *write* to any Senator—one has to see them." He would be back north in a week or so and would willingly go to Washington for that purpose.

Migel's trip to Washington bore fruit when the bill was reported out by the Senate Finance Committee. It now contained a brand-new section, Title X, that established aid to the blind as a separate assistance category. But the title's provisions were quite different from what Irwin had asked for. It merely appropriated $3 million for 1936 to match state expenditures "for aid to the needy blind," with a ceiling of $15 monthly per person on the federal share of such grants. Instead of paralleling the preventive and rehabilitative features of the crippled children's program, Title X was patterned after the straight relief features of old age assistance grants.

Workers for the blind were unhappy that the constructive elements of their proposal had fallen by the wayside. An eleventh-hour effort was made to change the nature of Title X so as to incorporate rehabilitative services. In June, Migel and Helen Keller went to Washington to call on three Senators: Wagner, chairman Pat Harrison of the Finance Committee, and Hugo Black of Helen's home state of Alabama. Their purpose was to persuade Wagner, as author of the bill, to amend it from the floor of the Senate; to dissuade Harrison from objecting to changes in his committee's recommendations, and to gain Black's support for the broadened title.

The outcome of their mission to Washington was that Senator Wagner offered, and the Senate passed, an amendment to the committee bill expanding Title X to include not only "money payments to permanently blind individuals" but also "money expended for locating blind persons, for providing diagnoses of their eye condition, and for training and employment of the adult blind."

In an excited bulletin sent to leaders of work for the blind the day after passage of the amended Senate bill, the Foundation noted with satisfaction that the amendments would mean federal money to match state expenditures for most of the activities carried on by commissions and agencies for the blind. However, the rejoicing was premature. Having passed the House and Senate in different forms, the bill had to be reconciled by a conference committee, and in the course of this process most of the features of the Senate version were knocked out. Title X survived, but only as a separate relief category for blind persons.

Robert Irwin's disappointment was tinged with suspicion. "I was unable to find out who was responsible for this change," he wrote Mervyn Sinclair, "but I have a hunch. I believe it was an inside job." He was alluding to the fact that the group of state public welfare officials who had drafted the overall provisions of the Social Security Act saw no justification for separate treatment of blind people. They were particularly resistant to any possibility that administration of federal funds might be diverted from state welfare departments. Only a few of the state commissions for the blind were tied to welfare departments; others were units of state education departments, and still others were independent bodies. Whether or not Irwin's hunch was justified in this particular instance, the years ahead were to bear out his belief that there would be a continuing tug of war between public welfare officials and the organizations promoting the interests of blind persons.

Sinclair, while sharing Irwin's disappointment, took a more optimistic view. The mere fact that a separate title for aid to the blind had been achieved was a crucial gain, he felt. The next step, he wrote Irwin, was to establish good working relations with the Social Security Board, which the Act established to administer its provisions.

There was also a lot of other work to be done, both nationally and locally, before the first dollar of federal money could find its way into the hands of blind people.

While the Social Security Act was signed into law on August 14, 1935, it failed to receive funding and its first appropriation was not enacted until Congress reassembled the following January. Even if the money had been available earlier, however, the Act's administrative regulations were such that not a single one of the 26 states which already had relief programs in effect for blind residents would have been eligible for the federal grant. Some states had residence requirements more stringent than those allowed by the statute. Others did not meet the stipulation that relief had to be a statewide program rather than on a county-by-county basis. And, of course, there remained 22 states and several territories that had yet to begin any sort of assistance program for the needy blind.

In virtually every state, therefore, legislative action was needed before the flow of federal money could begin. By mid-1936 the necessary measures had been taken by 20 states and the District of Columbia, and in August the Social Security Board reported that some 22,000 blind residents of these states had received an aggregate of $584,610 the preceding month. This came to an average of $26.27 per recipient, although the figures making up the average ranged from a low of $5.74 in Arkansas to a high of $34.05 in California.

There was a good deal of confusion over regulations. For the Social Security Act to get through Congress at all, the states had to be allowed wide discretionary latitude in the administration of their individual programs. Different states did things differently, and the impact of their actions affected their residents in different ways.

A random survey made by the Foundation in the summer of 1936 and published in the October issue of the *Outlook*, highlighted some of the problems. In Massachusetts the commission for the blind, which was a unit of the state welfare department, was required to turn over to the department's old age assistance division all cases of blind persons aged sixty-five and over. In Wisconsin, on the other hand, elderly blind people were given the choice of whether to register under Old Age Assistance or under Aid to the Blind, and many opted for the former category. Indiana reported that red tape and the complications of setting up an operating structure were delaying implementation of the law. Relaying this information, C.D. Chadwick made an observation that was echoed from Vermont and Pennsylvania:

> This assistance has improved the living conditions of some of our more needy or destitute blind; but the blind who are self-supporting or who are barely able to earn their support complain that [it is] more difficult for them because the general public is cognizant of assistance being granted and naturally assumes that all blind are being assisted. . . .

In New York City, the Greater New York Council of Agencies for the Blind made a valiant but futile effort to have Title X funds administered through the state's commission for the blind rather than its department of welfare. In a detailed account of this ultimately unavailing campaign, Peter J. Salmon, executive secretary of the Industrial Home for the Blind in Brooklyn, and one of the nation's staunchest spokesmen for the traditionalist view, concluded with this somber warning:

> If those of us who have lived with work for the blind have learned one thing, it has been this: that such progress as has been made has come only through specialized work for the blind, whether in the field of private philanthropy or in that of legislation. Granting the necessity of relief-giving, there is still nothing more dangerous than the administration of relief or assistance to the blind by those unfamiliar with the whole problem involved. . . .

Vivid illustrations of the initial effects of the Social Security Act came from individual blind people, whose views were also incorporated in the *Outlook* survey. Some had benefited, but many more had not, and almost all were bewildered.

One of the chief complaints was that in many states relief applicants were required to divest themselves of whatever property they owned before they could be eligible for assistance. Limitations on the amount of life insurance relief applicants were permitted to retain also caused a great deal of resentment.

In states like Massachusetts, that had long provided pension allowances for blind residents, the operation of the new law was a blessing to some, a blow to others. An elderly Massachusetts man, who had been receiving a small, state old age pension as well as a blindness stipend, was a victim of the new regulations. His letter capsulized the pathetic suffering that so many endured during the depression years:

> I am so worried I am near to a nervous breakdown as I cannot get by on what I am told I will now have for the future. I will only receive thirty dollars per month, old age pension and all, whereas I have been getting twenty-four dollars from the [state] old age pension and twenty dollars from the [commission for the] blind, so it is not satisfactory to me at all, this new system. I do not know what I am going to do. I am a man eighty-three years old, and all I ask is food to eat and fuel to keep me warm. The woman who looks after me and keeps my house has given me her wages to buy the coal for this winter. All I pay her is three dollars per week.

The bitterest pill of all was the requirement that all earnings, no matter how small, and even gifts from relatives or friends, were to be deducted from the relief allowance. While the same rule applied in the Aged and Dependent Children relief categories, the situation of blind people was not really comparable. The aged were too old to compete for jobs, the children too young, but many of the needy blind people were of an age where they were capable of doing something, however little, toward self-support. The guiding philosophy of all organized work for the blind was to encourage such activity. If every dollar earned meant a dollar lost in relief payments, the incentive to earn would be quenched.

One way out of the dilemma was suggested before the Social Security Act was a year old. It was outlined, with due regard for delicate political overtones, in the February 1937 issue of the *Outlook*. Under this plan only 50 percent of the blind person's earnings up to a given limit would be taken into account in computing his relief budget. The same plan could be applied in the Old Age Assistance category —and thus be less criticized as special favoritism for the blind.

However, no effort was made that year to incorporate such a solution into law. Nineteen thirty seven was a year in which federal spending reached such unprecedented proportions that Congress and the White House embarked on an economy drive. The following year, legislative efforts of workers for the blind were centered on the Wagner-O'Day Act, which gave a new lease on life to the sheltered workshops. It was not until 1939 that attention was once again turned to the Social Security Act. At the Foundation's persuasion, Senator Wagner, who by this time wore the mantle of national legislative champion for blind persons, addressed letters to the state commissioners of public welfare, urging them to use their discretionary powers and follow the 50 percent plan. Such an arrangement, Wagner noted, was already in effect in Michigan, North Carolina, and part of New York State, and had proven its worth.

The response he received was lukewarm; several welfare commissioners agreed to go along, but most were noncommittal. It seemed clear that the fastest route would be to write such exemptions into the Social Security Act. An opportunity to do so was at hand, for the Social Security Board, having completed its shakedown cruise, was preparing to correct the weaknesses that had shown up during the Act's four years of operation.

In the course of the Senate debate over these changes, Wagner introduced an amendment regarding earnings exemption, but it failed to pass. Worse yet, one of the changes proposed by the Social Security Board that did get through made it mandatory rather than optional for all income and resources to be taken into account in all categories of assistance. The few states that did exempt some earnings in administering Title X would no longer be able to do so.

Wagner was not the only senator responsive to the pleas of blind constituents. Various other legislators proposed amendments in an effort to revive two of the provisions voted by the Senate in 1935 but killed in House–Senate conference. These were 1) assistance to state agencies for the blind in carrying out programs of rehabilitation and employment, and 2) federal participation in financing the costs of eye care to ameliorate or prevent visual impairment. Such efforts were also doomed to failure. The only concrete benefit the 1939 amendments conferred upon blind people was to raise the ceiling on federal participation in individual relief grants to $20 a month as against the former $15. A number of the overall changes, however, were indirectly beneficial. The federal government would henceforward reimburse the states for a greater share of their costs for adminis- tration of categorical relief. This could mean reduced caseloads and more efficient performance. All states were required to set up merit systems for hiring welfare workers. This would divorce such jobs from political patronage.

Despite its numerous imperfections, workers for the blind felt, on the whole, that the Social Security Act had produced sizable gains for blind people during those first five years. One of the most worthwhile was the requirement that applicants for Aid to the Blind undergo eye examinations. These examinations revealed that many applicants were needlessly handicapped; with proper medical or surgical treatment their vision could be improved and even restored. In Kansas alone, it was reported, 125 blind persons were restored to sight in a single year.

Discussing this fact in an address to a convention of blind people in late 1939, Robert Irwin posed a logical question: "If eye examinations and medical service for restoration of sight are beneficial to needy blind people, why wouldn't they be equally beneficial to blind persons who are not eligible for Aid to the Blind?" There were many, he said, whose families barely managed to support them but could not summon up the additional resources for medical care. For blind adults of working age, this problem was met through passage in 1943 of the Vocational Rehabilitation Act. Where the elderly blind were concerned, it took longer, even for some of those on welfare. The last group consisted of people who were not getting assistance under Aid to the Blind but had been assigned to the Old Age Assistance category, where no eye examinations were required. Repeated efforts were made to correct this situation through legislation, but it was not until the enactment of the Medicaid and Medicare systems in 1965 that the idea was implemented.

Improving the Social Security Act was not a major item on anyone's agenda during the war years. Not only was the nation preoccupied with matters of more desperate import but the war economy erased the last traces of depression unem- ployment, with the result that all welfare rolls decreased. Thanks to full employ- ment, many more families could assume the support of their blind members, and able-bodied blind adults were themselves in demand for defense work. Moreover, due to the Wagner-O'Day Act, the sheltered workshops which had formerly been unable to yield more than the meagerest of earnings for their blind workers were now on double and triple shift, producing millions of dollars' worth of goods for the war effort.

The gratification felt by organizations for the blind at this turnaround was tempered, however, by concern over the future. World War I had also seen a boom in employment of blind workers, but the gains had not been retained in the postwar years. The knowledge that war's end would bring a drastic drop in the economy, that veterans would be given preference in employment, and that the large numbers of men being blinded in battle might also be competing for the limited kinds of work available to the blind—these were reality factors that could not be ignored.

It was primarily with disabled servicemen in view that steps were initiated in 1942 to enlarge the scope and depth of the Vocational Rehabilitation Act of 1920. Both the Barden-LaFollette Act for civilians, which became Public Law 113 of the 78th Congress, and the Clark-Walsh Act for veterans, which became Public Law 16 of that same Congress, opened a broad range of services for newly blinded adults. But neither measure could do anything for the many blind persons who were not suitable candidates for vocational rehabilitation either because they had already made a satisfactory vocational adjustment or because they were too old or too handicapped in other ways to qualify.

Since so few blind people commanded even moderate means, federal income tax was of no great concern to the field until, in 1943, the tax structure was revised to reach down into the lower income brackets. When this happened, many who were employed held that the extra expenses of blindness should be recognized in their tax obligations. A given income, they argued, did not represent as much purchasing power to a man who had to hire eyesight in the form of readers or escorts as it did to his sighted colleague at the next desk or factory bench. The argument carried sufficient weight with Congress for an amendment to be passed in 1944 permitting a legally blind taxpayer to take an additional personal exemption on his tax return. In 1948 a further amendment extended the exemption to a blind spouse.

Once the special expenses of blindness were acknowledged for those who earned enough to pay taxes, blind people were encouraged to hope that comparable recognition might be extended to all. The cost of living of even the relief recipients who were blind was higher than that of others: they could not shop as economically, they had to pay people to do chores and errands that sighted persons could do themselves, they could not always make use of inexpensive public transportation.

There was no general agreement, however, as to just how this end might be achieved. Some spoke of a handicap allowance in the form of a federal pension for the blind. Others thought in terms of an insurance system to protect against dependency due to blindness, along the same lines as the old age insurance feature of the Social Security Act. Still others maintained that the best chance for equalizing the status of blind people lay in federal support of the state agencies for the blind so that they could strengthen and extend their rehabilitative and medical and social services. Since the federal government was now sharing the costs of vocational rehabilitation services which would primarily benefit those of working age, why should it not give similar help, through the state commissions, to others whose needs were equally urgent?

Blind people were not alone, of course, in clamoring for more help from their government. Groups representing people with other physical disabilities were also insistent on the need for greater federal support. In the summer of 1944 the House Committee on Labor appointed a Subcommittee on Aid to the Physically Handicapped to study the aid given by public and private agencies to the physically disabled and to frame legislative recommendations based on their findings. The seven-member subcommittee, chaired by Congressman Augustine B. Kelley of Pennsylvania, took testimony from more than five hundred witnesses over a two-year period. Its recommendations, published at the end of 1946, were numerous and broad-ranging; many ultimately found their way into law.

Testimony before the Kelley Committee by spokesmen for the blind focused largely on the changes needed in the Social Security Act. Robert Irwin reopened the question of exempting part of blind people's marginal earnings from computation of their budgetary needs. He urged that exemptions also be made for occasional gifts, up to a maximum of $20 a month, from relatives and friends. He reiterated the importance of federal help to the states in defraying medical expenditures for the improvement or restoration of sight. He called attention to "the shockingly low relief grants" made by the poorer states, proposing that the federal reimbursement formula be made variable so that it could meet a greater share of the relief expenditures in states with low capital wealth. He pleaded that the $20 limitation on the federal share of a blind person's relief grant be raised; most states, he pointed out, were unwilling to go beyond an exact matching of the federal contribution, even in cases where the person's needs were admittedly higher than $40 per month.

Speaking for all organized groups interested in the welfare of the nation's blind citizens, Irwin took the opportunity to introduce the idea of a system for insurance against blindness. Under such a plan the cost of benefits for people who might become blind in the future would be met through a trust fund to which all insured workers could contribute. As for financing the cost of benefits to those who were already blind, a one-time federal appropriation to establish the trust fund would take care of things.

A few weeks later Helen Keller also addressed a hearing of the Kelley Committee, and used the occasion to enter a special plea for a handicap allowance for two subgroups, "the hardest pressed and the least cared-for among my blind fellows." These were the Negro blind and the deaf-blind. Of the former, she said:

> In my travels up and down the continent I have visited their shabby school buildings and witnessed their pathetic struggle against want. I have been shocked by the meagreness of their education, lack of proper medical care, and the discrimination which limits their employment chances. I feel it a disgrace that in this great wealthy land such injustice should exist to men and women of a different race—and blind at that!

Even before the Kelley Committee published its findings, the House Committee on Ways and Means began extensive hearings on new amendments to the Social Security Act. The principal measure before it was a bill introduced by Representative Aime J. Forand of Rhode Island which proposed a number of fundamental changes in the nation's public welfare system. The broadest of these was that the federal government participate financially in the total welfare package—not merely the special categories of aged, dependent children and blind covered by separate titles in the Social Security Act but also in what was called general assistance: financial aid to individuals and families in need due to the breadwinner's temporary unemployment, sickness or physical disability other than blindness. Under the existing Act, the full cost of general assistance was borne by the states.

A logical consequence of this proposal was the proviso that the states should have the option of establishing unified administration for all welfare grants, categorical and non-categorical.

Other proposed changes were that the federal government should share in the costs of social services designed to prevent or overcome dependency, and that a variable grant formula be established to help the poorer states raise their level of assistance.

Many facets of the Forand bill were welcomed by the organizations of and for the blind, but much concern was expressed over the idea of a comprehensive welfare system which would allow the states to do away with separate categorical titles. With Title X seemingly in danger of disappearing, much of the testimony presented at the hearings by the blind interest groups centered on the necessity for its preservation.

Representative Forand responded to these anxieties by voicing assurances that adequate safeguards had been introduced into his bill for the protection of blind assistance recipients. "As one of a large family [he had 15 brothers and sisters] of a father who went blind, I have more than an academic interest in the welfare of this group," he declared.

At the conclusion of Robert Irwin's testimony, Forand engaged him in a colloquy. Irwin had maintained that if the states were given the option of consolidating all welfare administration, "what we are afraid of is that there will be more advantage financially for the states to throw the blind into general relief than . . . to keep them under Title X." Any generalized relief program would penalize the blind because it would be administered by staff members not familiar with the special needs and problems of blind people.

When Forand demurred that his bill was intended "to help rather than hinder the cause of the blind," Irwin credited him with the best of intentions. "I think you are as good a friend as we have on the committee," he said, "only I am just afraid that some of these lawyers in Washington are going to misinterpret your intention in the bill." Experience had shown, he went on, that federal bureaucrats often interpreted laws differently from what Congress had in mind. "Let us write [the new bill]," he urged, "so that even a lawyer will get only one meaning out of it."

Neither the American Public Welfare Association nor the organizations for the blind got very much of what they wanted when the 1946 amendments to the Social Security Act were passed that summer. The public welfare directors failed to get their consolidated system; it was to be 16 years before they could achieve even part of this goal through an amendment giving the states the option of grouping all adult assistance programs in a single plan. Even here, however, advocates of Title X salvaged something; under these same 1962 amendments, states which had a separate agency for the blind could still designate that agency to administer Title X.

While Title X survived in the Public Welfare Act of 1946, none of the other gains organizations for the blind campaigned for got through: neither the handicap allowance, nor the exemption of earnings, nor federal support for state commissions, nor the blindness insurance system. However, a few grains of comfort were provided. The maximum individual monthly assistance payment for a blind person went up from $40 to $45 with the federal share slightly raised. Two years later the maximum was upped to $50 and the federal share was again raised. By this time—1948—there were 45 states rendering aid to the blind under the Social Security Act, but it was not until 1953, when Nevada came into the system, that all states and territories were covered.

In 1952, both the maximum and the federal share were again raised by $5. Additional increases were authorized in 1956, 1958, 1961, 1962, and 1966. By the end of the 1970 federal fiscal year, the national average monthly grant to recipients of Aid to the Blind was $102.

Groups pressing for legislation cannot afford to be discouraged by defeat. They merely wait until the next session of Congress and try again, modifying their demands in terms of what they may have learned the last time around. In 1948 two New York legislators, Congressman Daniel A. Reed and Senator Irving M. Ives, introduced amendments to effectuate the income exemption provisions that had failed to get through two years earlier. Their bill permitted states that wished to do so to allow a blind recipient of public assistance to earn up to $40 per month without having a corresponding reduction made in his benefits.

The Reed-Ives bill was unanimously passed by both houses of Congress, but to the astonished chagrin of the bill's advocates, President Harry S. Truman vetoed it. The detailed "Memorandum of Disapproval" gave as its main reasons that the bill contravened the principle of assistance rendered on the basis of need, that it discriminated unfairly against other assistance categories, that it would render large numbers of new blind people eligible for public assistance, causing the available funds under Title X to be spread thinner. What was needed in the Social Security Act, the memorandum asserted, was not special treatment for one assistance category but a substantial increase in all payment categories.

There was little question in anyone's mind as to how this veto had come about. Jane M. Hoey, director of the Bureau of Public Assistance in the Social Security Administration, had repeatedly voiced the position spelled out in the document signed by Truman, Irwin told Migel. In a letter to Ives on July 15, 1948, Migel declared that, where blind people were concerned, the veto was "one of the most disappointing legislative steps ever taken by a President." He reasserted the belief that people on public assistance must be encouraged to help themselves, otherwise: "This results in bitterness and subterfuge on the part of the industriously inclined and makes loafers out of the less courageous."

Two years later workers for the blind rallied to press once again for the changes they wanted in the Social Security Act. They had used the interval to seek an accommodation with the federal welfare officials and had found Arthur J. Altmeyer, Commissioner of Social Security in the newly established Federal Security Agency, somewhat more amenable than his predecessors to the income exemption plan. Early in 1950 H.R. 6000 was introduced in Congress. Among other things it contained a section giving each state the option of disregarding earned income of up to $50 a month in determining the relief budget of a blind assistance recipient in order "to encourage or assist the blind to prepare for, engage in, or continue to engage in remunerative employment to the maximum extent possible." It also contained a new provision: any worker registered with Social Security who lost his sight would have an immediate right to retirement benefits even though he was younger than sixty-five. This proviso was subsequently stricken, but the income exemption clause finally went through. When H.R. 6000 became Public Law 81-734, approved August 28, 1950, it provided that exclusion of earned income of up to $50 a month would be optional with the states for a two-year period; thereafter, it would be mandatory.

To achieve this long-sought breakthrough, organizations representing the blind joined forces as never before. One group, the National Federation of the Blind (NFB), a membership body of blind people organized a few years earlier, pressed hard for even greater liberalization; it asked that half of all earnings above the $50 exemption also be disregarded in calculating income. This demand threatened to upset the applecart. When, during the final hearings preceding passage of H.R. 6000, the NFB representatives insisted they would not compromise their stand, Commissioner Altmeyer had a private word with Peter Salmon, who had taken an active role in the negotiations with the Federal Security Agency. "Peter," he said, "you people can walk out of here with the $50 a month, but if you press for everything, you'll wind up with nothing."

Robert Irwin lived long enough to enjoy the triumph of the idea he had campaigned for since 1937, although by the time the law was signed he had already retired and his leadership role in the 1950 legislative drive had been taken over by M. Robert Barnett. Barnett was assisted by Hulen C. Walker, a member of the Foundation's field staff who, shortly thereafter, was appointed its first Washington-based legislative analyst. One of Walker's initial accomplishments was to secure a clarifying clause in the next set of Social Security Act amendments (1952) to insure that the earnings exemption applied to all blind people receiving public assistance, even if their aid came under a classification other than Title X. Since many were receiving help under Old Age Assistance, and others, who were family heads, were drawing benefits under the Aid to Dependent Children category, this move expanded the number of beneficiaries of the exemption allowance.

Walker, a blind attorney, resigned in 1958 to become the first full-time executive director of the American Association of Workers for the Blind. He was succeeded as the Foundation's legislative analyst by Irvin P. Schloss, who had been blinded in action in World War II. Schloss had been an active leader in the Blinded Veterans Association, serving as editor of its bulletin from 1948 to 1953 and then as its executive director until he joined the Foundation staff.

Walker began, and Schloss continued, the practice of issuing periodic newsletters on legislative developments to a large list of persons and organizations interested in the welfare of blind persons. Since the Washington office made it unnecessary for the Foundation's executive director to spend as much time in the nation's capital as his predecessor, the legislative analyst also took over the task of testifying for the Foundation before Congressional committees on routine matters. Appearances by Barnett were reserved for major episodes.

One such episode took place in 1956 when several issues were at stake. Title X was once more in jeopardy; a bill had again been introduced to lump together all categories of adult assistance under a single new title. On the affirmative side, an effort was under way to increase the income exemption allowance for the blind.

Stalled in committee was a separate proposal for the appointment of a temporary national advisory body that would study all work for the blind. Most urgent of all was the issue of disability insurance.

In 1954 amendments to the Social Security Act had set the stage for a disability insurance program by instituting a "disability freeze." This provided that a worker insured under Social Security who became totally and permanently disabled could have his wage record "frozen" at that point, so that subsequent periods of lower or non-existent earnings due to his disablement would not diminish the amount of his ultimate retirement benefit. The amendment proposed in 1956 inaugurated a cash disability program under which a disabled worker who met stringent standards relating to both the nature of his disability and his potential for gainful employment could begin, at the age of fifty, to collect retirement benefits equivalent to what he would have been entitled to receive on the basis of the same wage record upon retirement at age sixty-five.

While blindness per se constituted presumed disability under the "freeze" provisions, the 1956 amendment stipulated that, to be eligible for benefit payments, a blind person would have to prove that he or she was unable to engage in any "substantial gainful activity." This meant, for example, that an architect who lost his vision would have to prove not only that he could no longer pursue a career in architecture but that he was unable to earn anything "substantial" by opening a small business or taking employment in a sheltered workshop. What constituted "substantial gainful activity" was not defined and could easily constitute a booby trap. Moreover, the definition of blindness stipulated in both the "freeze" and the cash benefit regulations was not the accepted 20/200 standard for legal blindness but a much more restrictive 5/200.

In the Congressional debates over the 1956 amendments, the Foundation and others made strong efforts to preserve some incentive for persons who became blind to engage in as much productive activity as they were capable of. To assist toward this goal, Representative Jere Cooper of Tennessee introduced a bill that 1) established 20/200 as the definition of blindness for disability benefit purposes; 2) postulated that persons certified as blind should not be required to meet the "substantial gainful activity" test; 3) made blinded workers eligible for cash benefits from the onset of blindness instead of requiring them to wait until age fifty.

A further provision in the Cooper bill was that blind workers who did qualify for disability benefits should be permitted to earn up to $1,200 a year before their disability payments were reduced. The rationale behind this demand was that such an arrangement was already in effect for over-sixty-five workers receiving retirement benefits under Old Age and Survivors Insurance.

While the Cooper bill was not enacted in 1956, most of its proposals eventually became law. The blindness definition for disability purposes was broadened to 20/200 in 1967. Disability benefits prior to age fifty were instituted in the 1960 amendments. The requirement for the amount of covered employment needed to qualify (originally 20 out of the preceding 40 quarters), was modified in 1965 to as few as six quarters if a person lost his or her sight before age thirty-one. In that same year the "substantial gainful employment" stipulation was loosened for blind persons between the ages of fifty-five and sixty-five; they could now qualify for disability benefits by proving inability to work at the same occupation or one requiring similar skills. Two years later, the same concession was extended to sighted persons disabled by any type of handicapping condition.

Eventually, too, the more liberal earnings income exemption, for which the National Federation of the Blind had pressed so hard in 1950, was achieved. In 1962 the monthly exemption figure of $50 was raised to $85 and half the earnings over that amount were also excluded in calculating a blind person's public assistance grant. A further concession was wrung in 1964 when it was ruled that, for a Title X recipient enrolled in an approved plan leading to self-support, all income for a period of 12 months was to be disregarded; states were given the further option of extending this period to 36 months.

Along with all others receiving welfare assistance, blind persons benefited from across-the-board improvements introduced into the Social Security Act over the years. Among these were the gradual easing of state residence laws, culminating in the 1969 Supreme Court decision forbidding residence requirements as a condition of eligibility for public welfare aid; the enactment of the Medicare and Medicaid programs which helped cover the cost of eye care as well as general health maintenance; the widened scope of the child health program, which assisted with vision screening and remedial ophthalmic services for children; the broadening of survivor benefit regulations to make disabled widows, widowers and divorced wives eligible for cash benefits at an earlier age.

In retrospect it can be seen that virtually all of the goals sought by champions of the blind in relation to the Social Security Act were sooner or later attained. The demand for a flat pension or handicap allowance for needy blind people was one of the major exceptions, but hopes were aroused that it might yet be achieved in the guise of a guaranteed annual income for the poor—the "family assistance plan"—which the Nixon administration proposed as part of a set of welfare reform measures in 1971.

The compromise measure which finally passed Congress and was signed into law in late 1972 (Public Law 92-603), omitted the family assistance plan, but it did improve benefits in many categories, including the extension of Medicare to disability insurance beneficiaries. It also federalized the three adult public assistance categories (Old Age Assistance, Aid to the Blind, and Aid to the Permanently and Totally Disabled), effective January 1, 1974. One effect of this scheduled change would be to raise the monthly income of Aid to the Blind recipients in the many states which, under the previous federal-state funding formula, had made inadequately low grants. Another effect would be to finally put an end to Title X as a separate category.

Advocates of the family assistance plan were still hoping, at the end of 1972, that some form of guaranteed annual income might come into existence at a later date. Blindness would not be a factor in such a plan; blind persons would receive the same treatment as all others, handicapped or non-handicapped, whose incomes were below the poverty level. The days of preferential treatment for the blind were clearly coming to an end. Most of the new legislation introduced was framed on the theory that blindness should no longer be singled out from all other disabilities for special preference.

While professional workers and organizations for the blind came to accept and promulgate this concept, some membership organizations of blind persons continued for the most part to adhere to the opposite view. The point most frequently made in favor of special treatment was that, historically, once special legislation for the blind was in force, it tended to serve as an opening wedge for all handicapped groups as, for example, in the 1965 liberalized disability benefit provisions for the blind which were extended two years later to all disabled persons.

While granting the weight of this argument, many leaders in work for the blind held to the belief that since the ultimate desideratum for blind people was to become part of the mainstream of society, the seeking of preferential treatment in law defeated this end.

At the same time that thoughtful persons in work for the blind were executing this 180-degree turn, public welfare authorities were also reversing their stands on a good many formerly cherished principles. Their experience with welfare programs for the blind undeniably contributed to these changed viewpoints.

One example was the earnings exemption concept, which was resisted for so many years by welfare officials on the grounds that it contravened a basic tenet of welfare administration. In 1964 the Economic Opportunity Act, which launched Lyndon B. Johnson's "war against poverty," recognized the validity of a work incentive for all welfare recipients by including an earnings exemption clause.

Another basic change in thinking related to methods of administering welfare. From the inception of the Social Security Act, federal and state authorities were insistent that the heart of the relief system lay in the public welfare worker's determination of individual budgetary needs, case by case. On the opposite side, the spokesmen for blind people who sought to have Title X administered by state commissions for the blind maintained that this budgetary function was a more or less mechanical operation, devoid of rehabilitative assistance to the recipient. In the Seventies several state and municipal welfare departments assigned clerical workers to make the eligibility and budgetary determinations and reserved their professionally trained social workers to render constructive services designed to lead people out of poverty.

In these and comparable directions, workers for the blind were ahead of their time in identifying weaknesses and suggesting remedies for welfare programs. To the extent that they persisted until experience proved them right, their foresight benefited all the nation's people.

13

The Showcase of the Blind

"Give a man a fish," says an ancient Hebrew proverb, "he eats for a day. Teach him to fish, he need never be hungry again." A contemporary writer added a psychological dimension to this concept: "Work shapes a day, and so shapes a life."

It is only in recent years that blind men and women have been given the opportunity to do much about shaping their days or their lives. In past centuries blindness meant a life sentence, either to idleness or to the narrow range of occupations known as the "blind trades." For the more competent and the more mobile, these included musicianship, piano tuning, shopkeeping, house-to-house peddling, and a few small entrepreneurial ventures, one of which was street beggary. For most of the others, the "blind trades" were those involving semi-skilled manual operations: chair-caning, broom making, hand weaving, basketry. Some pursued such trades in their homes, while others worked at sheltered workshops established under community auspices and supported by philanthropic or tax funds.

There were, of course, exceptions: mettlesome souls who broke out of these confining molds and made places for themselves in the world at large. One of the earliest aims of the Foundation was to train a spotlight on these exceptional people in the belief that their example would not only encourage others but would persuade society to open new doors of opportunity to blind men and women. There was hardly an issue of the *Outlook for the Blind* during the Twenties that failed to feature one or more success stories. Two of the Foundation's first published pamphlets also dwelt on this theme: "Blind Women Who Have Conquered" and "Blind Dictaphone Operators and Typists in the United States and Canada." In succeeding years, similar brochures dealt with career opportunities in insurance underwriting, osteopathy, and organ-playing, and toward the same end the "Weeks for the Blind" local agencies were helped to organize centered around articles made by blind craftsmen and the craftsmen themselves at work.

An organized effort to expand vocational opportunities was greatly needed. In 1926 a Foundation report proposed a vocational study that would assess and attack the problem. The study would cover three major facets:

> employment of the blind side by side with the sighted in industrial and commercial concerns; employment in which blind people are engaged in more or less independent ventures; and employment in industries fostered by agencies for the blind, such as special shops, subsidized home industries, etc.

To organize the study, the Foundation employed Evelyn C. McKay, who held a degree in economics from the University of British Columbia, had done graduate work in industrial management, and had gained professional experience as a statistical analyst. Miss McKay, who was to remain on the staff for the next 24 years in a variety of responsible capacities, was given the title of research agent.

To develop a factual base, an ambitious questionnaire was sent to 50 leading state and local organizations for the blind with the object of building a "vocational clearing house system" that would provide "as complete a catalog as possible of the jobs engaged in by blind people of this country since January 1, 1926." By the end of 1927, job data had been received from 1,141 individuals: 171 factory workers, 153 professionals, 185 independent businessmen, 170 salesmen, 93 piano and organ tuners, 49 clerical workers, 80 handicraft workers, 49 household workers, and 191 miscellaneous. Not surprisingly, in view of the catchall nature of the inquiry, the information was frustratingly incomplete, particularly on the people in professional work, many of whom had no contact with agencies for the blind. Also missing were all-important details regarding the specific types of industrial operations performed by factory workers. The broad sweep of an overall study was clearly not the answer. If usable knowledge was to be gathered, individual employment sectors would have to be tackled one by one.

A Vocational Advisory Committee appointed in early 1928 selected for initial study the fields of insurance underwriting, clerical occupations, vending stand-keeping, osteopathy, and physical therapy (the last two fields were then open to blind practitioners but subsequently closed by action of their respective professional associations). It also proposed an examination of subsidized home industries and an inquiry into the question of workmen's compensation laws in various states and how these affected employment of blind persons. The need for a study of the sheltered workshops was noted, but deferred until resources were available to undertake what was sure to be a difficult and time-consuming project.

To stimulate interest in employment problems, a periodic bulletin, *Vocational News Notes,* was circulated among agencies for the blind. One of the early issues listed 84 different factory operations performed by blind workers in a dozen industries, from automobile manufacture to candy production. The list was designed to jolt into action some of the laggard agencies that were doing little or nothing about industrial placement work in their communities. In its 1928 annual report, the Foundation offered to assign a staff member to "conduct demonstration placement work in these communities and to train newly appointed placement agents to perform this difficult service."

By way of national action, an illustrated brochure, "What the Blind Do," was sent, early in 1929, to a large list of persons, organizations, and industrial firms. A special covering letter from Helen Keller accompanied the mailing of this brochure to Lions Clubs, asking that their members spread its message among potential employers.

By mid-1929 the clearing house operation had already registered close to 2,000 blind persons engaged in non-subsidized work, and the Vocational Advisory Committee was continuing to recommend new lines of investigation. Most of these necessarily faded from view a few months later, with the Wall Street crash. Although the register continued to be maintained for several years thereafter, active promotion of overall vocational opportunities for blind people was clearly futile at a time when so many of the nation's able-bodied workers were unable to find jobs.

The key to survival during the early Thirties was catch-as-catch-can, but once the Social Security Act came into force to safeguard the most helpless, the vocational needs of abler blind people could be returned to the spotlight. The Randolph-Sheppard Act of 1936 and the Wagner-O'Day Act of 1938 opened significant channels of economic opportunity to blind persons who were capable of operating small businesses, holding production jobs in open industry, or increasing their earning power in sheltered workshops. It took a third piece of legislation, the Vocational Rehabilitation Act amendments of 1943, to chip away at remaining barriers by providing federal funds to help the states finance an unprecedented array of vocational training, counseling and placement services for blind adults.

In pre-electronic days, when the printed word was the sole channel of public information, there were small numbers of blind people who earned their livings by operating newsstands in busy urban locations. Once the 1914–18 war aroused the public conscience to the needs of disabled servicemen, ordinances were passed in a number of cities and states giving such men preferential opportunities as licensed newspaper vendors. New York City was one of the leaders; a 1920 law gave veterans with service-connected disabilities preference in securing strategic newsstand locations at subway entrances, under elevated railroad stairways, and at high-traffic intersections. Under this law, second preference was given to blind civilians, and third preference to civilians with disabilities other than blindness.

The New York Association for the Blind, popularly known as the Lighthouse, seized the opportunity to initiate a program that would help blind persons gain access to these small businesses. It processed applications for newsstand licenses, supplied applicants with the required blindness certifications, negotiated with municipal authorities over locations. It made interest-free loans to applicants for the necessary initial investments: money to equip new vending stands or modernize old ones, to prepay insurance premiums, to meet suppliers' demands for cash deposits, etc. It initiated training programs to prepare applicants for their responsibilities through on-the-job clerking experience and sought to expand the available number of profitable locations by securing indoor stand concessions in municipal and commercial buildings.

Adoption of comparable laws in a handful of other cities and states prompted hopes that similar concessions could be achieved nationally. In 1921, at the request of the New York State Commission for the Blind (then chaired by M.C. Migel), Senator James Wadsworth of New York introduced a bill designed to open federal buildings to blind newsvendors. The bill failed to attract interest and never came to the floor. From time to time during the next few years efforts were made to approach the problem through administrative channels. Control over most federal buildings was then in the hands of the Treasury Department. All that was needed, it seemed, was to get that department to exempt blind persons from its general ruling against vendors in federal buildings.

When efforts to accomplish this proved unavailing, sights were once again trained on a legislative approach. Meeting in 1927, the American Association of Workers for the Blind adopted a resolution "to strongly recommend that the federal government open its public buildings to business stands to be operated by the blind." Not long thereafter, a blind senator, Thomas D. Schall of Minnesota, introduced a bill proposing the creation within the Department of Labor of "a bureau for the blind" whose functions would be to open government buildings— federal, state, and municipal—to stands to be operated by blind people. Reporting on this measure at the next AAWB convention, the association's Committee on Legislation declared that the Schall bill had provoked so much controversy "of a confusing and baffling character" that the committee had been unable to arrive at a consensus.

Most of the controversy centered on means, not ends. Everyone agreed that vending stand concessions in public buildings would open important new economic channels for blind persons, but there was sharp divergence over whether the creation of a federal bureau for the blind was a viable method of doing so. In November 1930, at a conference convened by the Foundation to consider the matter, a dozen specialists in employment thrashed out the question of strategy. The group concluded that revival of the Schall bill (which had meanwhile died in committee) did not hold the answer, that "the complete control of federal buildings lay with the Secretary of the Treasury" and that, as a first step, the Foundation should approach Treasury Secretary Andrew W. Mellon. Legislative action could be the second resort.

Mellon was not receptive to the proposal. Neither was his Republican successor, Ogden L. Mills, who served in the final year of the Hoover administration, nor William H. Woodin, who was Franklin D. Roosevelt's first appointee to the Treasury post. Migel, who called on all three with the help of introductions from influential friends in Congress, encountered stony indifference to every argument he put forward. In a letter to Secretary Mills following a personal meeting in March 1932, he noted among other things that if the Treasury Department was unwilling to bother with screening and selection of persons to operate vending stands in federal buildings, the Foundation, with the help of state agencies for the blind, "would cheerfully agree to assume the responsibility for determining the merit of applicants, their capacity and reliability."

None of these persuasions having prevailed, at Migel's request Senator Reed Smoot introduced a bill giving the Secretary of the Treasury optional, not mandatory, authority to grant vending stand permits to blind persons. Unwilling to be told what to do by Congress, the Treasury opposed the measure and the bill was never reported out.

In the first year of the Roosevelt administration a House bill introduced by Congressman Joseph W. Martin of Massachusetts revived the Schall plan for establishment of a bureau for the blind in the Labor Department to handle federal vending stand concessions. In the conviction that this measure, like its predecessors, would get nowhere, Migel decided to reach for the top. Accompanied by Foundation trustee Mary V. Hun, the old friend and political associate of Franklin D. Roosevelt, he called on the President, who responded with gratifying promptness by issuing an executive order to the Treasury Department directing that blind people be exempted from the general rule prohibiting vending stands in federal buildings. On May 18, 1933, a general order was sent out to building custodians by the Secretary of the Treasury permitting "blind persons to sell papers, et cetera, in such buildings where there is sufficient space to make this possible without interfering with the public business."

The long impasse was now seemingly broken, but rejoicing was short-lived. Just four weeks later the Treasury issued a supplementary order which imposed such strangling limitations on the newly granted concessions as to all but cancel them. The privilege extended to blind persons, this second order stipulated,

> is to be confined to the selling of newspapers and magazines, and is not to include candy, chewing gum, tobacco or any other commodities whatever.

Worse still:

> No rack, stand, counter, table or other fixture or furniture is to be permitted within the building for this purpose, but there is no objection to the use of a portable stool or chair, which, if used, must be taken away when the vendor leaves the building each day.

Migel fired off an indignant telegram to Assistant Secretary of the Treasury L.W. Robert, Jr., who had signed the order. He then had a conference with Robert, following which he reiterated his objections in writing. Not only was the amended order totally at variance with the Roosevelt directive, he wrote, but "the use of a chair or stool and a blind man sitting on it brings him down almost to the status of a mendicant (something that we have for years endeavored to get away from), whereas a stand, no matter how tiny, creates a sense of dignity and responsibility." All over the country, he went on, the first order had activated organizations for the blind to begin screening candidates for vending stand permits. "Rescinding of the original permission granted would mean a sad and bitter disappointment to the blind of practically the entire country."

Perhaps because the Treasury Department was in a state of disarray—Secretary Woodin's health had collapsed as a result of the banking crisis of the past spring; his successor, who was to be Henry Morgenthau, Jr., had not yet been appointed; there were basic reorganizational changes in the offing, under which post office buildings were to be transferred from Treasury Department jurisdiction to the United States Post Office—whatever the reason, Assistant Secretary Robert stood pat.

The reorganized postal structure led to the introduction of a new bill in the House of Representatives to set up a bureau in the Post Office Department to license blind persons "for the operation of stands in federal buildings, post offices, Army and Navy structures, and other governmental buildings throughout the United States for the vending of newspapers, periodicals, candies and tobacco" as well as other articles should these commodities fail to yield a sufficient volume of business. This bureau, the bill said, was to be headed by a director, "to be appointed by the President, by and with the advice and consent of the Senate"—a person with "practical business experience and social work [experience] pertaining to the blind." Preference in the appointment was to be given to a qualified blind person.

The bill, H.R. 5694, was introduced by Matthew Dunn of Pennsylvania, then serving his maiden term in Congress. Dunn, a graduate of the Overbrook School for the Blind, was known to Robert Irwin, who did not wholly approve of him. In private correspondence he described Dunn as "quite a champion of street beggars in Pittsburgh and Harrisburg, and during the several years he was a member of the Pennsylvania legislature, he always lined up with the more radical of the labor group." Nevertheless, Irwin recognized that Dunn's blindness would lend him weight in Congress on laws relating to the blind.

Disheartened by the bureaucratic undermining of the Presidential order to the Treasury Department, workers for the blind were sufficiently stirred up over the Dunn bill for the AAWB to ask the Foundation to call a nationwide strategy conference in December 1933.

The bill's most vigorous advocate was a blind Cleveland lawyer, Leonard A. Robinson, who headed a statewide organization of blind people. He was known to have drafted the Dunn bill, and it was generally believed that he hoped to be appointed to the directorship of the projected bureau. But at the strategy conference the consensus—with Robinson's the sole dissenting voice—opted once again in favor of a two-step plan. First, the Foundation was to continue its efforts to get more satisfactory administrative compliance with the President's executive order. If this approach failed, then legislation was to be attempted. Herman M. Immeln, then president of AAWB, appointed a seven-man legislative committee to draft a revised version of the Dunn bill should the legislative tack be called for.

Named to chair the legislative committee was Benjamin Berinstein of New York, a blind attorney who was a charter member of the Alumni Association of the New York State School for the Blind at Batavia. Berinstein, a short-tempered man with an eloquent, frequently acerbic tongue, soon found himself at loggerheads with Robinson who, while accepting membership on the committee, nevertheless chose to go his own way by campaigning in the name of Ohio groups for immediate legislation.

Worked out by the committee, the revised version of the Dunn bill which the Pennsylvania congressman introduced on March 7, 1934, differed in two important respects from his earlier bill. Dunn had originally proposed financing the cost of the bureau for the blind by charging annual license fees for vending stands; the revised version called instead for a modest federal appropriation to launch the bureau. A second change concerned the qualifications of the bureau's director. These now required, in addition to practical business experience, "not less than two years of experience in the work of placing blind persons in stands and dealing with the problems of such persons in the operation of such stands." The last requirement appeared to eliminate Leonard Robinson from the top job slot.

As it happened, neither part of the two-step strategy succeeded that year or the next. A meeting with Franklin D. Roosevelt and James A. Farley in February 1934 brought no results. The second Dunn bill failed to pass. According to Robert Irwin, the inability to make progress with the postal authorities was due at least partially to the disharmony in the ranks of spokesmen for the blind.

Neither side gave up, however. The Post Office having proved intractable, Migel and Irwin used the connections they had previously established in the Treasury Department to see what could be done about the buildings that remained within that department's jurisdiction. This brought about the Foundation's first contact with Mary E. Switzer, then assistant to an Assistant Secretary of the Treasury and destined to become, in the years ahead, the nation's most influential government official in rehabilitation of the handicapped. Migel met Miss Switzer in late 1934 and at her suggestion wrote to Treasury Secretary Henry Morgenthau, Jr., urging that at least an experiment be tried by establishing stands in a few buildings "with the full understanding that your Department would have absolute power to revoke the privilege." Several stands, including a most successful one in the United States Customs House in New York City, were established on this basis.

Robinson, on his part, was indefatigable in pursuit of legislative action. At a Lions' convention in 1934 he met Jennings Randolph, then a newly elected Congressman. Early in 1936 Randolph introduced a vending stand bill in the House. An almost identical measure was introduced in the Senate by Morris Sheppard of Texas. Following hearings, the House Committee on Labor recommended passage of the Randolph bill. The committee's report said in part:

> The Federal Government is spending billions of dollars to create employment opportunities for millions of persons, but not one blind person is benefitted thereby. The blind cannot build bridges, buildings, and do other kinds of work now being authorized by the Public Works Administration. . . . There is no definite or practical national system or plan whereby placement work for the blind can be done. . . .
>
> The committee believes that the speedy enactment of this measure into law would take care of a group of our people who are in distress and who are not being reached by any of the vast rehabilitation experiments which the government is conducting.

(The committee report, commendable in its zeal, was not quite accurate in its details. There were, in fact, a small number of blind people employed in public works programs—in hand transcribing of braille, making of embossed maps for students in schools for the blind, supplying home teaching and other personal adjustment services to housebound blind persons. And the WPA project for the manufacture of Talking Book machines was just getting started.)

Following passage by the House on March 16, 1936, the Randolph bill and the companion measure of Senator Sheppard came before the Senate Committee on Education and Labor, whose chairman, David I. Walsh, had solicited the written views of the affected government departments. Walsh's committee report reflected the negativism of the bureaucracies:

> This legislation would allow the setting up of stands by the blind in federal buildings for the sale of newspapers, magazines, candy, tobacco products, and so forth, and provides that these stands be licensed by the Office of Education. The bill further provides that a survey be made of concession stand opportunities for the blind in this country; second, that a survey be made throughout the United States of industries, with a view to obtaining information that will assist blind persons to obtain employment; third, that this data be made available to the public and especially to persons and organizations interested in helping the blind; and fourth, that licenses be issued to blind persons, to be approved by the custodian of the building and the Commissioner of Education.
>
> The Senate and House bills, as originally introduced, made mandatory rather than permissive the operation of stands by blind persons. . . . These provisions were objected to by the Department[s] of the Treasury, Interior, and Labor, and upon the suggestion of the Secretary of the Interior, the committee has amended section 1 of the House bill leaving "in the discretion of the head of the department or agency in charge of the maintenance of the building" whether such vending stands shall be operated by blind persons licensed under the act.
>
> The committee has omitted section 3 of the House bill, which section authorized the Commissioner of Education, with the approval of the Secretary of the Interior, to purchase vending-stand equipment for use in federal buildings, and also the purchase by the Federal Government, rather than by the State, of stands and stand equipment for loan by the states to the blind operators of such stands. . . .

The amended bill was signed into law on June 20, 1936, as Public Law 74-732. It was a pale shadow of what spokesmen for the blind had sought and it contained the seeds of much future discontent, but it was nevertheless recognized as (and subsequent events proved it to be) an important breakthrough in three different directions:

1. Vending stands operated by blind men in federal buildings served as showcase operations—public demonstrations, day after day, of the competence of blind persons to handle businesses efficiently and profitably. This not only raised the popular estimate of blind people's capabilities but encouraged the establishment of similar vending operations in state and municipal buildings and, even more significantly, in non-governmental office buildings and factories.

2. The provisions touching upon industrial placement opportunities opened new channels for employment of blind persons in factory and other production jobs.

3. It was an opening wedge in federal civil service for blind people. The nation's first blind civil servant was the man chosen to administer the Randolph-Sheppard Act with the title of special agent for the blind in the Vocational Education Board of the United States Office of Education, then located in the Department of the Interior. He was Joseph F. Clunk who, in turn, saw to the appointment of a number of other able blind men—including Leonard Robinson—to serve on his

staff, the Act having specified that at least 50 percent of those employed by the federal government to work on the vending stand program should be blind.

Clunk was sworn into federal service in June 1937. By every standard he was the right man in the right place at the right time. He had just completed nine years of creating, in Canada, a vending stand and industrial placement program for blind people that was the envy and admiration of United States workers for the blind.

Joseph Clunk had lost his sight in 1918, when he was twenty-three and a student at Western Reserve University in his native state of Ohio. A zealous, stubborn man of mercurial temperament imbued with exceptional courage and self-confidence, he started his new life as a blind person by proving he could fill a sighted man's shoes. Two months after leaving the hospital he began earning his living as a house-to-house salesman of toiletries, traveling alone. On the theory that anything he could do, other blind people could also do, he joined the staff of the Cleveland Society for the Blind to handle placement work and performed so effectively that he was soon offered the post of executive secretary of the Youngstown (Ohio) Society for the Blind.

His approach to industrial placement was simplicity itself. As he later recounted:

> It fell to me as a young newly-blinded man to develop the method of analyzing industrial jobs by working on each process for an hour or more in the same manner as though employed by the company. This procedure enabled the employer to understand that various machines did not require sight on the part of an operator, and that persons without sight but possessing adequate basic ability could be employed as easily as sighted machine operators.

Clunk regarded himself as a salesman whose product ("the commodity of blind labor") was worth "selling to industry on its merits and at face value." His viewpoint was bluntly practical:

> To appeal to an employer to give a poor blind man a job on basis of sympathy or charity is a waste of time and effort. . . . The employer must be shown . . . that our worker is not going to cost him any more in wages, in overhead or in liability insurance, and that his investment in space occupied by a properly placed blind worker will bring him just as much profit as any other employee. Placement workers must be as ready to condemn suggested jobs as to approve them, for it is folly to accept any job offered by an employer unless we are absolutely certain that it can be held by the worker we have to place.

He believed that should a blind worker fail at a particular job, it was the responsibility of the placement agency, rather than the employer, to remove him and substitute another blind person who could do better. By standing behind the placement, the agency could preserve the confidence of the employer.

So convinced was Clunk of his techniques that in 1926 he proposed that the Foundation establish a placement bureau with a capable blind man in charge to lead a nationwide movement. The Foundation was not ready for this, but soon enough an opportunity materialized north of the border. Ever since its founding in 1919, the Canadian National Institute for the Blind (CNIB) had sought to develop an effective industrial placement and vending stand program. In 1928 Clunk was invited to try. Within two years, the CNIB had more blind persons at work on industrial production lines and in vending stands than were employed by all five sheltered workshops in the Dominion. By 1937, when Clunk left to take the Washington job, seven hundred blind men and women had been placed in non-sheltered work in Canada and the CNIB was that country's largest operator of industrial lunch, canteen, and vending services.

The year's delay between passage of the Randolph-Sheppard Act and the appointment of Clunk to carry out its provisions was due to the lack of an initial appropriation. In the interim, the Office of Education used its existing staff to initiate some of the administrative steps needed to launch the program. John A. Kratz, who had been chief of the federal Vocational Education Board since its establishment in 1920, called a conference of interested parties in September 1936 to exchange views on how the Act could best be put into effect. This led, the following month, to issuance of a set of principles and procedures covering such basic points as selection of buildings and building locations, equipment, articles to be vended, selection and training of operators, and supervision of stand operation.

This final item was a touchy one, and was to remain so throughout the years. The opinion of many vending stand operators was that they were independent businessmen whose freedom of action was infringed by outside supervision. But Kratz had already discovered that, left to its own devices, the whole program could easily collapse. His conviction was borne out by evidence close at hand.

A few years earlier the Public Buildings Administration in Washington had given a local agency for the blind permission to install 17 vending stands in federal buildings. Lacking any sort of experienced guidance, 6 of these had already been abandoned and the remaining 11 were on a shaky footing. The Public Buildings Administration had told Kratz:

> There is nothing in our experience which leads us to believe that blind persons and retail merchandising are compatible, and we intend to close the 11 stands as rapidly as circumstances will permit. We do not believe in the program envisaged in the Randolph-Sheppard Act and we want nothing to do with it.

Since the Act called for designation in each state of a public agency to license stand operators, and invested the licensing agency with the responsibility for training, placing, and supervising the vendors and for providing them with initial stocks of merchandise as well as adequate equipment, there was an obvious need for such agencies to keep some degree of control. It was not the individual vendor but the licensing agency—usually the state agency for the blind—that had to persuade custodians of federal buildings to allow vending stands to be installed.

By the summer of 1937 a total of 27 state agencies had been approved by the Office of Education to administer vending stand programs; two years later, the number was 43. Describing the progress made as of mid-1941, Kratz told a convention of the AAWB that 316 vending stands had thus far been established in federal buildings and about six hundred others in non-federal locations.

He was particularly gratified to be able to report the complete turnaround in the nation's capital where, under the aegis of the District of Columbia's Vocational Rehabilitation Service—with a newly organized voluntary agency, the Washington Society for the Blind, serving as fiscal agent—there were now 29 stands in operation doing a gross business of $42,000 a month and yielding the operators an average monthly income of more than $200. Since the District of Columbia lacked civic autonomy and was run by the federal government, the District's Vocational Rehabilitation Service was a unit of Kratz's bureau in the Office of Education. Leonard Robinson, who was put in charge of the D.C. operation in 1940, and remained in that capacity until his retirement in 1971, had been largely responsible for the successful performance. (The Washington Society for the Blind was dissolved in 1971 and replaced by a new non-profit agency, District Enterprises for the Blind, which took over the licensing, managerial and fiscal responsibilities for the 75 vending stands then in Washington buildings.)

The District of Columbia operation was modeled after the Canadian system of "controlled management" under which the licensing agency held title to the stands, took responsibility for equipment, merchandise displays, bookkeeping, accounting, and general supervision of the operators. A number of states copied this system, despite the resistance of many operators who saw no need for supervisory and management services and saw no justification for paying the licensing agency a small percentage of their gross sales—known as the set-aside—for them.

At an AAWB meeting in 1951 Maurice I. Tynan, who a year earlier had succeeded Clunk as head of what had by then been renamed Services for the Blind of the Office of Vocational Rehabilitation, placed equal blame on what he called the selfish attitude of such operators who "are usually better off financially than any other group of blind persons," and on the inadequate performance of some of the state licensing agencies which were failing to give the operators the services that justified the set-aside. Exhorting his hearers to make new efforts to keep the vending stand program as "the show window of work for the blind," he continued: "We should build a reputation for having the best operated, best equipped stands to be found anywhere if we are to compete and overcome the inherent prejudices of the general public in dealing with blind persons."

Tynan was speaking in his capacity as a federal official. This may account for the fact that his remarks did not even touch upon a situation which was engendering mounting concern and anger among both the vending stand operators and the state licensing agencies, and which was the subject of a resolution adopted at the very convention he addressed. The resolution called for a law to "prohibit government employee welfare associations from sponsoring or placing vending machines in public buildings in competition with the business enterprise program for the blind."

The newly elected president of AAWB that year was Roy Kumpe, managing director of Arkansas Enterprises for the Blind. His state had shared honors with the District of Columbia in pioneering effective vending stand programs under the Randolph-Sheppard Act. On behalf of his own state, as well as in the name of AAWB, Kumpe brought the encroachment problem to the attention of Congressman Graham A. Barden of North Carolina, chairman of the House Committee on Labor and Education.

Following a fact-finding inquiry by his staff, Barden summoned a meeting on August 1, 1951, of members of the Arkansas Congressional delegation, representatives of the General Services Administration, members of the Office of Voca-

tional Rehabilitation staff, and Hulen C. Walker, the Foundation's legislative
analyst. Barden made a strong statement, and the other Congressmen concurred.
He said: "The intent of Congress to give preference to blind persons with respect
to vending stands in federal buildings is quite clear and places a definite responsibility on the various federal agencies . . . to see that no policies or procedures
circumvent or encroach upon it in any way."

But no action was taken, and the situation grew steadily worse. By early 1954, in
one of the strongest editorials ever to appear in its pages, the *New Outlook for the
Blind* called for an end to lethargy. It voiced alarm over "the insidious wedges into
the Congress-given right of blind persons" to earn a living as vendors in government buildings. Postal employee groups, the editorial said, were the main aggres-
sors in installing vending machines for the benefit of their own recreation or
welfare associations, in spite of the fact that there existed "absolutely no legal
authority for postal employee union groups to install vending machines for
something called their welfare."

To build a factual case for a legislative campaign, the Foundation conducted a
national survey of vending stand operations in government buildings. Simultaneously, a number of bills were introduced in the House of Representatives to
amend the Randolph-Sheppard Act. One of these called for removing the power to
decide on installation of vending concessions from both the custodians of federal
buildings and their parent agencies, and centralizing all such decisions in the
Department of Health, Education, and Welfare.

In his testimony before the House committee which held hearings on the various
vending stand and related measures in May 1954, M. Robert Barnett trained his
principal fire on the offending bureaucracies. The fact that the vending stand
program had "fallen upon evil times" was "the fault of the Government itself," he
said bluntly. Worse still, said Barnett, the offending groups were "openly bragging
about their victory over the blind and making it crystal clear that they do not
intend that they shall be prevented from continued expansion of their illegal
practices." The most recent encroachment had occurred

> as a result of the action of the Secretary of Agriculture who in his anxiety to
> dispose of surplus milk supplies has arranged for a commercial vendor to
> install milk vending machines in the Department of Agriculture building, in
> competition with a blind-operated vending stand whose hours of business
> have been limited by some official edict, in order "to divide business." The
> Secretary is further quoted as having said that if he could have his way,
> similar vending machines would be installed in all federal buildings.

Barnett asserted that while workers for the blind would prefer enactment of a
bill specifically designed to amend the Randolph-Sheppard Act, they would go
along with the omnibus administration bill, then before Congress, which dealt with
both the Vocational Rehabilitation Act and the Randolph-Sheppard Act and which
was subsequently enacted as Public Law 83-565. While the bill's principal importance was in accelerating vocational rehabilitation services, it also effected some
potentially significant changes in the vending stand program. By changing the
phrase "federal buildings" to "federal properties," it created additional opportu-

nities in national parks and reservations. It stipulated that vending machines were part of the vending stand program, reaffirmed in specific language that blind persons were to be given preference whenever a vending stand was to be installed on federal property, and required federal agency heads to issue regulations to that effect.

Although P.L. 565, which was enacted August 3, 1954, did not go along with the request that all decision-making power over vending installations be vested in the Department of Health, Education, and Welfare, it did transfer such power from the individual custodians of federal properties to their parent agencies.

The new law also reinforced both the obligations and the privileges of the state licensing agencies, which were now required to furnish the equipment and initial stock of new vending stands. The law permitted the agencies to take title to the stands, though not forbidding personal ownership. In this respect, it disappointed the National Federation of the Blind, which had urged mandatory decontrol of agency ownership. The Federation was also unhappy over the specific permission given in the law for the set-aside arrangement. And everybody was unhappy over what the amendment altogether failed to do: grapple openly with the problem of competition from federal employee groups. Nor did it really enforce a change in what the *Outlook* called the "ineffective if not dilatory attitude of governmental administrators."

In late 1954, and again in 1955, the Foundation held two national meetings to develop a unified point of view on the basic goals, problems, and opportunities of the vending stand program. It was hoped that clarification of the needs and wishes of both licensing agencies and operators would lead to prompt, helpful, and practicable regulations by the 12 federal agencies controlling property on which stands were located. The hope failed to materialize. It took nearly a year after passage of Public Law 565 for the first of the federal departments to issue regulations, and more than three years before the last of the 12 provided orders to custodians of its buildings. The vending stand program was stymied, not only by these delays but also by some of the regulations themselves, which were unhelpful.

It is perhaps too easy to cast the federal bureaucracy in the role of outright villain in this situation, although advocates of the blind did not hesitate to do so. The fact was that these bureaus were under considerable counterpressure from their own employees to protect the kind of squatter's rights by means of which the latter claimed vending machine income. The employee groups that installed vending machines in the buildings in which they worked vehemently denied, despite clear evidence to the contrary, that these machines invaded the income of the blind vendors in the same buildings. They insisted that the yield from the machines was essential to staff morale because it financed flowers for sick members, scholarships for employees' children, uniforms and prizes for bowling teams, annual picnics and the like.

The reluctance of the federal agencies to disturb relations with their workers evidently overbalanced their knowledge that not only was their action (or lack of it) in direct conflict with the obligations imposed upon them by Congress, it was also in violation of two rulings—in 1949 and again in 1952—by the United States Comptroller General. These had stated flatly that vending machine operation for the benefit of employee groups was without statutory authority and that any such proceeds should accrue to the United States Treasury.

While the potential for expansion of vending opportunities for blind persons in federal buildings was thus substantially throttled, the program made major strides in non-federal installations. In 1952, for example, there were 559 stands in federal buildings and 920 in non-federal buildings. Between the two there were employed some 2,100 persons whose aggregate net earnings were $3,690,000 on gross sales of $18,660,000. That the federal buildings were desirable from a profit viewpoint could be seen from the fact that the operators in these installations averaged $2,279 in income as against $1,761 for those in non-federal buildings. But nine years later, the number of federal stands had grown by only 97, while those in other locations had increased by 598. At the end of fiscal 1971, the overall figures stood at 3,142 vending stands (986 federal, 2,466 non-federal) with gross sales of just over $101 million. Annual earnings of vending stand operators then averaged $6,516.

One of the troublesome issues growing out of the regulations of the various government departments, once they were finally promulgated in the late Fifties, concerned the question of how to settle disputes between state licensing agencies and the bureaus in control of federal property. A state agency which applied for a vending stand location and was turned down had little recourse. In 1962 Jennings Randolph, who was by then in the Senate, introduced a bill calling for a Presidentially appointed appeals board to resolve such disputes. Hearings on the bill brought fervent assurances from the Bureau of the Budget and other federal agencies that no legislation was needed because departmental regulations could be amended to provide for internal appeals procedures. Such regulations were finally issued two years later, but they proved cumbersome and not readily applicable to the central issue of conflicting claims between agencies for the blind and employee welfare groups.

Other efforts were made in 1968, and again in 1969, to introduce corrective legislation. To present a united front against the employee associations, the Foundation convened the leadership of the five other national organizations concerned with the issue: the American Association of Workers for the Blind, the National Council of State Agencies for the Blind, the Blinded Veterans Association, the National Federation of the Blind, and the American Council of the Blind. The six groups reached agreement on what was needed (and also agreed not to disagree—in public at least—on the set-aside question which remained a major point of difference among them). They drafted a bill which was introduced as S. 2461 by Senator Randolph on the 33rd anniversary of the original Randolph-Sheppard Act.

The basic purpose of the bill was to establish more precise and binding definitions that would assure blind licensees preference in vending operations, including exclusive assignment of vending machine income. It also called for all new public buildings to include in their design a satisfactory site for a vending facility.

Hearings on S. 2461 were held in the summer of 1970 by a sub-committee of the Senate Committee on Labor and Public Welfare. The same hearings took testimony on a bill to amend the Wagner-O'Day Act, then also before the Senate. For reasons of strategy, the federal employee associations abstained from testifying at these hearings; should the Randolph bill die in the Senate, they could avoid the public obloquy of interfering with blind men's rights to earn a living. When, however, the bill achieved unanimous passage in the Senate, the employee associations—principally spokesmen for postal groups—took vigorous action at the subsequent House hearings. Enough of a crossfire was set up for the House committee, chaired by Congressman John Brademas of Indiana, to refrain from reporting out the bill.

Senator Randolph reintroduced substantially the same bill (S. 2506) during the next session of Congress, and hearings were once again held in the Senate in 1971 and in the House in 1972. They were for the most part a reprise of the testimony given at the earlier hearings—except for what one journalist, in a slashing exposé titled "Stealing from the Blind," called "perhaps [the] most remarkable achievement" of Senator Randolph: to produce the president of one federal union, the National Association of Internal Revenue Employees, who testified that its 47,000 members were firmly in favor of the bill.

In the election year of 1972, this union president's statement did not carry enough weight to offset the opposition of the other employee unions and associations whose combined membership added up to many millions—all of them voters, as one witness carefully reminded Congressmen at the House hearings. Although the Senate passed a modified form of the Randolph bill, its principal features disappeared in the compromise version that emerged from a House-Senate conference committee. The conference report noted that the omissions were not "due to any lack of concern for, or disregard of the need for, strong and forward-looking amendments to the Randolph-Sheppard Act" and that both House and Senate would "consider these matters in depth" in the next Congress. It added:

> The conferees are deeply concerned that the Congress has not been able to obtain any definitive information concerning legitimate uses of vending machine income on federally-controlled property [and] urge that the General Accounting Office conclude, at the earliest possible date, its audit and study of such funds. . . .

The few changes that did get through the conference committee were among the several titles incorporated in the omnibus Rehabilitation Act (H.R. 8395) which was vetoed in toto by President Nixon in October 1972. An even more ominous development surfaced the following month when the General Services Administration, in an effort to reduce the annual deficits in certain cafeteria operations in federal buildings, proposed regulations to prevent blind vendors in those buildings from selling hot foods prepared in microwave ovens. Final action on this newest restriction was still pending at the end of 1972.

In work for the blind, the Randolph-Sheppard Act evokes automatic association with the expansion of vending stand opportunities. Often overlooked has been the pivotal role of this piece of legislation in the development of pioneering techniques that enabled large numbers of blind men and women to earn their living as industrial workers.

It was a particularly timely role, one which shared with the Wagner-O'Day Act of 1938 the initial credit for the contribution made by thousands of blind produc-

tion workers when the nation needed their manpower in World War II. What the
Wagner-O'Day Act did for the blind men and women producing goods in
sheltered workshops is recounted in the next chapter. The program under the
Randolph-Sheppard Act was aimed at a diametrically opposite purpose: taking
blind people out of these workshops and into open industrial employment, side by
side with sighted workers. Its contribution to that goal was achieved through the
training of a group of blind placement agents in the practical demonstration
methods perfected by Joseph Clunk during the preceding two decades.

Clunk himself had had some notable forerunners. The first instance of industrial
placement by an American organization for the blind is said to have taken place in
Massachusetts in 1904 when Charles F. F. Campbell induced the Dennison
Manufacturing Company, producers of paper products, to employ a blind man to
cut box corners. At the time, Campbell headed what was called the Experimental
Station for the Trade Training of the Blind, a unit of the Massachusetts Association for Promoting the Interests of the Blind.

Campbell, whose missionary zeal was second only to his versatility, took photographs and made lantern slides of the box-cutter at work and showed them
throughout the East in a drive to popularize the idea that blind people could
function in other than the "blind trades." When he left New England, the
industrial placement program he had initiated, by then under the direction of the
Massachusetts Commission for the Blind, was carried on by his successors. Flor-
ence W. Birchard and Francis Ierardi both gained national prominence for their
achievements along this line in the Bay State.

Similarly intrepid souls had made inroads in the industrial Midwest. One of the
outstanding employers of blind labor was the Ford Motor Company, which
employed 41 blind men between 1914 and 1944, retaining many even during the
depression years when most plants let their handicapped workers go. Henry Ford
II was awarded the Foundation's Migel Medal in 1944, in recognition of his
enlightened labor policy toward the blind.

It was not, however, until Clunk joined the federal government as administrator
of the Randolph-Sheppard Act that any organized national program was launched
for the specific purpose of training vocational specialists in methods of placing blind
persons in open employment. Clunk's authority for this program derived from the
clauses in the Act that called for making national surveys of employment possibilities and passing on the information to organizations for the blind. A believer in
direct action, Clunk did not bother much with extended formal surveys and
reports. He dived at once into a training and demonstration program that would
indoctrinate a nationwide corps of placement counselors in result-getting methods.
The fastest road to this goal was to send likely blind men to Canada for field
training, where they could learn from first-hand experience just what was entailed
in locating jobs that blind men could do, persuading employers to give blind
workers a trial at such jobs, preparing the job candidates themselves, and following
through on such placements to make sure they stuck.

O. E. (Barney) Day, an Indiana mechanical engineer blinded at age thirty-one,
was the first person to receive such field training. After six months with the
Canadian National Institute for the Blind, he returned to the United States to take

on the job of placing graduates of the Overbrook School in Philadelphia and later became chief of the Pennsylvania State Council for the Blind. His characteristic approach was illustrated in a magazine article which related his experience with the Keebler-Weyl Baking Company.

Day had gone to J. Y. Huber, the company's president, and asked that he be allowed to scout around the plant looking for spots suitable for blind workers. Huber wondered how Day could tell, and Day asked him

> to speak to the workers as he and Barney walked through the plant. "If anybody looks up or turns around to answer but at the same time keeps working," said Barney, "that's the job I want to try." They had just started when Barney heard Mr. Huber say, "Hello, Marion, how are you?"
>
> "I'm fine," she said, and looked up and smiled. Mr. Huber nudged his companion.
>
> "By the way, Marion," Barney asked, "how long have you been on that job?"
>
> "Oh, two or three years, I guess."
>
> "Bet you could do it with your eyes closed, huh?"
>
> "Sure," she answered. "Want to see me?"
>
> The president laughed. "Come on," he told Barney, "let's get out of here before you fill the plant with blind people."

Similarly ingenious ploys were used by the many other blind men who, following Clunk's training program, achieved notable careers in industrial placement. Among those named by Clunk in a 1966 article recapitulating the pioneering days were Arthur Voorhees and Carl Hvarre in New Jersey, James Hyka in Cleveland, John McGettigan in Pittsburgh, August McCullom in Kansas, Kenneth McCullom in Connecticut, Floyd Lacy in Texas, Carston Ohnstead in Oklahoma, Carlos Gattis in Arkansas, John McAulay in Seattle, Hulen Walker in Tennessee, Walter Moran in Maine, J. Hiram Chappell in Oregon, Anthony Septinelli in California.

John McAulay, who had lost his sight in an accident during his college days, joined the federal staff in 1942 and was assigned to demonstrate that industrial placement of blind persons could be carried out in every part of the United States, whatever its economic complexion. He conducted whirlwind 30-day job-finding campaigns in each of three very different states: Louisiana, Colorado and Delaware. His accomplishments made the point. There were job opportunities everywhere.

McAulay also added a new dimension to the placement process by showing how the facilities of regular vocational and trade schools could be used to train blind people for industrial work. A manual he wrote on the subject was published in 1954 by the Foundation. Addressed to employment counselors, it spelled out the "live demonstration" technique he had perfected to induce shop instructors to take on blind students. It consisted of assembling the instructors around a piece of power machinery and then blindfolding one of them to prove how much could be done without sight, provided a "four-point pattern of safety" was followed to prevent accidents. In one such demonstration a blindfolded hygiene teacher, a woman who had never even seen a power lathe, performed perfectly.

McAulay's principles were given a practical test in the mid-Sixties when a three-year demonstration program enrolled groups of blind students in a full-scale machine shop course at a technical school in North Dakota and found that the graduates could more than hold their own in industrial jobs. The school's faculty, who began the experiment with an attitude of "we'll believe it when we see it," were soon able to see it:

> Class instructors have observed that the determination and initiative shown by the blind students often amazes and encourages sighted students in the same shop area to do better. "There's one thing about these [blind] boys," they note. "They don't goof off a bit. We can't find a job they can't do. Once we transmit a mental picture of the job to be done to their minds, your job is practically done."

In 1961 the AAWB established an annual award for excellence in vocational counseling in memory of McAulay, who died in 1957.

The availability of people like Day, McAulay and their compeers became extremely important when, with the passage of the Vocational Rehabilitation Act amendments of 1943, large new amounts of federal funds were appropriated for vocational training of disabled persons. With these men as instructors, intensive six-week group training classes for blind industrial placement officers were conducted in several cities. In 1944 and 1945, eight such courses were given. In each, after two weeks of instruction in theoretical concepts, the trainees spent the remaining time undergoing actual work experience in about a hundred different production processes commonly found in the kinds of plants that almost every community had: machine shops, laundries, dry cleaning plants, bakeries, department stores, textile and furniture factories, etc.

Comparable courses were given for vocational counselors specializing in vending stand programs. There was also a course in agricultural placement, the first organized effort ever made to provide vocational help to blind persons living in rural areas.

Those enrolled in these courses were primarily staff members of state agencies for the blind. In a later appraisal of the long-range impact of this pioneer training program, the point was made that not only did it set the pattern for preparation of vocational counselors, it also developed leadership material for the years to come. Some notable names could be found among the alumni of those early training courses. They included Douglas C. MacFarland, since 1964 chief of services to the blind in the Social and Rehabilitation Service, Department of Health, Education, and Welfare, and M. Robert Barnett, since 1949 executive director of the American Foundation for the Blind.

Joseph Clunk, the "husky fellow with the flashing teeth and a cherubic but leather-plated countenance" who spark-plugged the movement, resigned from federal service in 1950 to become director of the Philadelphia branch of the Pennsylvania Association for the Blind. Following retirement from that post, he was continuing to function as a consultant in 1972.

14

The Workshops

It is eminently logical that the nation's first school for blind children should also have been the first to confront the problem of what to do about graduates, equipped with wage-earning skills, who found every employment door closed to them. In 1840, eight years after founding what was then called the Perkins Institution and Massachusetts Asylum for the Blind, Samuel Gridley Howe established a "separate work department" at the school. It was the nation's first example of what later came to be called the sheltered workshop, an idea that came to provide succeeding generations of handicapped people not only with employment but with the gratification of self-support. As Howe put it: "In this department the blind feel perfectly independent, being assured of the bread they eat; and if any surplus remains to them, it is far more prized than would be ten times the amount of alms."

Howe hit upon one other basic characteristic that remained constant for well over a century. The workshop was "not intended to be a source of gain to the Institution; on the contrary, it must be a pecuniary loss at the outset; it is wholly for the benefit of the individuals who work in it. . . ."

The innovation was soon duplicated by several other early schools for the blind. They found, as did Perkins after a few years, that education of the young and an employment enterprise for adults did not really belong under the same roof. The workshops were ultimately separated from the schools and came under the management of voluntary organizations for the adult blind and, later, of state agencies. Perkins held out longer than most; its workshop, though moved to separate premises, did not close until 1952.

Because there was little public transportation in those early years, the men and women engaged in the workshops had to be housed nearby, so boarding homes were established for them. Then, too, newly blinded adults who had not attended schools for the blind had to learn the necessary personal adjustment and work skills, so the workshops took on a training function. They slowly turned into institutions. Tracing the development of the workshop movement in *As I Saw It*, Robert Irwin noted:

> In some instances those entering the institutions came with the under-standing that they would remain for only two or three years, while they were learning their trades. But when the training period was over, their home connection had often been broken and there was no place for them to go except to the county poor farms. Often they were permitted to remain in the institution for many years, so that it became difficult eventually to say whether the institution was a training school, a working home, or just a refuge for aged blind people.

This diffusion of focus troubled those who were attempting to modernize work for the blind; their solution was to establish day workshops. Irwin credited Eben P. Morford of the Industrial Home for the Blind in Brooklyn and Charles W. Holmes of the Massachusetts Commission for the Blind with leadership in this develop-ment. Eventually the combination boarding home and workshop all but disappeared.

For the most part, the early workshops produced simple, handmade objects that were in everyday use, could be manufactured out of easily obtained materials, and could be sold in local markets. A 1908 survey of the 16 workshops then in existence revealed that the majority were principally engaged in broom-making, with chair-caning and hand weaving the other two main activities. These 16 workshops did a gross annual business of $311,000. They employed 583 blind workers whose total wages came to $102,500—an average of just over $3.00 per week per person. It was hardly a living wage, even in those days. But then, workshops were not expected to yield a living wage; they were subsidized by their sponsoring agencies, and the blind person whose family could not supply the difference between his earnings and his needs usually received a small cash supplement from the agency.

The first sizable opportunity for blind people with good skills to move out of the workshops came during World War I, when several hundred were employed in war factories. Only a handful were kept on after the armistice, however, and many of those returning to the workshops were no longer ready to accept their condi-tions and wages. There was another problem, too. The workshops had kept going during the war with whatever personnel they could muster; these were, for the most part, low-skilled, often multihandicapped persons, many incapable of meeting even minimal production standards. One way or another, some people were bound to be crowded out once the wartime industrial workers came back to the shops.

This situation—which was to be repeated in heightened form following World War II—was at the heart of the dilemma that perennially troubled the leadership in work for the blind. What should be the basic function of a workshop? Should it be primarily a training school to fit people for employment in open industry? Should it be a self-supporting production unit, able to compete in the open market with commercial firms? Should it be an outright social service, a work therapy setting for those blind people who could never realistically be expected to pull their economic weight? Should it combine all three functions?

Opinion on these thorny questions was sharply divided during the Twenties and, to a certain extent, continues to remain divided despite the striking transformations that workshops for the blind have undergone in succeeding decades.

One transformation began in 1929 with the passage of the Hawes-Cooper Act (Public Law 77-669). This piece of legislation had been sought for twenty years by labor unions, citizen bodies, and manufacturers' associations who were attempting to halt the deadly competition of convict labor. Prison-made merchandise, often produced under contract with outside firms, was flooding a number of markets. With prisoners paid as little as 14 cents a day, their products could be profitably sold at prices far below anything free labor could afford. It was a substantial threat. Prison output in the late Twenties was valued at some $50 million a year.

One of the industries affected by convict labor competition was broom manufacturing. In joining the multi-industry drive that would keep the products of prison shops off the free market by restricting their sale to "state use" (i.e., use in governmental departments and institutions), the broom manufacturers thought it advantageous to enlist the support of the workshops for the blind. They were not overly concerned about competition from the workshops, whose cost of manufacture was not too different from their own and thus did not present the same price-cutting threat as prison labor. The Eastern Broom Manufacturers and Supply Dealers Association even sweetened the pot by declaring themselves in favor of having "state use" brooms reserved for manufacture by the workshops for the blind. Although this was a more or less self-serving action, to the extent that blind-made brooms would thereby be deflected from the open market, the workshops were willing enough to accept this industry concession. Many years later, a knowledgeable observer was to comment that, had the broom manufacturers had any conception of how large this "state use" business was destined to become during World War II and thereafter, they would not so readily have yielded it to the workshops for the blind.

The Hawes-Cooper Act, when it finally became law in January 1929, did not represent a complete answer to the convict labor problem, but it did divest prison-made goods of their interstate character by making them subject to the laws of the various states. The Act did not become effective for five years. As the deadline date neared, a national committee was formed to promote passage of the necessary state laws. These laws had to do two things: (1) provide that all goods produced by prisoners within the state would be used by the state itself and kept off the consumer market; and (2) prohibit the importation of convict-made goods from other states. The national committee, which had representation from the American Federation of Labor and the General Federation of Women's Clubs as well as from the various manufacturing associations, invited Peter J. Salmon of the Industrial Home for the Blind and Charles B. Hayes of the Foundation to become members.

Salmon, who at that time was also president of the New York State Federation of Workers for the Blind, had played a signal role in the passage of the Hawes-Cooper Act. His agency operated one of the nation's largest workshops for the blind; its major product was brooms. In the course of pressing for passage of the Act, he had met and formed a firm friendship with James V. Bennett, then federal commissioner of prison industries in the Department of Justice's Bureau of Prisons. It was a friendship that would stand the blind in good stead a few years later.

Salmon's appearance to testify before the Senate Interstate Commerce Committee's 1928 hearings on the Hawes-Cooper Act had had a dramatic effect. An affable, blue-eyed, fair-haired Irishman, whose open-faced countenance with its dimpled pink cheeks bespoke a genuinely gregarious personality, the witness—then in his early thirties—conducted himself like anything but the stereotype of a blind man. Using braille notes, he stood up confidently at a lectern to read a statement in his cheerful, Boston-accented voice. Seated behind him, the committee chairman, Senator James E. Watson of Indiana, dabbed at tear-filled eyes. The senator had a blind brother. It was not on the grounds of sympathy, however, that Peter Salmon made an impact. He was and would be a doughty fighter for the cause to which he had dedicated his career.

The Hawes-Cooper Act had specifically excluded goods manufactured in federal prisons from its ban on interstate shipments. The federal institution specializing in broom manufacture was Leavenworth Penitentiary; under an executive order, its entire broom output was purchased by federal departments, which then met any additional needs through purchases in the open market. Workshops for the blind were among the bidders for this open market business, and this gave rise to a serious problem. In their struggle to survive in the straitened economic conditions of the depression, the workshops were competing to a disastrous degree by undercutting each other's prices.

At its 1933 convention, the American Association of Workers for the Blind named Salmon to head a committee whose charge was to "work in cooperation with the American Foundation for the Blind for the purpose of establishing a code of fair practices [in] the various phases of work among workshops for the blind." The resolution was a follow-up to steps taken the previous year by the Foundation, which had convened two regional conferences of workshop managers in an effort to resolve the more serious causes of friction among them.

There was also another pressing reason for the adoption of such a code. The National Recovery Act (NRA), passed by Congress in the first year of the New Deal administration, had called for the establishment in all industries of fair labor practice codes, including minimum wages and maximum hours. The sheltered workshops, both those for the blind and those for persons with other handicaps, had taken the position that, as non-commercial organizations, they could not be expected to meet such minimum wage requirements. General Hugh S. Johnson, the National Recovery Administrator, named a special commission to examine the workshop question and subsequently issued an order which recognized the unique situation of the sheltered workshops as "charitable institutions . . . conducted not for profit but for the purpose of providing remunerative employment for physically, mentally or socially handicapped workers." The order granted all workshops exemption from the NRA industry codes on several conditions. Most important was that they agree not to engage in "destructive price cutting or any other unfair method of competition."

Although the National Recovery Act was later declared unconstitutional, the principle it established of exempting sheltered workshops from minimum wage laws was preserved in the Fair Labor Standards Act of 1938 and subsequent federal labor laws. In somewhat modified form, it was still in effect in 1972 despite the repeated efforts of organizations of blind people to have it overthrown.

Once the Randolph-Sheppard Act had embodied into law a precedent for granting some blind people special opportunities for self-support through vending stand operation, the time seemed ripe to seek federal help for the even larger group of blind men and women whose only source of livelihood came through the sheltered workshops. In March 1937 Peter Salmon wrote M.C. Migel: "I don't think that the Foundation could possibly do anything that would result in more jobs for the blind in a shorter period of time than to pursue this proposition of getting the Federal and State Governments to purchase brooms and possibly mops from the blind."

The most strategic approach was to use an already established entree. James V. Bennett had just been promoted to the directorship of the federal Bureau of Prisons. Salmon set up a meeting for himself, Migel, and Irwin at Bennett's office. Just how, they asked, could the workshops for the blind go about securing the federal broom business? Recognizing Bennett's obligation to protect prison interests, the trio explained that "first we would like to secure the open market orders, and later it [is] our hope that through the cooperation of the Department of Justice, we might gradually take over the entire requirements of the Federal Government."

Bennett was receptive to this approach. His opinion was that legislation would be the most feasible path to follow, and he gave helpful advice on how a law should be framed.

A measure along the suggested lines was drafted and, in July, introduced in Congress by two New York Democrats. In the Senate the bill's sponsor was Robert F. Wagner, then completing his second term as a senator following a political career that had begun with his election to the New York State Assembly in 1905. On the House side, the bill was introduced by Congresswoman Caroline O'Day, also a second-termer on the Hill. Both legislators had the ear of Franklin D. Roosevelt; Mrs. O'Day was also a close personal friend of Mrs. Roosevelt.

The Wagner bill was referred to the Senate's Committee on Interstate Commerce; Mrs. O'Day's went to the House Committee on Expenditures in the Executive Department. As a matter of routine practice, both committees solicited the views of the various government departments whose purchasing policies would be affected by the bills. Replies were slow in coming in, however, and Congress adjourned before they were all in hand, which meant that hearings on the bills would have to go over to the following year.

The interval was constructively employed by the bill's advocates. Migel, Salmon, and Irwin used the time to see to it that all key political fences were in good repair. They secured promises of cooperation from A.F.L. and C.I.O. representatives in Washington; they talked to members of Congress and to the heads of various federal bureaus, and constantly touched base with James V. Bennett.

The amended bill, as reported out by the Senate Interstate Commerce Committee and subsequently passed, was called "An Act to Create a Committee on Blind-Made Products and for Other Purposes." Its major provisions were these:

• The President of the United States would appoint a Committee on Purchases of Blind-Made Products, to be made up of one representative each of six government departments (Navy, War, Treasury, Agriculture, Commerce and Interior) plus "a private citizen conversant with the problems incident to the employment of the blind."

• The committee would "determine the fair market price of all brooms and mops and other suitable commodities manufactured by the blind and offered for sale to the Federal Government by any non-profit-making agency for the blind." It would make all necessary rules and regulations concerning such transactions, including "authorization of a central non-profit-making agency to facilitate the distribution of orders among the agencies for the blind."

• The bill mandated that "all brooms and mops and other suitable commodities hereafter procured in accordance with applicable Federal specifications by or for any Federal Department or agency shall be procured from such non-profit-making agencies for the blind . . . at the price determined by the Committee to be the fair market price," except when brooms and mops were available from the Federal prison industries or were procured for use outside the continental United States.

As originally drafted, the bill referred only to brooms and mops. It was the committee that added "and other suitable commodities" and it was this phrase that opened vistas workers for the blind had not dared dream of.

Just about the only opposition to the Wagner-O'Day Act came, not from any legislator or government bureau, but from one man who held a unique and more or less solitary position in the ranks of workers for the blind. He was Dr. Merle E. Frampton, principal of the New York Institute for the Education of the Blind, who wrote to Senator Wagner and to Senator Burton K. Wheeler, chairman of the Interstate Commerce Committee, expressing strenuous objection on several grounds.

He alleged that workers for the blind had not been adequately consulted about the measure. The bill's "most objectionable" feature was that it granted authority to a non-profit agency to centralize and distribute government orders. No one agency, he said, should be allowed such a controlling role; it would lead to "favoritism and malpractice." There was no reason, in his opinion, to change the existing system of open competitive bidding for government orders; if, however, a central allocation agency was indeed to be designated, it should be "an organization not immediately engaged in work for the blind." A few other arguments were advanced, all leading to the insistent plea that the bill be withdrawn and not reintroduced until a nationwide conclave of all agencies for the blind could consider it.

Frampton sent copies of his letters to Robert Irwin, who replied with a patient explanation of how thoroughly the proposed legislation had in fact been discussed by the field as a whole: at the preceding AAWB national convention, at a convention of the New York State Federation of Workers for the Blind, at meetings of the Greater New York Council of Agencies for the Blind, at conferences with workshop managers and with the legislative committees of both AAWB and AAIB. Irwin also detailed the repeated consultations held with the Bureau of Prisons, the federal Budget Bureau, the Treasury's procurement officers, the purchasing departments of the military services.

Just what Frampton was after was never spelled out. His position as head of a school for blind children hardly qualified him to be a spokesman for the workshops, which were operated by agencies for the adult blind. But Merle Frampton was not content merely to be an authority on education; he was unwilling to recognize that the torch of leadership in work for the blind had passed from the elite hands of the school superintendents to the control of wider and more representative groups.

Because Merle Frampton will be encountered again—almost always in an adversary role—a brief discussion of his background may prove enlightening.

In 1938, when he was attempting single-handedly to kill the Wagner-O'Day bills, Frampton was still relatively new in work for the blind. He had been appointed three years earlier to succeed Edward M. Van Cleve as head of the New York Institute, a large, influential, and venerable school for the blind. His background was in general education and theology. A graduate of Boston University, with a Ph.D. from Harvard and a LL.D from the College of the Ozarks, he had been associate dean of Boston University's School of Religious Education and Social Service and, later, vice-president of the College of the Ozarks. None of his past experience was in the field of blindness.

Frampton's usual public stance was that of a philosopher and theoretician whose lofty views transcended the narrow interests of his colleagues in work for the blind. His first appearance on the national scene had been unfortunate. Invited to give a paper at the 1935 AAWB convention, he had proposed an elaborate scheme for the creation of segregated colonies of blind people—"self contained communities" in which "all the economic functions which can be performed by the visually handicapped are performed by visually handicapped people, and where sighted competition is not permitted." Acknowledging that this plan would limit association of blind people with the sighted, he questioned whether

> the visually handicapped man needs as much so-called sighted intellectual and social contact as we sighted people assume. . . . Quite the contrary is probably the case. The visually handicapped person needs more and more to build his own world, which can be for him a much happier and more fruitful and probably quite a different world than that in which many of our sighted people live.

Propounded by a rank newcomer at a time when most leaders in work for the blind were moving ever more purposefully toward greater integration of blind people with the sighted, this proposal created a considerable uproar. It was to be thrown up at Frampton many times in the years to come, as he pursued his self-appointed role as dissenter.

Despite his unpopularity with co-workers, however, he ranked high with his school's board of trustees and retained his position as principal of the New York Institute until retirement early in 1971.

In any event, Frampton's effort to halt passage of the Wagner-O'Day Act proved futile. The bill had already been reported out by the Interstate Commerce Committee and on March 31, 1938, was passed by the Senate.

In the House of Representatives, Mrs. O'Day's bill encountered a rather different series of obstacles. To begin with, according to Robert Irwin's first-hand account:

> The Committee on Executive Department Expenditures was quite inactive. Few bills were referred to it. The chairman [John J. Cochran of Missouri] was not in good health and the committee seldom met. . . . It happened that the committee had before it a bill which the chairman did not like. It was sponsored by certain women's clubs, and required the Army to put its superannuated horses and mules out to pasture for life, instead of killing them as had been common practice. The chairman felt that this was sentimental, and would have none of it.
>
> [As a consequence, the O'Day bill] lay neglected in the files of the committee. The chairman would not say why he would not call a meeting, but everyone knew it was the superannuated horse bill. . . . If the committee met, the pressure from women's clubs would make it necessary for the committee to act on that bill. . . . Finally, however, sufficient pressure was mustered to get both bills reported out with a recommendation for passage.

By the time the superannuated horses were on their way to pasture, it was April 25, about six weeks before Congress was scheduled to adjourn. In the House there were two "unanimous consent" days left. The first time the O'Day bill came up on the consent calendar, obstacle number two arose from an unexpected quarter. Again from Irwin:

> Congressman Hamilton Fish, who usually favored bills benefitting the blind, for some reason did not like this bill—probably because it was sponsored by two New Deal Democrats from his own state. Therefore, when it came up he shouted from the back of the room something about the New Deal not being satisfied with regimenting everybody else "and now it's trying to regiment the blind." Illogical as the argument was, it constituted a vote against the bill.

What seemed to be the bill's last chance came two weeks later, on the session's final unanimous consent calendar. Congressional rules at the time were that a unanimous consent bill which had drawn a negative vote could be considered one more time. On that final consent day, the calendar was so crowded that the committee in charge ruled that no previously rejected bill would be allowed to come up.

There remained one parliamentary device that might work; on the last day of Congress, there could be a request from the floor for suspension of the rules in order that a particular bill could be taken up. Passage under such suspension had to be unanimous. It was the speaker of the House, William B. Bankhead of Alabama, who suggested this procedure when a distressed Irwin appealed to him for help in getting the O'Day bill passed before Congress adjourned. Bankhead, who never missed a public opportunity to "point with pride" to Helen Keller as a fair daughter of his state, promised that he would recognize a motion from the floor to suspend the rules before thumping his gavel to signal adjournment.

Came the last day of Congress, June 12, and Irwin was in the visitors' gallery at 9 A.M. Adjournment was scheduled for noon. Irwin was uneasy. Mrs. O'Day, absent because she was ill, had delegated her role to a freshman New York congressman, James J. Lanzetta. The latter, according to Irwin, "knew very little about the bill, knew less about this special procedure, and was very obviously nervous about the whole matter." As the morning wore on, Irwin sought out the then Democratic floor leader, Sam Rayburn. Suppose Bankhead forgot? Rayburn advised him to relax; if the Speaker had promised to get the bill through, he would deliver.

Bankhead had instructed Lanzetta he would signal him when to move for suspension of the rules. When, by eleven o'clock, no signal had been given, Irwin went back to Rayburn, imploring him to send a reminder to the Speaker. Irwin's published account says that he was "brushed off with the assurance that if the Speaker promised to take care of the bill he would not forget." What Irwin did not relate was the nature of the brush-off. Many years later Peter Salmon told a Congressional hearing that Rayburn had threatened Irwin with bodily harm if pestered one more time.

In any event, just before adjournment Lanzetta finally got his signal, was given the floor, and offered a somewhat muddled explanation of the O'Day measure. Clarifying assistance came from Congressman Matthew Dunn, but the greatest help came from Bankhead who, ignoring some commotion from anti-New Dealers in the back of the room, proclaimed: "Hearing no objection, I declare the bill passed." The Wagner-O'Day Act thus survived its somewhat ludicrous voyage through the shoals of Congress. It was signed into law by Franklin D. Roosevelt on June 25, 1938, as Public Law 739 of the 75th Congress.

Even before the President affixed his signature, the Foundation called a meeting of workshop managers to discuss how the new law was to be implemented. Two key conclusions were reached. The Foundation should act as the agency to handle distribution of federal orders to the workshops, and no workshop would try to beat the gun by expanding its facilities in anticipation of government orders until it was known just how much business would be available, and when.

A large advisory committee representing workshop interests was elected to work with the Foundation on the allocation question. One of its first decisions was to agree with the Foundation's executive committee that it would be more advisable for a separate corporation to be formed to carry out the provisions of the Wagner-O'Day Act than for the Foundation itself to undertake this function. In August 1938 the National Industries for the Blind, Inc. (NIB) was formed. Its founding officers were M.C. Migel, president; Robert B. Irwin, executive vice-president, Peter J. Salmon, vice-president, and William Ziegler, secretary-treasurer.

The Wagner-O'Day Act had made no provision whatever for funding either the Committee on Purchase of Blind-Made Products or the non-profit agency that would allocate orders among the workshops. The former organized itself as an interdepartmental committee of the federal government. The need to set aside seed money for the latter had been anticipated by the Foundation, whose budget for 1938 carried a line for an employee to be assigned to finding new outlets for the products of blind labor.

The Foundation had a well-qualified candidate in mind for this post: Chester C. Kleber, whose performance in managing the WPA project for the manufacture of Talking Book machines had impressed everyone. At an executive committee meeting in September 1938, C.C. Kleber was appointed vocational research agent of the Foundation at $4,000 a year. Once National Industries for the Blind got under way, the committee decided, half of Kleber's salary would be charged to the new corporation. An appropriation to give him a secretary was also voted. National Industries for the Blind was now in business.

A Pennsylvanian by birth, C.C. came to New York as a young adult and pursued a successful career in motion picture promotion until the depression cost him his job. It was then that his cousin, J.O. Kleber, introduced him to the Foundation and he was put in charge of the WPA project. A roly-poly extrovert endowed with ebullience and a promotional flair, C.C. also had the knack of working with others. There could hardly have been a more valuable quality in the man to whom was entrusted the delicate job of allocating government orders among hungrily competing workshops. As will be seen, he did an outstanding job until a fatal illness necessitated his resignation in June 1960. He died that November, just a month after being awarded the Foundation's Migel Medal for his accomplishments.

The question of how the new corporation should be financed was one of the earliest issues settled by the workshop advisory committee. A simple formula was agreed upon: a small percentage, not to exceed 5 percent, of the receipts from government orders would be charged to the participating workshops to pay for the cost of NIB's operations. The workshops would not be hurt by this arrangement, since it was expected that the fee would be regarded as an overhead expense to be taken into consideration by the Committee on Purchase of Blind-Made Products in its pricing determinations.

(In later years various other fee arrangements were developed for financing NIB, with the commission on government orders as low as 2 percent during periods of heavy volume, and with a different fee scale for NIB-generated commercial sales. At no point in the organization's history was the public ever asked for funds to support it.)

The men selected by Franklin D. Roosevelt to serve on the Committee on Purchase of Blind-Made Products came out of the top drawer of federal officialdom:

From the Treasury: Rear Admiral Christian J. Peoples, chief of the Procurement Division.

From the Navy: Rear Admiral Arthur H. Mayo of the Bureau of Supplies and Accounts.

From the War Department: Brigadier Augustus B. Warfield, the Quartermaster General.

From the Agriculture Department: Alexander M. Ashley of the Office of Budget and Finance.

From the Department of Commerce: Fletcher H. Rawls, assistant director of the Bureau of Foreign and Domestic Commerce.

From the Department of the Interior: Maurice I. Tynan, then assistant to (and later successor of) J.H. Clunk in the Office of Education's Bureau for the Blind.

As the "private citizen conversant with the problems incident to the employment of the blind": M.C. Migel.

At the committee's first meeting, Admiral Peoples was elected chairman. He appointed Robert LeFevre, a member of his staff with some thirty years of experience in federal procurement, as secretary. He named Warfield, Mayo, Migel, and LeFevre to serve as the subcommittee that would decide on the blind-made products to be purchased by federal departments, determine quantities and fair market prices, and devise regulations to govern the procurement process.

In both the committee and the subcommittee, LeFevre was to admit many years later, there was "an air of skepticism . . . an air of doubt that blind workers could produce according to standards of quality." To guard against the possibility of failure during the crucial early stage, one of the initial regulations prohibited workshops from attempting to supply articles with which they had had no experience. The first allocations would be made only to those shops that had produced and sold similar articles during the previous six months.

Another regulation specified that at least 75 percent of the workers engaged in the production of federally purchased articles be blind. This was later revised to refer specifically to labor used in direct production, exclusive of supervision, administration and shipping. The 75 percent ratio was designed to protect bona fide workshops for blind persons from competition with quasi-commercial organizations using a handful of blind workers as window dressing. Until 1971, when the Wagner-O'Day Act was amended for the first time, it also excluded non-profit workshops which served a few blind clients but were operated primarily for persons with other types of disability.

The committee's first schedule of approved orders for brooms and mops appeared on January 1, 1939. That year, sales to federal departments came to $220,000 with 36 workshops participating. It was a slow and careful start but one in which, as LeFevre said, "the ability of blind workers to produce suitable commodities was firmly established."

Probably no piece of legislation in work for the blind was more opportunely timed than the Wagner-O'Day Act. It came into being because, under depression conditions, the nation's blind people needed the support of their government. In very short order, however, the need became reciprocal, and the nation gratefully turned to blind workers for help in the massive World War II defense buildup. By then, many of the workshops had gained experience in meeting government specifications and had broadened the variety of products they could supply. At the end of 1939 these included cocoa mats, mattresses, pillow cases, whisk brooms and several different types of mops and swabs. The expanded opportunities were reflected in the volume for 1940; in this, the second year of NIB operation, federal business aggregating more than $1 million was shared by 44 workshops.

No more prescient than anyone else, NIB's principals decided, some two years before Pearl Harbor, that defense-related orders were bound to level off soon. It would be in the best interests of blind workers, they told one another, not to rely on a continuing heavy volume of government business but to expand workshop sales to commercial outlets. With this in view, NIB announced, early in 1940, that it would seek markets for blind-made products among such quantity consumers as railroads, steamship companies, and large manufacturing concerns. An experienced salesman, D. H. Schill, was employed to carry out this national sales plan and succeeded in gaining some important industrial customers (American Can Company, National Dairies, and similar firms) as well as such chain store outlets for consumer goods as Sears Roebuck, J. C. Penney, and F. W. Woolworth. Simultaneously, NIB kept an eye open for new types of consumer goods that the workshops could manufacture. One successful new product was a line of rubber link mats developed through cooperation with the United States Rubber Company. These Nib-Link mats, made from rubber scraps and short ends, required very little equipment and relatively simple skills.

One problem that surfaced early was that many of the workshops were not capable of handling the necessary quantities. In mid-1940 an Army order for 625,000 pillow cases could only be two-thirds filled because all the workshops with sewing departments were already operating at capacity. Such frustrations had a positive side, however; they were powerful spurs for enlargement and modernization.

With government business booming, and sales to national chain stores also showing healthy growth, the General Committee on Sheltered Workshops for the Blind, into which NIB's participating shops had organized themselves, met in Chicago early in 1941 to plot directions for future expansion. The principal thrust, they agreed, should be pursuit of retail sales. House-to-house canvassing operations were already successful in Wisconsin and in Pittsburgh. To help workshops in other parts of the country embark on similar programs, NIB employed Eugene D. Morgret, the man who had developed the Pittsburgh venture. Two years later he became assistant manager of NIB and remained in its employ until retirement in 1963.

Morgret, a graduate of the Western Pennsylvania School for the Blind, had perfected sales training methods. Once he joined NIB, the first community to request his help was Wichita, Kansas, where a workshop was employing 12 blind persons three days a week. Less than three months after Morgret organized a door-to-door sales team, this same workshop had enough business to put 20 men to work five days a week and could market the products of 10 blind homeworkers.

Morgret managed to get three other workshops started on such local sales programs before Pearl Harbor and its aftermath. Until then, federal business had represented about one-fourth of the workshops' total output. This changed almost overnight as they were called upon to exert the same maximum effort as the rest of the economy. From 1941 to 1945 they delivered to their government some $32 million worth of commodities: 14 million brooms, 21 million mops, 6.5 million deck swabs, 17 million mailing bags, 41 million pillowcases, etc. There were workshops that stayed open around the clock so that three shifts could keep going. Often enough, Kleber and his staff also worked far into the night, juggling allocations, pacifying impatient purchasing officers, rushing out into the field to clear production bottlenecks, keeping tabs on delivery deadlines, scrambling for priority ratings on the raw materials needed to keep the flow of goods moving.

If National Industries for the Blind had closed its doors at the end of World War II, it would still have earned an honored place in the history of work for the blind. As leader, catalyst, and unifying force, it ushered blind workers into a new and promising era. By 1945 a congeries of 60 separate workshops was scattered through 32 states. Many of them had once been fierce competitors (in pre-NIB days many a workshop would not allow the manager of another shop to set foot on its premises), but by 1945 this assortment of diverse organizations had learned to work together, to trust one another, and to pool their resources toward common goals with a degree of mutual cooperation never before experienced in work for the blind. Not the least of their motivations was the satisfaction of serving their country. Before the end of the war a number of workshops were proudly displaying the Army-Navy "E" pennant and the Maritime "M," awards for excellence in wartime production. NIB itself was given the Navy's Certificate of Achievement for its role.

Busy as the workshops were during the hectic war years, they looked ahead. In 1943 a Postwar Planning Committee was named by the General Committee on Sheltered Workshops for the Blind. It was chaired by M. Roberta Townsend, a social worker who was then head of the department for the handicapped of the Brooklyn Bureau of Charities (she later joined the staff of NIB as director of its Survey and Homework Department). After studying the results of a mail survey, the planning group came up with a series of recommendations designed to avert a disastrous drop in postwar employment of blind workers.

There was general agreement that the major problem was not production, but sales, and that the most promising avenue was retailing, both through local stores and door-to-door canvassing. The few workshops that had established sound pre-war retailing programs had managed, despite shortages of raw materials, to maintain and even increase those sales figures throughout the war years. Another well-received idea was for cooperative production and marketing arrangements, by means of which workshops could sell each other's products. Each shop could then concentrate on manufacturing only a few items and still be in a position to retail a full line of consumer goods.

There was also considerable potential in "state use" sales to local governments. Robert Irwin urged the workshops to pursue this potential:

> Steps should be taken immediately to secure laws in the states similar to the federal Wagner O'Day Act. Our competitors in the commercial field are so fully occupied with war orders, they are not likely to oppose state legislation of this kind just now, so the shops should act at the earliest possible opportunity.

At this same conclave in December 1943, Irwin also called attention to a new and promising development. Public Law 113, the Barden-LaFollette amendments to the Vocational Rehabilitation Act, had been enacted a few months earlier. Under its provisions, a new flow of federal funds would be available for vocational training purposes. Workshops for the blind had long performed a training function; now, for the first time, they were in a position to expand that service without the financial loss entailed in instructing novices whose output was necessarily minimal.

This line of opportunity was carefully followed up; in mid-1945 a formal agreement was reached between National Industries for the Blind and the federal Office of Vocational Rehabilitation, stipulating that OVR recognized "acceptable workshops for the blind as a facility from which appropriate rehabilitation services may be purchased or secured on a basis comparable to that of other types of facilities." For its part, NIB agreed that it would "encourage and assist its affiliated workshops to establish training and employment facilities and opportunities comparable to those of other existing private and public facilities."

As anticipated, the end of the war put the brakes on government purchases. Nearly $1.9 million worth of workshop contracts were cancelled. Federal business during the war years had averaged $8 million annually; in 1946, the first postwar year, the figure plummeted to below $600,000. Thanks to foresighted planning, most of the workshops were prepared for the transition. They were able to maintain about the same overall level of employment and wages because the nation's hunger for civilian goods was so great that commercial sales could largely fill the void left by the drop in federal orders. Also, wartime needs had given the workshops experience in producing a much wider variety of merchandise than ever before. Sewing shops that had made pillowcases for the military now switched to diapers and aprons.

One problem the workshops had in common with the rest of American industry during the postwar reconversion period was difficulty in acquiring needed new equipment. It was at this point that, to take up the slack, some began accepting labor subcontracts—sorting and assembling of parts, packaging goods, etc.—from nearby industrial firms and from such military installations as army camps and air force supply depots. Subcontracting became, in time, one of the most widely used methods of employing blind labor, but where government installations were concerned, this phase of workshop activity met with a setback a few years later, when the Comptroller General ruled that the Wagner-O'Day Act was not applicable to anything other than tangible articles produced by the blind. The ruling meant that workshops could no longer claim preference for subcontract work from military units, although they were free to enter bids on a competitive basis. It was not until the Wagner-O'Day Act was amended in 1971 that this ruling was reversed.

Regrettably, only a few of the workshops heeded the suggestion to follow through on enactment of "little Wagner-O'Day" laws in their own states. In New York, however, agencies for the blind succeeded in getting a "state use" law passed in 1945. To implement the law, the Foundation helped organize a state allocation agency, Industries for the Blind of New York State, and loaned it sufficient capital to get under way.

One of the most productive postwar ideas, initiated by NIB in 1948, was to open up the military commissary markets to blind-made products. The household items sold to the general public were entirely suitable for post exchanges. The idea was simple in concept but difficult of execution; it was not until 1955 that the program was able to thread its way around all the bureaucratic obstacles. Once in the clear, however, it proved a steady and profitable outlet. Commissary sales in 1971, secured through competitive bids, came to $3,350,000. The figure was expected to go higher in the future, since the Wagner-O'Day Act amendments of 1971 required the "non-appropriated fund instrumentalities" of the armed services—post exchanges and military commissaries—to give blind-made products the same preferential status as did all other federal departments.

Because the various federal reorganizations that followed the war changed many of the government's purchasing procedures, NIB decided in 1950 that it needed a permanent representative in the nation's capital to make sure that the Wagner-O'Day program did not get lost in the reshuffle. Robert LeFevre, who had just retired from the federal service, was engaged while continuing to serve, in an unpaid volunteer capacity, as secretary of the Committee on Purchase of Blind-Made Products. He maintained the dual role until 1962; two years later, he was awarded the Migel Medal for his accomplishments. LeFevre made a final contribution by writing a brief history, *The Story of the Wagner O'Day Act*, which NIB published in 1966. He died before the book came off the press.

The postwar period saw several other changes. One was the retirement in 1950 of M. C. Migel as the civilian member of the Committee on Purchase of Blind-Made Products. The Major was then eighty-four years old; five years earlier he had relinquished the presidency of the Foundation to become its board chairman. In 1948 he had also resigned as president of NIB and was named chairman of its board. Migel was succeeded in the presidencies of both the Foundation and the NIB by William Ziegler. (A similar pattern was followed in 1958 when Ziegler died; Jansen Noyes, Jr., took over both presidencies.)

When M. Robert Barnett succeeded Robert Irwin as the Foundation's executive director in 1949, one of his first acts was to clarify the respective areas of responsibility of the Foundation and NIB. Both organizations were getting requests for help with workshop programs. A memorandum of understanding worked out by Barnett and Kleber specified that NIB would handle all requests from existing workshops, but that it would be the Foundation's province to decide, on the basis of the total needs of a community's blind population, whether or not a workshop should be established in a territory where none existed. The agreement also regularized certain intramural relationships. NIB, which had begun with a two-person staff in a single room in the Foundation's building, had now expanded to occupy an entire floor. In 1962, when it needed even more space, the organization moved to a separate location.

Still another change during the postwar years was a two-way expansion of NIB services. Until 1950, membership was restricted to workshops qualified to produce goods that met federal specifications; now participation in NIB's commercial program was opened to shops that did not handle federal orders. The other direction of expansion was the inclusion of industrial homework programs in NIB's marketing services.

Industrial homework was differentiated from hobby pursuits through its definition as an agency service designed "to offer regular work training and remunerative work opportunity to those eligible blind persons who cannot for physical, psychological or geographic reasons leave their homes to travel to and from a place of business." By thus extending the workshop into the home, provision was finally made for the last group of blind workers: those incapable of employment in open industry, in independent business pursuits, or in workshop settings. While organizations for the blind had traditionally made efforts to market the handmade products of blind people working at home, it had been a pin-money proposition at best. The new plan aimed at giving the homebound blind worker a careful course of rehabilitation training, as similar as possible to what he would receive in a workshop, so as to provide him with "an opportunity for reasonably steady employment at a fair and regular wage."

The Fifties saw National Industries for the Blind embarked on a broad-gauged search for ever wider markets. One means toward this end was the development of the brand name "Skilcraft" for all consumer merchandise manufactured by NIB-affiliated workshops. The thought here was that the use of a uniform label on goods of uniform quality would help condition the buying public to choose blind-made products for their quality rather than out of pity.

By the time C. C. Kleber resigned in 1960, NIB was a thriving enterprise whose 62 affiliated workshops did an annual business of more than $24 million, of which $8,700,000 was federal procurement. Kleber's successor was Robert C. Goodpasture, an engineer whose background included a dozen years of business development activity with industrial firms. Goodpasture embarked on a fast-paced program to expand the sales horizons for blind-made products. By 1966 NIB's staff had grown to 70 employees and included industrial designers, engineers, purchasing and marketing specialists. The number of associated workshops was up to 73. Sales totaled more than $43.5 million, of which $19 million was to government departments. Workshop wages that year aggregated $7,700,000. The average hourly wage was $1.39. (By 1971, it had reached $1.75.)

Nineteen sixty-six saw the initiation of a new merchandising system. Display racks of Skilcraft products were installed in chain supermarkets, serviced through truck deliveries from local warehouses. This was a step into the bigtime; it was predicted that, in five years, the rack program, which began with a pilot effort in Ohio, would be expanded to 12 major market areas and produce annual sales in excess of $5 million.

Hard on the heels of this venture came two other innovations. A research and development center was opened in St. Louis to work on new products that the workshops could manufacture, and, for the first time in its history, NIB itself became the owner of a workshop. In late 1966 it bought the Mogdlin Company, a housewares manufacturing firm, with the object of converting its plant facilities into a demonstration workshop for the blind.

An original idea lay back of this purchase. No sheltered workshop had ever been started except on a tiny scale with a handful of workers. As a rule, it took years to acquire enough plant, equipment, and experienced management for a new shop to operate on more than a shoestring basis. It took at least as long to develop markets for its products. The Mogdlin-Maid venture was aimed at showing that an alternative route to growth existed through the purchase and conversion of an ongoing industrial enterprise. The idea had never been tried before.

Under the NIB plan, which was supported by a grant of $105,000 from the Social and Rehabilitation Service of HEW, the Mogdlin-Maid factory in Hazelhurst, Mississippi, would continue in production during a gradual conversion period. All new employees would be blind workers; the sighted employees remaining at their jobs would be trained to form a team with the blind co-workers. Equipment would be retooled, readjusted and automated to fit the capabilities of blind operators. The plant would not only continue to produce the items for which it had well-established sales outlets; it would also begin to manufacture new products, along with parts that could be used by other workshops in making similar new products. Thus the financial risk of new product development would not fall solely on a single pioneering workshop but would be shared by all through National Industries for the Blind.

Another key feature of the Mississippi experiment would be as a demonstration of new and more effective ways of collaborating with a state vocational rehabilitation agency to provide evaluation, training and employment for blind and multi-handicapped blind persons, particularly the latter.

All of these goals were met by 1970, when the Mogdlin-Maid (subsequently renamed Royal-Maid) operation achieved qualified status as a workshop for the blind; i.e., its 68 blind workers accounted for 75 percent of the plant's direct labor. But this was just about the only good news NIB had to impart in 1970. Like many a commercial firm, it had been badly hurt by the business recession and military cutback that began in 1969. It was financially overextended, having expanded too far and too fast in the mistaken expectation that fees from federal orders would continue to supply a firm budgetary underpinning. The decrease in defense spending instituted as part of the "winding down" of the war in Southeast Asia dropped government orders to $22,800,000 in 1970—down from a peak of $28.7 million three years earlier. More serious yet, federal business was scheduled to be even further reduced in 1971, and the rack program was in trouble. It was operating in more than 1,000 supermarkets in four states and aggregating nearly $2 million in sales, but NIB's costs in warehousing and servicing the racks created a substantial budgetary deficit.

Draconic measures were called for. Following a management survey, certain low-margin rack operations were discontinued and the remainder of the rack program was taken over by one of NIB's affiliated workshops, the Cleveland

Society for the Blind. Operation of the commissary sales warehouse in Maryland was transferred to another affiliate, the New York Association for the Blind. The research and development laboratory in St. Louis was closed. Staff was reduced by some 50 percent. Robert Goodpasture resigned and was replaced by Noel B. Price, who had been his first assistant since 1965. A simultaneous reorganization took place in NIB's board of directors. Jansen Noyes, Jr., board chairman since 1963 and president for five years before that, was succeeded by Thor W. Kolle, Jr., former president; the presidency went to Abram Claude, Jr., former secretary-treasurer.

To relieve some of the financial pressure on NIB, the Foundation made it a $200,000 grant to reduce the large bank loan which had financed purchase of the Mogdlin Company. It was the first time since NIB's earliest days that the Foundation had been called upon to supply funds to the agency it had voluntarily "spun off" at birth. Additional financial help came from NIB's affiliated workshops, which loaned it an aggregate of $87,000, and from the Seeing Eye, Inc., which made a grant of $38,000 to keep NIB's rehabilitation service program going. By the end of 1971, National Industries for the Blind appeared to be stabilized on a sounder operating basis.

What happened to NIB during this troubled period constituted more than operational and financial reorganization. There was a change in direction, away from the toe-to-toe competition with profit-making industry which had been the main thrust during the Sixties and back to the basic purpose of services aimed at giving blind men and women maximum opportunity for self-support through constructive use of workshop facilities for vocational training and employment. Leadership in this turnaround was credited to Noel Price, who was presented with the Migel Medal in 1972; in appropriate tandem, his fellow awardee that year was Senator Randolph.

Beginning with World War II, a gradual change had taken place in the types of blind people employed in the workshops. Stepped-up vocational rehabilitation services had enabled the most efficient workers to take their place in open industry. Increasingly, those who remained were the multihandicapped.

NIB's Mogdlin venture had as one of its essential purposes the development of methods that could fit such multihandicapped persons into workshop production, not only by introducing needed equipment modifications but by incorporating all the necessary collateral rehabilitation services as well. Brought into play were medical, psychiatric, and psychological testing; individual and group counseling; assistance with mobility and with skills of daily living; recreational services; social work help with family relationships, housing, and other problems.

To give leadership to this renewed focus on individual needs, in 1969 NIB employed, as director of rehabilitation services, Harold Richterman, who had held a similar post at the Industrial Home for the Blind in Brooklyn. Richterman's function was not limited to Mississippi but included helping workshops all over the country upgrade their standards and strengthen their rehabilitation programs to a point where they could qualify for accreditation by the National Accreditation Council for Agencies Serving the Blind and Visually Handicapped and/or certification by the General Council of Workshops.

Emphasis on standards was a keynote of the Sixties in all areas of human services. That sheltered workshops for all types of handicapped persons needed help in meeting minimum standards of quality was recognized in the 1965 amendments to the Vocational Rehabilitation Act, which provided financial support for modernization and expansion of facilities and equipment, for construction of new facilities, for innovation in training methods and techniques, and for employment of qualified staff.

Improvement of workshop operating policies and practices was long overdue. Even during the period when NIB was being hailed as a success story in the annals of American industrial progress, thoughtful critics were pointing out, with equal justice, that conditions within the workshops as places of employment left much to be desired.

There had always been philosophic differences over operating policies and practices. To the sponsoring agencies and the taxpaying or contributing public which financed the workshops, the people who worked in them were subsidized clients of a non-profit social service. Many of the people, however, thought of themselves as employees who earned by means of their labor and were therefore entitled to the same rights and benefits as all other workers: minimum wages, unemployment insurance, paid vacations and various other fringe benefits. While many of the more enlightened workshops did, in fact, provide such benefits, others were guilty of substandard work practices if not outright exploitation. Even these, it should be said, were not necessarily acting callously but out of differences in viewpoint as to what workshops were designed to accomplish. Those who believed workshops should operate as self-supporting entities, neither making a profit nor requiring subsidy, attempted to hold on to their best and most productive workers, making little or no effort to move them out into open industry. In such shops the less capable workers who could not earn their keep were left to fend for themselves; they were given little help in improving their skills or output and were the first to be laid off during slack periods.

Most workshops for the blind compensated their workers on a piecework basis comparable to competitive industry, but some undercut prevailing wage rates, particularly when vying for industrial subcontracts. Some were paying low trainee wages to persons employed under a vocational rehabilitation plan and kept such persons in trainee status for unduly long periods. The charge was frequently made that state vocational counselors collaborated in this process by "dumping" clients who represented difficult rehabilitation problems into the workshops and leaving them there indefinitely.

If a few workshops for the blind were indeed guilty of these practices, the situation in sheltered workshops for other groups of handicapped people was often infinitely worse. This was the principal reason why, when the National Federation of the Blind initiated legislation in 1960 seeking an amendment to the Fair Labor Standards Act that would introduce a mandatory minimum wage scale in workshops for the blind, the Foundation and the AAWB opposed the bill. Although fully sympathetic to the intent of the legislation (which subsequently died in committee), these two national bodies held that it was discriminatory to focus such a bill on workshops for the blind, which were paying demonstrably higher wages than the sheltered shops for people with other disabilities. Four years later, when a similar measure—again sponsored by the National Federation of the Blind—was introduced that would apply to sheltered workshops for all types of handicapped people, it received the firm support of the Foundation and the AAWB.

Passed in 1966 over vigorous opposition from most organizations in the sheltered workshop field, the Fair Labor Standards Act amendments established, for the first time in history, a statutory minimum (50 percent of the going minimum wage) for people employed in all sheltered workshops. While exempting certain classes of workshop clients from this wage standard, it introduced safeguards to require annual certification by a state vocational rehabilitation agency that the exempted persons were either in a work evaluation or training status, or were so handicapped that their earning capacity was severely impaired, or were employed in a new category of facility, called a work activities center. A work activities center was not really a workshop but a therapeutic program for persons with little productive capacity.

While the organizations for and of the blind succeeded in overcoming the pressures of other interests in the sheltered workshop field with respect to minimum wages, they met with failure when it came to unemployment insurance. The Employment Security Act amendments of 1970, which mandated such benefits for all regular employees of non-profit organizations nationwide, specifically exempted clients of sheltered workshops from coverage.

The argument that prevailed with Congress in this instance was as much sheer weight of numbers as anything else. Sheltered workshops for all types of physically, mentally, emotionally, and socially handicapped persons grew tremendously during the Fifties and Sixties; in 1970, the number of such workshops exceeded 1,500, with an aggregate of 100,000 clients. In comparison, the blind workshop field was tiny: approximately a hundred shops employing 5,000 people. Insistence that non-profit organizations would be subjected to ruinous financial burdens if they had to carry the cost of unemployment insurance coverage for 100,000 people induced Congress to classify handicapped people employed in the workshops as recipients of vocational rehabilitation rather than as workers entitled to the same protection as other labor groups.

Over the years, repeated but unsuccessful efforts were also made by organizations of blind people to gain collective bargaining rights in the workshops. Even without the right of unionization, strikes occurred now and then. A report on the public reaction to a sit-down strike in Pittsburgh in 1937 observed that the press was "more impressed with the oddity than the gravity of the situation." In 1961, however, a strike in the St. Louis Lighthouse for the Blind over the issue of union recognition was treated more seriously. It went before the National Labor Relations Board which, in a split decision, refused jurisdiction. The two-month stoppage was finally settled by an arbitrated agreement in which union recognition was ruled out but two local labor leaders were added to the Lighthouse board of directors.

There was one other philosophic disagreement over workshop employment of blind men and women that arose from time to time. As has been noted, the overall sheltered workshop movement expanded greatly after World War II. While many of the newer shops served only people with a specific handicap (cerebral palsy, mental illness or retardation, alcoholism, cardiac weakness, etc.), others were set up as community workshops that served people with a variety of disabilities.

In work for the blind, the traditional position was that blind men and women were best off in their own shops, where conditions and equipment could be adapted to their particular needs. It was further argued that blind workers tended to be "lost" in the community workshops, where they were sure to be greatly outnumbered by people with other disabilities, and where those in charge lacked experience in how to deal with the emotional, psychological, and practical problems of blindness. Whatever the merits of these arguments, they seemed to contravene the more modern philosophy that blind people could best gain public acceptance through integration with the sighted in all phases of life.

This moot point was one of several issues raised during the Congressional hearings in 1970 and 1971 that preceded passage, in July 1971, of a sweeping set of amendments to the Wagner-O'Day Act. The major changes effected by Public Law 92-28 were these:

• Blind workers lost the exclusive preferential position they had held for 33 years in relation to federal procurement. The Wagner-O'Day umbrella was extended to all sheltered workshops for the handicapped. As a concession to the *status quo ante,* workshops for the blind were given priority (after the prison industries, which retained their traditional first-preferred status) on the manufacture of products for federal use; orders that the workshops for the blind were not in a position to handle would then go, as a second priority, to workshops serving persons with other disabilities.

• The provision of services as well as products was written into the law for the first time. Workshops for the blind were given a five-year priority on service contracts for federal agencies on the same "fair price" basis as the sale of products.

• Commissaries, post exchanges, and similar "non-appropriated fund" operations of the armed services were required to abide by the same Wagner-O'Day rules as all other government agencies. Workshop sales to these outlets, previously handled through competitive bids, were brought under the "fair price" provisions.

• For the first time, a budget was provided to staff the federal committee, whose membership was doubled to 14 and whose title was similarly enlarged to become the Committee for Purchase of Products and Services of the Blind and Other Severely Handicapped.

This bill to extend the provisions of the Wagner-O'Day Act to workshops serving other handicapped persons was introduced in April 1970 by Senator Jacob K. Javits of New York, with Senators Jennings Randolph of West Virginia and Warren Magnuson of Washington as co-sponsors. A companion measure was introduced in the House by a group of Congressmen led by Representative Craig Hosmer of California. The legislation was initiated by the International Association of Rehabilitation Facilities with the support of the National Association of Sheltered Workshops, the Federation of the Handicapped, Goodwill Industries of America, the National Association for Retarded Children, and the National Rehabilitation Association.

From the field of blindness, endorsement came from AAWB, the Foundation, NIB and the Blinded Veterans Association, all of which took the position that it would be poor public policy to refuse to share the Wagner-O'Day Act privileges with persons handicapped by disabilities other than blindness, so long as adequate safeguards protected the needs and rights of blind persons. Testimony in opposition to the bill came from the National Federation of the Blind and the American Council for the Blind, mainly on the grounds that administrative changes under the amended Act might operate to the detriment of blind workers.

Some witnesses at the Congressional hearings preceding the bill's passage described the expanded program's potential in euphoric terms, with predictions that the four-hundred-plus items on the 1971 federal Schedule of Blind-Made Products would soon grow to 75,000 items involving astronomical sums. The experience after one year gave greater credence to the assertions of other witnesses, who said the workshops newly admitted to the Act's provisions would first have to experience the same "learning curve" that began for workshops for the blind in 1938. Still, the newcomers were expected to have an easier time of it; here, as elsewhere, blind men and women had blazed a trail for others to follow.

15

The Magna Charta of the Blind

The Randolph-Sheppard Act of 1936 and the Wagner-O'Day Act of 1938 lit helpful hearthfires of economic security for particular groups of blind men and women, but it took the Vocational Rehabilitation Act amendments of 1943 (the Barden-LaFollette Act) to kindle the steady flame at which tools of wider opportunity could be forged.

Few blind persons benefited from the original Vocational Rehabilitation Act, which became law in 1920. This was due partly to lack of imagination on the part of the state vocational education boards, which considered blindness so severe a disability as to constitute a hopeless impediment to employment. It was also due to the limitations of the Act itself, which made no provision for medical intervention that might remove or ameliorate the disabling condition.

The Barden-LaFollette Act changed all that, and a good deal more besides. People in the field illustrated its effect this way: before 1943, if a man lost a leg, a rehabilitation agency had to train him for a job that could be done by a one-legged man; after 1943, the agency had the funds to buy an artificial limb and turn the man into a two-legged worker.

The same analogy applied to clients blinded by cataracts or other medically correctable eye defects. Thousands of operations were successfully performed with funds made available under the Barden-LaFollette Act; thousands of other people who did not need surgery were fitted with low-vision aids to overcome much of their visual limitation.

Funds were not the only factor accounting for the momentous turnaround that took place after 1943. In the effort to cope with the casualties of World War II, American military hospitals became laboratories for bold medical techniques which pioneered new ways of dealing with visual restoration. Significant strides were made in mobility training and other rehabilitation techniques. Of at least equal importance was the ever-mounting body of evidence that blindness was by no means an insuperable obstacle to attainment of many kinds of vocational goals.

Because little of this progress would have taken place without the specialized skills of the organizations working with and for blind people, one of the most important contributions of the Barden-LaFollette Act was the way it legislated these organizations into partnership with the federal government. The Act specifically provided that any state with a legally constituted commission or agency for the blind could assign to it the administration of the federal-state vocational rehabilitation program for visually disabled persons. For the first time, state agencies for the blind, some of which had been in existence for more than thirty years, were no longer solely dependent on the capricious ups and downs of annual legislative appropriations. For the first time, they had sufficiently firm financial backing to plan, staff, and organize their work on a systematic, comprehensive basis. It was no wonder that some called the Barden-LaFollette Act "the Magna Charta of the blind."

Why would a nation, in the midst of the most devastating war in its history, pause to concern itself with a social problem unrelated to the war effort? One answer is that the Barden-LaFollette Act, as originally conceived, did have a direct bearing on the war. When, in 1942, legislation was proposed to amend the 1920 Vocational Rehabilitation Act, it sparked little interest in Congress and none whatsoever in the House Committee on Education, which had jurisdiction over such legislation, until the committee's chairman was informed that it was designed to take care of disabled veterans as well as civilians. Although the civilian and veteran components were later divorced, by the time the separate law for veterans' rehabilitation was signed on March 24, 1943, the bill for vocational rehabilitation of civilians had gathered enough momentum to roll forward on its own.

In the history of work for the blind, the events surrounding the evolution of the Barden-LaFollette Act might correctly be considered a daring gamble. As originally drafted, the bill proposed federal-state sharing of the costs of vocational rehabilitation service for all disabled persons *except* the blind. Where the blind were concerned, a separate title stipulated that the federal government would pay the entire cost. This was surely a boon—or was it? Not a boon but a boomerang, concluded the leaders in work for the blind, who rejected it out of hand. The same spokesmen who had successfully pleaded for special treatment for blind persons under the Social Security Act, the Randolph-Sheppard Act, and the Wagner-O'Day Act took the position that this time there should be no whit of difference between the financing of rehabilitation services for the blind and the financing of similar services for persons disabled by other conditions.

The reasoning behind this about-face was explained in special bulletins issued by the American Foundation for the Blind in late 1942. State agencies for the blind, these said, "feel that a system by which a large proportion of their work will be financed by the Federal government . . . will jeopardize if not destroy all local initiative and independence." Also, should the impression be created that the federal government was taking total responsibility for the blind, private philanthropy might no longer support voluntary agencies.

The almost panicky tone of these communications reflected an understandable flurry of alarm. Workers for the blind had been taken by surprise by the move to amend the Vocational Rehabilitation Act. Apparently the attitude of the government authorities who initiated the measure was that blind persons constituted so small a proportion of the disabled, there was no need to consult them or their spokesmen. Indignantly, the leadership set about correcting any such notion.

Companion bills to amend the Vocational Rehabilitation Act of 1920 were introduced on August 13, 1942. The House bill was sponsored by Graham Barden of North Carolina, the Senate's by Robert M. LaFollette, Jr., of Wisconsin. Barden, a member of the House Committee on Education, chaired a subcommittee which held a series of hearings on his bill a few weeks after its introduction. The session on the separate title dealing with the blind was scheduled for October 15.

On October 14, the Foundation convened a strategy meeting in Washington at which officers of the AAWB, the AAIB, and a goodly number of executives of state and voluntary agencies sought to reach agreement on the changes they would press for. The group agreed there were only two basic issues to be pursued: first, the bill should specify the use of state agencies for the blind in the delivery of vocational rehabilitation services to blind persons and second, the formula for federal-state support of these services should be identical with the formula applicable to the rehabilitation of other disabled persons.

Because of a backstage power struggle between the Veterans Administration and the Federal Security Agency, the 77th Congress wound up without action on the Barden and LaFollette bills. The replacement measures introduced at the opening of the 78th Congress incorporated the two changes sought by workers for the blind, whose only remaining concern was how the legislation, when passed, would be administered. At the instigation of M.C. Migel, Senator Robert F. Wagner put a direct question to Paul V. McNutt, administrator of the Federal Security Agency. "If this bill passes," Wagner wrote McNutt on February 1, 1943, "is it your intention to delegate to the state commissions for the blind responsibility for carrying out all rehabilitation work for the blind?"

The reply he received was most reassuring:

It is my intention . . . to work to the greatest possible extent through blind commissions or comparable organizations set up under State administrative or legal structures. It is not my intention to establish Federal facilities for any of the services [for] the blind, unless it becomes absolutely necessary through failure of the State bodies or organizations to do the job effectively.

McNutt's statement provided the final evidence that the workers for the blind had won their gamble. They had been fully aware that insistence on parallel treatment for those disabled by blindness and those disabled by other conditions entailed a real risk. If the two programs were to be dealt with identically, why should they not become one? It was no secret that control of the entire rehabilitation package was sought by the state vocational boards. To avert this, Irwin had visited, and Helen Keller had written to, a number of key legislators during the Congressional recess. Local and state agencies had also made it their business to contact their own representatives in Congress, and so had numbers of blind individuals stimulated by the Foundation's frequent bulletins.

The amended bills, as finally reported out, "gave us all we have ever asked for," Irwin wrote Migel jubilantly on March 9, 1943. Three months later, the Barden-LaFollette Act became Public Law 78-113. These were its basic features:

• The federal government would make grants to the states covering the total costs of vocational guidance and placement of physically disabled civilians.

• There would be fifty-fifty federal-state sharing of the costs of providing medical and psychiatric examinations, hospitalization and medical treatment, prosthetic appliances, vocational training, transportation, occupational tools and equipment, and maintenance payments to clients while they were undergoing rehabilitation.

• Certain of these services would be provided to all clients without charge: counseling and guidance, physical examination, vocational training and placement. If financially able to do so, clients would meet all or part of the cost of all other services. Whatever costs they were unable to meet would be defrayed by the vocational rehabilitation agency.

• State agencies were permitted to contract with qualified public or voluntary bodies for the provision of part or all of the rehabilitation services. This brought into the picture almost the entire spectrum of community agencies engaged in work with the handicapped.

To qualify for participation in the program, each state had to submit a detailed plan outlining how its vocational rehabilitation services would be set up and administered. Such plans had two parallel sections, one dealing with disabled persons other than the blind, the other with blind persons. The Foundation lost no time getting busy on the latter. A bulletin went out to the state agencies spelling out the necessary procedures and offering help in developing sound plans; in the course of the next few months, 14 states took advantage of the offer.

There was also a public relations problem to be met. Ever since passage of the Social Security Act, workers for the blind had had to cope with resentment on the part of welfare officials over separate treatment for blind persons. They were aware that this spilled over to state legislatures and to the public at large. As a precautionary countermeasure, the Foundation sent out a statement detailing the reasons why blind persons needed separate handling. Its principal emphasis was that only agencies for the blind had the specialized knowledge and experience to deal with the social and psychological factors which constituted essential elements in vocational rehabilitation of blind persons.

The precaution proved largely unnecessary. Public Law 78-113 provided more than enough work for all in terms of scope, responsibility, and steadily increasing caseload. Five years after its enactment, the federal head of vocational rehabilitation reported that in the previous year (1947) some 44,000 disabled persons had been rehabilitated, 115,000 persons were currently being prepared for employment, more than 1.5 million disabled Americans were in need of rehabilitation services, and newly disabled persons were accruing at the rate of 250,000 a year.

While the figures for blind rehabilitation clients kept pace proportionately, they were minuscule by comparison. Of the 44,000 persons rehabilitated for employment in 1947, for example, 2,155 were blind and an additional 3,000 were visually impaired. Modest as these numbers were, they nonetheless signalled the birth of a vigorous forward thrust in work for the blind.

What may well have been the most far-reaching effect of the Barden-LaFollette Act was the impetus it gave to the establishment of rehabilitation centers, which brought together under a single roof the interdisciplinary battery of personal adjustment and vocational preparation services that could enable a blind man or woman to function with minimal limitation. It was not only new muscle that the Act afforded, but new blood as well. In a 1970 review of the Act's long-term effects, Burt L. Risley and Charles W. Hoehne, executive director and assistant director respectively of the Texas Commission for the Blind, made the point that "many people who have spent the greater part of their careers in work for the blind entered into the profession as a result of the staff recruitment spurred by this legislation."

With vocational rehabilitation funds serving as financial anchor, most state programs were able to develop and maintain a wide range of other services for blind people not involved in vocational rehabilitation. Risley and Hoehne de scribed the state agency programs of the Seventies as delivering

> a configuration of various services. In addition to vocational rehabilitation, a state agency for the blind normally will be the licensing agency for the Randolph-Sheppard Vending Stand Program within the state; the agency will offer home teacher services for the elderly or other homebound cases; some sort of prevention of blindness program, usually directed toward children, will be found; and the agency will in one way or another be involved with the talking book machine program of the Library of Congress.

> A number of state agencies . . . have responsibility in the administration of the public assistance program for the blind. In some states, the agency is responsible for the operation of sheltered workshops, and increasing numbers of state agencies are establishing and operating comprehensive rehabilitation centers.

On the federal level, too, work for the blind gathered new momentum with the Barden-LaFollette Act. Recognizing that vocational rehabilitation now embraced a much wider sweep of activities than in the past, a new federal unit, the Office of Vocational Rehabilitation (OVR), was created within the Federal Security Agency. Its nucleus was the staff which had formerly administered these services in the Office of Education. Named to head the new unit was Michael J. Shortley, who had served with the federal Board for Vocational Education, with the Veterans Administration, and with the Social Security Board in various administrative capacities. John A. Kratz, who had headed the vocational rehabilitation program in the Office of Education, became OVR's assistant director under Shortley.

The transfer from the Office of Education also involved the Services for the Blind unit under Joseph Clunk. With the administration of the vending stand program now part of the new OVR, Clunk had the opportunity to use funds provided by the Barden-LaFollette Act for rapid expansion of the industrial placement program that had begun under the Randolph-Sheppard Act.

The frequent reorganizations of the federal government's executive branch in recent decades, accompanied by name changes and interdepartmental transfers, make it difficult to trace the development of particular functions. The problem is further complicated by the custom of using initials as short-cut identifications. The following capsule summary is provided to guide the reader through the balance of this book,

Under the Smith-Fess Act of 1920, vocational rehabilitation was placed under the federal Board for Vocational Education, which was subsequently placed in the Office of Education. The latter was one of the units which became a component of the Federal Security Agency (FSA), an umbrella superagency created in 1939 to bring together a number of domestic social programs formerly located in separate federal departments.

With the passage of the Barden-LaFollette Act, vocational rehabilitation was taken out of the Office of Education and given separate status within the FSA. The change was reflected in its new name, Office of Vocational Rehabilitation (OVR). Ten years later the Eisenhower administration added new spokes to the FSA umbrella; along with broadened responsibilities, it acquired a new name, the Department of Health, Education, and Welfare (HEW). In 1963, as part of an internal HEW reorganization, OVR was reconstituted as the Vocational Rehabilitation Administration (VRA). Yet another HEW reorganization took place in 1967, under which all of its service-giving units were brought together in a single agency, the Social and Rehabilitation Service (SRS). This involved more name-changing. What had been VRA now became known as the Rehabilitation Services Administration (RSA).

Thus the initials OVR, VRA, and RSA all refer to the same federal unit at different periods in time. Under OVR and VRA, that segment of the unit concerned with blind persons was called the Division of Services for the Blind; in 1969 the title was expanded to Division of Services for the Blind and Visually Handicapped. In 1970 a further administrative reshuffling within HEW established a new overarching structure in SRS, the Division of Special Populations, and the blindness unit, now renamed Office of the Blind and Visually Handicapped, was placed under it. This demotion to less than full divisional status evoked so strong a protest from the leading organizations in the field of blindness that the order was subsequently rescinded and the Office of the Blind and Visually Handicapped was restored to its former divisional status in the Social and Rehabilitation Service.

The foregoing digression from a chronological account of vocational rehabilitation history might also serve to introduce the major federal personalities who shaped it. Michael J. Shortley, the first chief of OVR, was succeeded in 1950 by Mary E. Switzer, under whose tenure vocational rehabilitation grew from a lusty infant to giant stature. The year she took over, the overall rehabilitation budget was $20.5 million; when she retired 20 years later, the budget had multiplied 25-fold to over $500 million.

Mary Elizabeth Switzer was a career civil servant who entered federal employment in 1922, a year after graduation from Radcliffe College. She began as a junior economist in the statistics section of the Treasury Department and was steadily promoted until, by 1934, she was in an upper administrative echelon of the Public Health Service, then located in the Treasury Department. When the Federal Security Agency was created in 1939, the Public Health Service was one of the programs moved into it, and Miss Switzer was promoted to the job of assistant to the FSA administrator. Her superior performance in this post led to her appointment as director of OVR when Shortley resigned.

The 1963 reorganization that changed OVR's name to VRA also changed Mary Switzer's title from director to commissioner. The crowning success of her career was her selection in 1967 as administrator of the comprehensive Social and Rehabilitation Service, which broadened her jurisdiction to include the public welfare programs as well as rehabilitation. She retired in 1970 and died a year later at the age of seventy-one.

To the achievement of her outstanding record Mary Switzer brought a unique blend of personal qualities. She was a surefooted and knowledgeable administrator with a deserved reputation for always doing her homework. This fact, plus the ability to articulate her deeply-felt convictions about the value of rehabilitation, inspired bipartisan confidence in her in key Congressional committees and in top bureaucratic circles. A lifetime of government service gave her a shrewd and sophisticated insight into political currents. She also made it her business to know the strengths and weaknesses of her colleagues on the national, state, and local levels. Thus armed, she could be a powerful friend or a formidable foe.

Mary Switzer's acknowledged bias was in favor of innovative research. During her tenure, 184 research and demonstration grants in blindness alone were made by her agency. When she received the Shotwell Award from the American Association of Workers for the Blind in 1962, the citation acclaimed her "action to liberate humanity from . . . the tyranny of physical disabilities." The Foundation's Migel Medal, which went to her in 1965, paid tribute to "the breadth of her vision and the warmth of her heart." At the end of 1972 preparations were being made to name one of HEW's headquarters structures in Washington the Mary E. Switzer Memorial Building.

Within the federal vocational rehabilitation unit, Joseph Clunk initiated services for the blind in 1937. In 1950 he was succeeded by Maurice I. Tynan. A graduate of Perkins, Tynan spent his entire career in work for the blind, beginning as an instructor at the Maryland School for the Blind. When the Canadian National Institute for the Blind was founded in 1919, he moved to Toronto to initiate their vocational adjustment program. He returned to the United States two years later to work with the Veterans Bureau, then became superintendent of Evergreen, where he remained until its closing in 1925. Then he went to Minnesota to head that state's services for blind residents. He joined the federal vocational rehabilitation service in 1938 and had become assistant chief of its services for the blind when Clunk's resignation brought him the top post in 1950.

On Tynan's retirement six years later, he was succeeded by Harmon Burton Aycock, who had spent the 13 previous years as head of the Louisiana state agency for the blind. Aycock, the only sighted person ever to head the federal services for the blind, resigned in 1958 and was succeeded by his assistant, Louis H. Rives, Jr.

Totally blind since the age of two, Rives held a degree in law from the College of William and Mary in his native state of Virginia. He spent his first four years after graduation on the legal staff of the Federal Security Agency; in 1947 he transferred to the rehabilitation service, where he served in various administrative capacities. Rives resigned as director of the Division of Services for the Blind in 1964 to become program planning consultant for the overall VRA. He was followed in the blindness post by Douglas C. MacFarland, who was still the incumbent in 1972.

MacFarland came to the federal agency from the Virginia Commission for the Visually Handicapped, where he had spent two years as assistant director and eight years as director. Born in 1918 and blind since the age of nine, he attended the public schools of his native New Jersey and earned a bachelor's, a master's, and a doctoral degree in vocational rehabilitation from New York University. He pursued his professional specialty in work with three state agencies for the blind—New Jersey, Delaware, and Virginia, successively—amassing a total of 22 years of experience in these posts before being named to the federal office. Unassuming, articulate, and gregarious, MacFarland enjoyed great popularity with his colleagues. He was elected to the presidency of AAWB in 1963 and again in 1969.

Compared with World War II, the war in Korea was a minor social earthquake, but it, too, had the effect of refocussing the nation's attention on manpower utilization. A report issued by a high-level task force on the handicapped on how to make more effective use of disabled persons in the nation's labor pool became a springboard for the enactment, in 1954, of Public Law 83-565. This law introduced basic changes in the Vocational Rehabilitation Act. The most significant was replacement of the system of all-purpose grants to the states with separate grant programs for research, personnel training, demonstration projects, and facilities expansion. Separate budgeting for each of these gave the OVR the flexibility to put its money where the needs were.

Rehabilitation is a skilled person-to-person service requiring special knowledge and training. P.L. 83-565 made it possible to give tangible recognition to the need for properly equipped personnel. It was a coincidence, but a revealing one, that the very first research and development project supported by the OVR under the new grant program was to the American Foundation for the Blind for a 1955 survey of the functions, qualifications, and compensation levels of professional and administrative personnel in work for the blind. The findings, published in 1958, had an immediate impact in stimulating improved salaries and personnel practices. It had a longer-range effect as well, serving as one of the basic documents in the later work of the Commission on Standards and Accreditation of Agencies Serving the Blind. Two follow-up personnel studies were made in 1961 and 1966.

While much of the research in work for the blind sponsored under the 1954 Vocational Rehabilitation Act amendments dealt with specific aspects of placement and vocational training, it was not confined to these subjects. It was Mary Switzer's view that "the real challenge in the field of work for the blind is . . . how one can compensate for loss of sight in a seeing world," and the federal agency financed a staggeringly wide spectrum of projects. It sponsored early sensory research to explore development of ultrasonic mobility devices, electronic reading machines, and other technological substitutes for sight. It established 30 optical aids clinics that pioneered new ways of overcoming the handicaps caused by partial blindness. It supported demonstrations in orientation and mobility training services. It moved into the field of medical education through grants to develop teaching programs for residents in ophthalmology in university hospitals. It supported research in computerized translation of inkprint into braille. It funded psychological investigations into attitudes toward blindness on the part of sighted people and among blind people themselves. It paid for publications and educational films to interpret and promote public interest in rehabilitation. It assisted in sponsorship of international conferences on worldwide problems of blindness.

The projects on aspects of vocational preparation, training, and placement were equally far-ranging. They included pilot programs to examine employment opportunities in agricultural pursuits, in industrial homework, in professional occupations, in computer programming, in hospital service jobs, in hotel and motel work, in recreational services. They enabled Arkansas Enterprises for the Blind to establish a training program that taught blind persons to work as taxpayer service representatives; by the end of 1971 there were 60 such persons working in Internal Revenue Service offices in 35 states. They developed guidelines for manual arts instruction and the use of trade schools for vocational training of blind students. There were numerous projects related to prevocational services of all types, ranging from braille instruction to psychiatric testing.

To attract qualified personnel, training grants went to universities and other teaching institutions for courses in the several rehabilitation disciplines; support was also given for student traineeships and research fellowships.

Predictably, not all of these projects landed on target, but even those that failed were useful in identifying unproductive lines of inquiry, while those that attained their objectives sometimes exceeded their initial promise. One such was the set of three successive projects conducted by the Industrial Home for the Blind in rehabilitation and training of deaf-blind adults. The results achieved over a ten-year period at an aggregate cost of some $700,000 in grants led directly to the creation in 1967 of the National Center for Deaf-Blind Youths and Adults.

Launched by P.L. 83-565, vocational rehabilitation grants in blindness research and demonstration accelerated at a steady pace. Beginning with five projects aggregating $32,000 in 1955, the year after the law was passed, by 1964 the cumulative total was just over $4 million. Five years later, the $10 million mark had been exceeded.

The 1960s saw the United States grow increasingly aware of flaws in its social fabric. Poverty in the midst of affluence. Racial discrimination and oppression of minorities in the midst of democracy. In a nation proud of its medical skill, unmet health needs in millions of people. Youth in ferment. Most bewildering and divisive of all, the United States had somehow stumbled into a war nobody wanted and nobody seemed to know how to stop.

Before long terms like consumerism, community control, welfare rights, black power, student revolt, began to vie in newspaper headlines with other catch phrases signifying the nation's efforts to attack some of these problems: War on Poverty, Economic Opportunity, Medicare, Medicaid, Welfare Reform, Great Society. Many of these measures took as their prototype the successful experience of the Vocational Rehabilitation Act.

It was generally acknowledged that the nation's investment in vocational rehabilitation had paid handsome dividends not only in human restoration but in the cost-benefit ratio, i.e., the financial cost of rehabilitating a handicapped person to the point of self-support as against the taxes then paid by him as a wage-earner. It was this recognition that paved the way for the ever larger scope of the vocational rehabilitation program. The 1965 amendments lifted appropriation ceilings for the three succeeding years from $385 million in 1966 to $526 million in 1968. Subsequent amendments brought the ceiling up to $800 million for 1972.

The 1965 amendments did more than authorize higher spending. For the first time, federal funds could be granted toward construction of new rehabilitation centers and workshops, toward expansion, remodeling and renovation of existing facilities, and toward defraying much of the cost of staffing. Washington's share of the basic federal-state partnership was raised from 50 percent to 75 percent, and its share of project grants to 90 percent. Vocational rehabilitation agencies were authorized to furnish reader service for blind students and professional persons without charge. A new clause permitted a severely handicapped individual to receive up to six months of diagnostic rehabilitation services before a decision was reached on his potential for ultimate employment.

When the Act was amended once again in 1968, a disturbing new element was introduced through a clause extending its provisions to people who were not physically or mentally handicapped but were socially disadvantaged. The 1968 law authorized the setting aside of $50 million in 1969, $75 million in 1970, and $100 million in 1971 to finance a new program for "comprehensive evaluation of the rehabilitation potential of the disadvantaged."

In the hearings that preceded passage, John F. Nagle, representing the National Federation of the Blind (NFB), spoke for the entire field when he urged that, given the greater difficulty of working with the disabled, any service for non-disabled persons should be separately financed, staffed, and administered. He asserted that, should the same vocational counselor be assigned to work with both disabled and disadvantaged clients, the counselor,

> pressured by the need to show the results of his work by the numbers of persons served, would find it much too advantageous to concentrate his attentions and labors upon the relatively simple and soluble problems of the socially and culturally and educationally disadvantaged, rather than [on] the difficult and seemingly insoluble problems of the physically and mentally disabled.

While these fears turned out to be premature—this particular clause in the 1968 amendments was never funded—the possibility that rehabilitation services for the disabled and the non-disabled might be combined continued to be a source of concern. In May 1971 H.R. 8395, a bill calling for radical revision of the Vocational Rehabilitation Act, was introduced by Congressman Carl Perkins of Kentucky at the request of the National Rehabilitation Association. One of the changes proposed by this measure was its definition of handicapped workers as including people with a variety of social and behavioral disorders "who have unusual and difficult problems in connection with their rehabilitation. . . . Such classes include but are not limited to alcoholics, drug addicts, migratory farm workers and public offenders."

At about the same time Senator Jennings Randolph put before the Senate a bill, co-sponsored by 49 Senators, which had been initiated by the six national organizations representing the blind. An identical measure was subsequently sponsored in the House by Congressman Perkins. In introducing the Senate measure, Randolph pointed out that although much legislation existed for the benefit of elderly people, no federal program—neither Medicare, Medicaid, public assistance, Old Age Survivors and Disability Insurance, the Older Americans Act nor the Public Health Service Act—brought to elderly blind persons the non-medical adjustment services available to younger blind adults as part of vocational rehabilitation. These adjustment services, designed to reduce dependency, included training in orientation and mobility, in activities of daily living and in communication skills.

The effect such training could have on the welfare of the older blind person was spelled out by Irvin P. Schloss when, as spokesman for the Foundation, the AAWB, and the Blinded Veterans Association, he testified before the House committee on the Randolph-Perkins bill. It could mean, he said,

> that an elderly blind diabetic won't have to become a leg amputee as well, because he will be trained in orientation and mobility skills to avoid repeated bruising and the possibility of gangrene. It could mean that an elderly blind person will be taught to avoid falls and the fractured hip which results in long-term invalidism and shortens life . . . [that he] will be taught mobility and personal management skills so he can go to the bathroom by himself, bathe and dress himself, fix himself a cup of coffee and a snack, go for a walk when he wants to, be a substantially independent member of his family group, not a burdensome dependent who has to be waited on for his every little need.

The basic purport of the bill, where blind persons were concerned, was that the factor of employability should no longer be the sole criterion for delivery of rehabilitation services. Men and women over forty constituted by far the largest percentage of the blind population. Of those newly blinded each year, three out of four were middle-aged or older. It was the newly blinded who most urgently needed training in how to live without sight, yet in a youth-oriented society people over forty were seldom regarded as "feasible" for employment and were thus denied access to vocational rehabilitation services.

A good many other bills were introduced in 1971 and 1972 to make substantive changes in the Vocational Rehabilitation Act scheduled to expire on June 30, 1972. One, sponsored by Representative John Brademas of Indiana, was aimed at keeping the Act focused on the needs of the group it was originally designed to serve—the physically and mentally disabled. The bill was, in effect, a countermeasure to the movement that would dilute the Act through coverage of non-disabled, socially disadvantaged people.

H.R. 8395 was the bill finally passed by Congress in October 1972 after extensive hearings and many modifications, but it was pocket-vetoed by President Nixon after Congress adjourned. Its sponsors planned to reintroduce it as soon as Congress reconvened in January 1973. In the meantime, the existing Act was authorized to continue without change for an additional year.

In 1902, a man named Robinson Pierce began a professional career as a teacher of mathematics at Stevens Institute of Technology. A dozen years later, having gradually gone blind, he moved to the country and started over again as a chicken farmer. Toward the end of his life, he had this to say:

> When my sight went all I knew, literally, about blind people was that they read with their fingers and felt their way about with a cane. I had never known a blind person and I knew of no one who was familiar with their ways of life. . . . Someone suggested that I go to the Commission for the Blind and see what they would say. I went and told them my idea of living in the country. They agreed heartily that it was a grand scheme, and encouraged me in it. Not one word was said to the effect that many people, blinded in adult life and having been established in a profession, kept on with their work and led much the same life as before. I had been teaching in a technical school when my sight began to go. If I had had a little good advice at that time, I imagine the last thirty years would have been different.

Latter-day Robinson Pierces have had access to far more than "a little good advice." With the services available under the Vocational Rehabilitation Act, they can be taught enough of the skills that mitigate the limitations of blindness to be able to resume their professional careers with hardly a missed beat. But there remain extraneous factors to cope with.

Although substantial progress was made in the teaching field in the Fifties and Sixties (a 1969 survey showed more than 300 blind teachers employed in elementary and secondary schools; in 1972 there were more than 150 on the college and university level), only a fraction of the potential was being realized. Studies of teaching opportunities for blind persons universally emphasized the continuing existence of impediments, some solidly realistic but others rooted in stereotypical attitudes held by school administrators.

The main realistic factor was that unless would-be teachers possessed superior personal adjustment and mobility skills, as well as competency in their subject areas and instructional techniques, their job chances were slim. Surveys of blind teachers emphasized another reality: they had to purchase certain amounts of sighted assistance to fulfill their faculty responsibilities. Overcoming uninformed and prejudicial attitudes in school boards and administrators was a problem that yielded more readily to example than to persuasion; the successful blind person was always the best salesman for his fellows.

Different sets of obstacles existed in other professions. One of the most discouraging was the closing of the doors in osteopathy and physical therapy. In each instance the ban came about in the course of professionalization of the discipline.

Where physical therapy was concerned, the United States in 1972 continued to be far more restrictive than many other countries. In Japan, massage, the forerunner of physical therapy, was an acknowledged and popular occupation for blind persons and had been so for centuries. In Great Britain blind physical therapists had been functioning successfully since World War I; as of 1970, about a hundred trained and accredited therapists were active in hospital and private practice there. In the hope that the British example might influence the American Physical Therapy Association to modify its position against opening schools of physical therapy to blind persons, the Foundation went so far as to finance the attendance of two blind British physical therapists and their instructor at the Second Congress of the World Confederation for Physical Therapy when that body met in New York City in 1956. Although the visitors gave impressive demonstrations of their competence in all areas of practice, the attempt was in vain. A further effort was made in 1961, when OVR gave a demonstration grant to a rehabilitation center in Hartford, Connecticut, to finance a year's employment of a blind British physical therapist whose work could be observed by officials of the American schools. This also failed to achieve the desired change of policy.

During the Sixties an occupational field whose potential for blind persons aroused great enthusiasm was computer programming. The explosive initial growth of the data processing industry called for huge quantities of personnel. The educational requirements were modest; not even a college degree was a prerequisite for the technical training that could produce programmers in a few months of intensive study. Moreover, the personal qualities needed to master computer science were those that well-adjusted blind persons had had to cultivate in order to function in daily life: the ability to concentrate and to think in logical, sequential steps. The discovery, in 1963, that computers could be adapted to produce their printouts in braille apparently removed the final barrier. Financed with the help of federal grants, studies at the University of Cincinnati and elsewhere proceeded to develop a body of knowledge concerning the needed techniques and aids that would enable blind computer programmers to do their jobs without the need for sighted assistance.

Pioneering efforts to place blind persons in the data processing field were then undertaken by a handful of state agencies for the blind. With tuition and training grants paid under the Vocational Rehabilitation Act, students were enrolled in a number of the computer schools that sprang up all over the country to feed the new, manpower-hungry industry. A joint committee of the AAWB and the Association for Computing Machinery was established in the mid-Sixties to evaluate these schools for their ability to provide blind students with a solid grounding; seven such schools had been screened and approved by the end of 1969, at which time there were 350 visually handicapped people employed in data processing, with approximately 150 additional persons being trained each year.

As had been the case with every new endeavor for blind persons, there was much initial skepticism on the part of employers. It began to be overcome, but as data processing technology evolved, job classifications for blind people were narrowed down to coders (which involved low-paid clerical operations), and systems analysts (which involved sophisticated skills and knowledge of advanced computer language). The intermediate job levels more or less disappeared. The basic problem, some authorities asserted, was the tendency of many placement counselors to pursue "vocational fads" long after the demand for certain types of jobs had peaked. While this affected the non-handicapped equally, it worked special hardships on blind students.

One of the most satisfactory advances in employment of blind persons following World War II occurred in government work. In the federal civil service, the breakthrough came in 1937 with the appointment of Joseph Clunk and his staff under the Randolph-Sheppard Act. Later, federal civil service jobs gradually opened up at many levels. A law passed in 1948 forbade discrimination against physically handicapped persons in civil service examinations, employment, or promotion. While this facilitated jobs for such blind clerical workers as typists and stenographers, and also removed barriers to employment of blind persons in top professional positions which entitled them to secretaries, it left a gap in the intermediate grades, where positions were not normally accorded secretarial services and blind persons were consequently ruled ineligible. Applicants who sought to overcome this limitation by offering to pay for their own reading assistants were prohibited from doing so because of a regulation forbidding any person to work in a government agency while receiving compensation from an outside source. The problem was solved in 1962 when a law was enacted to exempt reading assistants from this regulation.

Other special provisions put into effect by the United States Civil Service Commission included the designation of coordinators for the employment of the handicapped and a special appointing authority which allowed a severely handicapped person to have a 700-hour trial period on the job before permanent appointment. For blind applicants there were also arrangements for administration of oral tests in place of written examinations.

As of 1972, an estimated six hundred blind men and women were working in federal civil service positions; no figures were available as to the number in state, county, or municipal posts.

Texas workers for the blind enjoy pointing out that their state once had a blind chief executive. This was technically true: as president pro tempore of the Texas State Senate, Criss Cole of Houston was for a single day—January 10, 1970—that state's acting governor. No technicality was involved, however, in the elections and re-elections that put Thomas D. Schall and Thomas Gore in the United States Senate from Minnesota and Oklahoma respectively, or Matthew W. Dunn in the House of Representatives from Pennsylvania. And, thanks to the horizons expanded by the Magna Charta of the Blind, there is no barrier, technical or otherwise, to a blind man's occupying a governor's mansion or, for that matter, the White House.

16

The War-Blinded, World War I

War-blinded. Few phrases evoke a stronger response, a response in which shock, pity, and guilt seek release through a passionate desire to make amends.

Even during the centuries when wars were fought by professional soldiers and the crippling consequences of conflict were regarded as occupational risks, men blinded in battle were special objects of concern. When, however, the men in the field were not mercenaries but conscripted citizens, public reaction reached new heights. It took a brilliant Briton, Arthur Pearson, to devise a way of channeling this reaction into a boldly original experiment.

A self-made publishing tycoon, Pearson suffered from progressive glaucoma. Surgery proved unavailing, and in 1913, when he was forty-seven years old, his sight failed altogether. With characteristic brio he told his wife, "I will never be *a* blind man. I am going to be *the* blind man."

What is now England's Royal National Institute for the Blind was then an old-established but fiscally faltering institution whose chief activity was braille publishing. Pearson used his press connections and his promotional flair to put the Institute on its financial feet. His reward was the presidency of a strengthened body, and it was in this capacity that, when World War I broke out a few months later, he began to give thought to what the war's consequences might be. That there would be men blinded in battle was a certainty; as to numbers, no one could guess. How could such men be helped to avoid feelings of hopelessness and uselessness? Pearson came up with an answer: a temporary hostel where men could "learn to be blind." Thus was born St. Dunstan's, an organization unique in its time. Some of its features were to serve as prototypes for rehabilitation centers the world over.

The Blinded Soldiers' and Sailors' Hostel, as it was called when its first two charges arrived, was established in a private residence in London in February

1915. Six weeks later, when the number had risen to 16, it moved to St. Dunstan's Lodge, a palatial estate in Regent's Park belonging to the American financier Otto H. Kahn. In one of the hands-across-the-sea gestures that preceded America's formal entry into World War I, Kahn had placed at Pearson's disposal—free of charge—the house, gardens, grounds, and outbuildings whose 15-acre spread was said to make it the largest single piece of property in London next to Buckingham Palace.

Kahn's villa was called St. Dunstan's Lodge because, when the mansion was built by the third Marquess of Hertford in 1830, its most distinctive feature was a mammoth clock adorned by lifesized carved figures which raised and lowered wooden clubs to strike each quarter-hour. This mechanical marvel had once been part of the ancient Church of St. Dunstan in the West, situated on Fleet Street in the City of London. Just as the Marquess' new home in Regent's Park neared completion, the church had been destroyed. The nobleman bought the clock, had it installed on the premises of his new home and christened the estate after it.*

St. Dunstan's physical quarters may have been rooted in an elegant past, but its mental outlook was fixed on the homely future. It was not enough, Pearson reasoned, to train men in self-care, in the techniques of daily living, and in vocational skills, and then leave them to their own devices. He set up a settlement department whose tasks included finding jobs for men who had been prepared for open employment as masseurs, typists, or telephone operators; furnishing initial capital and equipment to those who wanted to start small shops or farms; providing tools and raw materials to others who proposed to engage in home handicrafts like basketry, shoe-repairing or woodworking; and setting up a central marketing system for products they did not sell locally.

Even this extended service did not represent the end of the line. In launching a worldwide campaign to raise funds for St. Dunstan's, Sir Arthur Pearson (he was knighted in 1916) pledged that the organization would look after the welfare of every war-blinded man to the day he died. This meant that aftercare would be carried on for the next forty or fifty years and that the St. Dunstan's financial structure would have to be geared accordingly. Thirteen hundred blind men had already passed through St. Dunstan's by the time of the armistice in 1918, while two hundred more—still in military hospitals—had yet to be admitted for rehabilitation. What could not be predicted was the number whose sight had been injured during the war and who would eventually go blind. When the first actuarial survey was made in 1922, that figure was seriously underestimated at about three hundred; on this assumption, the survey calculated that there would still be fifteen hundred St. Dunstaners alive in 1935, nearly thirteen hundred in 1945, and just under eight hundred by 1955. The one factor that no one foresaw was that a second world war would necessitate opening the doors of St. Dunstan's to more than a thousand newly blinded men, and that the delayed blindness growing out of

---

* The person for whom both church and villa were named had no connection with blindness. St. Dunstan was an Archbishop of Canterbury in the tenth century. The church and its clock are today both back on Fleet Street, the former having been rebuilt and the latter restored to it when the Regent's Park house was torn down.

the eye injuries of both wars would bring the overall count of beneficiaries to some sixty-five hundred by 1972.

The man chosen by Sir Arthur to head the aftercare department was a tall, handsome young South African, Captain Ian Fraser. A sniper's bullet had gone through the eyes of the nineteen-year-old officer (later knighted as Lord Fraser of Lonsdale) during the battle of the Somme in 1916. Like other blinded British soldiers, his first contact with St. Dunstan's came soon after he was brought to the special eye ward of a military hospital in London. It was Pearson's practice to visit and talk with each new admission to this ward. At the time Fraser was admitted, however, Pearson was out of the city. Instead his personal assistant came, bearing a braille watch and a letter of cheer and encouragement from her chief. Both the message and the gift did a great deal to lift the spirits of the youthful officer; even more inspiring was the messenger, a young woman named Irene Mace who later became Mrs. Fraser. Miss Mace, like many others who staffed St. Dunstan's, was part of the Voluntary Aid Detachment corps whose members were popularly known as V.A.D.'s.

By the time Ian Fraser was medically fit and ready for admission to St. Dunstan's, its quarters had been greatly expanded to include additional buildings in Regent's Park and annexes in Brighton and Torquay. Blinded officers lived on Portland Place, not far from Regent's Park, in a house where Sir Arthur Pearson and his wife had also taken up residence. It was this proximity that gave Pearson the opportunity to spot the lively minded young South African as a promising assistant. When Pearson met an accidental death in 1921, Fraser was chosen to be his successor. A half-century later he was still chairman of St. Dunstan's, having maintained active interest and leadership in its work throughout a productive career in industry, in politics (he spent 34 years in the House of Commons before being made a Life Peer in 1958) and in distinguished public service.

Not only did St. Dunstan's succeed in achieving its basic purpose of preparing war-blinded men for productive lives, it proved to be a fertile spawning ground for leadership in work for the blind throughout the British Empire. After rehabilitation at St. Dunstan's, Captain Edwin A. Baker, the first Canadian officer to be blinded in World War I, played a key role in founding the Canadian National Institute for the Blind in Toronto. Clutha MacKenzie, blinded at Gallipoli, was the son of a former Prime Minister of New Zealand. When he returned home, he launched a campaign to raise the funds which transformed a small local school for blind children into a comprehensive service organization—the New Zealand National Institute for the Blind. During World War II, Sir Clutha (he had been knighted in 1935) established a St. Dunstan's outpost in India for men blinded in action in that war zone and then, at the urging of the Indian government, drew up plans for a postwar organizational structure to serve the country's numerous blind men, women and children.

In greater or lesser degree, all these men shared the outlook of St. Dunstan's founder, who referred to his institution as "the Aladdin of the modern world— going through the streets of Baghdad offering new lamps for old." The basic idea, Arthur Pearson said repeatedly, was "just this—a refusal to accept blindness as anything but a handicap."

So firm an organizational and financial structure was built by St. Dunstan's during and after World War I that England was ready to serve its men blinded in World War II. There were, of course, problems to be overcome. Temporary new quarters had to be found away from the Brighton seacoast where St. Dunstan's had established its principal residential training facilities after the Regent's Park property had been reclaimed by its owners. Provisions had to be made for a new, large-scale admissions program. Outposts were needed in war zones far from Britain—the Middle East, Australia, South Africa, India—so that preliminary rehabilitation treatment of newly blinded men could begin at once. New funds were needed to finance all of these efforts. It was Britain's good fortune to have a strongly established, ongoing body able to meet and surmount these challenges.

Not so the United States. Its World War I equivalent of St. Dunstan's was not perpetuated once the last war-blinded American serviceman had completed his rehabilitation training. With Pearl Harbor, the United States had to start all over again.

Compared with its European allies—and, for that matter, with the enemy countries—the United States had a small number of blinded casualties in the first war. Varying reports cite figures ranging from under 300 to nearly twice that many. The commonly accepted estimate was 450.

In 1924 the United States Veterans Bureau reported that it had given some form of rehabilitation service to 800 men with visual defects, of whom 480 came within its own rather narrow specifications for blindness. Among the latter group, 185 had been blinded in action and 162 by diseases contracted while in service. Pre-existing diseases and congenital defects aggravated by service accounted for the blindness of the others. The remainder of the 800 men on the Bureau's rolls still had too much sight to be classified as blind, but more than 200 of these subsequently suffered ocular deterioration, so that in September 1941 the Veterans Administration (successor to the Veterans Bureau) had on its register 726 World War I veterans receiving disability compensation for service-connected blindness.

The United States declared war on Germany on February 28, 1917. Shortly thereafter, the Council of National Defense appointed a Committee on Ophthalmology to advise the Surgeon General on problems resulting from eye wounds. An officer of the Surgeon General's staff, Major James Bordley, a Baltimore ophthalmologist, was assigned to survey the work being done for war-blinded in England and France and to seek the opinions of leading American workers for the blind on potential plans for America's war-blinded. The assembled information was presented to a ten-member Advisory Committee summoned by the Surgeon General's office to a conference in Washington in October 1917.

The members constituted a fairly representative Who's Who of contemporary and future leadership in work for the blind. There were the heads of the three pioneer schools for blind children: Edward E. Allen of Perkins, Olin H. Burritt of Overbrook, and Edward M. Van Cleve of New York. Another residential institution, the Ohio State School for the Blind, was represented in the person of Charles F.F. Campbell, then its superintendent, although Campbell was less important as an educator than as an idea man, placement specialist, and editor. The "progressives" in education—those who favored keeping blind children at home and having them taught in local public schools—were represented by Robert B. Irwin, then supervisor of classes for blind children in Cleveland and other Ohio cities.

Also on the committee were two experts in work for the adult blind: Liborio Delfino, field officer of the Overbrook school, who specialized in job placement of its graduates and alumni, and Frederick H. Mills, superintendent of a sheltered workshop, the Pennsylvania Working Home for Blind Men. Non-vocational interests were reflected in the membership of Gertrude T. Rider, then in charge of the Library of Congress' Reading Room for the Blind in Washington, and Walter G. Holmes, who probably had more direct contact with blind people all over the country than any of the others, through his editorship of the *Matilda Ziegler Magazine for the Blind.* The tenth member of the Advisory Committee, and its only layman, was M.C. Migel, designated in his capacity as treasurer of the Commission on Uniform Type for the Blind.

In two days of strenuous work the Advisory Committee drew up a detailed set of "Plans of the United States Government for Soldiers Blinded in Battle." These called for a two-step operation, beginning with the establishment of a special hospital center in France where preliminary rehabilitation training could be started as soon as the eye-wounded were brought in from the battlefields. The function of the center's staff—which was to include "at least one capable blind man for the inspirational value of his example"—would be to provide the newly blinded soldiers with "games, amusements of suitable kinds and physical and mental occupation" in various forms, including introductory "training in self-helpfulness": eating, dressing, shaving, etc. without benefit of sight. These activities were to be sustained during the transfer to ports of embarkation, on the homeward voyage, and at the American ports of entry until the men could be dispatched to a "Station for Re-Education of Blind Soldiers" to be established, equipped, and operated by the government on the eastern seaboard.

Here phase two would begin. From three months to a year would be required, the committee estimated, for completion of instruction and training

> in such subjects as reading and writing the approved uniform embossed system, writing with the pencil and the typewriter, transcribing from the dictaphone and telephone switchboard operating; in such trades and occupations as are suitable for the blind. . . . in physical training through gymnastics, athletics, swimming, bowling, tramping, boating, etc.

The committee's document was nothing if not thorough. It contained a table of organization for the "re-education station" and a comprehensive syllabus detailing the personal adjustment and manual training skills to be taught, a list of the occupations open to blind persons, the range of recreational pursuits to be offered, even a percentage breakdown of the types of literature to be embossed for the instruction and diversion of the men as they acquired competence in finger-reading.

Looking beyond the training period, the plan called for the appointment of a placement agent to find employment for those completing their reeducation, and for establishment of a follow-up system to work with the blinded veterans and their families in the years to come.

Much of the plan was based on the two years of experience the British had already gained at St. Dunstan's. There were, however, two important differences. One was operational. The British, whose war-blinded could be transported to London overnight, had no need for a preliminary hospital center in France. The other was more fundamental. St. Dunstan's was a voluntary organization supported by private funds. In the United States, the program was to be conducted and financed by the government.

The Advisory Committee had no say on this last point, which was a government decision. At Dr. Bordley's instigation, the American Red Cross had volunteered to act as "the American St. Dunstan's" and had placed a formal proposal to that effect before the United States Surgeon General. The offer had been promptly refused on the principle, according to a diary kept by Dr. Bordley, "that the Secretary of War was not inclined to accept financial aid from civilian agencies."

Even before the Advisory Committee met, Dr. Bordley had located eminently suitable quarters for the proposed training school. He had suggested to a wealthy Baltimore woman, Mrs. T. Harrison Garrett, that she offer Evergreen, her 99-acre suburban estate, for this patriotic purpose, and she did so at a rental of one dollar a year. The Surgeon General accepted the offer in November 1917, but delays in appropriation of the funds needed to convert the estate's facilities to government use and to build additional needed structures put off the actual opening for six months.

In April 1918 the first trainees were admitted to Evergreen, whose official title was U.S. Army General Hospital No. 7. The term "hospital," used because the facility was under the direction of the Surgeon General, was a misnomer. Men still in need of medical treatment were cared for at a military hospital in Cape May, N.J., until they were physically fit for training. But their discharge from medical care did not mean discharge from military service.

Therein lay another essential difference between the American and British systems. For war-blinded Tommies, entrance to St. Dunstan's was voluntary; as soon as they were medically fit, they were discharged from the British Army and could begin to collect their disability allowances. So long as Evergreen remained under War Department control, however, the blinded American doughboy was obliged to remain in military status until a medical survey board decided that he had reached "the highest point of medical and physical restoration." This meant, among other things, that the enlisted man would sleep in a 20-bed dormitory at Evergreen, that he would eat Army-style in a mess hall where metal plates clanged on bare wooden tables, that officers would be separately housed and differently treated, and that—of paramount importance to a man who had a dependent family—he would continue to receive $30 a month in military pay instead of the far larger disability compensation he would be entitled to on discharge.

A complex set of circumstances governed the compensation question. In 1914 Congress passed the War Risk Insurance Act (subsequently amended in 1917), which introduced two novel ideas. One was indemnity through insurance, rather than pensions from public funds, for men disabled in line of duty in the armed forces. Total blindness, under this Act, called for a lifelong compensation payment of $100 a month; lesser degrees of disability were compensated according to the extent to which they reduced earning power. The other new feature was government-financed vocational training and rehabilitation for men invalided by military service, with the object of enabling them to function as productive members of the community.

What was unique about the War Risk Insurance Act was that compensation payment was keyed to the severity of the disability rather than to the military rank of the disabled person. This concept differed radically from systems then in existence in other western countries, where rank was the determining factor. In France, for example, the annual disability pension paid at the time of the Armistice for service-connected total blindness ranged from 975 francs ($195) for privates, to twice that amount for top-ranking noncommissioned officers, to a scale that went as high as 12,600 francs ($2,520) for commissioned officers. The British system also differentiated between ranks, although less sharply (40 shillings, equal to $10 weekly, for privates; 60 shillings for warrant officers). In addition Britain took into account a man's family obligations, making small extra payments for wives and children.

America's initial effort to establish a single disability standard for the war injured was short-lived. The War Risk Insurance Act was superseded in mid-1918 by the Smith Hughes Vocational Education Act. It created a Federal Board for Vocational Education to administer the task of providing vocational training for all war-disabled men, finding them jobs on completion of training, and maintaining follow-up services until they achieved financial independence.

Under this legislation, men in training status were to receive the same pay and family allowances as they had while in the service, which meant differential payments for varying ranks. But veterans were protected against arbitrary reduction in benefits. A man could elect to receive either the Federal Board's training allowance or the War Risk Insurance Act's disability benefit, whichever was greater. For a fully insured enlisted man, the latter could be as high as $157 a month. No wonder, then, that the men at Evergreen chafed at being kept in the service at one-fifth that amount. And no wonder, either, that the confusion of dealing with separate branches of the government added to their demoralization. A disabled veteran had to cope with the medical department of the Army for certification of his disability, with the United States Public Health Service for continuing medical care and treatment, with the Treasury Department's Bureau of War Risk Insurance for his disability compensation, and with the Federal Board of Vocational Education for his training and employment needs. It was not until 1921 that some of this bureaucratic red tape was simplified when the last two functions, plus all of the veterans' hospitals formerly supervised by the Surgeon General, were consolidated in the newly created United States Veterans Bureau.

These were some of the factors that, even allowing for all the plusses, made the first year at Evergreen disappointing to its trainees and to the leaders in work for the blind who had pinned such great hopes on an American version of St. Dunstan's. Disappointing, even though the plusses were many. Evergreen's surroundings were idyllic, dotted with magnificent gardens, groves, meadows and walks. The enlisted men occupied the stately main house, whose paneled entrance hall, with its beamed ceiling and carpeted floor, served as their lounge. Another fine old building housed the blinded officers, the military staff in charge of the installation and the civilian instructors. There were six new buildings, erected by the government at a cost of some $250,000. They included a schoolhouse, manual training shops and a recreation building with a fully equipped gymnasium, two bowling alleys, and a 60-foot swimming pool.

The teaching staff was also of high quality. More than half the faculty were experienced teachers on leave of absence from various schools for the blind. But they were civilians, half of them women, and they lacked status in a military establishment. The trainees were said to resent their presence; they came to classes late or not at all, and were generally uncooperative. Adding to the low morale was the fact that military bureaucracy took little account of individual educational needs. According to a man who taught at Evergreen during those early days: "A high school student sat next to a man who had finished only the fourth grade of grammar school some ten years ago. A boy who was hard of hearing was there with a man who was so nervous that he jumped whenever you spoke above a whisper."

Although the American Red Cross had been turned down on its original offer to operate Evergreen, it took the position that as handmaiden to the armed forces in time of war, it had an obligation to serve blinded soldiers and sailors in whatever way it could. While the school was being fitted out by the government, the Red Cross acquired a building on adjacent property and installed a special unit called the Red Cross Institute for the Blind.

At that point in time, in March of 1918, the Federal Board for Vocational Education had not yet been legislated into existence and no provision existed for post-training aftercare of blinded veterans. The Red Cross saw its overall function as providing that essential bridge: "to supply the necessary economic and social supervision of blinded marines, sailors, and soldiers, after their discharge from military service." This would be done through individualized social service so that when the blinded man went back into civil life, he would "be helped to establish himself, with the greatest possible expedition, in his new field of endeavor."

In addition to casework, there would be practical research. The Institute would make "a scientific study . . . of occupational possibilities for the blind in industry, commerce and agriculture." It would explore new occupational fields. It would find, test and install such special devices as would enable blind men to work efficiently and safely in factories and would then undertake the industrial placement of men trained in the use of these devices with the help of a commission of manufacturers. It would get around the reluctance of industry to hire blind men by standing behind each placement; should a man fail to make good on a particular job, the Institute itself would remove him, "thereby relieving the employer of all embarrassment."

There was more, much more. The Institute would establish sheltered workshops and would act as purchasing and sales agent, respectively, for the raw materials and finished products of such workshops, as well as for the handcrafted articles made by blind workers in their homes. It would train men for work in commerce and agriculture and supply them, if necessary, with the tools and materials of their trades. Men capable of professional or technical education would be helped in these directions. Sighted readers would be supplied to facilitate their studies, and placement service would follow.

A cottage would be opened near Evergreen where, prior to a man's discharge from training, his wife or parent or other close family member would be instructed in how to help him in his occupation as well as in his home life. If a man proved too incapacitated to work, his wife would be "taught some vocation from which she can add to the family income."

Had this staggeringly ambitious program ever come to fruition, it could have become the nucleus of an integrated, nationwide welfare service for blind people—something that does not yet exist in the United States and probably never will. There would have been no need, after the war, to organize the much more modestly conceived American Foundation for the Blind, which ultimately undertook many of the broad research, planning, and coordinating functions embodied in the Institute's prospectus.

That the Red Cross Institute's grand design never materialized was due to several major factors:

First, World War I ended a few months later. Not only did the number of blinded American servicemen prove to be thankfully small, but a good many of them had been discharged from service and were back home before either Evergreen or the Red Cross Institute got under way.

Second, most of the Institute's proposed vocational training, placement, and aftercare activities were ostensibly preempted by the United States Government once the Federal Board for Vocational Education was legislated into being.

Finally, existing state and local organizations for the blind were by no means willing to see their work overshadowed and perhaps eventually swallowed up by a national program with the prestige and money-raising power of the American Red Cross. While there was no way of knowing how many men from a given state or community might return blind from the war, the local agencies felt that any such men should be cared for in their own homes and by their own communities rather than by a national group. Power, authority, and fund-raising potential were all at stake from the viewpoint of the local agencies, and their leaders worked intensively behind the scenes to avert any possible threat to their dominion. This was why, when the American Foundation for the Blind was launched three years after the war's end, Dr. Bordley warned against overloading its policy structure with the professional workers for the blind whose self-interest, he charged, had thwarted the development of the Red Cross Institute as a national body.

In preparation for the role it hoped to assume, the Institute equipped and staffed its building next door to Evergreen with the help of a public fund drive. By the time Evergreen was ready to begin operations, however, the Institute was left with a far more limited function: "to do anything that would help make the life of the soldiers and sailors better and more effective while at Evergreen and also after their discharge."

The Institute found a number of useful ways "to do anything." It installed a library and club room that could serve as an off-post center. A braille transcribing service was started to provide light literature for the beginning finger-readers.

Large numbers of volunteers were recruited and trained to serve as educational aides to the Evergreen teaching staff. Housing facilities were provided for visiting families. The Red Cross also sent a nine-person unit overseas to assist in the preliminary adjustment of war-blinded men, and to carry out some additional reconstruction assignments in France. This was the unit headed by M.C. Migel.

The Institute's first director was Dr. Bordley (by then promoted to Lt. Colonel), who simultaneously held the official post of Officer in Charge of the Reeducation of Blinded Soldiers, Sailors and Marines in the Surgeon General's Physical Reconstruction Division. The assistant director was Charles F.F. Campbell, who had taken a leave of absence from the Ohio State School for the Blind.

It was fortunate for all concerned that the Red Cross did not quit in frustration when its master plan was blocked. By early 1919, less than a year after Evergreen admitted its first trainees, the Army recognized that it was not fulfilling its purpose. It was operating under capacity—no more than fifty or sixty men were in residence at any time and, with the cessation of hostilities the preceding November, no great future influx was to be expected. The men in training were restless, largely unmotivated, and eager to leave. The blend of military administration and civilian instruction was not working well. So when the Red Cross renewed its offer to take charge of the school's operations, the War Department was more than willing to reverse its previous attitude. An agreement was reached, and on May 25, 1919, the installation formerly known as General Hospital No. 7 changed hands and was renamed the Red Cross Institute for the Blind. Simultaneously, the military status of the men at Evergreen was terminated; they were now veterans, entitled to receive their disability benefits and eligible to receive their Evergreen training at the expense of the Federal Board of Vocational Education.

The Federal Board's view was that Evergreen should be used primarily to provide prevocational services, equipping men with the basic skills that would help them achieve a degree of adjustment to a life without sight. To furnish specific vocational training, as well as education for the professions, the Board used a variety of other schools, workshops, and local agencies for the blind. It did, however, approve Evergreen as a vocational training center for a few trades and occupations.

Once the military regime was out of the picture, the program at Evergreen took on new life. Flexibility and experimentation became the keynotes. Each student was individually appraised and provided with a course of instruction tailored to his ability and his needs. More than half the men had had little formal education; classes were given in spelling, business arithmetic, American history, civics, and literature. Men who had had a high school education took advanced courses in cultural subjects. Manual training was seen as important for all, since all had to learn to make greater use of the tactile sense, but the men who had been mechanics or factory workers were given more advanced training in woodworking or machine shop operations.

Men who had come off the farm and wanted to go on living in rural surroundings were given a full year's training in commercial poultry raising, followed by three months on a model farm. Another vocational sequence was in massage;

those with the necessary academic backgrounds were taught anatomy and all of the technical skills that would qualify them for hospital jobs in what was later called physical therapy. Vending stand operation was taught at the school's canteen, which was operated as a model store. Cigar-making was also taught, but proved a commercial failure.

All Evergreen students, whatever their vocational goals, were given access to a variety of avocational skills to prepare them for rounded social and personal lives. Discussion groups and activities involving music, athletics, dancing, and games were shaped toward that end. Evergreen's "Braille Orchestra" played at the weekly dances; some of the more able musicians performed in community concerts, and several developed enough expertise to lead small commercial ensembles.

With the Federal Board for Vocational Education furnishing referrals, Evergreen flourished under the management of the Red Cross Institute. There had been about sixty men in residence when the Army bowed out; half of these stayed on, and new men sent by the Federal Board brought the population to 104 a year later. But it was not always easy for the Board's field staff to persuade men who had been discharged before Evergreen came into being, or those whose sight had deteriorated into blindness since their discharge, to invest the time and effort involved in undergoing vocational rehabilitation. The Board's 1920 report to Congress contained passages such as this: "In one instance, an agent of the Board was told by the mother of one of the men that her son would never be given vocational training except over her dead body. . . . The father of one of the men refuses to be convinced that his son should receive training. 'My boy will always have enough money, and all he needs now is a good wife.'"

The Federal Board paid Evergreen $106.50 per month for tuition and board of each registrant. The remainder of the necessary funds was raised by public subscription. Approximately $4,500,000 was said to have been spent by the Institute, much of it for structural changes to erase the traces of military rule. The 20-bed dormitories were partitioned off into separate rooms for two. The bare wooden dining trestles were replaced by cloth-covered oval tables seating companionable groups of six or eight. Out went the metal dishes and in came chinaware and attractive cutlery. Now that everyone was a civilian, teachers and students could and did dine together. These gracious touches helped to lift morale, but the most potent factor in the new spirit at Evergreen was, of course, that no man was there against his will.

At the conclusion of its first year of operating the school, the Red Cross Institute had accomplished such affirmative results that it once more had visions of an expanded future. And at this point Evergreen did indeed have a potential. It was groping toward a formula for the rehabilitation of blinded adults that might have served as a model for such facilities all over the nation, and had in fact taken a tentative step toward testing out the practicability of such a program by admitting nine non-veterans. But Evergreen was due for another change in administration.

When the Veterans Bureau was created in the summer of 1921, that part of the work of the Federal Board for Vocational Education which dealt with ex-servicemen was transferred to the newly created umbrella organization while the Federal Board, its scope enlarged by the Smith-Fess Act of 1920, remained in charge for civilians. The jurisdictional split meant that the Red Cross Institute had a new partner at Evergreen. It was a partnership that lasted only a few months; on January 1, 1922, the Veterans Bureau assumed full control, the Red Cross Institute for the Blind went out of existence, and the establishment on Mrs. Garrett's spacious acres acquired its third and final name, the Evergreen School for the Blind.

With the change of jurisdiction came changes in personnel. Dr. Bordley had returned to private practice in Baltimore in mid-1919, but had remained in a volunteer capacity on the Institute's Committee of Direction. Originally just on leave of absence from the Ohio State School for the Blind, Charles Campbell had burned his bridges by resigning from the school once the Red Cross Institute took over from the Army. When Bordley left the directorship of the Institute, Campbell had hoped to be appointed in his place. But the Red Cross passed him over and gave the job to L.W. Wallace, keeping Campbell as assistant director. Wallace later resigned and Campbell succeeded to his post, but his tenure was brief; at this point Evergreen was about to be handed over to the Veterans Bureau. When the transfer took place, Joseph E. Vance became Evergreen's new director. He resigned a year later and was succeeded by Robert B. Reed, former head of the school's academic department. Maurice I. Tynan was next in line, and he presided over Evergreen's disbandment in June 1925. By then the school had pretty well exhausted the supply of potential students among blinded veterans and Veterans Bureau regulations ruled out continuation of the experiment of admitting civilians. Hopes for a national body to give leadership in work for the blind were now centered in the new American Foundation for the Blind.

Those who had known Evergreen intimately and were reluctant to see its pioneering efforts eradicated without a trace made a few efforts at salvage. Vance, when he resigned at the end of 1922, wrote Migel, suggesting that Congress might be willing to enact a law transferring Evergreen's equipment to a more permanent institution that could move ahead with development of rehabilitation methods. The Foundation, which had yet to open an office, was not in a position to follow through on the suggestion.

Not long thereafter some of the Evergreen graduates, who had formed an organization called the United States Blind Veterans of the World War, proposed that the Foundation join forces with them in a fund-raising campaign to establish a permanent national training school for blind adults. This, too, was premature where the Foundation was concerned; it had not yet started raising funds for its own basic program. The veterans group then proceeded to establish a separate corporation, the U.S. Blind Veterans' Memorial Fund, which lobbied successfully for a bill appropriating $350,000 in federal funds to the Veterans Bureau for a national training school. But the money was never spent; the blind veterans group was torn by dissension, some members insisting the money should be used only to benefit ex-servicemen while others were willing to share with blind civilians.

The Veterans Bureau was indifferent, to say the least; it had far more serious troubles of its own at the time and was pursuing a policy of strict economy under a new director, General Frank T. Hines. Hines was replacing Charles B. Forbes, the first director, who had been thrown out of office (and was eventually imprisoned) for complicity in corrupt and wasteful practices that were alleged to have cost the taxpayers more than $200 million.

To the bitter disappointment of Philip N. Harrison, a blinded veteran from Pittsburgh who, as president of the Memorial Fund, had been largely responsible for inspiring passage of the bill, the $350,000 appropriation lapsed a year after it had been voted and one more opportunity to begin an adequate rehabilitation program for the adult blind was lost. Harrison himself, like several others who went through the Evergreen program, took up work for the blind as a profession. Eventually he became executive secretary of the Pennsylvania Association for the Blind, whose work was greatly expanded under his leadership. When he retired in 1960 he received the AAWB's Shotwell Award.

If Evergreen itself could not be salvaged, could not at least the fruits of its experience be preserved? In May 1925, just before the school closed its doors forever, Robert Irwin wrote to James L. Fieser, vice-chairman of the American Red Cross, asking whether that organization could appropriate $10,000 to finance a study and evaluation of what had been attempted at Evergreen. "If we were to go into a war ten years from now," he said, "we would be about as much in the dark as to how to proceed as we were eight years ago."

Unfortunately, the Red Cross had no spare research money either, and Irwin's prophecy proved all too accurate when the United States once again went to war.

17

The New Breed

One of the lasting by-products of World War II was the coining of a colorful word that proved so useful it remained in the language. The word was "snafu" an acronym for "situation normal, all fouled up." It was as good a term as any to describe what happened when a well-intentioned government tried to do its best for 1,400 American servicemen blinded in the European and Pacific war zones between December 1941 and August 1945.

That—in spite of bureaucratic bungles, intramural rivalries, incessant red tape—the end result was more triumph than disaster, was due in great measure to the blinded men themselves. They were a new breed: smarter, tougher, better educated, more sophisticated than the men who had fought in France a generation earlier. The best of them were realistic and determined not to succumb to self-pity, and it was their unflagging morale that helped inspirit the rest.

There were other factors in their favor. The blinded men of World War II had the benefit of advances made since the preceding world war. There was now a firm and experienced leadership structure in work for the blind, a structure equipped to act as authoritative spokesman and influential advocate. Prominent in it were men who had known from personal experience the weaknesses of Evergreen and who set out to prevent their recurrence in caring for the new wave of war-blinded.

Early in 1941, as defense mobilization got under way in the United States, the American Association of Workers for the Blind appointed a committee with a cautiously worded title: "Committee on the Care, Training and After-Care of Persons Becoming Blind as a Result of the United States Defense Program and Possible Participation in the Present World War." Robert Irwin chaired the committee, whose twelve members included three blinded veterans of World War I: Colonel Edwin A. Baker of Canada, Rabbi Michael Aaronsohn of Cincinnati, and Dr. J. Francis Smith of Philadelphia. Three other members had had direct experience in working with the men blinded in that war: Maurice I. Tynan, former director of Evergreen and now a field agent of the Service for the Blind of the Federal Security Agency; Grace S. Harper, director of the Bureau of Service for the Blind of the New York State Department of Social Welfare; and Irwin himself, who had served on the 1917 committee which drew up the plan for care of the American war-blinded.

The other six members represented various phases of work for the adult blind on local, state, and national levels: Alfred Allen, who then held the dual jobs of executive secretary of AAWB and executive secretary of the Hadley Correspondence School for the Blind in Illinois; J. Robert Atkinson, managing director of the Braille Institute of America in Los Angeles, which provided a range of social services for the blind in Southern California; Francis B. Ierardi, executive director of the National Braille Press in Boston, an agency which combined publishing activities with social services; Peter J. Salmon, then assistant director of the Industrial Home for the Blind in Brooklyn; Louis L. Watts, executive secretary of the Virginia Commission for the Blind; and Joseph F. Clunk, supervisor of the Federal Security Agency's Service for the Blind. Of the 12 committee members, only Alfred Allen and Grace Harper were sighted.

The committee had just begun to formulate a set of principles when Pearl Harbor was struck. When, in March of 1942, the President of the United States directed Federal Security Administrator Paul V. McNutt to draft plans for the rehabilitation of men disabled in combat, a delegation from the committee called at McNutt's office to offer assistance in planning for the war-blinded.

Central to the committee's thinking at this stage and throughout was the belief that the federal government and not private philanthropy should assume responsibility for the rehabilitation of men blinded in military service. A public declaration to this effect was issued by the committee in September 1942, in an effort to halt what it called a "brand of war-racketeering"—the spurious fund-raising drives that claimed to serve the war-blinded. The warning was not altogether effective; phony appeals along these lines persisted, particularly in California, for the duration of the war and even thereafter.

One factor that held up formal submission of the committee's recommendations to the government was uncertainty over whether Congress would adopt a single rehabilitation service for both war veterans and civilians, or whether the two programs would be separately administered. August 1942 saw the introduction of companion measures (the Barden bill in the House, the LaFollette bill in the Senate) to expand the Vocational Rehabilitation Act of 1920, but these bills languished in Congress because they were not seen as pertinent to the war effort. To make the legislators aware that rehabilitation did have relevance to war goals Franklin D. Roosevelt delivered a special message to the Senate on October 9, 1942. That message supported a comprehensive rehabilitation plan that would embrace both veterans and civilians and enable physically handicapped persons to "become a national asset ready to serve in war industries, agricultural and essential occupations."

Although the message made clear the White House's preference for a unified rehabilitation service, pressure from veterans' groups for separate legislation and a separate program prevailed. March 24, 1943, saw passage of Public Law 78-16, authorizing the Veterans Administration to provide vocational rehabilitation for disabled veterans, increasing disability compensation rates, and providing other benefits that would assist war-disabled servicemen to make a new start. The Barden-LaFollette Act for rehabilitation of disabled civilians was enacted three months later.

Even before formal passage of P.L. 78-16 it was apparent that the Veterans Administration would be given charge of men blinded in service. Accordingly, a delegation from the AAWB committee, now retitled the United States Committee on the War Blind, called on the VA administrator, Brigadier General Frank T. Hines, in January 1943 to deliver a revised version of the plan that had been submitted to the Federal Security Agency a year earlier. The plan outlined a three-stage program:

1. *Services in the hospital,* including first steps in rehabilitation of the blinded soldier—learning independence in eating, dressing, walking, etc., and possibly a beginning in the use of special devices for reading and writing. Such services provided at the earliest practical moment will do much to alleviate the despondency common to newly blinded persons.

2. *Services in a temporary rehabilitation training center,* to which the blinded soldier should be sent on leaving the hospital. A short intensive training course is proposed, in which the man would continue the adjustment begun in the hospital. . . . During this period each man should be studied intensively with a view to determining the proper vocational retraining and employment program for him.

3. *Services for return to the home community and placement in employment.* While this phase of the work should be under the direction of the Veterans Administration, it is suggested that so far as practicable the services of existing State and private agencies for the blind be utilized. . . .

The document went on to urge that the program make use of "personnel specially trained and experienced in work with the blind," and that it include "the employment of trained blind so far as practicable, since blind persons can, on the basis of common experience, enter into the difficulties of the newly blind to an extent seldom achieved by the seeing." It listed a set of fifteen basic principles, among them that service to the blinded should be separate from the program for the war-wounded with other disabilities. It emphasized that this separate program should be headed by an experienced administrator "who has kept pace with the progress in services for the blind over the past quarter of a century [and] who has the complete respect and support of organization executives, of blind persons, and of the community he now serves."

Soundly and carefully drafted, the committee's plan worked better on paper than in actuality. "We have complications," Irwin explained to a British colleague,

growing out of the fact that the Veterans Administration, which is responsible for the rehabilitation of disabled veterans, has no jurisdiction over the men until they are discharged from the Army. Blinded men who may be kept in the hospitals for months are under the Surgeon General of the Army or of the Navy.

Moreover, the plan's key element, a temporary rehabilitation training center, was encountering opposition in the Veterans Administration. One reason, Irwin noted, was that in World War I Evergreen had been "a headache, and all the government officials are a little bit leery of it." Another factor was the open struggle among several agencies for the blind to be awarded the VA contract to operate such a training center.

Where did the War Department leave off and the Veterans Administration begin? This, too, was clearer on paper than in practice. In July 1943 the Office of the Surgeon General issued a detailed directive to all of its service commands. For a military communication, it was a surprisingly human document, infused with sensitivity and worded with stylistic grace.

The directive designated two Army hospitals for medical treatment of the eye-wounded: Valley Forge General Hospital in Phoenixville, Pa. and Letterman General Hospital in San Francisco (the latter subsequently replaced by Dibble General Hospital in nearby Menlo Park). They would be staffed with physicians who were specialists in eye disease, in facial and plastic surgery, and in ophthalmic surgery. Rehabilitation of the blinded casualty would be started in these two eye centers "instead of awaiting the casualty's arrival in a Veterans Administration facility, where rehabilitation and vocational programs are properly centered." The reason? "Unless facilities for rehabilitation are placed in Army hospitals, long months of convalescence, made necessary by complicated wounds or other conditions, may postpone the early beginning in re-education of the blind, which is so essential to a successful result."

However, the directive also made a point of saying, "it is not the intention of the Medical Department of the Army to take over the entire rehabilitation program; that still remains in the hands of the Veterans Administration." The Army program would be modeled after St. Dunstan's in England. Drawing on the latter's "high order of special service to the blind,"

> . . . it is intended that contact be made with the blind soldier at the earliest possible time, by a blind worker, before the psychological aspects of the deprivation of sight may make any deep inroads on the personality. . . . The possibility of a happy life must be presented by one familiar with the hardships of that experience.

It was the Army's intention "to keep the soldier in a military hospital until maximum therapeutic benefit has been obtained" and to begin rehabilitation training during this period. There was to be "a full daily program which leaves little time for self-pity." Psychological support was to be given by all personnel in contact with the blinded men so as "to build some measure of optimism." All personnel were to give the patients tactful guidance in personal habits: "neatness of dress, erect posture, mannerisms devoid of groping." There was to be individual instruction in such special techniques as braille reading and writing, typing, and motor skills to assist in mastering the environment.

Perhaps the most astonishing passage in this military document was captioned "A Philosophy":

> There was a time when those handicapped by blindness might only look forward to selling shoelaces on a corner, or to begging, or to making brooms, or to caning chairs, or to tuning pianos, without regard to educational background or personal fitness. Each individual, we believe, has potentialities that fit him for a particular kind of activity. Some possess the ability to achieve professional distinction in the fields of law, medicine, education, etc.; others possess the technical skills and adaptability to fit them for industrial assignments; still others may look forward to clerical work, vending stand sales, or agricultural activities. It is our feeling that every opportunity should be given the patient to discover his own capabilities and what he would like to do and to give him the assistance to achieve that objective.

To put this philosophy into practice, each eye center would be staffed with one or more vocational counselors to advise on opportunities for self-support, and with social workers to counsel the patient and to assist in preparing his family. The last function was crucial: "A sympathetic family may, through its pity, destroy much of the self-confidence and reliance that the patient will learn, unless they are prepared to meet the situation wisely."

Another staffing provision was that persons trained in work with the blind would be rounded up from among a number of such men serving in various military units. A key role in the total program would be assigned to "a blind man who can get about easily and who has a pleasing personality . . . [a person] well adjusted to his blindness and capable of imparting that philosophy of life so essential in creating proper psychological support by demonstrating in himself its operation."

Finally, transfer to the care of the Veterans Administration for continuation of rehabilitation measures and for specific vocational training and placement services would take place when the patient had secured maximum hospital benefit and was discharged from the armed services.

The only trouble with this admirable prospectus was that it failed to anticipate how rapidly the number of war-blinded would grow, and how slowly the VA would move to pick up its end of the job. In a matter of months the two Army eye centers grew crowded with new casualties. But if the men ready for medical discharge were to move out and make room for new arrivals, where were they to go?

The question was thrashed out at the highest government level and formalized in a four-party agreement approved by Franklin D. Roosevelt on January 8, 1944. The signatories to this document—Secretary of War Henry L. Stimson, Secretary of the Navy Frank Knox, War Manpower Commission chairman Paul V. McNutt, and VA Administrator Frank T. Hines—agreed:

1. "Each blind person should have such social adjustment training during hospitalization as may be feasible." However, since few would achieve enough adjustment during hospitalization to prepare them for vocational training or em-

ployment, additional help should be given under military auspices until the blinded patient had made "the best adjustment he is capable of making."

2. Blinded personnel would therefore be retained in the service until social adjustment training was completed. It was expected that this would take about four months.

3. During this extended training period, the Veterans Administration was to "initiate and complete as early as possible . . . the vocational advisement of each case" so that "the blind person will know precisely . . . not only his ultimate vocational objective but also the vocational training program by which the objective is to be attained."

4. Social adjustment training would consist of specific instruction in:

Mental adjustment as may be necessary to develop a proper attitude and a will to overcome his handicap; use of the braille watch; use of the Talking Book; perception of objects by sound; recognition of people; use of the cane; how to get about indoors and out of doors; assistance with personal problems, shaving, eating, posture, etc.; pencil writing; typewriting; braille reading; braille writing with slate and machine; aid in learning how to study; hand training, hand tools, machine tools; use of leisure time—games, checkers, cards, etc.; recreation, theatres, parties . . . and such sports as may be feasible.

5. To execute this plan, all blinded personnel of both the Army and Navy would become the responsibility of the Army Medical Department for training in a rehabilitation center to be made available by the Army.

The center established in fulfillment of this agreement was located in Avon, Connecticut, and bore the official title of Old Farms Convalescent Hospital (Sp.). Colonel Frederick H. Thorne, an Army ophthalmologist, was named commanding officer. As had been the case with Evergreen, "hospital" was a misnomer; it was used because the installation was under medical direction. Nor was "convalescent hospital" an accurate description. Old Farms, which opened in June 1944, was a training school with a specific curriculum and specific goals.

The physical setting to which men now began to be transferred from Valley Forge and Dibble was unique. Old Farms occupied the premises of a former private preparatory school of the same name, located on a 2,000-acre tract of rural land in Connecticut's Farmington River valley, about 11 miles from the state capital of Hartford. The school, which had been built in 1926, was the creation of an eccentric and talented woman architect, Theodate Pope Riddle, heiress to a bicycle-manufacturing fortune. Mrs. Riddle had designed Old Farms to simulate the appearance of centuries-old English schools. Its buildings had three-foot-thick stone walls, red slate roofs, hand-hewn beams and doors, a good deal of hand-wrought ironwork. Its plant comprised 26 irregularly shaped buildings, the principal structures arranged around a quadrangle and connected by a complex maze of passages and pathways. In the words of one of the blinded veterans trained there, Old Farms was "a good substitute for an obstacle course. The ceilings are of various heights, none of them very high; the stairways are winding and uneven, and the floors are uneven, too."

The Army took an affirmative view of these navigational hazards. If a blind man could learn to cope with the topography of Old Farms, he could get along anywhere. It was this approach to the shaping of self-confidence that led the staff to adopt a policy which became the target of considerable criticism.

This policy was to take away from the blinded man arriving at Old Farms "the thing on which he had come to place the most confidence—his cane. . . . During the 18 weeks he remains at Avon, while on our grounds he gets about without a cane, without a dog, and without a guide—completely on his own."

The criticism stemmed from the fact that this approach represented an abrupt about-face for most of the men coming to Old Farms. It was generally agreed that one of the most valuable accomplishments of the preliminary adjustment program at Valley Forge was the "long cane" foot travel system, developed by Sergeant (later Lieutenant) Richard E. Hoover, who was one of the soldiers brought to the Valley Forge eye center when the Surgeon General's office spread a net through all Stateside Army service commands to locate men with experience in work for the blind.

Before the war Hoover had been a teacher and physical training coach at the Maryland School for the Blind. He was convinced that the "white cane" customarily used by blind people was too short, too heavy, too cumbersome, and not a sufficiently good sound conductor to be really helpful as an aid to mobility. Moreover, it was employed in the wrong way and for the wrong purpose. The most serious problem of all was that no system existed for teaching blind people how to use a cane to maximum advantage. The assumption had always been that each person could learn for himself.

A man of scientific bent (after the war he entered medical school and became a distinguished ophthalmologist), Hoover came up with the "long cane." It was made of metal with a plastic tip, was six to ten inches longer than the usual wooden cane, had a shaft about half the thickness of the latter, and weighed only six or seven ounces.

What came to be known as the Hoover cane was topped by a shepherd's crook that protected the hand. Designed for use as a bumper and a probe, the cane had to be employed in a definite technique, sweeping a low arc in front of the user in a rhythmic, cross-body pattern in which it lightly touched the ground in front of the foot that was about to be brought forward, insuring that this foot had an unobstructed spot on which to land. As it described the arc from one side to the other, the long cane struck any obstruction (a wall, the edge of a half-open door) directly in front of the blind man. It was long enough to keep the user from stooping while executing the arc or changing posture when going down or up a step. Its metallic body was a good sound conductor which provided important orientation clues to the presence of walls, open spaces or changes in terrain.

Skill in the use of the cane was acquired only through careful teaching and rigorous practice. At Valley Forge Hoover trained a group of instructors in the systematic and orderly method by means of which they, in turn, could train the newly blinded men.

The hundreds of men who passed through this preliminary training were startled to discover that at Old Farms the canes were banned on the premises. This arbitrary rule also dismayed leaders in work for the blind, who deplored the absence of continuity between the two programs—an absence which left those in charge at Old Farms free to devise their own theories and methods of teaching mobility.

It is difficult to say which of many possible reasons was responsible for the discontinuity. To the trainees, it was simply one more example of "the Army way" of doing everything. To the Surgeon General's staff in command at Old Farms, it was at least partly a question of making use of human laboratory subjects to pursue independent lines of scientific inquiry. One of those lines was the subject of facial vision, then very much in the news by reason of the just-published Cornell study of echolocation. A number of experiments were conducted at Old Farms with various "crickets" or other noise-making devices, whose echoes helped blind men to orient themselves in space.

Exaggerated press reports about the experimental work at Old Farms led to the false impression that cane travel had been totally abandoned there. The men did use canes when they went on field trips to Hartford, where they were given practice in street travel and in the use of busses, trains, and other public conveyances and facilities. However, further refinement of cane travel technique, which might logically have been pursued, was put off, and it was not until the Veterans Administration eventually opened its rehabilitation center in Hines, Illinois, in 1948 that the technique was perfected.

The basic 18-week training program at Old Farms had four separate aspects. One concentrated on self-care and other personal adjustment activities. Another dealt with physical exercise, particularly sports, to prove to the trainees that they could continue to enjoy many of the same outdoor activities they had engaged in when they had sight. They bowled, swam, rode horseback, roller-skated, fished, boated, played golf and thus came to realize that they were by no means sentenced to a future of physical torpor. A third aspect—social recreation in the form of dances, dinner parties, and other entertainments—made the same point.

The heart of the program lay in the several dozen courses which occupied most of the men's time. Each man was free to choose what he wanted or needed. There were three types: courses in braille, typing, and manual dexterity designed to help the trainees live as blind men, courses in English, music, public speaking, and creative writing designed to help them live as full human beings; and courses in industrial and commercial skills aimed at discovering vocational interests and aptitudes.

One of the most constructive aspects of this last group was their extension into actual practice with the cooperation of some large business and industrial firms in the area. Men who had learned to operate power machines were given brief tryout placements in factories, holding down regular production jobs for which they earned regular salaries. Others worked as paid employees in stores, garages, filling stations, and insurance companies. These tryouts were the capstones of the Old Farms training program; they were both practical prevocational tests and important confidence builders.

All told, 850 men went through the Old Farms program during its three years of existence. A study made by Colonel Thorne after the first 200 men had completed their training showed four out of five to have achieved adjustments rated satisfactory or better. The other 20 percent were men who showed consistent immaturity or irresponsibility; men who were mentally retarded, brain-injured or suffering from severe emotional disturbance; or men who were chronic alcoholics or sociopaths. An even higher degree of success—90 percent—was later claimed by a ranking military medical officer who termed the Army's rehabilitation of blinded soldiers "one of the greatest achievements in military ophthalmology."

While evaluations by outside observers produced a less roseate picture, the overall judgment was "that newly-blinded persons could learn to be blind in a time-limited period if there were sufficient personnel, equipment and services available." Mounted at substantial cost (the Old Farms program alone was said to have involved over $6 million), this demonstration helped give the final impetus to postwar development of rehabilitation centers for all newly blinded adults.

Where was the organized field of work for the blind in this largely military picture? Except for a few special circumstances, and even more special personalities, the professional experts on blindness played only a peripheral role. In the initial planning for the Army program, the Surgeon General's office refrained from seeking advice from leaders in work for the blind. It did not get around to asking for help from specialists in blindness until the beginning of 1945, when it invited Robert Irwin to recommend a small group of "honorary advisory consultants" who would "visit our blind hospitals from time to time and give us counsel and advice as to the working of our program." The group suggested by Irwin, which was given the official title of Honorary Civilian Advisory Committee, Program for the War Blinded of the United States Army, held its first meeting with the Surgeon General's chief consultant in ophthalmology, Colonel Derrick T. Vail, on March 21, 1945.

Colonel Vail told the ten men and two women who met with him that day that they were there as individuals and not as representatives of agencies or professional associations. He was blunt in his criticism of some of the interagency and interpersonal rivalries he had observed while setting up the Army program. At least part of his negative impression, it became clear, had grown out of contact with Dr. Merle E. Frampton who, as a reserve officer in charge of special services for the Navy's department of rehabilitation, had been instrumental in the Navy's last-minute decision not to participate in the Old Farms program. Instead, the Navy established its own rehabilitation service for blinded sailors and marines at the Philadelphia Naval Hospital; the program incorporated a two-week period at Dr. Frampton's school, the New York Institute for the Education of the Blind.

Vail was equally outspoken in his criticism of the Veterans Administration which, he said, had dragged its feet to the point where the Army had been forced to go much further into the work of rehabilitation than it had wanted or expected. He made it clear, however, that he and his colleagues in the Surgeon General's office were pleased and proud over their accomplishments and that, while they were willing to heed criticism given in a constructive spirit, the basic pattern had been set and would continue.

In addition to Irwin, who was elected chairman, the Army's honorary civilian advisory committee consisted of Canada's Colonel Baker; Reverend Thomas J. Carroll, then assistant director, Catholic Guild for the Blind, Newton, Mass., and an official chaplain at Old Farms; Joseph G. Cauffman, principal, Pennsylvania Institution for the Instruction of the Blind (Overbrook); Dr. Roma S. Cheek, executive director, North Carolina Commission for the Blind; Dr. Gabriel Farrell, director, Perkins School for the Blind; Philip N. Harrison, executive secretary, Pennsylvania Association for the Blind; R. Henry P. Johnson, executive director, Florida Council for the Blind (who was replaced, after his sudden death a few months later, by Dr. Richard S. French of the California School for the Blind); Mrs. Lee Johnston, executive director, Missouri Commission for the Blind; W. L. McDaniel, executive secretary, Washington Society for the Blind; Eber L. Palmer, superintendent, New York State School for the Blind (Batavia); and Peter J. Salmon, who by that time had become executive director of the Industrial Home for the Blind, Brooklyn.

The committee agreed that it would not be feasible for all of its members to visit the Army rehabilitation units, and three were selected to serve as the official consultants. In the course of the next weeks they made their first round of visits to Valley Forge, Dibble, and Old Farms. The reports they submitted were, on the whole, favorable, but they also pinpointed specific areas of weakness and offered suggestions on how these might be overcome.

One observation made by the consultant group was that the Army's standoffish attitude toward the established organizations for the blind was being passed on to the trainees. This was shortsighted, Peter Salmon warned Colonel Vail on his return from the first tour. For many of the men, he pointed out, the grandiose hopes for professional or commercial careers encouraged at Old Farms would prove empty dreams. They would need the more down-to-earth approach taken by agencies for the blind.

When the consultants made a second round of visits early in 1946, they found that most of their earlier recommendations had been followed, but that a host of new problems had arisen, many of them due to rapid changes of personnel now that the war was over. One by one, the military ophthalmologists and key staff people at Valley Forge, Dibble, and Old Farms, as well as those in the top echelons of the Surgeon General's office, were returning to civilian life. The guns having been silenced, no large new influx of blinded men could be expected. The military rehabilitation units were beginning to retrench and prepare for shutdown. If the Veterans Administration was ever to take hold of its end of the job, now was the time.

The Veterans Administration was then undergoing a vast reorganization following the retirement of General Hines and the appointment of General Omar Bradley as his successor. In the circumstances, the Army's Honorary Civilian Advisory Committee disbanded in mid-1946, but not before its members had volunteered to take on a comparable role with the VA. Their offer was promptly accepted by General Bradley. The VA's Advisory Committee on the Blinded Veteran was formally appointed in March 1946, with the same 12 members as the Army's advisory group, plus three additional persons: Navy Captain Howard H. Montgomery, commanding officer of the U. S. Naval Hospital in Philadelphia;

Colonel Charles A. Pfeffer, successor to Colonel Thorne as commanding officer of Old Farms, and Raymond T. Frey, a blinded World War II veteran who, following his own rehabilitation at Valley Forge, had been employed as the "blind consultant" there. (Frey was subsequently replaced on the committee by another blinded veteran, Major John F. Brady.)

The driving spirit in the new advisory group was Father Carroll, whose first-hand knowledge of the blinded men exceeded that of any of the others except Frey's. A frequent visitor to Valley Forge and the Philadelphia Naval Hospital in addition to Old Farms, Thomas J. Carroll was a tall, Hollywood-handsome young cleric endowed with a logical mind, a fighting spirit, and so deep a capacity for empathy with the problems of blindness that the men in the rehabilitation centers fondly called him "Father Tom," while others, disregarding the fact that he was sighted, spoke of him as "the blind priest."

Born in Gloucester, Mass., in 1909, Carroll was a graduate of Holy Cross University and St. John's Seminary. His first assignment, following his ordination in 1938, was as assistant director of the small, newly founded Catholic Guild for the Blind operated under the aegis of the Archdiocese of Boston. In 1947 he was made director of the Guild and went on to become a commanding figure in the overall movement for the rehabilitation of the adult blind when the Guild established its St. Paul's Rehabilitation Center in 1954. Under his active guidance the center's 16-week residential program won a nationwide reputation for creativity and standard-setting; its governing principles were subsequently set forth by Carroll in a challenging book, *Blindness: What It Is, What It Does and How to Live with It.* Although his heavily psychiatric approach was regarded by many people in the field as extreme, particularly his emphasis on accepting blindness as "a death" which had to be followed by a conscious psychological rebirth, the book became one of the resource materials used in educational programs preparing students for work in the field of blindness.

Despite its sectarian auspices, Father Carroll's agency served blind people of all faiths; to reflect its nonsectarian nature, the name was changed in 1964 to Catholic Guild for All the Blind. It was changed once again on July 1, 1972, to the Carroll Rehabilitation Center for the Visually Impaired, in memory of Father Carroll, who had died in 1971.

Through his work with the war-blinded Father Carroll grew into positions of leadership in a variety of national movements for the welfare of blind people. That his keen insights were already present in 1946 became clear when, at the very first meeting of the VA's Advisory Committee, he posed a list of 51 specific questions on VA services for the blinded and asked the agency's officials for their answers. He then analyzed the responses in a cogent 21-page report which bluntly identified the areas of weakness, confusion, and malfunction that needed immediate attention if the VA were to fulfill its mandated responsibilities toward men who had lost the use of their eyes in the nation's service. Following review by the entire committee, the Carroll report was forwarded to General Bradley on October 3, 1946.

The basic problem in the Veterans Administration was neither ill-will nor indifference but generalized disarray. Brigadier General Hines, who had been appointed in 1923 to head the predecessor Veterans Bureau, had succeeded in 22 years in building a tight and tamper-proof organization. The price of this probity, however, was the psychological paralysis that so often accompanies an entrenched bureaucracy. When Hines retired in 1945, two Army officers who had distinguished themselves during the war were persuaded to invest a couple of years in updating and reorganizing the sluggish structure to cope with its swollen postwar responsibilities.

A formidable job faced General Bradley as VA administrator and General Paul R. Hawley as chief medical director. More than 16 million men had served in the armed forces during World War II; some 400,000 had died, three-quarters of them in battle, and some 650,000 men had been wounded. The task was so gigantic that the problem of blinded veterans held a low priority. Although classified as among the most seriously disabled, the war-blinded represented only 2 percent of the disabled men for whose rehabilitation the VA was responsible. A complicating factor was that the services needed for blinded men fell athwart the administrative divisions of the VA: proposals endorsed one day by the Medical Department were frustrated the next by the Training Department; measures approved at headquarters were ignored, misunderstood, or misapplied in the regional offices if, indeed, news of their approval ever managed to get through the choked channels of communication.

A rueful account of the administrative snarls that delayed the Veterans Administration in moving ahead with a viable program for rehabilitation of the war-blinded was given in 1969 by C. Warren Bledsoe, a pivotal figure in the frustrating paper chase. An affable, articulate man with unmistakable relish for the role of fascinated observer and discursive chronicler, he was literally born into work for the blind. His father, John Francis Bledsoe, was superintendent of the Maryland School for the Blind when the son, baptized Charles Warren but universally known by his middle name, was born in 1912. Following graduation from Princeton in 1934, Warren spent the next six years teaching at the Maryland institution, taking a year's leave of absence during this period to attend the advanced teacher-training course given at the Perkins School for the Blind. The writing and publication of a successful novel then occupied him until he joined the Army Air Corps in 1942. He was a technical sergeant stationed at Craig Field in Alabama when the call went out for servicemen with experience in work for the blind to be transferred to the eye center at Valley Forge Hospital. There Bledsoe spent two years working with his old friend and former colleague, Dick Hoover, in the cane travel program.

On discharge from the Army, Bledsoe accepted a position with the American Foundation for the Blind as editor of the *Outlook*. Simultaneously, however, he was asked to become a part-time consultant to the Veterans Administration in activating its program for blinded veterans. After a year of dividing his time between the Foundation and the VA, Bledsoe accepted a full-time appointment at VA headquarters as coordinator of services for blinded veterans. The establishment of such a post had been one of the major recommendations of the VA Civilian

Advisory Committee, some of whose members also played a part in having Bledsoe appointed to the job after Hoover, the universal first choice, declined in favor of attending medical school.

It was during Bledsoe's year in this post that the VA's trailblazing center at Hines for treatment and training of blinded veterans was finally activated. He subsequently reverted to a consultant role and organized a comprehensive survey of the status of war-blinded veterans. In 1952, when the war in Korea brought about a new wave of blinded men, the VA reinstated a full-time position at headquarters and Bledsoe became chief of services to the blind in the central office. The position was abolished during a 1958 economy wave (it was reinstated the following year), but a comparable job opened at that point in the Office of Vocational Rehabilitation and Bledsoe joined Mary Switzer's staff in developing rehabilitation services for non-veterans. As of 1972 he was continuing in the service of the Department of Health, Education, and Welfare as a special assistant in the Office of Services for the Blind and Visually Handicapped.

Warren Bledsoe's employment history accurately reflects the period's on-again, off-again course of events in the Veterans Administration. That agency's vacillating attitude during the immediate postwar period was enough to cause Robert Irwin to write a testy letter in the spring of 1948 to Major General Carl R. Gray, who had just succeeded General Bradley as VA administrator. Announcing his decision to resign as chairman of the VA's Advisory Committee, Irwin's letter said: "Although this committee has been in existence for two years, we have very little in the way of concrete evidence that the VA is interested in our recommendations. The Veterans Administration service to the blinded veteran is about as ineffective as it was two years ago."

The letter drew a soothing overnight reply from Gray. "I am only here some 100 days," the new VA chief wrote. "This is the first indication that I have had that there isn't complete understanding between the Administration and your committee." He promised a prompt investigation. The general was as good as his word. Two weeks later he wrote that the medical department under Dr. Paul A. Magnuson, whom he had appointed to succeed General Hawley, was reorganizing the VA's program for the severely handicapped, including the blinded, in a way that would "straighten out this problem to everybody's satisfaction." Agreeing to defer his resignation, Irwin reiterated that success hinged on "selection of personnel—top personnel especially—who really believe that blind people can be rehabilitated."

This ultimately came about, but by then the Advisory Committee on the Blinded Veteran had dissolved through disuse and passed into history.

At the same time that leaders in work for the blind were reaping a harvest of disappointment in their efforts to influence policy through advisory committees, the war-blinded men were nonetheless benefiting on the operating level from the experience, goodwill, and resources of the professional organizations in work for the blind. In large measure this was due to the energy, brains, and personality of a remarkable woman named Kathern F. Gruber.

There were slow-moving bureaucrats who called her "hell-on-wheels." Less intimidated officials called her "amazing" and praised her "pleasing personality [which] made everyone relax." Bledsoe, who worked in close partnership with her over a number of years, termed her "most gloriously militant." As for the men who were the focus of her efforts, they later named her "Sweetheart of the Blinded Veterans Association" and renewed the title at annual conventions by toasting her to the tune of "Let Me Call You Sweetheart." The one thing nobody called her was Kathern; it was always Kay.

A handsome woman in her late thirties, whose wardrobe drew admiring comments from men and women alike, Kay Gruber found her true metier when, at the beginning of 1945, she joined the staff of the Foundation to initiate its Service for the War-Blinded department. She had spent 15 years as a teacher of the blind in Minneapolis high schools, where her effective system of vocational placement and post-graduate followup of students foreshadowed the kind of personalized interest she was to take in the "graduates" of the rehabilitation centers for blinded servicemen.

A desire to do something for the war effort led Miss Gruber to write Robert Irwin in 1944, asking him how to go about getting a job that would make use of her experience. The letter came at a propitious moment. Irwin had already alerted his trustees to the need for a staff member to work with the war-blinded. "As an entirely civilian organization we are free to go to anyone from the Surgeon General down and make representation in behalf of the men."

The job Irwin offered Kay was one she would have to shape as she went along. "I am not quite sure just what is needed," he wrote her just before she reported for duty. "For quite a while your job is going to be to find out what the government is not doing and why not. You can then accumulate the facts which we can lay before the proper government officials and get things going [in] the right way."

It was not totally virgin territory Kay Gruber was expected to plow. The Foundation was already well and favorably known at Valley Forge, Dibble, Old Farms, and the Philadelphia Naval Hospital because two years earlier it had initiated the policy of presenting each blinded serviceman with a braille watch. The rationale for this service was reported by the Foundation president at the 1943 annual meeting:

> Learning to tell time on these watches is almost the first step in the re-adjustment of these boys to their new life. We feel this is extremely important because time weighs heavily on their hands. Some of them report they "look" at their watches a hundred times a day. To meet this need the Foundation has placed orders for watches which will necessitate an investment of $8,000.

That first $8,000 investment was more than quadrupled in the years that followed. By 1950 the Foundation had presented 1,464 blinded servicemen with personalized braille watches. (It had also "redeemed" three such watches which had found their way to pawnshops in different sections of the country.)

Finding the money for the watches was in some ways the least of it. During the war years, there were few watches for sale to civilians and many of the first to be distributed were dredged out of bureau drawers and attic trunks by sympathetic citizens in response to public appeals. They were then cleaned and repaired, and tiny metal or glass dots were added around the face.

A few of the war-blinded men could not use the brailled timepieces, having lost hands as well as eyes. For them, repeater watches were procured and specially adapted. The design for encasing these in a special frame, which a handless man could keep in a shirt pocket and activate by depressing a plunger with his stump or prosthesis, came from St. Dunstan's. The watch operated by means of a two-tone chime; the deeper tone struck the hour, while a higher tone told the quarter-hour so a man could ascertain the time within a 15-minute range of accuracy.

A braille watch had great meaning to a newly blinded man, and it also had special meaning for the Foundation. "We expect to set up a follow-up service with all these men, and the watch makes an excellent original contact," Irwin explained to an official of the Army Surgeon General's office. Kay Gruber expounded on this point when she told VA officials that "the boys will need most of our services after . . . they are back in civilian life making a living in competition with the sighted."

The Foundation continued to present every blinded serviceman with a braille watch throughout the Korean War and into the early days of Vietnam. The practice was terminated in 1963 as part of the policy decision to discontinue using Foundation funds for personal services or equipment that could be supplied through other sources. Once the Veterans Administration got a workable program under way for blinded veterans, men discharged from military service became eligible to receive braille watches and other devices from the VA.

In point of fact, blinded servicemen had been entitled to receive all types of tangible aids from the VA under the provisions of Public Law 78–309, enacted in 1944. The reason they didn't was that the VA could do nothing until they became veterans, and as has been noted, they were kept in military status until after the completion of basic rehabilitation training. Recognizing the importance of the earliest phase of rehabilitation, the Foundation stepped in to fill the gap not only by means of watches but through supplying typewriters, braille equipment and other aids. It succeeded in persuading the Army and Navy to buy some of this equipment for teaching purposes; other types of equipment were given to the military eye centers on loan, and still others, such as portable typewriters, were sold at less than half the Foundation's cost to men who wanted to buy their own machines.

Public Law 78-309 had a curious history. In the first wave of concern over war-blindness, eager legislators introduced bills calling for the appropriation of $5 million to supply dog guides to blinded men through the Veterans Administration. These early bills died in committee, but in early 1944 a fresh bill, reducing the amount to $1 million, was introduced by Hamilton Fish in the House and James J. Davis in the Senate. Even this sum, in the opinion of those who knew how small a percentage of blind people could make practical use of dog guides, was "about fifty times as much as [the] VA will probably need." However, since the bill seemed sure to pass, Robert Irwin decided it could be made really useful if its scope was enlarged to include money for "mechanical and electronic equipment." There was no difficulty in getting the bill amended along the lines of this suggestion, and it was enacted May 24, 1944.

The VA's administration of this law was one of the chief points of dissatisfaction among blinded veterans and those attempting to help them. Interpretation of the bill's provisions varied from one VA regional office to another. On the grounds that the VA's rehabilitation function was purely on vocational lines, some offices made grants only for specific occupational equipment, ruling out such objects as typewriters, braille writers, recording machines, even the $2.50 aluminum braille slates which blind men used to make notes.

Perhaps the source of greatest distress was an early administrative ruling that P.L. 309 was applicable only to totally blind men, rather than to all who met the commonly accepted legal definition of blindness. While this was eventually corrected in a revised ruling early in 1947, there had been a two-and-one-half-year delay between the law's passage and its usefulness to those it was intended to benefit.

During the war years, procurement of typewriters and braillewriters presented the same problems as the watches; there were simply none for sale on the open market. The public appeals that had succeeded with watches were also used to obtain an initial supply of used typewriters. About a hundred were donated and, after reconditioning, contributed to the adjustment centers. An effort was also made to collect used braillewriters, but there were few to be had, so with Army help the Foundation obtained priority ratings from the War Production Board to have a moderate supply manufactured. Priority ratings also helped to procure the new portable typewriters which the blinded men in the hospitals were eager to buy for their personal correspondence.

Initially, it was thought that the typewriters should be gifts, like the braille watches, but this idea was modified on the advice of the social workers at the military eye centers. The men were "hanging on to every ounce of self-respect permitted," a social worker at Valley Forge wrote the Foundation, so the policy adopted was to charge a nominal $25 for a personal portable, with the Foundation defraying the additional $30 cost of the machine. By the end of the war, more than five hundred portable typewriters and a smaller number of braillewriters had been furnished to war-blinded men on this basis.

There was one other way the Foundation had paved the road that it employed Kay Gruber to travel. It had sent Helen Keller and Polly Thomson on two "Purple Heart circuit" tours during 1944 and 1945. Helen, who began by visiting the centers for blinded men, was invited by the officers in charge to tour other wards in the same hospitals. Out of this experience came her wish to tour all the hospitals for the nation's war-wounded, and the Foundation agreed to defray the costs of the cross-country journeys that eventually took her and Polly to 70 Army and Navy hospitals in a six-month period.

The impact of these visits was little short of sensational. In one hospital after another, Helen Keller was hailed as the ultimate morale builder. The twenty-year-olds who filled the beds were astonished that this woman, whom they had read about in their history books, was still alive, and not only alive but vibrant, cheerful, and indefatigable. Helen did not spare herself. As Polly Thomson wrote to a friend in November 1944:

It's hard work, the hardest we have ever done, but it's worth it. We walk miles up and down corridors and wards. . . . We get up sometimes at 4:30-5:30 and begin at the hospitals by 9 o'clock and stay in until around 5 P.M. We literally tumble into bed exhausted. Don't speak to each other, too weary—our voices are tired. Up again following morning to start all over again. . . . Helen never did a finer work and I'm proud she has been privileged to do it.

Not only the wounded men but the hospital staffs appreciated these visits. Brigadier General W.R. Dear, commanding general of the Northington General Hospital in Tuscaloosa, Ala., put his thanks in terms that really appealed to the sixty-five-year-old Helen. "You are the most impressive and stimulating visitor we have had at our hospital and that puts you ahead of the Hollywood blondes, brunettes and play boys."

Helen herself reacted in equally exhilarated terms. "To be permitted to kindle even one light for the wounded or the despondent is an event as blessed as if I had my sight restored," she wrote Migel at the conclusion of her first tour. The trip inspired her as much as she inspired the men who came in contact with her. A visit to the gymnasium of an amputee unit led her to write the commanding officer that the men's "gaiety carried me back to my girlhood and almost before I knew it I was throwing a ball for them to catch, rowing in the boat and punching the bag as light hearted as the merriest of them."

The glow kindled in Helen Keller's heart by such experiences lasted a long time. This recharging of her spiritual batteries was assuredly a key factor in enabling her, in the years ahead, to undertake the exhausting overseas tours of war-stricken lands that climaxed her lifetime of work for the blind people of the world.

Kay Gruber wove these strong strands of good will into a tight and durable fabric. Unlike some other emissaries from the field of work for the blind, she came not to criticize the staffs of the military medical and rehabilitation units, but to help them do the best job they could. She took infinite pains to listen to their problems and furnish useful clues and helpful suggestions: the names of potential candidates for staff vacancies, lists of books on blindness, information on where to procure equipment, tips on rehabilitation techniques successfully tried out in other centers. Careful note was also made during her field trips of the blinded men's personal requests, and items large and small were followed through conscientiously. A voluminous correspondence resulted from these visits as well as from the many office interviews conducted with blinded veterans or members of their families.

Beginning in 1946, with the hostilities at an end and most of the blinded men discharged and back home, the Foundation's activity focused increasingly on the Veterans Administration. An offer to help indoctrinate the staffs of the VA's regional offices, to which veterans now had to apply for all services, was readily accepted, and four intensive training courses, each three weeks long, were given to acquaint regional personnel with the necessary philosophy and techniques. A total of 127 VA employees attended these courses, which were held in New York and included, in addition to lectures and discussions, field trips to a typical voluntary agency for the blind, a sheltered workshop, the Foundation's technical laboratories, the Seeing Eye dog guide school, the Army's rehabilitation center at Old Farms, and the Navy's program at the New York Institute for the Education of the Blind.

The courses did an excellent job; unfortunately, much of the effect was dissipated when a number of VA staff members who had attended were transferred to assignments not involved with the war-blinded (one such transfer took place less than two weeks after completion of the course) and their replacements were not offered the opportunity of similar orientation. Efforts were made with the Veterans Administration to have the course repeated for newcomers, or to establish other methods of familiarizing regional office staff with the special needs of the blind, but these came to naught. This situation constituted one of the major complaints of the VA's Advisory Committee.

Another complaint was that ignorance, indifference and internal pressures caused by heavy workloads were resulting in inequities in the VA's treatment of war-blinded men. One, which was still in force in 1972, had to do with the arbitrary distinction made between men who had suffered anatomical loss of both eyes and those who were equally sightless but whose eyes had not been enucleated. The first group received appreciably larger disability compensation awards.

An additional flaw in disability compensation payments concerned the eight thousand or so men who had lost the sight of one eye in the service. Men in this category were awarded compensation on the basis of 30 or 40 percent disability. Long experience prompted workers for the blind to alert the VA to the likelihood that some would sooner or later lose the sight of the remaining eye. Even though this might come about through a wholly unrelated accident or illness, the resulting total blindness was entitled to be adjudged and compensated as service-connected. By 1947, when more than 15 such cases had already occurred, the men were still receiving compensation for only partial disability. Eventually, legislation straightened out this inequity.

The terms "disability compensation" and "pension" are often used interchangeably, but they actually represent two different ideas. Disability compensation is paid for a service-connected injury which impairs a man's earning capacity; it is not a reward for services rendered but an effort to insure that the injured veteran's future standard of living will not suffer by reason of his diminished earning ability. Disability compensation is not related to economic need; a veteran disabled in service is entitled to receive it whether or not he is gainfully employed.

Pensions, which are regarded as recompense for services to the nation, are paid to men who have served in the armed forces and who, by reason of non-service-connected illness or disability, or because of advancing age, are in temporary or permanent need of financial assistance.

The laws governing rates of payment for both disability compensation and pensions are complex and have been subject to frequent upward revision. Thus the disability compensation rate for anatomical loss of both eyes, which was $265 per month in 1945, was $371 in 1954 and $770 in 1972.

Troublesome as individual inequities might be for the affected veterans and for people like Kay Gruber and Father Carroll who were trying to help straighten them out, they ranked second in importance in the opinion of leaders in work for the blind to the need for the Veterans Administration to formulate and execute a permanent plan for the future social adjustment of blinded veterans. The Army and Navy rehabilitation units were closed down by mid-1947. A large number of blinded men had been discharged from military service without any sort of rehabilitation training, an even larger number had not derived sufficient benefit from such training as they did receive, an unpredictable number had marginal vision at the time of discharge that would undoubtedly deteriorate into blindness in future years, and a similarly unpredictable number might be expected to incur blindness-producing injuries during peacetime military service. At this point no one even dared to think about the possibility of future wars.

Obstacle after obstacle impeded the VA's initiation of a rehabilitation program for blinded veterans and, one by one, they were cleared away. In the spring of 1947 the federal Budget Bureau raised a question over whether the VA was legally empowered to give anything other than vocational services. To settle this point an executive order was issued by President Harry S. Truman on May 31, 1947, specifically assigning responsibility to the Veterans Administration for social rehabilitation training of blinded veterans. This, Bledsoe was to write, "should have been enough to make the most inveterate shilly-shallyer shamefaced." But it wasn't. There was still resistance in some of VA's top administrative echelons to getting a rehabilitation center under way. "Why all this fuss about the blinded veteran? He will be just as blind three years from now," was the cynical comment of a ranking executive at VA's central office on one occasion.

There was also uncertainty over where a VA rehabilitation center should be located. At one point it was to be Fort Thomas in Kentucky; a little later, Framingham, Mass. For a time, too, there was talk that the Federal Security Agency might set up a national rehabilitation center for the blind that could serve both veterans and civilians; although the idea failed to materialize, it served as one more excuse for deferring VA action. In the closing days of 1947, however, the VA finally decided to establish a training center for blinded veterans that would be located in a suburb of Chicago at Hines Hospital, which had a strong physical medicine and rehabilitation service in operation.

What may have tipped the scales was the fact that Carl Gray, the VA administrator, was himself functionally blind. According to the memoirs of Dr. Paul Magnuson, whom General Gray appointed as the agency's medical chief: "Carl Gray could not see. In one eye he had only a little lateral vision, and he had not been at the head of the Veterans Administration long before he developed a block of central vision in his other eye. He was unable to read a typewritten word."

In any event, 1948 saw the turning point. With the appointment in late February of Russell C. Williams under the title of Chief, Physical Medicine Rehabilitation of the Blind, Hines Hospital, there at last came into being a permanent government facility where blinded veterans could be trained in personal and social adjustment through a carefully designed, time-limited program which utilized and improved on everything that had been learned at Valley Forge, Dibble, and Old Farms.

The initial program at Hines was designed to be very small and very selective. Only nine men at a time were to be trained in an 18-week program, and for these there was to be a nine-person staff, a one-to-one ratio. Finding and training staff and equipping the center took several months. The first patients were admitted in July.

Within a year, the Hines program was recognized as a model of excellence, its quality of which was due largely to the unwavering standards established and maintained by its chief. Once again history had provided the right man in the right place at the right time.

A few months away from his thirtieth birthday when he came to Hines, Russell Williams was a blinded veteran who had achieved his own rehabilitation at Valley Forge and Avon and had then returned to Valley Forge as blind consultant when Raymond Frey left to begin the study and practice of physical therapy. A Hoosier by birth, Williams held a degree in education from Indiana's Central Normal College and was a teacher and athletic director at the Dillsboro, Indiana, High School when he was called up for military service in 1942. In August 1944, two months after his field artillery unit landed in France, an exploding shell tore across Williams' face, destroying both eyes.

Although neither a psychiatrist nor a psychologist by training, Williams was endowed with an instinctive understanding of human behavior that was constantly enlarged and enriched as he developed the program at Hines. His empathy for the men who came to the rehabilitation center as patients was more than that of one blind man for another. He regarded himself and every other blinded veteran as a person struggling for growth, and was able to communicate this kinship of need not only to the trainees but to every member of his carefully chosen staff.

These were all sighted men, some with a few years of experience in work with the physically handicapped, but none specifically knowledgeable about blindness. With help from Kay Gruber and Warren Bledsoe, who spent months at Hines assisting in the personnel screening and indoctrination process, Williams looked for "sincere, healthy minded, emotionally balanced persons, with varied interests, sufficient security to respect their fellow workmen and the patients with whom they would come in contact."

It is doubtful whether Williams could have articulated, at this early stage, just what he meant by "sufficient security." Many years later, after he had moved to Washington to become VA's national chief of blind rehabilitation, he was able to formulate this essential quality as the subordination of the staff member's emotional needs in favor of building the client's ego.

To motivate such an attitude, the indispensable element was what Williams called "a pivot person"—a leader who firmly believed "that when sight is diminished or lost, life can be pursued in effective ways and pleasure gotten out of it." His unremitting personal demonstration of this belief was what enabled the rehabilitation therapists at Hines to push on despite seeming stalemates or setbacks and to become believers themselves.

Williams trained his staff "as thoroughly as a coach trains a team for a big game" by emulating the methods developed at Valley Forge—methods which became the core of teaching programs for rehabilitation therapists. Training took place under a blindfold, and encompassed both self-care functions and orientation and mobility skills. The blindfolded instructors (called "orientors") were taught how to orient themselves in space by touch, smell, and hearing; how to travel erectly, rapidly, and safely with the use of the long cane; how and when to ask for sighted help. It wasn't easy. According to John D. Malmazian, one of the first staff members at the Hines center and later its chief:

> There were numerous occasions during mobility lessons when they became disoriented and walked into the streets. One man walked into an open garage and was unable to get out without assistance. . . . The men frequently were anxious and occasionally panicked when they were confused and lost but did not remove their blindfolds. Instead, they shouted for assistance. . . . Each experience taught them better to appreciate and use their newly acquired skills and command of their remaining senses to select and interpret environmental clues.
>
> By the time the first patient arrived on July 6, 1948, all the orientors . . . had acquired enough experience to believe that the techniques were valid and would, if used properly, enable a blind person to travel safely, efficiently and independently in almost any type of environment.

Flexible but firm in his judgments, Williams was capable of resisting the outside pressures that in any way threatened to impede the work of the center. And pressures there were. Some were trivial. Residents of the nearby community of Maywood who saw the trainees and their orientors practicing mobility techniques on the streets called to complain that the latter were heedlessly risking the safety of blind men. Now and again a citizen, sure that something sinister was afoot, would notify the police that a blind man was being followed by a mysterious stranger.

More serious was the fact that many people in influential positions regarded the center's omission of specific vocational training as a mistake. Williams, however, held to the principle that the blind rehabilitation unit at Hines was essentially "an environmental therapy in which the patient learns how to deal with the effects of blindness" and that specific vocational preparation could and should take place only after this fundamental goal had been attained.

Still a different set of problems arose when regional VA offices referred men who lacked the necessary emotional or physical strengths to benefit from such environmental therapy. "Our program is tough," Williams explained over and over. "Its keynote is hard work." Only men in sound health, able to undergo a regimen of physical reconditioning after years of inactivity, could be considered. Good physical tone was essential for successful training in independent travel. "A blind man needs extremely strong feet and ankles if he is not to be thrown by the pebbles, sticks and unexpected depressions the ordinary person unconsciously sees and avoids. Even though the cane weighs only six ounces, its use requires a strong, flexible wrist and an untiring arm," he told a reporter for the Chicago *Herald-American* in one of the few newspaper interviews he permitted.

Avoidance of publicity was deliberate. During the first year or two, while the Hines program was being refined and shaped, very few visitors were permitted. The only welcome exceptions were Bledsoe and three consultants appointed by the VA's Department of Medicine and Surgery who came regularly to advise and assist. These consultants were Kay Gruber, Richard Hoover (by then an M.D.) and Harry Spar, an able blind man who was the industrial training specialist of the Industrial Home for the Blind in Brooklyn. Spar, who later became IHB's associate director and in 1972 held the title of associate director of the IHB-operated National Center for Deaf-Blind Youths and Adults, helped set up the manual arts shops in which the Hines trainees developed their sense of touch through manipulation of various materials and machines.

The greatest challenge to the Hines staff lay in the trainees themselves. They were different from the eager, enthusiastic, newly blinded men, so many of whom had succeeded brilliantly at Valley Forge and Old Farms and had gone on to establish themselves in new life patterns. The men who came to Hines in 1948 and 1949 had been blind for four or five years and had not yet learned how to come to terms with that fact. Some had tried and failed; others had not even tried but had spent the years in debilitating inactivity and mounting despondency as the glamor of being war heroes wore off. Williams made it his business to get to know these men intimately; he came to know their family situations, their personal hangups and the behavioral defenses they had erected to protect their damaged egos. He spent time every day with every man, sensing when to soothe, when to encourage, when to challenge. He was kind and understanding but at the same time strict in his insistence that a man respect the discipline of the training program and that he work ceaselessly to rise to his own potential.

The one eventuality not foreseen when the Hines program was established on such a miniature scale was that American servicemen would soon be fighting on a new battlefield. When the Korean conflict began to produce its tragic harvest of blinded men, the United States was prepared at last to do something about them without having to start all over again.

Early in 1951 authorization was given for the capacity of the Hines program to be tripled to 27 beds, and for a 13-bed preliminary adjustment unit to be established in the hospital's ophthalmology ward. This expansion, which also meant 20 new staff members to be recruited and put through blindfold training, was accomplished within the year. The nature of the Korean War, with its close hand-to-hand fighting, resulted in many more multihandicapped casualties than World War II. The Hines program's emphasis on physical fitness had to be modified. The staff, by this time, had acquired sufficient expertise to tackle the adjustment of men who had sustained serious injuries in addition to blindness. Adaptations of training procedures and prosthetic devices were evolved to enable amputees and neurologically impaired men to learn how to cope with lack of sight. The Korean toll ultimately came to 500 men, the highest ratio of blindness—more than 5 percent of all casualties—in any American war up to that time.

Sadly, the Foundation reactivated its Services for the War-Blinded department. At the request of the Defense Department Kay Gruber, now one of the Foundation's three assistant directors, once again went to military hospitals treating the eye-wounded and provided their administrators with information about Hines and other facilities and services which could be of help to the men. There was, however, an important difference in the Foundation's approach to its responsibility for this new group of blinded veterans. It no longer tried single-handedly to untangle the men's individual problems. Many were turned over to a new and increasingly potent ally: the Blinded Veterans Association.

From a psychological viewpoint, the men who went through the World War II program of social adjustment fell into three categories: (1) those who accepted their blindness and strove to overcome its limitations; (2) those who refused to accept the fact of blindness and were confused and depressed as a result; (3) those who sought to escape the reality of blindness through resort to alcoholism and other denial mechanisms.

It was the men in the first category who genuinely profited from the training that taught them the techniques of living as blind men, and it was this group that realized that, no matter what benefits and assistance might be offered them by society, the key to successful rehabilitation lay within themselves. This was the motivating force that led to the establishment of the Blinded Veterans Association, which adopted as its motto: "that the blinded veteran may take his rightful place in the community of his fellows and work with them toward the creation of a peaceful world."

The Blinded Veterans Association was born at Old Farms in March 1945, when about a hundred able and determined men, knowing they would soon be dispersed to their homes, agreed they could help one another in the future. They sensed that the true battle for acceptance in a sighted world would begin only after they had left the protected environment of Old Farms and faced the personal, social, and economic realities of making a place for themselves in society. In this struggle they could not only draw moral support from one another but, through exchanging experiences, learn from one another.

Several midwives assisted in the birth of the BVA. Two, Father Carroll and Kay Gruber, were predictable. A third, who came from outside the professional field of work for the blind, was the mystery writer Baynard Kendrick.

Kendrick's interest in war-blinded men stemmed from a World War I experience at St. Dunstan's, which he had frequented as a volunteer while stationed in London as an American enlistee in the Canadian Army. One Saturday afternoon a young blinded Tommy had astonished him by fingering the emblems and insignia on Kendrick's coat and then rapidly and accurately reconstructing his entire war service record.

Kendrick had originally called at St. Dunstan's to see an old school friend, also a volunteer with the Canadian Army, who had been blinded in action. On returning home, this friend turned into what Kendrick later described as "an alcohol-soaked cabbage," who became utterly lost following his over-protective mother's death. The contrast between the helpless friend and the British soldier who had so deftly demonstrated what a blind man could discern with his fingers stayed in Kendrick's memory for twenty years and ultimately led to a series of mystery novels featuring Captain Duncan Maclain, a blind detective, who, as Kendrick said, "would never perform any feat . . . that couldn't be duplicated by someone totally blind, always presuming they had the necessary brains and will power to train themselves and try it." To make sure he knew just what blind people could and could not do, Kendrick read extensively in the literature and visited a number of schools and organizations for blind people.

As author of the popular mystery series, Kendrick was invited to speak to the war-blinded in the military hospitals; his speech at Old Farms made such an impression that the commanding officer urged him to accept a dollar-a-year job conducting a writing class there. He also arranged for Kendrick to receive an official assignment to write a history of the Army's blind rehabilitation program, but what Kendrick wrote instead was his first serious novel, *Lights Out,* which, using Valley Forge and Old Farms as its setting, told in fictional form the story of one young soldier's struggle to overcome the fear and despair of finding himself suddenly plunged into blindness. Later made into a successful motion picture titled *Bright Victory,* the novel was dedicated "to Lt. Lloyd Greenwood, U.S.A.A.F., who has vision."

A B-24 pilot flying over Vienna when he was blinded by flak, Greenwood was one of the nucleus of spirited men at Old Farms who founded the Blinded Veterans Association. Kendrick, rightfully regarded as the association's prime catalyst, was named honorary chairman of its board, the "honorary" reflecting the fact that, unlike all the other board members, he was not a blinded veteran.

The other catalytic force in establishing the BVA was Kay Gruber, who interested the Foundation in supporting it. As an initial step, Robert Irwin agreed to furnish the BVA with office space and the services of a secretary. He went further after Kay read the galley proofs of *Lights Out* to him on a train journey from New York to Washington. Impressed by the novel and assured by Kay that Kendrick was selflessly interested in the cause of the BVA, Irwin proposed to the Foundation board that a grant be made to get the organization on its feet. The board accepted his recommendation and, at its November 30, 1945, meeting, voted $10,000 to help BVA through its first year. The money was personally contributed by M.C. Migel, a lifelong believer in self-help.

It may have been at Migel's instigation that Irwin then addressed a cautious inquiry to Kendrick's publisher, William Morrow & Company, as to the writer's reliability. The reply was reassuring: "There is no question about Kendrick's complete sincerity and integrity. Any cause that he is interested in becomes a holy cause to which he devotes himself with passionate intensity." Forwarding this letter to Migel, Irwin observed that Kendrick's business responsibility seemed sound enough. "I think Mr. Kendrick is a little temperamental," he added, "but that goes with being an author, I guess."

The reason for checking on Kendrick was that the Foundation grant was to be used to pay him a salary while he went about the tasks needed to get the BVA started: mailings to blinded veterans inviting them to join, founding a monthly publication, the *BVA Bulletin,* to serve as the organization's channel of communication with its constituency, speeches to community groups and on radio programs, applications for financial support in various quarters. Kendrick was a whirlwind, but, like other tempestuous forces of nature, he left a certain amount of destruction in his wake. An internal squabble over his role resulted in his resignation from the BVA post in June 1946.

Fortunately for the infant organization, Kendrick had done an excellent job of training two of its key members. Working side by side with him during those early months were Lloyd Greenwood, who served as *BVA Bulletin* editor beginning with its first issue in April 1946, and Raymond Frey, the association's first president. Greenwood, who aspired to a writing career, continued issuing the *Bulletin* after Kendrick's resignation; following the BVA's first convention in September, he was hired as its executive director. The funds to pay his salary and that of a small staff came from the BVA's first outside "angel"—the Women's International Bowling Congress, which pledged $25,000 a year for three years. With this, plus some other funds from philanthropic sources, the Blinded Veterans Association was on its way.

That first convention also elected new officers, with John F. Brady of Brooklyn succeeding Frey as president. It voted Father Carroll into the position of official chaplain * and heard the eloquent priest, in his address to the closing banquet, urge the men of the BVA to serve as "a flying wedge" to effect change in the "unreasonable and unreasoning attitude of the sighted public" toward blind people. people.

By the time BVA held its second annual convention in September 1947 there was impressive progress to report. It had been authorized by the VA to represent blinded veterans in formal appeals and claims; it had moved to larger quarters; the staff had been expanded; a number of state and regional chapters had been established and more were in formation. Elected to a second term as president, John Brady—a cavalry major blinded in action in Munich—took an extended leave of absence from his job, which was then that of employment specialist on the staff of the Industrial Home for the Blind (he later became its executive director), and spent the next years formulating a plan for the BVA to bridge the vital gap of actual job placement in services to blinded veterans. A survey had shown that, three years after the war's end, nearly half the nation's blinded veterans were neither employed nor in vocational or educational training. In some parts of the country, Brady reported, job-ready veterans had been waiting for over a year for the VA to place them.

Brady's proposed solution was a five-year program, estimated to cost $1 million, in which BVA would place ten men in the field, each serving a specified region, to seek out every unemployed blinded veteran, get him into training if necessary and then find a suitable job for him. It was a bold dream—too bold for a few hundred young people who were not only inexperienced but had scruples about how they would raise the needed funds "quietly, without general appeal, because of the maudlin sympathy such a drive would excite."

The BVA moved to Washington in 1948. It saw legislative advocacy as one of its major roles, and gradually gained experience and sophistication in the ways of

---

* Later, two other chaplains were added to reflect BVA's interdenominational nature: Rabbi Michael Aaronsohn of Cincinnati, a blind veteran of World War I, and the Reverend Harry O. Anderson, a Baptist minister in California, who had served as chaplain to the men at the Dibble eye center.

lawmaking and government. It testified before Congressional committees, developed contacts with the policy makers at the Veterans Administration, and worked closely with them, cajoling or prodding as the occasion demanded. Its membership grew; there were 900 dues-paying members in 1960 and 1,200 in 1971.

The one respect in which the organization fell short of its goals was in fundraising. The optimistic plan to raise $1 million proved unattainable, and the BVA had to turn back to its original sponsor, the Foundation, for survival grants. These ranged from relatively small sums—$5,000 in 1949 to pay for publication of the *Bulletin*—to larger subsidies. It was a Foundation appropriation of $30,000 in 1954/55 that furnished the seed money which finally launched the BVA's field service program; the sprouting money came from the federal Office of Vocational Rehabilitation as a demonstration grant to show how the services of federal, state and community agencies could be coordinated on behalf of individual blinded persons.

In the course of the next ten years or so, BVA's six field representatives contacted some two thousand blind veterans. Men who had never undergone adjustment training were persuaded to apply for admission to the Hines rehabilitation center. Jobfinding efforts, which included on-the-spot demonstrations of how blind people could perform in specific tasks, opened up a number of vocational opportunities. Hundreds of veterans were made aware of the variety of benefits and services available and guided through the red tape involved in making use of them.

Lloyd Greenwood remained as BVA executive director until 1954; he was succeeded by Irvin P. Schloss, who had previously been editor of the *Bulletin*. When Schloss resigned in 1958 to join the Foundation staff as its legislative analyst, the BVA saw a series of short-term executives come and go until chronic shortage of funds left the position vacant and the program attenuated.

However, like the men it represented, BVA refused to allow financial and organizational reverses to weaken either its sense of purpose or its determination to prove that blind men could shoulder both the rewards and the burdens of participation in society. It continued to be governed by a board of directors made up of 10 blinded veterans and to receive guidance from a national advisory committee whose membership in the early Seventies included Senator Jennings Randolph, M. Robert Barnett, and Kay Gruber. Miss Gruber, who left the Foundation staff in 1963, moved to California, where in 1972 she was maintaining a consultant practice and continuing to be actively involved in BVA work. Over the years American bowlers continued their financial support of BVA; the initial three-year grant from the Women's International Bowling Congress was followed by sizable annual contributions from the Bowlers Victory Legion and, later, the National Bowling Council.

The first follow-up study of World War II veterans was made in 1952-3 by the Veterans Administration, when social workers in 70 regional offices conducted structured interviews with 2,000 veterans whose service-connected blindness had been incurred in that war and in Korea. The demographic and social data accumulated in the interviews were set forth in a book edited by Bledsoe, *War-Blinded Veterans in a Post-War Setting,* issued by the VA in 1958. The findings amply supported the conclusion that rehabilitation training had "paid dividends, both psychologically and economically." While approximately half of the total group was employed, a much higher employment percentage was found among those who had completed rehabilitation training. Other criteria used to evaluate adjustment and acceptance into society were marital status, family structure, home ownership, social activities, attitudes to self and toward society. These, too, not only substantiated the conclusion that rehabilitation had paid off, but helped demolish the oft-expressed opinion that liberal compensation awards to wounded veterans were bound to destroy motivation for normal, job-centered lives.

Ten years later a second follow-up study was launched. This project, executed by the American Foundation for the Blind with VA financial support and with the Blinded Veterans Association serving as technical consultant, dealt with a smaller sample and used different research techniques. Its outcome was proclaimed in the title of the volume which reported its findings: *851 Blinded Veterans: A Success Story.* Bearing out the title were conclusions such as these:

> The group is relatively well educated. Those who took advantage of the GI Bill—especially in college training (mostly whites) and vocational training (mostly Negroes)—have increased their employment opportunities. Their general socioeconomic status is high because they are well educated and upward or laterally mobile occupationally (those in the labor force, that is) and because they receive generous disability compensation payments. . . .
>
> Age is a problem, especially in employment, as it is for the all-veteran population. Those in the labor force are unemployed in about the same numbers as all unemployed males in the labor force. Like most American males of their age [the median age was 46], they own their own homes, don't move much, live with their wives in small primary family units averaging about 3.5 persons per household, and consider themselves heads of their households. . . . [They] would probably be indistinguishable if it were not for their visual and other impairments; they are middle-age, middle-class American family heads who live "next door" in a comfortable average neighborhood.

Like the previous survey, this one also yielded discoveries that called for action. One of the most important was that half of the men studied had not had an eye examination in five years, that a substantial group had hearing loss, and that others were neglecting a variety of other health problems. Since regular eye care to halt further deterioration was essential for those not totally blind, and hearing loss clearly constituted a serious threat to people who had to depend on their ears for environmental clues, these findings helped jolt into existence an outreach program the Veterans Administration had been considering for several years.

Under the Visual Impairment Services Teams (VIST) program initiated in 1967, the names of all veterans receiving disability compensation or pensions for any degree of visual impairment were sent to regional VA outpatient clinics, which were instructed to make personal contact with those within their jurisdiction and arrange for periodic reviews of their medical conditions and needs. Each multidisciplinary team—consisting of a physician, a social worker, and other appropriate personnel as needed—scheduled an annual physical examination for each of these blind veterans. The physical, which included ophthalmic and audiological tests, also served as the occasion for the social worker to review with the veteran the full range of aids, equipment, benefits and resources to which he was entitled. As of 1972 there were 71 such VIST units in operation with 5,500 visually handicapped veterans on their registers.

The year 1967 also saw the opening of the Western Blind Rehabilitation Center, comparable to Hines, at the VA Hospital in Palo Alto, California. Two years later a third unit, the Eastern Blind Rehabilitation Center, was established at the West Haven, Connecticut, hospital. The three centers, with a combined capacity of 70 beds, were all professionally affiliated with nearby universities and served as clinical training centers for graduate students in various rehabilitation disciplines. They also participated in field-testing the various electronic reading and mobility devices developed under sponsorship of the VA's Prosthetics and Sensory Aids Research and Development Division.

In the late Sixties the three VA Blind Rehabilitation Centers launched programs designed to overcome the problem of transition back into society. As described by John Malmazian, director of the Hines unit,

> a month before the veteran leaves, the wife or mother is invited to the center. They come on a Sunday night with the travel, the motel, meals and local expenses paid. The veteran then stays with his wife at the motel. On Monday the wife arrives at the center. She is put on a program which includes observation, going to classes with the veteran, observing the veteran in his activities, discussing with the staff members the veteran's progress, his potential and his limitations. She then meets with the psychologist, the social worker and the veteran. Another part of the program is training for the family member in basic skills. The family member is taught how to use a sighted guide, how to familiarize a person with an area. They put a blindfold on the family member, and then the next day the family member instructs a staff member, who blindfolds himself.

The $200 cost of this five-day program of observation, consultation, and direct experience was defrayed through non-VA funds; in the case of the Hines center, the subsidy came from the Military Order of the Purple Heart.

At all three VA centers, priority for admission was given to Vietnam veterans, whose number was estimated in early 1972 to be 550 to 600. Concern that a discouragingly large percentage of these newly blinded young men seemed uninterested in social adjustment training prompted a two-day conference jointly sponsored by the Foundation, the BVA, and the VA in April 1972. Various approaches were explored as to how to serve this badly battered group of men, who had suffered a higher percentage of multiple disabilities than the men in any previous war.

Many of the Vietnam veterans, it was recognized, would have been fatalities instead of casualties were it not for the airborne rescue teams which brought them in for prompter medical care than was possible in pre-helicopter days. Of the 363 blinded Vietnam veterans who had passed through the VA's rehabilitation centers as of early 1972, 235 had one or more additional disabilities, ranging from bilateral leg amputations to hearing loss and brain damage. They also bore the psychological burden of public attitudes toward the war in Vietnam. As one VA social worker noted: "Instead of the respect and acclaim given to World War II veterans upon their return home, the Vietnam veterans are oftentimes met with indifference or derision."

Paralleling this rejection by the community was hostility felt toward "the Establishment" by some of the veterans themselves, often exhibited in a refusal to have anything to do with government agencies. The prevalence of disenchanted viewpoints in a wide spectrum of American youth, veterans and non-veterans alike, offered perhaps the severest challenge of all to those concerned with helping the newest group of war-blinded men find satisfying roles in society.

One positive approach took shape in November 1972, when the Veterans Administration awarded a one-year contract to the Blinded Veterans Association to revive the outreach program which would send three BVA representatives into the field to seek out newly blinded veterans and encourage them to take advantage of the rehabilitation and other helping services available to them. This, it was hoped, would help to instill in the men who gave their eyes in the least popular war in American history the determined spirit that enabled so many blinded veterans of a previous generation to rise above their disabilities.

18

The Three-Wheeled Cart

The soldier suddenly stripped of sight by an enemy bullet might have been the most dramatic example, but the exacting challenges he had to overcome were essentially no different than any other newly blinded adult's. Understandably, therefore, the military rehabilitation programs were watched with close attention by the agencies concerned with the welfare of all blind people. Even though newly blinded adults constituted a relatively small part of their caseloads, it seemed reasonable to suppose that the techniques that succeeded with men blinded in battle might well be adapted for those whose blindness was of years-long, even lifelong, duration.

Although, thanks to the Barden-LaFollette Act, the federal government was prepared from 1943 onward to become a partner of the states in the vocational training and placement of employable blind adults, no realistic leader in work for the blind was under the delusion that rehabilitation programs for civilians could be mounted on a scale comparable to what took place at Valley Forge or Old Farms. The military centers commanded unlimited resources of funds, personnel and authority. There were no quantitative ceilings on manpower to staff the centers or to create and maintain the necessary facilities.

Of equal importance were the psychological differences. The war-blinded constituted a largely homogeneous group of youthful and vigorous men whose hopes for the future were not vitiated by memories of failures in the past. In a state-operated rehabilitation center for blind civilians a few years after the war conditions were very different:

> Our students are a most heterogeneous group. What they have in common is that they are all legally blind. . . . Their ages vary from 16 to 65; their I.Q.'s from 65 to 145; their visual handicaps, from congenital blindness to partial

sight with travel vision. Their heterogeneity is accentuated by wide differences in ethnic, social, educational, and cultural backgrounds.

Our present group of eight, for example, consists of the following clients: a 25-year-old congenitally blind college graduate; a 44-year-old divorcee who has been blind only a few months; a 42-year-old congenitally blind borderline mental defective who was recently released from 15 years in a state hospital for epileptics; a 40-year-old mechanic who retains vision sufficient for travel—his visual handicap is the result of a self-inflicted gunshot wound eight years ago; a 32-year-old congenitally blind male who, until recently, was spoonfed by his mother; a 30-year-old man with travel vision who is a borderline schizophrenic; a 20-year-old man with practically no vision but who likes to drive cars and whose I.Q. is 80.

Agencies for the blind were not lacking in experience in working with persons so diverse in background, need and potential. What was new, in the rehabilitation center movement that began just after World War II, was bringing them together under a single roof for a concentrated period of adjustment services. It was the exact opposite of the traditional home teaching method which delivered such services to blinded adults one by one.

As was the case with many other forms of social service, the movement for home teaching of the blind stemmed to a great extent from religious motivation. In 1855 Dr. William Moon, the well-to-do Englishman blinded in young manhood who devised the linear type system named for him, founded a charitable organization, the Moon Society, to promote and distribute the devotional works he was publishing. The society's emissaries toured the British countryside, seeking out blind persons who could be instructed in the reading of the books and benefit by the religious consolation they offered.

Twenty-five years later Dr. Moon, accompanied by his daughter, crossed the Atlantic to introduce his type and the program of his society to the United States. He did not make much headway in New England, where Howe's Boston Line Type was flourishing. Philadelphia, however, proved more receptive. It was there, in 1882, with the active help of John P. Rhoads, who headed the local branch of the American Bible Society, that there came into existence the Pennsylvania Home Teaching Society and Free Circulating Library for the Blind, which pioneered home teaching of the blind in the United States.

William Moon died in 1894. Soon after his death, his son, Robert, an ophthalmologist, came to the United States, married a girl from a prominent Philadelphia family, and settled in that city to become secretary of the home teaching society his father had founded. Supported by private philanthropy, the society remained in existence until 1945. Although Moon type lasted longer and in 1972 was still being produced in England, it was home teaching that proved to be Dr. Moon's most enduring legacy.

A few years after the program's successful start in Philadelphia, the Perkins school began a similar effort in Massachusetts, partly as a way of providing useful employment for its intellectually gifted graduates. There was no question in anyone's mind, then and for many years thereafter, but that home teaching of blind adults could and should be performed by other blind persons. In 1900 the Massachusetts legislature was induced to appropriate public funds in support of the home teaching service, which Perkins had financed up to that point and which it continued to administer until 1916, when the program was taken over by the state commission for the blind. As established by Michael Anagnos, the first criteria for selection of home teachers were graduation from Perkins, followed by graduation from a normal school and some experience in teaching.

Connecticut preceded Massachusetts in financing home teaching through public funds; its first appropriation was made in 1893. Other states launched similar services soon after the turn of the century; by 1926, home teaching programs existed in 25 states under such varying auspices as state commissions, voluntary agencies and libraries for the blind. It was hardly an expensive service, which may partially account for the fact that although two of the first four home teachers appointed by Anagnos were men, the field evolved as one almost exclusively staffed by women. The early home teacher was paid as little as $1 a day, out of which she had to defray her expenses as well as some of the expenses of the sighted guide who accompanied her (few were capable of traveling alone, nor was it the custom, in those days, for respectable women to go about unescorted).

The duties of the pioneer home teacher were far more extensive than the title implied. She instructed homebound blind adults in one or more finger-reading systems, in handicrafts whose sale might yield a small income, and in methods of coping with the demands of daily living. But before she could fulfill these basic tasks, she had to turn to local officials, clergymen, educators, even newspaper advertising, to locate an area's blind residents. If, as often happened, her case-finding efforts turned up a blind child, she became the referral link between the child's parents and an educational resource. Some other essential parts of the job, as described in 1919 by Kate M. Foley, California's first home teacher, were

> to conduct a campaign for the prevention of blindness and conservation of vision in adults and children; and . . . to set forth the need of the blind, convince the public that its attitude toward them is often an added affliction, and correct a few of the many mistaken ideas concerning those deprived of eyesight, and, when possible, to find employment for them.

To fulfill these added responsibilities the home teacher had to have a sound working knowledge of eye diseases, their causes, prognoses, and possible cures. She had to be familiar with existing resources for help to blind persons. She had to be an accomplished speaker and a persuasive advocate. Above all, at no time could she forget that she herself was exemplar and symbol.

It was a tall order, one that could hardly be filled by the average young woman newly graduated from a school for the blind, which was all the prerequisite needed in some states for appointment as a home teacher. Recognition of the unrealistic nature of such assignments was what motivated Olin Burritt of Overbrook to initiate, in 1922, a two-year course in cooperation with the Pennsylvania School of Social Work and Health. His choice of a social work school as partner in this area of vocational preparation reflected his and others' growing awareness that the home teacher's job had at least as much to do with social service as it did with instruction.

During the Twenties and Thirties social work was emerging as a profession with rapidly evolving standards of advanced education and training. The dilemma thereby created in work for the blind was a painful one. If home teaching was a social service, and social service could only be properly administered by the educationally qualified, should blind people be content with less than the best? Should they not have the benefit of service from professionally equipped social workers even though such persons were apt to be sighted and thus lacking in empathetic understanding of the special problems of blindness? This was one side of the coin. On the other was the question of how blind home teachers could attain recognition and status in the burgeoning social work profession.

"Home Teachers—Sightless or Seeing?" was the title of a symposium organized by the *Outlook* and published in its issue of March 1932. The three participants—Burritt, Murray B. Allen, executive secretary of the Utah Commission for the Blind, and A. Siddall, chairman of the Northern Counties Association for the Blind in England—were unanimous in their conclusions that any handicaps imposed by blindness on the efficient execution of the home teacher's job could be largely overcome by adequate training and preparation. All three deplored the fact that such preparation was not universally demanded in the employment of home teachers. But, as Burritt blandly observed, the identical problem existed among those engaged in general welfare work: "Some have less than a grammar school education; some are high school graduates; a few have college degrees, and a very small number of these have done graduate work." Not only were most welfare workers unequipped to meet professional standards of social work but, knowing little or nothing about the problems of blindness, they were doubly incapable of serving as home teachers of the blind. Given equal qualifications of training and experience, Burritt maintained, the blind home teacher would invariably outperform her sighted counterpart.

Most of the arguments he advanced in support of his position centered on the confidence a capable blind person inspired in the client, the client's family, and in the community. There was also a practical consideration: "Under present conditions the blind home teacher can be secured for lower compensation than a seeing welfare worker of equal ability." The dollar-a-day era was past, but an agency's outlay for salaries and traveling expenses for two persons—home teacher and sighted guide—was only some $50 a week, "which would not be considered excessive for a thoroughly trained and experienced [sighted] welfare worker."

Burritt's tone was dispassionate. Not so Allen's, whose article dwelt on the emotional impact of the blind home teacher: "There is a freemasonry set up when blind and blind stand face to face. When one is teacher and the other pupil, the pupil's resistance is already half gone...." The first blind graduate of the University of Utah, Allen was a dedicated champion of home teaching, credited with initiating work for the adult blind in his own state and also in neighboring Arizona, Nevada and Wyoming.

The British contributor to the symposium added still another facet. How could agencies for the blind expect to persuade industry and commerce to employ blind workers if they themselves did not set the example by hiring the capable blind?

Clearly, blind home teachers would have to be instructed in the principles and methods of social work, and sighted social workers whose jobs brought them into contact with blind clients (which became more and more the case as the nation's public assistance network grew) would have to be taught about blindness.

In 1932 the Eastern Conference of Home Teachers appointed a committee to develop minimum standards of practice. The committee's report, presented two years later, analyzed the responses to questionnaires it had sent out to home teachers and employing agencies across the country and concluded that the needs in the field varied so widely that "it is to be doubted if any one code of standards would meet them all, but it is to be hoped that the time is not far distant that such a code can be formulated."

The time came five years later. The 1939 amendments to the Social Security Act stipulated that all persons employed in administering welfare programs financed by federal funds be placed under a merit system. Since, in many states, the commission for the blind was part of the state welfare department, home teachers would have to meet the same civil service standards as the sighted social workers employed in other facets of welfare assistance.

The worrisome element here was not only that a great many blind people were in danger of being ruled ineligible for jobs they had long held, but that they might be replaced in the home teaching posts by sighted workers who, while possessing the required education and training, lacked knowledge of how to deal with blind people.

In 1937 a number of short-term training programs in the special problems of blindness were conducted for state and county social workers in Colorado, Maryland, Florida, South Carolina, and New York City. Kansas, Michigan, Arizona and South Dakota were added to the list in 1938. In addition to assigning staff members to participate in these training sessions, the Foundation produced a book, *What of the Blind?*, which was a collection of papers by specialists on various aspects of blindness and services to blind people. A supplementary volume, *More of the Blind*, was issued three years later. Both became standard reading resources in graduate schools of social work.

Throughout this period, promising young blind people were urged to prepare for a career in social work. The Foundation's 1942 annual report noted that of the 19 scholarship recipients that year, five were full-time students at graduate schools of social work and three others were enrolled in the home teacher training course at Overbrook. The next sentence was printed in italics for emphasis: *"At present all of the former Foundation students who have completed training in social work are employed."*

Provisions for professional education and training might solve the problems of the next generation of home teachers, but what was to be done about the three hundred or so persons already employed in the field? In 1938, following a conference of specialists convened by the Foundation to work out the philosophy and principles of home teaching, the AAWB established a committee on professional standards, which in turn appointed a board of certification for home teachers. The recommendations of these groups were presented to and adopted by the 1941

AAWB convention. The certification system had two levels. The Class I requirements called for two years of college work, including courses in social work and teaching, plus proficiency in braille, typing and six handicraft skills. Four years of experience could be substituted for the two years of college attendance. Class II was reserved for those who, in addition to meeting the Class I academic, experience, and skills requirements, were college graduates with at least one year of postgraduate study in a school of social work.

When the certification board's chairman, Murray B. Allen, reported to the AAWB convention in 1947, he stated that 60 Class I certificates and three Class II's had been granted; that, under a one-time "grandfather clause" arrangement, 52 home teachers with 20 years or more of experience had been certified in a separate classification; and that 73 new applications were pending.

All but a few of the first certificate holders were women. But in 1956 a partial survey of home teachers employed by 60 agencies found 64 men among the total group of 241. The same survey also made it clear that home teaching continued to be dominated by blind workers; 204 of the 241 were legally blind, with the remainder about equally divided between the sighted and the partially sighted.

A key factor in the certification of home teachers was the establishment, in 1942, of a six-week summer training program, cooperatively conducted by the Foundation and a graduate school of social work, that enabled practicing teachers to earn the academic credits they needed to qualify for Class I. Initiated at AAWB request, the program was conducted in 1942 and 1943 at Western Reserve University in Cleveland, and then transferred to the University of Michigan at Ypsilanti where it continued under Foundation sponsorship for the next ten years until federal funds became available for training grants.

Another important source of aid for those seeking certification came through the college-level correspondence courses offered by the Hadley School for the Blind in Winnetka, Illinois. This unique organization was founded in 1920 by Dr. William A. Hadley as an avocational pursuit when he lost his own sight in middle age. A former high school teacher, he worked out a series of correspondence lessons to teach braille to a newly blinded woman in another state. The success of the experiment led him to devise courses in various other subjects. When word of the one-man enterprise reached local citizens, a group of Winnetka businessmen and educators raised funds to supply the professor with an office, secretarial help and a braille press. The school, originally known as the Hadley Correspondence School for the Blind, was incorporated as a non-profit organization in 1922.

From a handful of courses in such subjects as reading and writing braille, English grammar, business correspondence, and biblical literature, the Hadley program grew over the years to embrace more than a hundred subjects on grammar school, high school, and college levels, as well as vocational and avocational subjects. Its tuition-free courses served 4,700 blind youths and adults all over the world in 1972.

AAWB certification requirements and classifications were substantively revised in 1959, with the former Class II being retitled Home Teacher Specialist. Two years earlier, the number of certificate holders had reached an overall total of 261. The statement of philosophy issued by A.N. Magill, chairman of the board of certification, in connection with the revisions, underscored what was already accepted reality: "that professional home teaching embraces counseling and casework as well as instruction" and that it "should be the basic field service for the blind which begins the process of rehabilitation."

It was in these words that the link was finally forged between the century-old home teaching function and the newly emerged rehabilitation center idea. The connection was more tightly drawn a few years later when, after a lengthy semantic wrangle, home teachers were renamed rehabilitation teachers. Official status was given to the new job title at the point when the Commission on Standards and Accreditation of Services for the Blind (COMSTAC) adopted its standards in late 1965. Three years later the AAWB accepted this change in terminology for certification purposes.

As with the other rehabilitation disciplines, the trend toward professionalization of home teaching was greatly accelerated when the 1954 amendments to the Vocational Rehabilitation Act provided a separate grant program for personnel training. The discipline took a further step into professional status in 1963 when Western Michigan University used a federal training grant to inaugurate a two-year master's program for home teachers. A major impetus for the establishment of this graduate program was the Cosgrove report, *Home Teachers of the Adult Blind: What They Do, What They Could Do, What Will Enable Them to Do It.* This report, published by the AAWB in 1961, was the product of a year-long federally financed study to evaluate the role of the home teacher and provide guidelines for improved services.

Elizabeth Cosgrove, who directed the study with the help of a 22-member advisory committee, disclosed its findings with unsparing candor. Because of caseload pressures, ill-defined intake policies, lack of clarity as to the place of home teaching in an agency's overall service structure, administrative indifference or unawareness, many home teachers were being left with "a diffusion of activities," some of which they were not qualified to execute. In too many instances home teachers were treated as appendages who were not functionally integrated into the agency's program. Two out of five teachers interviewed in the course of the study did not even have desk space in the agency office but operated out of their homes. Even fewer had adequate access to clerical help. Personnel practices and salary scales tended to reflect this nebulous, not to say inferior, status.

Boldest of all, Miss Cosgrove said out loud what for years had only been whispered: that many pursued home teaching not because it was their choice but because it had been presented to them as the only type of position available to educated blind persons. This was a note that had seldom been struck in the published literature. One of the few exceptions had been in 1951 when Sophy L. Forward, home teaching consultant for the Pennsylvania Department of Public Welfare's Office of the Blind, told the AAWB that vocational counselors had "misdirected many blind young people into the home teaching profession. Home teaching has been too ready a solution to a placement problem."

The recommendations made by the Cosgrove study flowed from its criticisms: agency policies to be clarified, intake procedures to be placed in the hands of those professionally qualified to make competent decisions, personnel practices to be standardized, home teaching functions to be clearly delineated and educational curricula to be developed in relation to those functions. Most of the recommendations were subsequently embodied in the COMSTAC standards.

No longer a jack-of-all-trades, the rehabilitation teacher came to operate on a level that was deeper but narrower than that of his nineteenth-century forebears. No longer invariably referred to as "she," any more than was the modern classroom teacher, the rehabilitation teacher employed up-to-date tools and techniques of both education and social casework in his operations, some of which began to take place in such group settings as convalescent care and geriatric institutions. Even electronic technology was seen to have a potential role. In 1968 an experimental effort was made in "teleteaching" homebound blind adults in California. Using a telephone console unit hooked up to the phones of nine clients of the Braille Institute of America, a rehabilitation teacher gave simultaneous lessons on braille reading to the nine, switching to recorded tapes with part of the group while working individually with other members.

While the auxiliary duties once discharged by the old-time home teacher— case-finding, public education, etc.—were transferred to others, his core responsibility remained essentially unchanged. As one teacher put it: "The newly blind adult will always need someone to search him out at his home, sit down by his rocking chair, allay his fears and show him how to live a fuller life." The home teacher himself also remained essentially unchanged, continuing to command those unique personal qualities that started generations of blind adults on the road to rehabilitation.

There were two members of the civilian advisory committee on the war-blinded who followed the developments at Valley Forge, Dibble and Old Farms with particular interest. They were the heads of their respective state agencies for the blind—Dr. Roma S. Cheek of North Carolina and R. Henry P. Johnson of Florida. Both enjoyed sound political connections in their states, with the result that within a few months after the war ended, both managed to secure legislative authorization to establish state rehabilitation centers for blind civilians.

North Carolina was first off the mark. With a $15,000 appropriation, matched by an equal sum from the Lions Clubs of North Carolina, the State Commission for the Blind opened what it called a Pre-Conditioning Center for the Blind in November 1945. Using as its initial quarters a handful of vacant buildings that had formerly housed a National Youth Administration facility in Greenville, it was developed into a substantial establishment under the leadership of the energetic Henry A. "Pete" Wood, who eventually succeeded Roma Cheek as state commissioner. The Florida operation, named Holly Hill Diagnostic and Pre-Vocational Training Center, was opened in Daytona Beach in April 1946 as a unit of the state agency then known as the Florida Council for the Blind.

The first center to open under non-governmental auspices was in Little Rock, where the Adjustment Center for the Blind began operations in March 1947 as a project of Arkansas Enterprises for the Blind. The project had been initiated the preceding year when Roy Kumpe, founder and executive director of Arkansas

Enterprises, persuaded a statewide convention of Lions Clubs to sponsor a civilian rehabilitation center and to raise $10,000 for its first quarters.

By 1950, when about thirty units of one kind or another were in existence and calling themselves "rehabilitation" or "adjustment" centers, it became apparent that these terms meant different things in different places. The length of training in some was six weeks, in others, four months, and in one, nine months. Costs varied correspondingly: from as little as $102 in one center, which conducted a six-week summer program on the premises of a state school for the blind, to sums ranging up to $650 for three-month programs in residential centers operated by voluntary agencies.

In the great majority of cases, costs were borne by the state vocational rehabilitation unit, financed by a combination of federal and state funds under the Vocational Rehabilitation Act. There were also some trainees whose tuition and maintenance were paid by the Veterans Administration, and rare occasional instances in which the needed funds came from private sources.

A 1950 Foundation survey of 11 centers highlighted the diversity of services, techniques and philosophy that then existed under the rubric of "adjustment." Definitions ranged from Dr. Howard Rusk's aphoristic statement that rehabilitation meant "to help the disabled to live within the limits of his disability but to the hilt of his capabilities" to the detailed tripartite formula evolved by the Baruch Committee on Physical Medicine, which analyzed a center's services in three separate categories: physical medicine, psycho-social treatment and adjustment, and vocational-educational programs.

Apart from differences in sponsorship among the 11 centers (5 were newly established by state agencies, 6 were units of long-established voluntary agencies which also operated sheltered workshops), there were also important variations in program, emphasis and execution. All 11, for example, made use of psychological testing, but the tests were administered and interpreted by personnel with such differing degrees of professional competence that some of the results were viewed with doubt. Craft training was given in all, but for different purposes and under different types of supervision, ranging from occupational therapists in some centers to self-taught instructors in others. Mobility lessons of one sort or another were also given in all, but here the differences were even sharper. The report noted:

> The greatest variation in travel training lies in the use of the cane. All concede that the cane is the extension of the hand and is a tool with more uses than to show the sighted public that the blind have a visual disability. Two centers use the long metal cane but of varying lengths. Some insist upon the length of the cane being measured from the waist, others from the middle of the forearm, and again, others recommend no specific length but consider the comfort of the student. All centers use some variation of the Valley Forge training technique. Two of them follow it almost to the letter. . . . Much needs to be done to develop more uniform techniques based on past experience.

Since the ability of a blind person to travel independently depended on more than the use of a mobility device, whether cane or dog guide, all 11 centers offered help in the development of the auditory, olfactory, and kinesthetic senses. Here, too, they used different techniques. In one center, the only formal practice in using the sense of smell was through not telling trainees what was on their dinner plates. Kitchen odors plus sensations in the palate were considered sufficient clues to olfactory training. In others, practice in distinguishing odors took the form of a game in which trainees tried to guess the identity of vegetables, spices, and various woods by smelling them without touching them. All the centers emphasized olfactory alertness in teaching outdoor travel orientation, calling attention to the environmental clues offered by distinctive odors emanating from bakeries, shoe repair shops, restaurants, or laundries.

Makeshift techniques and trial-and-error methods were a feature of most programs, but this was to be expected in what was essentially a new form of service. But there were also some genuine positives, particularly in the training for daily living which every center offered. More concrete teaching techniques might be needed, but the real key was something both more intangible and more important than technique: the atmosphere built by staff attitudes and relationships. The survey report devoted a pregnant paragraph to this aspect:

> The student usually comes from a protected environment where he has absorbed the fears of his family and friends and has never had an opportunity to develop independence and self-confidence. The casual attitude of the entire staff toward blindness, observed at all centers, is perhaps the thing that makes the training click. . . . There is no one there who says "Don't do this" or "Be careful." He can try and adventure as far as he feels he is capable.

It was awareness that "the best and only authorities with practical experience were the people who were doing the job" that led to the convening of a unique six-day meeting in early 1951. The Spring Mill Conference, co-sponsored by OVR and the Foundation, took the form of a workshop featuring no speeches, no outside "experts" and no participants other than 29 persons actually engaged in full-time work at 12 different rehabilitation centers for the blind. The location—a small hotel in a state park in southern Indiana—was chosen for its isolation; here the participants could concentrate on just what they did that "made the training click."

They succeeded in getting the heart of it down on paper. Fortified with a good deal of background material (including a 136-page document giving detailed profiles of nine different center programs, along with a set of case records from each of the nine, selected to show failures as well as successes), the workshop members produced the first organized body of basic methods and techniques for rehabilitation center programs. The product of their combined thinking was incorporated in a report, *Adjustment Centers for the Blind*, which became what amounted to a comprehensive operating manual.

In the next five years enough changes took place to warrant a second look at the national picture. Good programs had been made better, marginal efforts had been strengthened, and some of the weakest had either closed down or had stopped claiming to be rehabilitation centers. The number of centers had grown and would probably continue to expand under the incentives offered by the Vocational Rehabilitation Act amendments of 1954 and another bill enacted the same year, the amended Medical Facilities Survey and Construction Act, which enlarged the Hill-Burton hospital building program to make funds available for construction of rehabilitation facilities that did not have to be part of a hospital complex.

The New Orleans Seminar of February 1956 was convened, again under joint OVR-Foundation sponsorship, to develop principles and standards that could guide the proliferating growth along constructive lines. It, too, was attended by a small and carefully selected group, some of whom had been at Spring Mill. Their assignment this time was not to deal with specific operating methods or procedures, but to think along broader conceptual lines. Out of the work of the 17 persons who spent five days in subcommittee and general sessions came a set of precepts that largely foreshadowed the standards later adopted by COMSTAC.

In addition to evolving criteria for assessing the need for a center in any given community, state or region, the conferees dealt with staffing patterns and personnel qualifications, with physical plant requirements and essential elements of finance and budget. Their conclusions, published by OVR in *Rehabilitation Centers for Blind Persons*, propelled work for blind adults a considerable distance toward professionalization by putting new stress on the psycho-social aspects of rehabilitation and differentiating more sharply than ever before between the needs of center clients as persons and their needs as potential jobholders. A basic concept was that a rehabilitation center existed "for the specific purpose of assisting blind persons to meet their individual reorganization needs" and that eligibility for its services "need not be limited to those with remunerative employment potential."

The standards and principles evolved at New Orleans proved too lofty to be realized in a few years' time. That vital differences continued to exist in policies, procedures and philosophy became evident in 1960 when a third national conference in Washington brought together the administrators of 25 centers. Their major conclusion was that an accreditation procedure was needed for ongoing evaluation and review of the centers and their performance. At a fourth national session in Chicago in April 1965 the standards for rehabilitation centers proposed by COMSTAC were critically examined and approved. These leaned heavily on principles developed at a 1961 conference, whose findings had been published as *The Grove Park Report*. That report broke down into discrete categories the many services lumped under the general heading of rehabilitation, presenting differential definitions and criteria for personal adjustment services, prevocational diagnostic evaluation, and actual vocational training.

Although some rehabilitation centers continued to be much more vocationally-oriented than others, this form of service became a permanent feature of work on behalf of blind adults. Many centers expanded their physical facilities with the help of federal funds. Arkansas Enterprises for the Blind estimated the 1969 value of its five-building rehabilitation complex at more than $1,500,000. Constructed in 1970 by the Texas Commission for the Blind, the Criss Cole Rehabilitation Center in Austin, Texas, incorporated architectural features specifically tailored to training needs: corridors in three contrasting floor surfaces to help develop the kinesthetic and aural awareness required for orientation and mobility exercises, various types of doors and stairs, different kinds of walls in outdoor courtyards to help in differentiating echoes.

By 1972 the rehabilitation center for the blind had come a long way since the early days of hasty improvisation in North Carolina, when Henry A. Wood scrounged trucks from the State Highway Commission, equipment from Army surplus stocks, money from the state legislature, and free labor from volunteers to transform the nation's first civilian rehabilitation center from a makeshift affair in an abandoned NYA camp into a landscaped complex with housing for eighty clients at a time and a headquarters building named for Wood after his 1965 retirement as executive director of the state commission for the blind.

One of the principles enunciated at the New Orleans Seminar and reaffirmed by the Washington administrator's conference was that rehabilitation centers for the blind should also serve persons with additional handicaps, provided these handicaps did not pose insuperable obstacles to the rehabilitation of the trainee or to the progress of others simultaneously undergoing training. Perhaps the most venturesome effort in this regard was made by the Industrial Home for the Blind in Brooklyn which, in 1962, undertook an extended regional project in rehabilitation of deaf-blind adults. Noteworthy rehabilitation programs serving other types of multihandicapped blind persons also came into existence in many parts of the country, making use of group therapy and individual psychotherapy to cope with emotional and personality maladjustments.

Even with the most expertly refined techniques, no rehabilitation process can hope to achieve its goals without sufficient motivation on the client's part. The ophthalmologist has a crucial role to play in imbuing the visually impaired person with the will to go on despite blindness, and it has been a source of deep concern to workers for the blind that many eye specialists are slow to reach out beyond purely medical concerns. Writing in the *Archives of Ophthalmology* in November 1967, Dr. Richard E. Hoover noted: "It is difficult to tell a person he is irrevocably blind. It is easier to insinuate or hold out a hope that the person may some day see again through a miracle of medical or surgical triumph. Hope for recovery, so important therapeutically in most aspects of medicine, is a cruelty to the permanently blind. . . ."

A similar point had been made a decade earlier by the psychiatrist Louis Cholden who wrote that maintaining hope for the return of vision was "the wrong kind of hope." Cholden, who for three years served as psychiatric consultant to the Kansas Rehabilitation Center for the Blind, drew his insights from work with the trainees at that center, for whom he conducted a group therapy program. A lucid speaker and writer, he had begun to attain a nationwide reputation in the field of work for the blind when a 1956 automobile accident cut his life short at the age of thirty-seven. A posthumous collection of his papers, *A Psychiatrist Works with Blindness*, published by the Foundation in 1958, became a standard reference work in illuminating the emotional impact of blindness.

How much did the practicing ophthalmologist actually know about rehabilitation possibilities for persons who lost the use of their eyes, and to what extent was this knowledge being employed to start blind patients on the road to rehabilitation?

A study seeking the facts was jointly sponsored by the Foundation and the Seeing Eye, Inc., and conducted by Professor Samuel Finestone and Dr. Sonia Gold of the Research Center of the New York School of Social Work, Columbia University. The study, whose findings were published in 1959 in *The Role of the Ophthalmologist in the Rehabilitation of Blind Patients*, analyzed the responses of 180 randomly selected eye specialists to a questionnaire probing their attitudes and practices. It found that relatively few were doing as much as they could in referring blind patients to sources of rehabilitation service: that a large number, particularly those in private practice, admitted to inadequate knowledge of community resources that could give such services and therefore made few referrals, and that among the latter were a significant percentage who did not themselves feel optimistic about a blind person's chances for a useful life.

Blind people themselves had long been vocal on the question of the eye doctor's role. Addressing a conference of ophthalmologists in 1950, M. Robert Barnett said bluntly that a patient's adjustment to blindness would be much easier if the process began "in the doctor's office and at the hospital bed."

No matter how skillful and supportive the ophthalmologist, what Barnett called "the will to carry on" does not come easily to the person confronted with blindness. The extent to which emotional reorganization is involved in adjusting to a new kind of life situation is generally acknowledged, but the form that this adjustment takes has long been a subject of controversy.

At one end of the spectrum were psychiatrically oriented authorities such as Dr. Cholden, who wrote in 1953 that a patient's initial reaction to blindness was apt to fall into a pattern in which a stage of shock is followed by a reactive depression, "a period of mourning for his dead eyes." It was Cholden who, in the same paper, first voiced the belief that "the patient must die as a sighted person in order to be reborn as a blind man"—a theme put into practice the following year by Father Thomas J. Carroll when he founded the 16-week program for newly blinded adults at St. Paul's Rehabilitation Center. As elaborated by Father Carroll, the death-and-rebirth rehabilitation theory involved acceptance and resynthesis of 20 separate losses of function ranging from the tangible—vocation, financial security, freedom of movement, activities of daily living—to the psycho-social: sense of physical integrity, social adequacy, self-esteem, etc.

This dire view was vastly different from the equally extreme denial mechanism of intrepid blind people who dismissed loss of sight as a mere inconvenience, easily overcome by "learning to use the other gateways to the mind." One of the most extraordinary statements along these lines was made by Helen Keller who, lacking both sight and hearing, wrote that "the language of the senses is full of contradictions, and my fellows who have five doors to their house are not more surely at home in themselves than I."

It remains a moot question whether there is, in fact, a specific personality pattern that enables some blind persons to overcome their handicap more readily than others. Efforts continue to be made to explain the mechanism of adjustment. The death-and-rebirth theory was set forth during a period when Freudian psychoanalytic concepts dominated much of professional thinking. Two decades later, computer-age thinking found expression in a concept that compared the human organism with an information system in which the sensory organs were the source of input while the brain acted as a processing and storing mechanism that determined behavioral response to various physical and social situations. The author of this viewpoint was the psychologist Emerson Foulke, director of the Perceptual Alternatives Laboratory at the University of Louisville (Kentucky), according to whom there was no "personality of the blind" and the Cholden-Carroll interpretations were "a non-valid concept."

From the earliest efforts of home teachers to coax people out of rocking chairs, to the contemporary social service, recreational, and vocational programs for young and old, rehabilitation principles and techniques were always inherent in services for blind persons. Although practiced in their most structured form in the rehabilitation centers, these principles guided the work of all organizations that strove to equip blind persons with skills that lessened dependency on others.

A multidisciplinary national task force on independent living, appointed by the Foundation in 1971 to work out guidelines for service agencies, recommended a number of areas of further investigation and action, including study of the delivery of health services to the visually handicapped and development of a university curriculum for homemaker education.

Earlier the same year the Foundation issued a comprehensive manual, *A Step-by-Step Guide to Personal Management for Blind Persons*, that drew on the large body of practical experience accumulated by rehabilitation teachers, therapists and blind persons themselves to spell out in sequential form the easiest and most effective methods of self-care and homemaking without sight. The manual covered techniques of personal hygiene, grooming, cooking, and household management, shaving for men and application of cosmetics for women, tying shoelaces, coding and identifying clothing by color and style, vacuuming floors, pairing socks, sewing buttons, defrosting refrigerators, separating eggs, cutting pie, frosting cake, bathing and diapering babies, handling money, dialing a telephone, and dozens of other tasks that sighted persons perform without a second thought. Supplementary manuals of the same type dealing with home mechanics and repair were scheduled for the future.

Taking the manual one step further, a series of public demonstrations of how blind women could use the same cosmetic techniques as others was begun in 1969 in a cooperative endeavor with the Helena Rubinstein Foundation. In two years, 20 "cosmetology workshops" were conducted across the country.

Another Foundation project in partnership with a commercial firm, Thomas J. Lipton, Inc., was organized in 1972. This, it was announced, would consist of a series of short-term training workshops in food preparation and nutrition at which teachers, rehabilitation personnel, public health nurses, county agricultural demonstration agents and others could learn the techniques that would enable them to instruct blind people in modern home economics. Those attending the workshops would also be introduced to some of the specially adapted aids and appliances developed to enable blind persons to function efficiently as homemakers.

Rehabilitation is a complex process. But its basic theory is simple and perhaps best expressed by the analogy of the four-wheeled cart that loses one of its wheels. Is the vehicle permanently out of commission? Not at all. Move the wheel that has lost its partner to the middle, and you have a three-wheeled cart perfectly capable of moving forward.

19

Mobility, Key to Independence

Once upon a time, it is said, there lived in a German village a blind old woman who was led to church every Sunday by a gander, which seized a fold of her skirt in its bill, conducted her to a pew, remained in the churchyard until it saw people leaving the service, made its way back to the pew, and brought its mistress back home again.

"It seems scarcely credible," was the comment of the man who reported this possibly apocryphal tale in a "treatise on the science of typhlology" published in London in 1872. What is more incredible is that the context in which this citation was offered contained a series of trenchant observations and recommendations it took the world the better part of a century to put into practice.

The author was William Hanks Levy, an articulate and energetic blind man who was credited with a dynamic role in establishing home handicraft industries and workshops for the British blind. Just before he died, he summed up his life's experience in his "treatise," titled *Blindness and the Blind*. It contained a chapter captioned "On the Blind Walking Alone, and of Guides" in which Levy said:

> The importance to every blind man of acquiring the power of walking in the streets without a guide can scarcely be exaggerated. Loss of sight is in itself a great privation, and when to it is added the want of power of locomotion, the sufferer more nearly approaches the condition of a vegetable than that of a member of the human family.

What could blind people do to avoid turning into vegetables? Levy thought it "desirable to offer a few hints." The first was to use a cane, and his description of how the cane should be constructed and employed uncannily foreshadowed the modern "long cane" technique. He wrote of desirable posture for the blind person: "Perfectly erect, that his face may not be injured by coming in contact with various objects." He wrote of how to judge step-downs and step-ups, of when and how to ask for sighted assistance in crossing heavily traveled streets, of how to use hearing and smell as clues to the environment, of why thick shoes were undesirable because they interfered with using the "muscular sense as exercised through the feet."

Levy also had something to say about guides, two-footed and four-footed. As to human guides, his chief comment was a reflection of the times he lived in: a warning against a blind father keeping his children out of school to help him. Dogs were another matter: "To lead his master through the most crowded thoroughfares unhurt, to turn to the right or left when bidden, to cross roads only when quite safe . . . and to refuse to quit his charge for the choicest bone even when pining with hunger, are but a few of the virtues of this most instructive quadruped."

Two generations earlier, Johann Wilhelm Klein, whose pioneering work in the Hapsburg Empire earned him a stature comparable to that of Valentin Haüy in France and Samuel Gridley Howe in the United States as one of "the three great founding fathers of the education of the blind," had described in his *Lehrbuch zum Unterrichte der Blinden* ("Textbook on the Education of the Blind") a type of rigid harness for a dog guide which closely approximated the basic principle of what is used today. Moreover, Klein, whose book was published in 1819, outlined a method of training both dog and master that is also not essentially different from modern procedure.

In no aspect of work for the blind is there greater unanimity as to need—or greater controversy as to method—than in mobility teaching. Loss of the power to move about freely and safely is unarguably the greatest deprivation inflicted by blindness. The problem was less acute in earlier centuries, when not only blind people but the great majority of others seldom ventured far from their native soil. Life patterns grew less static with the industrial revolution, as great sections of the population shifted from farm to town, from town to metropolis, from one part of the country to another, in search of economic betterment. The greatest acceleration of all has taken place in the twentieth century, thanks to the automobile and the airplane and the changed socio-economic climate which brought about a surge of social mobility. For blind people to be members of the larger society, freedom of movement has become a "must."

It is no easy task. Mobility is keyed to a knowledge of the immediate environment, and vision, it is said, provides 80 percent (some authorities put the figure even higher) of the information needed for a person to move securely through space. The other senses also supply data, but vision is so dominant in its range and power that it assumes control of the total sensory apparatus.

That it is, in fact, possible to overcome the absence or loss of this integrative sense by means of efficient command and determined reorganization of the remaining senses is an idea so difficult for the sighted person to grasp that it has given rise to the mistaken theory of automatic "sensory compensation" which figures so largely in the popular mystique of blindness.

The term "reorganization" is not really applicable to the person born blind since, never having had the sense of vision, he must create rather than revise a structure based on his other senses. The blind child thus confronts a somewhat different set of problems from the person who could once see. But there are similarities as well. In 1946 Hector Chevigny, a writer who lost his vision in early middle age, provided a vivid description of what those problems are:

> The newly blinded man taking his first steps is very much in the position of a child doing the same thing. His need for orientation is all but absolute. Like the child, the problem is one of ascertaining his exact relation to the physical world of stationary and moving objects. . . . Taking his first steps, it seems as if the loss of sight has also taken from the man all but the power of touch as a means of relating himself to things. But touch is no good at a distance; he has to find things to touch them and finding them seems impossible. On his hearing he places no dependence. In time he will learn to judge the size, shape and even the contour of a room as soon as he enters it by the "feel" and the sound within it, but right now he fails to note even the loud clank of a passing streetcar on one side of him and the ticking of a clock on the other. That smell, too, may become a factor in orientation doesn't occur to him either. For the moment there is only what he can encounter with his hands and—confound it!—his shins.

Chevigny learned to spare his bruised shins with the help of a dog guide. So did several thousand others. A much larger number mastered the cane. The largest group of all, however continued to depend on human guides to navigate safely. Partly this was because the majority of blind people were elderly and had less need and less capacity to undergo the rigors of mobility training. There was also another, somewhat subtler, reason that contributed to the decades of delay in the development of independent mobility skills. It was the self-denigrating belief that blindness should be made as inconspicuous as possible, and that the use of a dog guide or a distinctive cane attracted undesirable public attention.

That remnants of this viewpoint lingered well into the contemporary era could be seen from the initial resistance of some leaders in work for the blind to the proposal for a dog guide movement in the United States. Even so imaginative a man as Robert Irwin was unable to perceive the potential at first.

(To Irwin's credit, he not only kept an open mind but soon lent the movement his active support, even though he personally "would not be caught using one of the blooming things." He was also big enough, in later years, to tell colleagues, as a joke on himself, that his greatest mistake in office was to have turned down the opportunity to sponsor the nation's first dog guide school, an opportunity that proved to be a financial bonanza.)

Irwin and his contemporaries knew that for centuries blind people had used dogs to lead them, but their image of this procedure was of "a dirty little cur dragging a blind man along at the end of a string," an image that another early doubter, Edward E. Allen, called "the very index and essence of incompetence and beggary." It took a wealthy Philadelphia woman socialite and a hot-tempered, rebellious blind youth from Nashville, Tennessee, to change the minds of the dubious and to capture the hearts, imagination and generosity of the American people.

Both the scientific training of dog guides and the invention of braille were offshoots of ideas originally developed for military purposes. The German army effectively employed search dogs on the battlefields of World War I. German shepherd dogs were trained in Oldenburg under the direction of Dr. Gerhard Stalling, a town privy councillor, who conceived the idea that these intelligent and responsive canines could also be educated as guides for war-blinded soldiers. A branch school was opened in Breslau and several more founded in other German cities. A decade after the end of the war it was estimated that close to 4,000 dogs were in use in Germany as guides for both veterans and civilians. The former received their animals as a government-issued "prosthesis" and the latter through organizations for the blind supported by voluntary contributions as well as by state and municipal welfare grants.

French military authorities also experimented, during and after World War I, with training dogs to lead blinded soldiers. Their approach, however, was a narrow one, centered on familiarizing a dog with his master's daily routes so it could obey commands to proceed to specific destinations. Neither specialized breeding of animals suited to the guiding task nor the use of trained instructors figured in the French system, which soon died out.

These European developments were no secret to American workers for the blind. The 1923 AAWB convention in Janesville, Wisconsin, heard a talk by a German dog trainer on "the training of the shepherd dog to act as guide." Apparently neither the talk nor the accompanying demonstration aroused much interest, for when an article on the same subject appeared four years later in the *Saturday Evening Post*, it took the field by storm.

The author of the *Post* article was an American woman of impeccable social standing (she was the daughter of Charles Custis Harrison, a former provost of the University of Pennsylvania) whose motives were clearly philanthropic. Dorothy Harrison Eustis was the owner of the large estate "Fortunate Fields" on the slopes of Mount Pelegrin in Vevey, Switzerland, where she and her husband, George, had spent years working on the scientific breeding and training of dogs for police work, guard duty, army communications, and other practical duties. They specialized in German shepherds, a breed which, Mrs. Eustis claimed, had been "overbred, overfed and underexercised" as show dogs in the United States. The shepherd, she wrote, was "a Niagara of energy going to waste, an intelligence waiting to be used intelligently, a public servant and useful citizen."

In 1926 the Eustises had visited Germany. What they observed in Potsdam, in one of the schools where dogs were trained for use by the blind, led to the November 1927 *Post* article, and this, in turn, brought the author a number of letters, one of them an almost incoherently excited note from Nashville, Tennessee. The writer was Morris Frank, who had lost his sight three years earlier and coped with his blindness by using paid helpers to get to and from his home to the office where he sold insurance and to Vanderbilt University where he was taking courses. What distinguished Frank's letter from all the others written by blind people wanting dogs for themselves was his statement, "I should like very much to forward this work in this country." There was also something Mrs. Eustis found irresistibly appealing in his statement that blind people "do not require sympathy but a laughing word and pat on the back."

Her response, some months later, was in the form of a challenge. Would he be willing to come to Switzerland to be trained with a dog? She would provide the transportation and have him as her house guest if he would contribute the time and effort. By early April of 1928, two weeks after his twentieth birthday, Morris Frank was on his way to Switzerland.

Bringing a blind youth across the Atlantic was a compromise. At about the time her article appeared, Mrs. Eustis had visited the States and made contact with a number of organizations for the blind, including the New York Lighthouse. With a letter of introduction from Daisy Rogers of that agency, Mrs. Eustis came to see Robert Irwin in mid-January of 1928 to ask whether the Foundation would be willing to launch a program to train dogs as guides for blind people. She offered to come to America with her husband, possibly accompanied by some of their own dogs, and to spend four months training the animals, teaching instructors how to train both the dogs and their masters, and instructing an initial class of blind people in how to work with dog guides. The Eustises would put on this demonstration free of charge, provided the Foundation agreed to continue the work. Two instructors, working full time, could "turn out 60 to 70 dogs and their blind masters a year." The cost, she estimated, would come to about $150 per dog, irrespective of whether already trained animals were imported and taught to follow commands in English, or suitable dogs were bought from American kennels and trained from the beginning.

Irwin presented this proposal to the Foundation's executive committee the following week without recommendation pro or con. In the absence of an affirmative staff endorsement, it is not surprising to read in the minutes of January 24, 1928: "The Committee expressed sympathy and interest in the idea. It was the consensus of opinion, however, that the budget for 1928 would not permit our taking on any additional activities for the year."

The minutes show that only three of the five members of the executive committee were present on that occasion: Prudence Sherwin, vice-president; Olin H. Burritt, secretary; and Herbert H. White, treasurer. M. C. Migel, a devoted animal lover, might well have made a difference in the decision, but he was absent, as was the committee's fifth member, H. Randolph Latimer, and three members out of five constituted a quorum.

Although the decision was undoubtedly influenced by Irwin's lack of enthusiasm, it was by no means capricious. Explaining that the Foundation had "taken on so many new activities during the past year," Irwin also voiced some of his own hesitancies over the dog guide proposal in a letter to Mrs. Eustis:

> As I see it we would not only have to conduct our dog training establishment properly but we would also have to do a certain amount of educational work among the blind people of the country and their friends. We would also have to sound out the blind people as to just how many would wish to use such a dog and how many could afford to buy one if they wished one. . . . The Committee also seriously questioned whether there would be a demand for eighty or ninety dogs a year at the price of $150. As you know blind people are usually quite poor and to most of them $150 looks like a fortune.

He tactfully refrained from adding his private conviction that anyone who could afford such a sum could afford to hire sighted guides, a practice he himself followed when traveling unaccompanied to other cities.

Nevertheless, Irwin was impressed with Dorothy Eustis and willing to help her in any way short of taking on her project. Soon after her visit he had a letter from Robert I. Bramhall, director of the Massachusetts Division of the Blind, indicating that some local philanthropists were interested in sponsoring the training of dog guides. His answer: "If Massachusetts will undertake the job, I should be delighted." He also informed Bramhall that, quite apart from Mrs. Eustis, the dog school in Potsdam had recently been in direct touch with the Foundation, offering to supply thirty or forty trained dogs plus the services of trainers, but that the prices quoted were high and the offer had been rejected. This, in point of fact, was the second approach from Potsdam; an earlier one had been made in 1925.

By this time Mrs. Eustis had embarked on her alternative course of action and issued her invitation to Morris Frank.* He called on Irwin before embarking on the transatlantic trip, and again in mid-July, upon his return. Irwin described the two encounters in his memoirs:

> The author well remembers Morris Frank calling him on the phone when he arrived in New York on his way to Europe. He expressed a desire to call on the writer but was appalled by the terrors of New York traffic. However, arrangements were made for him to come to the American Foundation for the Blind in a taxi with an escort. Four months later Frank again called the author on the phone from the same hotel two miles away and made an appointment to come to the Foundation an hour later. Accompanied only by his dog, Frank traveled across the city on foot to the Foundation offices and after a chat of an hour or so returned alone with his dog to his hotel.

Dorothy Eustis' article in the *Saturday Evening Post* had been titled "The Seeing Eye," a phrase drawn from Proverbs 20:12—"The hearing ear, and the seeing eye, the Lord hath made even both of them." Frank's return from Switzerland on the Cunard liner *Tuscania* was extensively covered by the press, and he took the occasion to announce that he and the Eustises would organize a Seeing Eye Association in the United States.

Now it was Morris Frank's turn to be flooded with mail from blind people and their friends. When would dogs be available? When could training begin? In December 1928 Elliott S. (Jack) Humphrey arrived in Nashville from Fortunate Fields accompanied by two trained dogs. The first class could now begin in a few weeks.

A student of animal genetics with long experience in breeding and training animals of all types, Humphrey had worked with the Eustises in Switzerland and, in preparation for launching the program in America, had spent some time ob-

---

* She also extended the same invitation to another blind man, Dr. Howard Buchanan of Colorado Springs, Colo., a physician who had lost his sight three years earlier while serving as a medical missionary in Sudan. He was unable to make the trip but did become one of the first two people to receive a Seeing Eye dog once the program got under way in the United States.

serving the dog guide schools in Germany. The two dogs Humphrey brought to Nashville were German; they had not been secured from Potsdam but from one of the other German dog schools. The Potsdam school, which viewed Mrs. Eustis' enterprise as commercial competition, refused to supply her with animals and followed up the refusal by sending an indignant letter to the Foundation in January 1929 challenging Humphrey's ability to teach dogs the specific techniques of leading the blind merely on the basis of a few weeks of observation. This might have been a valid enough doubt in relation to an ordinary man, but it underestimated Humphrey, whom an enthusiastic admirer described as having "a mind that absorbs information like blotting paper."

George Eustis was now out of the picture; he and his wife had just been divorced. But Dorothy Eustis soon arrived in Nashville, and stayed long enough to have Seeing Eye incorporated in Tennessee with herself as president and Morris Frank as managing director, to secure pledges of $2,500 a year for three years from each of three friends, and to watch the first two blind men taught to work with Humphrey's dogs.

Before long another personality came into the picture. A retired business executive who bred dogs on his New Jersey farm, Willi H. Ebeling became, first, a supplier of shepherds for Humphrey to train, then a fascinated spectator of what the dogs were able to do with and for blind people, then a volunteer participant in the work, then a host to Seeing Eye trainers and dogs when the New Jersey climate was deemed better suited than Tennessee for all-weather training and, finally, the first executive vice-president of the organization once it had established permanent quarters in New Jersey. Ebeling served as Seeing Eye's executive head from 1934 to 1954; following his retirement he became a trustee and remained a member of the board until his death in 1961 at the age of seventy-nine.

When Ebeling retired he was replaced as executive director by George Werntz, Jr., who had been his understudy since coming to Seeing Eye in 1950 from Colgate University, where he had been director of admissions. Werntz, who was continuing in office at the end of 1972, was a protégé of Henry A. Colgate of the soap manufacturing family, whose philanthropic interests included not only the university which bore the family name, but also Seeing Eye. Colgate became a trustee in 1934 and in 1940 followed Dorothy Eustis into the presidency, a post he occupied until his death in 1957.

Seeing Eye's fifth founding figure came upon the scene a little later. As soon as the program was under way in the United States, Dorothy Eustis returned to Switzerland to establish a Seeing Eye School *(L'Oeil qui Voit)* to educate instructors who could initiate dog guide movements in other European countries. Of the three elements that made up a dog guide program—dogs, trainers, and blind users—the trainers were the hardest to come by, due to the unique combination of qualities needed to work successfully with both dogs and people, the long and arduous nature of the apprenticeship and the exceptional degree of physical stamina required. Ebeling wrote in 1949 that in the 15 years he had been head of Seeing Eye "55 men have started on the road of apprentice instructors and only five have proved able to attain the goal."

The high fallout rate described by Ebeling was typical. In 1931 Mrs. Eustis had reported that "in Germany, a nation of dog lovers, dog trainers and dog educators, they have been able to retain as competent instructors of dog guides only between 5 percent and 8 percent of the selected apprentices who started the work." Of the many instructors she attempted to train at *L'Oeil qui Voit* until she closed it down in 1933, only three men ultimately made the grade. One went to England, one to Italy, and the third, William Debetaz, came to the United States.

Debetaz was a twenty-three-year-old French-Swiss whom Morris Frank described as "wiry and as full of bounding energy as the animals under his command." He not only stayed the course but in 1942 was placed in charge of instructors at Seeing Eye after Humphrey resigned to train dogs for military use in World War II. Humphrey later moved to the west to work at cattle breeding; he was eighty-two years old and living in Arizona in 1972. Debetaz was elevated to vice-presidency of Seeing Eye in 1946 and remained in charge of training until he retired in 1971.

If Dorothy Eustis was disappointed in the international aspirations she had held for *L'Oeil qui Voit,* her disappointment must have been assuaged by the extraordinary success of the American movement. By the time she died in 1946 at the age of sixty, Seeing Eye had supplied close to a thousand blind Americans with working dogs. It had acquired a large property in New Jersey where students and staff could be housed, kennels maintained, breeding and training facilities created. It had won so handsome a measure of public support, both moral and financial, as to inspire the flattery of imitation. Most meaningful of all, the sight of a blind man confidently striding along with his dog guide had come to evoke public admiration rather than pity.

While Robert Irwin never overcame either his personal aversion to dog guides or his skepticism that they could be the answer to mobility for most blind people (and in the latter belief he was right, for no more than a small fraction, 2 percent at most, have ever been able to make use of dog guides), he did not stint his cooperation during Seeing Eye's formative years. Article after article appeared in the *Outlook* describing the successful experiences of blind people with dog guides. When an experimental effort was made to consider a training program in New York City instead of Nashville, the event was fully reported in enthusiastic terms. When similar local trials were then scheduled for California, Irwin induced the railroads to grant half-fare transportation for two trainers and 12 dogs. He wrote cordial letters of introduction for Mrs. Eustis to officials in Canada and in England to pave the way for programs there. In what was probably an ultimate expression of confidence, he urged that she be put on the program of the World Conference on Work for the Blind held in New York in April 1931.

A few months later, Dorothy Eustis spent $30,000 of her personal funds to buy Seeing Eye's first permanent quarters, a spacious old house and outbuildings on 56 acres of land in Whippany, New Jersey, where all the needed training facilities for both dogs and people could be centered. At this point, demonstration classes in various cities were discontinued. Instead, Seeing Eye sent Morris Frank out on the road as a field agent, to crisscross the country addressing groups of blind people, talking to agency and school executives, and encouraging suitable candidates to apply for admission to the program that could make them as mobile as Morris himself.

Frank carried on this field service for more than two decades. When he retired in 1956 he was succeeded by Robert H. Whitstock, a youthful graduate of Harvard Law School and of Seeing Eye itself. Whitstock was elected Seeing Eye's vice-president for field services in 1967. In 1971 he was named president-elect of the American Association of Workers for the Blind, to take office following the 1973 AAWB convention.

There was one more element Seeing Eye needed to round out its initial organization, and that was someone who knew as much about the field of work for the blind as Jack Humphrey knew about dogs. In 1934 Mary Dranga Campbell came on staff as head of the social service division. A member of the redoubtable Campbell family to be described in a later chapter, she remained with Seeing Eye until retirement in 1945. Her experience with the problems of blind people antedated World War I.

Once the program at Whippany was well under way, Dorothy Eustis devoted herself to using her Social Register connections to build a circle of influential supporters for Seeing Eye. At a public banquet sponsored by leaders of New York's business and financial community, Alexander Woollcott's story-spinning imagination was captured by the combination of two irresistible subjects: dogs and blindness. He became one of Seeing Eye's most devoted fans and used his journalistic and broadcasting outlets to spread word of its work far and wide.

Within a remarkably few years, considering the depressed state of the economy, Seeing Eye built a membership constituency whose annual contributions met its operating expenses. By 1936 it was on sufficiently firm ground to think about the future. The average working life of a dog was eight years. The average working life of the blind man who depended on a dog could be three times, four times, even five times as long. Just as St. Dunstan's in England had felt itself obligated to accumulate enough capital to insure lifelong care of its war-blinded men, Seeing Eye felt it had a moral responsibility to insure that a person whose dog guide died would not be plunged back into dependency because of inability to obtain a replacement.

Calculations made in 1936 indicated that if a capital fund of $1,600,000 could be raised, its yield would assure the organization's continued ability to serve those it had liberated. A "security fund" of that size seemed a remote goal at the time, but in two decades, thanks to legacies and increasingly successful membership campaigns, the goal had been so far exceeded that, in 1958, Seeing Eye announced its reserves made it unnecessary to ask members to renew their annual gifts. That same year saw it take its first step toward becoming a donor rather than a recipient of funds. It initiated a grants program to support research and training in ophthalmology, in mobility and other rehabilitative services for blind people, and in veterinary medicine. Beginning with a $30,000 construction grant to the Retina Foundation of Boston University's School of Medicine in 1958, the grants program grew from year to year. By the end of 1972 the 15-year cumulative total was $5,886,000.

Recognition that these impressive contributions to the welfare of blind persons owed much to the initiative of George Werntz, Jr., was given tangible form when he received AAWB's Shotwell Memorial Award in 1968. It was under Werntz' administration that in 1965 Seeing Eye moved from Whippany to a 120-acre site on the outskirts of Morristown, New Jersey. As of 1972 the organization could point to totals of 6,300 dogs serving upward of 3,800 blind persons since its founding. Its annual report showed a net worth in excess of $21 million. Its income for the year was close to $2,250,000, of which less than $35,000 was unsolicited membership contributions and about $14,000 came from student payments.

The last figure reflected the philosophy, initiated in 1934, that there were positive psychological and rehabilitative values in asking each person who acquired a Seeing Eye dog to pay a small part of the cost. The fee, $150 for a first dog, $50 for a replacement, was to be paid by the person himself, not by a sponsoring group or benefactor. If need be, it could be paid in small installments. In the early days, Seeing Eye also defrayed part of the trainee's transportation costs to and from New Jersey if necessary; it later liberalized this policy to pay full transportation expenses from all parts of the country without regard to financial need.

The sole exceptions to the fee policy were the war-blinded veterans. The day after Pearl Harbor, Seeing Eye announced it would supply dog guides to the war-blinded without expense to either the veteran or the United States Government. Its trustees adopted a similar resolution in 1950, at the outbreak of the Korean conflict, and maintained the same policy with respect to servicemen blinded in Vietnam.

The year 1958 was historic in a third sense. It saw completion and publication of *Guide Dog Training for Blind Persons*, a segment of a three-year study made under Seeing Eye sponsorship by the Research Center of Columbia University's New York School of Social Work. The authors asserted that only about 3,500 people, representing 1 percent of America's legally blind population at the time, used dog guides; they estimated that another 3,500 blind persons had the requisite capacity, motivation, need and desire for dogs, and that there were at most 8,000 additional persons who might constitute a "secondary reservoir" of potential users, but who were not apt to enter a training program for one reason or another.

After surveying all of the nation's then existing dog guide schools, the study concluded that their "estimated current capacity is slightly in excess of the estimated immediate potential. . . . Expansion of dog guide training facilities is not supported by the evidence."

A number of factors had led to this study and gave its findings importance. One was the intense interest in mobility; "the new religion of the Fifties," one observer called it. The more immediate pressure was that new dog guide schools might continue to spring up unchecked at a time when none of the schools, not even the best-known and oldest-established, was operating at capacity.

As of 1972, there were nine dog guide schools in operation in the United States. Three decades earlier there had been thrice as many—19 in California alone. Most of these were one- or two-man operations, launched by dog breeders and others to take advantage of wartime emotions and of the federal law (P.L.309) which appropriated funds to supply war-blinded veterans with dogs. The California

situation in particular reflected such blatant abuses of public confidence that the
state legislature acted in 1947 to require licensing of dog guide schools and their
personnel on the basis of specific criteria. So strict were these criteria—the trainer's
license, for example, required that the candidate "be able to demonstrate by actual
blindfold test under traffic conditions his ability to train a guide dog with whom a
blind person would be safe"—that 16 of the 19 California schools soon disappeared.
The California law was still on the books in 1972; no other state had as yet enacted
a comparable statute.

California License No. 1 was awarded to Guide Dogs for the Blind in San
Rafael. Founded in 1942, this school was the nation's second largest dog guide
training establishment in 1972. Originally organized to serve blind people living
west of the Mississippi, it later expanded its coverage to the entire United States.
While not as heavily endowed as Seeing Eye, the San Rafael school was
sufficiently well financed (its 1971 annual report showed assets in excess of $4
million) to have completed a $600,000 building and modernization program to
accommodate 32 trainees at a time. Much of the organization's growth was
attributable to the forceful leadership of William F. Johns, who was its executive
director from soon after its inception until his death in 1969.

Another of the three licensed California schools in operation in 1972 was
International Guiding Eyes, Inc. in Hollywood, established in 1948 under the
aegis of a socially minded labor union, the International Association of Machinists.
The third school was Eye Dog Foundation for the Blind in Topanga, incorporated
in 1952. The westernmost American dog guide school was also the youngest: Eye
of the Pacific Guide Dogs, established in Honolulu in 1955.

Two schools were located in the Middle West although they, like the others,
served people from all over. Next in seniority to Seeing Eye was Leader Dogs for
the Blind in Rochester, Michigan, which was founded in 1939 at the initiative of a
group of midwestern Lions Clubs. Following an initial period in which dogs were
trained in a local kennel, Leader Dogs obtained the services of an experienced
trainer formerly employed by Seeing Eye and mounted an essentially similar
program. During the wartime period of proliferating dog guide schools, officials of
Leader Dogs appealed to the American Foundation for the Blind to establish
standards and an accrediting body that would protect blind people, and particularly
blinded veterans, from profiteering operators in the field. The Foundation agreed
that the problem existed, but confessed itself unequipped to offer a solution at the
time. He was not even convinced, Robert Irwin wrote, that there was need for
more than one such school to serve the nation. This was hardly encouraging to the
operators of the country's second school, and the matter was dropped.

Leader Dogs went on to gain a firm foothold; at the end of 1972 it reported it had
equipped 2,200 blind persons with nearly 3,500 dogs since its founding. Its 1972
budget was close to $600,000, more than half of which came from Lions Clubs in
midwestern states.

The other midwestern school, Pilot Dogs, Inc., in Columbus, Ohio, was incorporated in 1950 but was, in fact, the outgrowth of a much earlier effort,
antedating even Seeing Eye and begun by a Minnesota dog breeding enthusiast
named John L. Sinykin, who had started his kennels as a hobby in the early 1920s.

Sinykin had imported a trained German dog, retrained it to obey commands in English, and in 1926 presented the animal to United States Senator Thomas D. Schall, who used it for a good many years. When Lux, the Minnesota senator's dog, died in 1933 he was eulogized by his disconsolate master in the *Congressional Record* of May 23.

Sinykin later incorporated an organization in Minnesota under the name of His Master's Eye Institute. He imported a trainer from Germany to begin a large-scale breeding and training program, but this was cut short when fire destroyed the kennels in 1935. A decade later, a new Master Eye Foundation was established, this time in Illinois, under the direction of Bishop Bernard J. Sheil. It used dogs trained under contract by Sinykin in Minnesota. The contract was eventually terminated and the Illinois organization changed its name to Pilot Dogs, with offices in Chicago but training facilities in Columbus, Ohio. One of its fund-raising methods was through an arrangement with a dog food company, which redeemed labels from cans of its products by contributing funds to Pilot Dogs.

Leaders in work for the blind were uneasy over this commercial tie-in, not because they begrudged funds to Pilot Dogs but because of the troubles they periodically experienced as the result of unfounded rumors that collections of various useless objects—empty match folders, tin foil, cigarette wrappers, cellophane strips from cigarette packages, tea bag labels—would "buy" guide dogs for blind people. Hoaxes of this type were reported as early as 1938 and continued to crop up intermittently thereafter. In 1971 the Foundation issued a public warning against the newest manifestation, this one involving the ring-top pulls of aluminum cans, and repeated the message, delivered every time such rumors got under way, that no blind person was denied a dog guide for lack of funds.

The arrangement between the dog food company and Pilot Dogs continued throughout the years; its 1969 financial statement showed income of about $50,000, or one-third of its annual budget, derived from the tie-in.

In the eastern United States two dog guide schools were in operation in 1972 in addition to Seeing Eye. The Guide Dog Foundation for the Blind (also known as Second Sight), with headquarters in Forest Hills, New York, and a training center in Smithtown, Long Island, was organized in 1946 by a blind attorney who grew impatient over the long waiting list at Seeing Eye that resulted from the preference then being extended to blinded veterans.

Guiding Eyes for the Blind, also headquartered in New York City but with its training center in Yorktown Heights in Westchester, was organized in 1954, utilizing the services of a former Seeing Eye employee to organize its training program.

The two New York schools survived the uncomfortable limelight in which they were placed during the mid-Fifties in the course of widely publicized state legislative investigations of fund-raising practices. These investigations resulted in the state's Charities Registration Act, adopted in 1954 and amended two years later, a measure designed to prevent fraudulent or inordinately costly drives conducted in the name of philanthropy.

Despite their diverse origins, all nine dog guide schools pursue essentially similar patterns in preparing dogs and blind persons to work together as mobility partners.

Animals of suitable breed—no longer exclusively German shepherds but Golden and Labrador Retrievers, Boxers, Collies, and other canines of appropriate size and characteristics—are either bred in the school's own kennels or secured through purchase or donation. Several of the schools place their puppies in foster homes (youngsters enrolled in the 4-H Clubs of America are a valuable source of such cooperation for some of the schools), where they grow accustomed to family atmospheres until they reach the age, about a year-and-a-half, when they can begin to be trained as guides for blind people.

The dogs' active training period lasts three or four months, during which they are taught to obey basic directional commands, to halt at sidewalk curbs, to circumvent obstructions, to function in heavy pedestrian and vehicular traffic, to ignore lamp posts and the presence of other animals while in harness, to retain self-control even when startled by sudden loud noises. After learning obedience to commands, they are then taught what is described as "intelligent disobedi-ence"—e.g., to refuse a "forward" command when obeying it might risk the safety of the person being guided.

(It is only in such instances that the animal does anything other than follow a specific command. Contrary to public impression, it is the master and not the dog guide who decides when to cross a street or in what direction to proceed. The dog does not distinguish between red and green traffic lights—dogs are color blind—nor does it respond to such commands as "take me to the bus stop.")

Training the dog is only half the job. The more critical half is training the blind person in how to use the animal, and teaching the two together to work as a team. This takes about four weeks' residence at the school, during which the dog's fidelity has to be transferred from the trainer to the new master, while the master has to learn to trust his canine guide and to develop confidence in his own ability to travel safely with the animal's help.

The most arduous and extensive training is the lot of the instructor who works with both dog and master. An outline of the apprentice training program for dog guide schools, which was included in standards published in 1966, called for a three-year program during which the apprentice, under supervision, would gradually learn to take responsibility for preparing a string of dogs for assignment to a class of six or eight blind students, for matching students and dogs, and for instructing the students in how to work with their dogs. Part of the apprentice's training was to be performed under blindfold, so that he could more fully under-stand the blind person's problems in effecting a man-dog partnership.

Although the dog guide movement in and of itself has never served more than a small fraction of the blind population, it has nevertheless exerted a major influence by demonstrating the necessity for a formalized course of mobility training. This concept proved equally applicable to the cane travel technique initiated by Richard Hoover at Valley Forge and brought to advanced stages of development by Russell Williams and his staff at Hines.

The use by blind people of some form of cane or staff to guide their steps goes back to antiquity. A stout tree branch was probably the first such object; later, as man mastered the use of cutting tools, straighter and smoother staffs came into use.

The traditional method was for the blind man to tap his way along, warning others out of his path and simultaneously setting up echoes which he used, consciously or unconsciously, as clues to the environment. The clatter of horse hooves or iron wheels was usually loud enough to prevent highway accidents. When, however, rubber-tired automotive vehicles took over the roads at ever higher speeds, the unaccompanied blind pedestrian faced increasing peril.

In 1930 the Lions Club of Peoria, Illinois, decided it could help out in this situation by having motorists share the responsibility for safe crossing by blind persons. At its urging the city of Peoria passed an ordinance making it mandatory for motorists to yield the right of way to persons who identified themselves as blind by carrying red-tipped white canes. The following year a statewide White Cane Law was enacted, and the Lions proceeded to adopt the white cane movement as a national program, successfully pressing for passage of similar laws in all states. Some of these laws called for the cane to be held aloft or extended horizontally so as to be more readily observable.

Added impetus was given to the white cane movement when Senator Schall, who had not yet acquired a second dog guide, was run over and killed by a car while crossing a Washington street just before Christmas of 1935. In the wake of this accident the Foundation issued a bulletin urging all agencies for the blind to support the white cane movement and offering to supply such canes at wholesale prices. The fact that white canes represented conspicuous labels of blindness was now considered of secondary importance.

Twenty-five years later, in 1961, the Foundation issued a policy statement that more or less reversed its earlier position. Experience with the white cane had shown, the statement noted, that "the great majority of motorists are unaware of [its] meaning" and "there is no confidence that the percentage of drivers who recognize the white cane as a 'stop signal' will ever be very great." Moreover, white cane laws were not being widely enforced, and those state laws that called for holding the cane aloft or extended at arm's length from the body not only made the cane dangerous to other pedestrians but precluded its more practical use as an obstacle detector. The white cane laws, the statement averred, simply deepened the public's belief that blind persons "are unskilled in their ability to transport themselves, and, as a consequence, are socially or vocationally unacceptable." The essential value of any cane was in its skilled use as a mobility tool; its color was unimportant.

In this final point lay the crux of the matter, for by 1961 formal criteria for mobility instructors had been evolved, two graduate educational programs in orientation and mobility had been initiated, and a specialized discipline was on the verge of becoming a profession.

Few periods in history were as fertile as the Fifties in providing blind people with opportunities and incentives for economic and social progress. The decade was dotted with landmarks of liberation: expanded educational, vocational and cultural programs, a greater choice and availability of jobs, improved financial security, new resources for personal adjustment and growth through rehabilitation centers. To take advantage of these widened horizons, however, blind people had to forgo the comfort of sheltered lives and move out into the bustling traffic of their sighted peers. That it could be done, to a degree theretofore considered unattainable, had been demonstrated by the example of the World War II veterans and the cane travel techniques that had freed so many of them from immobility.

One of the first efforts to share the lessons learned at Valley Forge with agencies serving the civilian blind was a training manual prepared for the "orientors" at that Army hospital. As a service to its readers, the *Outlook* published the document in full in its issue of December 1947. It was a well-intentioned gesture, but it backfired. All over the country impulsive workers for the blind who read and clipped the article concluded that they now had all they needed to know to go and do likewise. The more thoughtful among them recognized that there was more to it. Some, taking advantage of the fact that Hoover, then living at the Maryland School for the Blind while studying medicine, was giving summer courses in the long cane technique, sent staff members to learn his methods.

Other agencies, aware that the long cane method was being refined at the Hines VA center, applied for permission to send staff members there for a week or two of observation. A number of such requests were granted, but those agency heads who hoped that a brief visit would enable the observer to return fully equipped to introduce a mobility program were disappointed. Instead, a former member of the Hines staff was to recall, the visits "served chiefly to whet the appetites for a much more thorough indoctrination and training."

One effort to satisfy these whetted appetites was the VA's production in 1952 of a training film, *The Long Cane*. Shot on location at Hines, the thirty-minute film used no professional actors; the man who took the role of the blind trainee was Lloyd Greenwood, on leave of absence from his post as executive director of the Blinded Veterans Association. Greenwood convincingly reenacted the mobility training experiences he had himself undergone some years earlier. The film also had Russell Williams, playing himself, as well as members of his staff and veterans who were actually undergoing training at Hines during the shooting.

In releasing *The Long Cane* for borrowing by civilian agencies, Dr. A.B.C. Knudson, director of physical medicine and rehabilitation for the VA, acknowledged that differences between civilian clients and the men at the VA center would make it difficult to use the Hines techniques without adaptation. He used the occasion to make an oblique but unmistakable point: "The war blind at the outset know nothing about being blind and as a rule know that they know nothing. They are willing to learn from seeing instructors because their self-esteem has not yet become involved with a concept of themselves as authorities on the subject."

Dr. Knudson was alluding to the resistance, both silent and vocal, that traditionalists in work for the blind were showing toward the idea of sighted mobility instructors. For decades, whatever travel techniques blind people learned had come to them through home teachers, most of whom were themselves blind. What they taught was "the way I get around," a hit-or-miss proposition at best, satisfactory enough for indoor orientation and mobility but hardly adequate for safe unescorted movement on unfamiliar city streets.

It was to plan ways of outflanking this resistance, and to prevent watering down of the laboriously evolved mobility discipline, that Father Thomas J. Carroll and

Kathern Gruber met in Chicago in November 1952 with Russell Williams and several members of his staff. What they worked out, in an off-the-record conference, was a set of guidelines outlining the overall responsibilities of a "mobility technician" whose function was "to be both teacher and coach in instilling into the blinded person knowledge of a science and skill in an art on which his personal safety and perhaps his life may depend."

The work of the mobility technician, a memorandum summarizing the group's conclusions declared, extended beyond "mere instruction in the proper use of a cane or of a guide dog." These were simply tools. The technician's work was

> with the sensorium of the blind person, making use of all the senses which remain when sight is gone; . . . with the intelligence of the blind person, giving knowledge of objectively evaluated methods of travel without sight; . . . with the will of the blind person, stimulating confidence in his ability to move without dependence.

The memorandum was unsigned, but its language would suggest Father Carroll's authorship. Whether or not he wrote this particular document, it was unquestionably he who took the next step to translate its ideas into action. Not quite a year later, he assembled, in his own home in Gloucester, Mass., a group of 24 persons to participate in a workshop sponsored by his agency, the Catholic Guild for the Blind. The occasion for the conference, the invitees were informed, was "the increasing recognition of the danger involved in allowing untrained persons to set themselves up as [mobility] experts." Those asked to participate included not just practitioners in work with blind adults and children but also specialists in physical education, physical medicine, general rehabilitation, ophthalmology, clinical psychology and psychological research.

No report of the workshop's findings ever appeared in print. It was later said that the field of work for the blind was not yet ready to accept the advanced principles and standards the participants were eager to promulgate. Quite possibly this was the final spur which led Father Carroll, the following year, to launch St. Paul's Rehabilitation Center, where he uncompromisingly put into practice the concepts he believed should be universally adopted.

By 1958 the vanguard thinkers of the Gloucester conference had succeeded in finding a powerful ally in the person of Louis H. Rives, then chief of the Division of Services to the Blind of the federal Office of Vocational Rehabilitation. Training of mobility instructors was adopted as an OVR program priority that year; to get things started, the American Foundation for the Blind was given a grant to convene a national conference of specialists. At this conclave, held in June 1959, much of what had been said years earlier in Chicago and Gloucester was reiterated, and the first step toward professionalization was taken in the form of a recommendation that at least one year of graduate study be required for mobility instructors.

The conferees also came out firmly, although not unanimously, with what they knew would be an inflammatory stand: that "the teaching of mobility was a task of a sighted, rather than a blind, individual." The concept of the blind mobility instructor was "bankrupt," the group insisted, if only because that instructor was just as incapable of seeing danger as his trainee, and was therefore unable to protect the latter in a hazardous situation.

As drawn up by the group, minimum standards for mobility instructors included good vision, hearing, and physical condition, an academic bachelor's degree, and those personal characteristics that could lend themselves to the exacting process of building trusted relationships with trainees. A tentative curriculum for graduate study and supervised practice was also proposed. The areas to be covered went well beyond technical training procedures, embracing psychology, dynamics of human behavior, anatomy, and physiology, with particular emphasis on the sensorium.

Coming as it did during one of the most dynamic phases of OVR's thrust toward expanded research and training in the field of vocational rehabilitation, the committee's report won prompt acceptance and action on the part of the federal agency. By June 1960 the nation's first graduate program in mobility was inaugurated at Boston College for 8 students (the number was doubled in ensuing years), and a year later the second opened at Western Michigan University for 12. Money was not a problem; the students were eligible for OVR traineeship grants. What did constitute an obstacle was finding qualified faculty, but Father Carroll and Russell Williams, the most ardent advocates of professionalization, met the challenge by volunteering the use of their own agencies for clinical practice, and releasing members of their staffs to teach and supervise.

To validate the usefulness of professional mobility instruction as soon as graduates of these first courses became available, OVR supported a cluster of demonstration projects in voluntary and state agencies, residential and day schools. Between 1963 and 1971, it funded 30 such demonstrations.

Apart from their tangible results, these grants helped defuse some of the negative reactions that followed the initiation of professional standards for mobility instruction. But protests there were, as has ever been the case when a new group struggles to wedge its way into established structures. Spokesmen for long-accepted professions questioned whether there was a sufficient body of knowledge or experience in mobility instruction to warrant awarding it professional status. Practitioners in related disciplines that were simultaneously seeking professional recognition feared their chances for acceptance might suffer from competition. The most vehement outbursts came from blind workers—home teachers and others—who felt themselves threatened.

A good-natured effort to mollify the doubters and dissenters was made at the 1960 AAWB convention when the leading proponents of the new discipline presented a humorous recorded skit contrasting the safety of trained long-cane users with the physical risks taken by those who scorned its use. The skit was followed by an informal demonstration in which four men experienced in teaching cane mobility techniques gave a "three-minute wonder course" to blind members of the audience who volunteered.

The standards for orientation and mobility services published in the 1966 COMSTAC report endorsed the concept of professionally qualified sighted teachers. As a practical matter, the COMSTAC standards also proposed that a certifying body be established that would "give formal recognition to those whose years of experience may be considered a substitute for graduate academic training."

This proposal was implemented in 1969 when AAWB appointed an Orientation and Mobility Certification Committee which, until the end of 1971, honored a "grandfather clause" in certifying applicants qualified by experience. By January of 1972 the committee had granted permanent certificates to 137 applicants and provisional certification to 138. By this time, too, four additional graduate programs had been established: at San Francisco State College, California State College at Los Angeles, University of Northern Colorado, and University of Pittsburgh, and a pilot effort on the undergraduate level had been set up at Florida State University. All told, however, no more than fifty to sixty mobility instructors per year were emerging from these educational institutions; demand far exceeded supply.

At the end of 1972 the question of what constituted qualification for teaching orientation and mobility remained hotly controversial. Two large local service agencies, the Greater Pittsburgh Guild for the Blind and the Cleveland Society for the Blind, which had undertaken a combination of in-service training and university courses, were under attack by members of the certified mobility group for diluting standards. The attackers were being attacked, in turn, for their "crusading attitude" by means of which the long cane had "become a fetish and the associated technology a ritual."

The mobility discipline itself had not yet fully coalesced. One of its minor problems was what to call itself. "Orientor," the term used at Valley Forge and Hines, was rejected; "mobility technician" did not sound sufficiently professional; "orientation and mobility specialist" was awkwardly lengthy. Back in 1953, at Gloucester, the term "peripatology" had been coined [from the Greek *peri,* meaning around or surrounding; *patein,* to walk; *ology,* the science of], but it was not widely used.

The major schism involved graduate training. Both the extent of the schism and a possible approach to straddling it were recognized in two policy statements issued by the Foundation in late 1969 and early 1970. The first of these, "The Science of Peripatology," declared:

> The American Foundation for the Blind believes that the professional training of peripatologists must be carried out at the graduate level. . . . and supports their professional group . . . in calling for proper certification of peripatologists. It also believes that these matters should be reviewed by the Foundation, together with the peripatologists, at least once every five years.

The second statement, "Delivery of Orientation and Mobility Services for Blind Persons," said:

> The Foundation recognizes that under circumstances of manpower availability and the pressing needs of blind persons, it may be necessary to train aides or other certified personnel to work under the direction of a peripatologist . . . once the latter has made a diagnosis and given a prescription in the individual case.

It seemed reasonable to suppose that this multi-level approach was the path that would have to be followed in years to come. In an era of expanding demand for all types of human services, it was a path already well trodden by other disciplines—social work, law, nursing and other health professions, even medicine itself—all of which had accepted the reality of trained aides working as junior partners to professionals.

The modern movement for scientific mobility techniques began with the war-blinded, who were adults. Instruction of children in the newer methods of independent travel arose somewhat later in the game.

Although orientation and mobility are customarily linked in a single phrase, they are separate functions. Orientation is the process by which a person locates his position in space and his relationship to surrounding objects. Mobility deals with actual locomotion from one position in space to another. Obviously, orientation is a prerequisite for mobility, but it is also an essential in itself, as when a blind person seated in a chair reaches out for the glass he knows is on a nearby table, or determines, by using his other senses, whether people have entered or left a room.

Blind students were traditionally taught basic elements of orientation in the residential schools and, to some extent, in day school programs for the visually handicapped. They also discovered a good deal about their surroundings in the same trial-and-error way as all growing children.

What they did not learn, until recent times, was how to navigate securely through unfamiliar environments. Richard Hoover, who had been a pre-war instructor at the Maryland School for the Blind, was concerned over the difficulties that confronted the older students, particularly those attending a community high school, in taking advantage of opportunities for growth-producing experiences "downtown." When, at war's end, he returned to live at the school for a time, he secured the consent of its superintendent, Francis M. Andrews, to introduce a few of the older pupils to the long-cane technique developed at Valley Forge.

The lessons were a great success. Superintendent Andrews warned against efforts to teach travel without adequate preparation, but he was genuinely enthusiastic. "Within reasonable limits, travel is safe; it is successful; it is an added means of independence for our blind."

Still, the idea was slow to catch on; the main drawback was that there was no school to teach the teachers who could, in turn, instruct the children. In 1953 the Foundation's specialist in education, Georgie Lee Abel, could list only nine schools for blind children in which any sort of travel instruction was given, and much of this was substandard. "There seems to be a great feeling of need," she noted, "but so little actual know-how."

The feeling of need gradually gave way to action. At summer workshops for teachers of blind children, representatives of cane travel programs and dog guide schools were invited to acquaint teachers with the potentials for independent movement. These workshops were not intended to make their participants instant experts on mobility, but to increase their awareness of the subject and supply them with reliable information that would enable young people and their parents to exercise intelligent choices at the proper time. One of the things made clear, for example, was that dog guides were not suitable for young children, who could not be expected to have either the physical strength or the maturity of judgment needed to work with dogs. A statement subsequently issued by a dozen authorities on the subject recommended that training with a dog guide not begin before the middle teens at earliest. It acknowledged the value of dogs as pets, but pointed out that dog guides were not pets but working animals. With rare exceptions, most reliable dog guide schools do not accept applicants under sixteen.

Once cane mobility instruction reached the master's degree level, a considerable demand arose among both residential and day schools for graduates of these programs. The United States Office of Education stepped in to assist in this process by granting funds for the formulation of educational principles in teaching orientation and mobility skills to children. The usual practice came to be instruction of younger children in various phases of orientation, with cane training beginning at the junior high school level. An important function of a certified orientation and mobility specialist working in a school was to determine when each individual blind child was physically, mentally and emotionally ready for cane travel.

The cane, the dog, the friendly elbow of a human guide—were these the only answers to greater freedom of movement for blind people? Could modern technology offer no more efficient solutions? Millions of dollars and uncounted man-hours have been invested in exploring the second question with relatively few usable results. At various times since World War II, the Army, the Navy, the Air Force, the Veterans Administration, the Rehabilitation Services Administration, the National Institutes of Health, and other government bureaus have all sponsored and financed research efforts to find effective substitutes for the information provided by the human eye. Private philanthropy, which ventured early money and effort in exploratory work, soon found its financial and manpower resources outstripped by the demands of technological research and invention. Consequently it reshaped its role to serve as the bridge from laboratory to consumer, as liaison agent among separate ventures, as stimulator of new efforts, as consultant and evaluator of experimental approaches and as the medium for field testing of laboratory products.

Many of these last functions were assumed by the Foundation once it decided, in 1959, to discontinue its independent efforts at invention of guidance devices and to concentrate its research role on enabling tasks. In 1961, 1962, 1964, and 1971 it took the leadership in convening national and international conferences on technology at which high-level experts in physics, engineering, electronics, automation, biophysics and optics exchanged ideas with equally high-level specialists in psychology, sociology, physical medicine, rehabilitation, and social services. At each conference, progress was assessed, new technological approaches disclosed and discussed, and ever-closer lines drawn between theory and application. The latter came to assume greater and greater weight in the thinking of those engaged in the hard sciences. As a psychologist associated with Massachusetts Institute of Technology put it at one of the international conclaves:

> I would like to encourage you to pay more attention to the organism you are trying to help, and less attention to the tools you are using. I think to begin

with a transistor and make a man adapt to it is not probably the best way to proceed. . . . it might be a little better to exploit some of the more subjective properties of human beings.

A blind student once put the whole issue even more succinctly when he said, "I walk with my head as well as with my feet."

20

The Watershed Years

Globally speaking, the decades beginning with the Forties were watershed years. Their events permanently altered the political geography of all five continents, the social and economic structures governing the lives of much of the world's population, the psychological climate of humanity's thinking, the very prospect of man's survival on earth.

In different and less drastic ways, the same era was one of major change in the world of work for the blind. The time had come for the generation of dedicated pioneers to relinquish their leadership. They would not be leaving a void, for they themselves had planted the seeds and cultivated the soil that produced a crop of sturdy successors. Decades of determination to turn work for the blind into a soundly based profession were now ready for harvesting.

When the guns of World War II were silenced, the American Foundation for the Blind was on the verge of its 25th anniversary. The ranks of its founders, already diminished by death, were about to be thinned still further by the toll of advancing years. By 1945 the permanently missing among the founding trustees included Henry Randolph Latimer, the insurance executive Herbert H. White, the Baltimore attorney William H. Hamilton, the banker William Fellowes Morgan, the blind Chicago heart specialist Robert H. Babcock, the Pittsburgh industrialist Captain Charles W. Brown, the financier-philanthropist Felix M. Warburg.

Gone, too, were two of the three founding trustees whose donations of $1,000 each salted the Foundation's treasury with its initial cash: the piano manufacturer Sir Charles W. Lindsay of Montreal, and Prudence Sherwin, a member of the Cleveland family whose fortune was made in paint manufacturing. The third member of the trio, Mabel Knowles Gage of Worcester, Mass., was to live another three years but had already retired from the Foundation board.

All but one of the remaining early stalwarts were nearing the end of long life spans. The retired Philadelphia educator Olin H. Burritt was seventy-seven; William Nelson Cromwell, international lawyer and philanthropist, was past ninety; the New York banker Harvey D. Gibson was sixty-three. Gustavus A. Pfeiffer was seventy-three; he was to survive another eight years. Sherman C. Swift, the blind Canadian librarian and literary critic, was sixty-seven; his life had just one more year to run. Mary Vanderpoel Hun maintained a reticence about her age; it was a matter of record, however, that she had held public office since 1914. She, William Ziegler, Jr., and M. C. Migel were the only three of the early trustees who were still in office in 1945. Ziegler was the baby of the group; he was fifty-four.

For M. C. Migel the war's end was also an opportune moment to withdraw from the firing line of work for the blind. He was approaching his eightieth birthday when, in November 1945, he felt free at last to resign the Foundation presidency and turn it over to Ziegler. The Major would probably have taken this step earlier, were it not for the war. He was not the kind of man to feel comfortable about slacking off when younger men were devoting their lives to the nation's defense.

As personalities, Moses Charles Migel and the man who succeeded him as president were a study in contrasts. Where Migel's commanding presence tended to overwhelm his associates, William Ziegler, Jr., was a shy and soft-spoken man, not given to self-assertion, who sought consensus through accommodation. Migel's dashing personal style made him a center of attention in any gathering. Ziegler, a stocky figure of middle height, the roundness of his face emphasized by rimless eyeglasses, had the benevolent look and reserved demeanor of a country doctor. He shrank from the spotlight; public appearances necessitated a genuine effort of will on his part.

Different as they were, Migel and Ziegler also had much in common. Their business interests consisted largely of managing their own investments, which left time and energy to devote to philanthropic and civic causes. They shared a decades-long concern for the welfare of blind people, a concern that had brought them into association as early as 1916, when New York State Governor Charles S. Whitman appointed Migel chairman of the state's commission for the blind and named Ziegler as one of its members. Both men had political interests and connections; Ziegler was at one point treasurer of the New York State Republican Committee. Both were sportsmen. Ziegler bred gun dogs and race horses, had his own racing stables and was prominent in yachting circles.

The name Ziegler was probably better known than any other to America's blind citizens. This was not due to William but to his adoptive mother, Electa Matilda Ziegler, whose generosity had founded and financed the embossed magazine bearing her name. Young Billy Ziegler was only sixteen when the magazine put out its first issue in 1907, but he already knew a good deal about the problems of blindness, having grown up in the same household as Charles Gamble, Matilda Ziegler's son by an earlier marriage, who had been blind since boyhood.

Born William Conrad Brandt in Muscatine, Iowa, in 1891, Billy was not yet five years old when he was adopted by his father's half brother, William Ziegler, and brought to New York to live. The senior Ziegler had made his fortune as founder of the Royal Baking Powder Company; when he died in 1905 his adopted son inherited $16 million. William Jr., on completion of his education at Columbia and Harvard universities, succeeded his adoptive father as president of the baking powder firm and went on to expand his business and civic interests. In World War I he served his nation first as executive secretary of the War Credits Board and then as company commander of an Army motor transport corps overseas.

At the time he became president of the Foundation, Ziegler was a director of Standard Brands, Inc., which had bought out Royal Baking Powder in 1929. He was chairman of the board of American Maize Products Company, held a similar post in a large manufacturing concern, and presided over a personal holding corporation. Ever since his mother's death in 1932 he had administered the trust fund she had set up for the *Ziegler Magazine.* In the course of his more than twenty years on the Foundation board, he had also assumed officer responsibilities in its affiliated organizations.

Ziegler was not one of the founding trustees named at Vinton in 1921; when, however, the bylaws were amended the following year to enlarge the number of trustees to 25, of whom 15 were to be "persons of influence," he was a natural choice. He was thus a member of the board when the Foundation opened its office early the following year and, in his unassuming manner, took an interest in every phase of the growing organization, particularly the area he knew best, financial management. When Herbert H. White, the first treasurer, died in 1934, Ziegler took over the post. Two years later, when Olin H. Burritt retired as principal of the Pennsylvania Institution for the Instruction of the Blind (Overbrook), he also withdrew as secretary of the Foundation board. To fill the void, Ziegler served in the combined role of secretary-treasurer until, in 1939, the death of Prudence Sherwin left the board without a vice-president. The secretaryship was assigned to another trustee and Ziegler, occupying the dual offices of vice-president and treasurer, became the Foundation's second in command.

When he became president, the post of treasurer went to Richard L. Morris, a member of the Wall Street brokerage firm of Hayden, Stone and Company. Morris, an elderly man who had been a trustee since 1935, agreed wholeheartedly when Ziegler, in his address accepting the presidency, urged that younger people be brought into work for the blind. He proposed two young Wall Street colleagues for trusteeship: twenty-eight-year-old Jansen Noyes, Jr., and thirty-year-old Richard H. Migel, M.C.'s younger son. Both were elected the following June and Noyes promptly followed Morris into the treasurership. Richard Migel became assistant secretary a few years later, and then secretary in 1958.

The process of rejuvenation in the Foundation's governing body was gradual but noticeable in the succeeding decades. The added ingredients were younger laymen and a more dynamic group of professionals in work for the blind, chosen not because they stood for particular segments of work but because they contributed broad spectra of experience to the board's thinking. Changes in the bylaws enacted in 1951, 1958, and again in 1971 first loosened, and finally eliminated, the stipulation that board composition include an arbitrary number of persons to represent specific segments of work for the blind. The updated bylaws reflected the Foundation's position as an independent, nonpartisan body accountable only to the public that supported it.

One of the earliest problems faced by the trustees in these watershed years was the necessity for a change in the Foundation's professional leadership. Robert Irwin reached the age of sixty-five in June 1948. Under the mandatory staff retirement system he himself had set up a dozen years earlier, it was time to make way for a successor. But Irwin, not yet psychologically ready to step down, persuaded the trustees to let him continue on a month-to-month basis while they pondered the problem of what sort of man should take the helm.

It was not a simple question. The Foundation, now a complex enterprise with assets in cash, securities, and real estate in excess of two million dollars, a staff of over a hundred to be directed, a budget close to $350,000, and a far-flung program that stood on the threshold of sizable expansion, would need an experienced and vigorous administrator with an unusual array of talents. The job called for a man accustomed to handling large sums of money who also knew his way around the intricacies of the federal and state laws and regulations that had come to govern major services for blind people. He would have to have sufficient professional prestige to win acceptance in the field of work for the blind, but not be so closely identified with any one ideological faction as to antagonize those with opposing views. Moreover, the Foundation itself stood in need of basic internal reforms. The circumstances of its growth—improvising solutions to unforeseen problems, responding to opportunities as they arose—had not been conducive to orderly planning or the development of an integrated organizational structure.

The issue facing the trustees, and troubling some of them, was whether even the most capable blind man would be able to cope with these diverse challenges, or whether the time had come to seek a sighted executive from the wider world of commerce.

Word that this question was even being contemplated was not slow in filtering down to the Foundation staff. On March 11, 1949, eleven staff members in key professional and administrative posts addressed a joint letter to the agency's president urging that preference be given to a blind man. They said that blindness was "an indispensable link" between the Foundation executive and those he would serve, and that "the inspiration of a dynamic blind leader" not only spurred the staff to higher achievement but also won an extra measure of support and cooperation from legislators and others in high places.

One of the signatories was Alfred Allen, who had joined the staff five years earlier as assistant to Irwin, and who simultaneously functioned as unpaid secretary-general of the American Association of Workers for the Blind. The same day as the staff letter, Allen sent a communication to the AAWB's board of directors, enclosing a draft of a proposed resolution to be endorsed and sent posthaste to Ziegler. The resolution echoed the staff's arguments in favor of naming a blind person to succeed Irwin.

As it happens, most of this concern was needless. Jansen Noyes, Jr., one of the five members of a committee assigned to the executive search, later said that the committee had never seriously considered appointing a sighted person. But the committee did not voice this view publicly, which may be why Dr. Francis J. Cummings, AAWB president, told his membership at their convention in Boston in July that one of the "proudest accomplishments" of the year was the influence the AAWB's board had exerted on the Foundation to choose a blind man as their new executive.

Cummings himself, it was rumored, had been one of the candidates considered by the search committee. A man of exceptional scholarly achievement who had been executive secretary of the Delaware Commission for the Blind since 1942, he held a Ph.D. from the University of Pennsylvania, where he had made history by becoming the first blind person to be named to the university faculty. His subject was French, which he had studied at the Sorbonne. He also taught foreign languages at Overbrook, of which he was a graduate. Later elected a trustee-at-large of the Foundation, he served until his death in 1962 at the age of fifty-eight.

By the time Cummings mounted the podium at Boston, the Foundation had already made its decision public. Its new executive director, as of September 1949, would be thirty-two-year-old M. Robert Barnett, executive director of the Florida Council for the Blind.

The announcement took many by surprise. Barnett was very young for a post of such national stature. He had behind him only five years of experience in work for the blind. He hardly qualified as a member of the old-line "establishment," having attended his very first AAWB convention only two years earlier. Nor could he lay claim to an "old school tie" relationship with graduates of one of the Ivy League schools for the blind.

The more perceptive of the leaders in work for the blind realized that these potentially negative factors were, in fact, a plus. Barnett's feet were not entangled in traditional ideologies, attitudes or loyalties. He was attuned to the future, not the past. In selecting him, the Foundation had given realistic recognition to a fundamental shift in the balance of power in work for the blind. The long-established voluntary agencies which had for so many years set the pace were rapidly being overtaken by the state bodies through which were funneled ever larger quantities of federal money for services to blind men, women, and children. The tools of progress were no longer the sole property of private philanthropy.

In the preceding decade virtually every piece of federal legislation—the Social Security Act, the Randolph-Sheppard Act, and particularly the Barden-LaFollette amendments to the Vocational Rehabilitation Act—had vested added degrees of power in the state agencies. As the head of one such agency, Bob Barnett had administered large sums in creating dynamic and imaginative programs. He had opened the nation's second adult rehabilitation center, patterning it in an original mold which emphasized rapid placement results. He had been elected president of the National Council of Executives of State Agencies.

Barnett had other assets as well. He was personable; the official photograph taken for his new job showed a handsome, youthful face topped by a wavy pompadour of dark hair, the broad forehead and cleanly etched features accentuated by heavy black eyebrows. He was quick-thinking and articulate, a good writer, and a fluent public speaker. He combined the pleasant manners and social ease of a Southerner with a ready sense of humor and the confident air of a man who, mainly through his own efforts, had surmounted both a difficult boyhood and the trauma of sudden blindness. In many ways, Bob Barnett was himself a symbol of the achievement workers in the field strove to make possible for all blind people.

M. Robert Barnett (his birth certificate read that way but Barnett assumed the first initial was intended to stand for Marvin, his father's name) was born in Jacksonville, Florida, October 31, 1916. His mother succumbed to a flu epidemic when he was a year old, and he spent his early years in the home of his paternal grandparents, then shared a bachelor apartment with his father until the latter, a commercial printer, died in 1931. After that he lived with various relatives while attending high school.

Shortly before his 16th birthday, Bob and two other teenagers went joy riding; as they drove past an orange grove, a prankish notion struck them. They would climb the fence, pick as many oranges as they could stuff into their shirt fronts, then drive on in search of further amusement. While they were in the grove an unexpected noise sent the boys scrambling for the fence. Two made it; the third was stopped by two bursts of buckshot that tore across his face. The grove's owner, who had been troubled by poachers, had decided to teach the next trespasser a lesson. The victim of this lesson was Bob Barnett, who would never see again.

During the next two years a series of operations gave rise to a faint hope that some sight might be restored, but there came a day when Bob's surgeon advised him to enroll in a school for the blind to finish his high school education. January of 1935 saw him a student at what was then the Florida State School for the Deaf and Blind; June 1936 marked his graduation. It was during his senior year at the school that he met with his first stroke of good fortune. Through an acquaintance, he was introduced to Mrs. Alfred I. DuPont, who maintained a winter home in Florida. She had been informed about Bob's family circumstances and his good academic record. He was definitely college material, but could never make it without help. Florida had yet to create a state agency for the blind or a vocational rehabilitation program that would finance a blind youth's college education. In the tradition of personal philanthropy characteristic of her generation, Mrs. DuPont volunteered to pay his tuition.

Barnett chose to attend a small denominational school, Stetson University, in DeLand, Florida. To earn pocket money he got a work scholarship editing the campus magazine. He managed his studies with the help of student readers paid by the National Youth Administration, one of the New Deal's depression agencies; the paid readers were supplemented by girl volunteers, one of whom he married a year after graduation.

Majoring in history and political science, Bob also took an elective course in journalism, which led to his joining the staff of the weekly student newspaper. Teaching was the career he had in mind, but during his senior year he discovered, after applying to every high school in Florida, that blindness automatically disqualified him under the physical criteria stipulated by school boards. (One of his later satisfactions, as executive director of the Foundation, was helping to circumvent this particular barrier; the first blind person to secure a teaching appointment in a Florida school got the position when a Foundation field consultant persuaded the local school board to give her a tryout.)

What helped Barnett land his first job was the wartime need for manpower which claimed Stetson University's journalism teacher, who also doubled as its public relations director. When the manager of the local Associated Press county bureau was drafted, there arose an opportunity to become a full-time journalist.

Using a Seeing Eye dog acquired during a college vacation, Barnett covered his journalistic beat to the satisfaction of his employers. A by-product of this job was meeting some of the state's political leaders, among them R. Henry P. Johnson, a Tampa lawyer prominent in Lions Club work, who was spearheading a campaign for a bill to establish a state agency for the blind.

It was a long-sought goal. As early as 1929, the Foundation, asked to help press for such a bill, had sent Helen Keller to Tallahassee. Although her reception by the state legislators left nothing to be desired, they failed to act. A dozen years later Johnson and his fellow Lions took up the cudgels and asked for the Foundation's help once again. Helen Keller made another trip to the Florida state capital and appeared before a joint session of the legislature in April 1941. This time the bill was passed.

Johnson was named by the governor to head the new agency, the Florida Council for the Blind, but he had only a $45,000 appropriation to work with. One service he could not afford was public relations; when he prepared his first annual report, he invoked Barnett's help, as a newsman, to publicize it. When the Barden-LaFollette Act was passed the following year, the Council gained access to new and substantial funds—some $200,000 in federal money plus $125,000 as the supplementary state grant required under the bill's formula. Money meant staff, and one of the first staff members to be employed was M. Robert Barnett.

Bob was ready for the change. His first child was about to be born, and he needed a post with a future. There was no assurance he could keep his Associated Press job once the war was over; the man who had been drafted would have first claim on it. What weighed even more heavily was his conviction that the Barden-LaFollette Act could open tremendous new vistas for blind people. He could not help but think how many of the new services might have made a difference in his own life, had they existed when he lost the use of his eyes.

It was thus an eager and enthusiastic young man who came to work as a placement counselor for the Florida Council for the Blind in September 1944. Like other recruits into this new program, he was sent to Canada for a few weeks to learn from that country's well-established vocational program for the blind, then to Washington to be instructed by Joseph Clunk and his staff in the basics of vending stand operations. Once back in Tampa, he was made supervisor of employment and worked with Johnson in getting the Florida legislature to authorize the Holly Hill Diagnostic and Pre-Vocational Training Center. He was so clearly the Council's second in command that when Johnson died suddenly in the summer of 1945, Barnett was the logical choice as his successor.

When he became executive director of the Foundation in September 1949, Barnett's first challenge involved a thorough internal housecleaning. In the last years of Robert Irwin's administration, the Foundation had succumbed to a certain degree of balkanization. Several little departmental clusters had grown up, each jealous of its autonomy and reluctant to surrender authority for the sake of a more coordinated whole. Staff rivalries as well as cliques were in evidence.

Some awareness of this situation existed among the trustees, particularly the younger men who had been taking a hard and objective look at program planning and budgeting practices and had called in outside consultants for expert advice. They made it clear Barnett would be given a free hand. His initial move was to consolidate allied types of service and carve out clear channels of command. Alfred Allen, who had been one of Irwin's two assistant directors, was assigned responsibility for administrative services. Two other assistant directorships were created, one for professional services, to which Kathern Gruber was appointed, and the other for technical and production services, to which Barnett named C. H. "Dick" Whittington, a man he had brought north with him from Florida. Whittington remained only a few years; in 1954 he was succeeded as technical chief by John W. Breuel, manager of the Talking Book Department.

These moves were the first of a series of internal reorganizations over the next two decades, each part of a continuing effort to shape an administrative structure responsive to expanding needs and evolving program priorities. Major milestones included:

—Building a field staff of six professionally trained community organization specialists to provide year-round consultation on all aspects of work for the blind, with each field consultant assigned responsibility for a specific region. Originally headquartered in the Foundation's New York office, the Community Services Division was geographically decentralized in 1966–67 when regional offices were established in Chicago, Atlanta, Denver, and San Francisco so as to place the field consultants in closer proximity to the areas they served.

While the Foundation had from its inception provided help in program development, administration, staffing, policy formation, and legislative action to state and local organizations requesting guidance in these or related functions, the requests for service had been sporadic, usually initiated by an agency or a community in crisis. The continuous availability of full-time regional consultants made possible ongoing assistance of a more planned and constructive nature. The regional staff also served as conduits through which national programs for strengthened services could move rapidly into the communities where those services were delivered.

—Building a parallel staff of program specialists, located at headquarters, to lead in spurring progress in their respective spheres of competence and be on call for expert advice when agencies or communities needed help in specific program areas. In 1972 the Program Development Division was staffed by seven professionals whose respective specialties were independent living, aging, early childhood development, personnel training, educational aids, child education, and career education.

During the Sixties, the two professional units were combined into a Program Planning Department which, at the end of 1972, was headed by William F. Gallagher. Directing the department's Program Development Division was Marion V. Wurster; the Community Services Division was directed by Doris P. Sausser.

—A gradual transition in the Foundation's research functions from in-house exploration, invention, and engineering to the multifaceted role of catalyst, coordinator, evaluator, information disseminator, and consultation center. These successive shifts in approach to both technological and psycho-social research took place under the guidance of advisory committees of ranking scientists.

—Streamlining the Foundation's manufacturing and sales units to keep pace with changing technology in the manufacture of Talking Books and mounting demands for development and distribution of aids and appliances for use by blind persons.

—Steady expansion of public education activities designed to produce a continuous flow of information aimed at three principal goals: (1) alerting blind people to the availability of goods and services for their use; (2) keeping organizations for the blind aware of professional developments and techniques that could help them upgrade their programs; (3) shaping more constructive public attitudes toward blindness and blind people.

—Heavy investment in expansion and modernization of offices and plant: new buildings, new recording studios, automated manufacturing equipment for Talking Books, computerized recordkeeping, and other facilities designed to promote efficiency of operation.

The administrative restructuring that accompanied such basic alterations in the Foundation's program involved more than reshuffling of existing personnel. A substantial increase in professional staff was called for, along with revised lines of authority. In 1959, ten years after Barnett took over as Foundation executive director, he reported to the board that while in that decade the total staff had increased 27 percent to 179, the number of professional staff members had grown 57 percent, from 28 to 44; when five budgeted vacancies were filled in the ensuing months, the rate of professional increase would mount still further. At the end of 1972 the professional staff comprised 56 persons out of a total complement of 204. Professional personnel were organized into seven departments, three of which (Program Planning, Research, and Information) reported to Barnett's associate director for service, Harold G. Roberts, and the remaining four (Business and Office Management, Manufacturing and Sales, Finance, and Program Support) reported to the associate director for administration, a post which was vacant at the time.

In many ways Harold G. Roberts personified one of the basic changes in program direction that began in the Fifties. When he joined the Foundation staff in 1959, his experience included seven years as chief of social services for a VA regional office, followed by six years as executive director of a community service council in New Jersey. Holder of a master's degree in social service administration from the University of Pittsburgh, he had taken additional graduate studies at the University of Michigan and the Columbia University School of Social Work and had been an adjunct faculty member of the Rutgers University Graduate School of Social Work. His first Foundation assignment was as director of field services; he later became director of the Division of Community Services and in 1967 was named to the newly created post of associate director.

Roberts personified the strong strand of professional social work thinking that had entered the Foundation's concept of its role. If it was to succeed in encouraging the field of work for the blind to move from paternalism to professionalism, it had to set the example. The first significant move in this process had taken place in 1954, when Alexander F. Handel was employed as consultant in community planning. Handel, who held a master's degree from the University of Chicago's School of Social Service Administration, had a solid background of professional practice in public and voluntary agencies and had also been dean and professor of social work at the Adelphi College School of Social Work. In addition to his specialized initial assignment, he carried major responsibility for manning the Foundation's field service staff with qualified social workers.

The first few years of Barnett's administration also saw important strengths added to the staff of program specialists. One of the first appointees was Georgie Lee Abel, consultant in education, whose ten-year stay helped the Foundation exert a powerful influence during a volatile era in the field of special education. Miss Abel, who brought to her job nearly twenty years of experience in teaching at residential schools for blind children, resigned in 1960 to join the faculty of San Francisco State College.

In 1952 another education specialist, Pauline Moor, joined the staff as consultant on services for preschool children. With a background that included teaching in elementary and nursery schools, direction of day care programs, and participation in a research team studying infant blindness, Miss Moor was in a position to offer expert guidance to parents, agencies, and schools struggling to cope with thousands of small children blinded by retrolental fibroplasia.

The following year saw a youthful blind man, J. Albert Asenjo, become the Foundation's specialist in vocational education and adult rehabilitation. For six years he had been chief instructor at the Florida Council's rehabilitation center in Daytona Beach. Asenjo's expertise led to his twice being detached on loan to foreign governments to design rehabilitation programs for their blind populations. In 1972 he was serving as the Foundation's specialist in independent living. A second expert in vocational rehabilitation, Arthur L. Voorhees, joined the staff in 1957. Blind since birth, he had begun his career with the New Jersey State Commission for the Blind in 1939 and had subsequently spent 13 years in the federal Division of Services for the Blind. He retired in 1972.

In a different area of specialization, Dorothy D. Bryan, who had directed the department of service to the deaf-blind for four years, resigned in 1950 and was replaced by Annette B. Dinsmore, who had been the department's assistant director since 1948. Miss Dinsmore's past experience as a teacher of the deaf and as a social welfare worker, together with her personal knowledge of blindness from having lost her own sight in adulthood, made her uniquely equipped to head a national program for the deaf-blind. She retired in 1971.

Shortly after Barnett took charge at the Foundation, Evelyn C. McKay, director of social research, resigned. On staff since 1926, Miss McKay had carried a variety of additional responsibilities during the organization's formative years, including major editorial duties on the *Outlook* and a number of special field assignments. January 1952 saw Nathaniel Raskin appointed to head a restructured research department. Raskin was a young psychologist who had taught at the University of Chicago, where he earned his Ph.D., and at Hunter College. His basic assignment was to initiate a research fellowship program as part of a plan to interest the nation's institutions of higher education in research bearing on blindness. These efforts also produced some needed spadework in surveying the state of research throughout the country, an overview which convinced the Foundation that its own research required a different and more sophisticated approach than before.

Raskin resigned in 1957 to become chief psychologist at Children's Memorial Hospital, Chicago, and the following year the research function was once again reorganized, with Milton D. Graham named as its head. Graham, whose background included direction of a research project at Yale University and classified work with the United States Defense Department, had received his Ph.D. in social psychology from the London School of Economics, which he attended as a Fulbright fellow after graduation from Antioch College. One of Graham's former associates at Yale, Leslie L. Clark, joined him at the Foundation in 1959 and, in 1964, took on direction of the newly created International Research Information Service (IRIS).

One other change in senior personnel took place in 1951, when Howard Liechty was named editor of the *Outlook*. For some years previously, the principal editorial responsibility had been in the hands of Philip Clive Potts, whose main interests were in the field of education. Potts, who held a Ph.D. in educational administration from Johns Hopkins University, came to the Foundation in 1937 from the Idaho State School for the Blind and Deaf, where he had been superintendent following a number of years as principal at the Maryland School for the Blind. At the Foundation, where he succeeded Eber L. Palmer as Irwin's assistant executive director, his role as educational specialist included editing a periodical, the *Teachers Forum,* which was later merged into the *Outlook*. When editorial responsibility passed into Liechty's hands, Potts was able to devote full time to educational consultation. He retired at the end of 1958.

In June 1950 Robert Irwin severed his last tie with his former colleagues and moved back to Puget Sound, the scene of his boyhood. He had spent the year following his retirement in semi-harness, serving as Barnett's associate director of the Foundation's sister agency, American Foundation for Overseas Blind. In this capacity he presided over the postwar international assembly of workers for the blind convened at Oxford University's Merton College in England in August 1949 under the joint auspices of AFOB and Britain's National (later Royal National) Institute for the Blind.

The Oxford assembly initiated the steps leading to the creation of a permanent body, the World Council for the Welfare of the Blind, which was formally incorporated in June 1951. At the meeting marking this event, Irwin was nominated as the Council's first honorary life member. Before this distinction could be formally conferred upon him, however, a heart attack ended his life on December 12, 1951. He was sixty-eight.

At the time of his death Irwin was working on a history of work for the blind for which he had received a Guggenheim Fellowship grant; his partial manuscript was subsequently published by the Foundation under the title *As I Saw It*. The first copies of the slim volume were distributed in May 1955 at a ceremony marking the dedication of the Robert B. Irwin Memorial Room at Foundation headquarters. The room, located just inside the main entrance and originally used as a repository for Irwin's personal library as well as a small museum of early artifacts associated with work for the blind, was later converted to more practical use as a display and sales room for aids and appliances.

Among other posthumous honors was the naming in Irwin's memory of a newly constructed academic building at the Washington State School for the Blind. In 1952 his role in the conception and passage of the Wagner-O'Day Act was memorialized by National Industries for the Blind through the Robert B. Irwin Award "for outstanding achievement in the field of workshops for blind persons."

Irwin did not lack for recognition during his lifetime. In 1943 he received an honorary degree from Western Reserve University; two years later, the University of Washington bestowed upon him the title of *Alumnus Summa Laude Dignitatus*, and in 1947 he was made a Chevalier of the French Legion of Honor, the first blind American to be so honored, for his leadership in restoring services for blind people in France following World War II.

The man who had been Robert Irwin's commander-in-chief outlived him by seven years. October 24, 1958, saw the passing of Moses Charles Migel, 11 days short of his ninety-second birthday. With him died the brand of paternalistic philanthropy that had been the hallmark of his generation of leadership. Because Migel had a passion for privacy where his personal benefactions were concerned, there exists no accurate record of how much of his wealth was poured into work for the blind. Some of the larger gifts, however, were too conspicuous to be kept under wraps. Outstanding among these was the $130,000 he gave in the early Thirties to provide the Foundation with its first headquarters building. His original pledge had been $100,000, but when quicksand and water in the subsoil made for additional expense, he insisted upon meeting the additional $30,000 cost himself.

All told, Migel's philanthropies may well have exceeded a million dollars during an era when that was a genuinely commanding sum. Almost all of this generosity took place during his lifetime; he was enough of a hedonist to want to enjoy the pleasures of giving. The sum he left the Foundation in his will was relatively modest—just enough to perpetuate the annual custom of bestowing what was originally called the Foundation Medal but later became known as the Migel Medal.

Initiated in 1937, the medal was designed by its sponsor's daughter, Parmenia Migel Ekstrom. One side was inscribed "For outstanding service to the blind" and the other showed a smiling angel shielding the lighted torch held in her left hand.

The first awardee was the lawyer-philanthropist William Nelson Cromwell, for his leadership in both international and American work for the blind. From 1937 through 1972 the number of recipients totaled 57 and embraced both laymen and professional practitioners. They included Henry Ford II of the Ford Motor Company and Thomas J. Watson of International Business Machines for the exceptional record of their companies in employment of blind workers; Major

General Melvin J. Maas for crusading leadership on behalf of the disabled through the President's Committee on Employment of the Physically Handicapped; Mrs. Aida da Costa Breckinridge, founder of the Eye Bank for Sight Restoration; Dr. Jules Stein, chairman of the Music Corporation of America, for his role in founding Research to Prevent Blindness; Mary E. Switzer for her accomplishments in federal vocational rehabilitation programs; the actress Katharine Cornell for her years of personal participation, through various media, in creating greater public understanding of blindness; the playwright William Gibson for *The Miracle Worker;* Dr. Jerome B. Wiesner, professor (and later president) of Massachusetts Institute of Technology for his encouragement of sensory aids research in the field of blindness; Dr. Richard E. Hoover, both for his pioneering work in mobility and his later leadership in ophthalmology; Senator Jennings Randolph for decades of legislative leadership to augment the welfare of blind Americans.

During his lifetime, the Major was a recipient as well as a giver of honors. A man who never went beyond high school, he was awarded an honorary Master of Arts degree from Wesleyan University in 1935. Both the French and Italian governments recognized his services to their people by making him a Chevalier of the Legion of Honor in the one instance, and awarding him the Order of the Crown of Italy in the other.

A posthumous tribute came five years after the Major's death when the Foundation's professional library was housed in spacious new quarters and rededicated as the M.C. Migel Memorial Library. At one end of its handsomely paneled reading room was placed Mario Korbel's bronze portrait bust of Migel, which William Ziegler, Jr., had commissioned and presented to the Foundation. An idealized likeness which smoothed over the crags and fissures of advanced age, the sculpture nevertheless captured the serene and courageous spirit of the man who, in his 90th year, used as the theme of his annual New Year's message to friends the words from an old hymn: "Safely led by His hand thus far, why should we now give way to fear?"

Migel's bronze likeness sits just east of the plot at 13-15 West 16 Street on which the Foundation's first building was erected with his $130,000 gift. The three-story red brick Federal-style building was designed to give the Foundation a permanent home which, the Major said, "would add greatly to its stability, permanence and the confidence of the public generally." Confidence was so scarce a commodity in the depression-ridden early Thirties that considerable public attention was paid when the cornerstone-laying ceremony for the new building took place on December 5, 1934. Helen Keller wielded the symbolic trowel; Dr. John H. Finley, associate editor of *The New York Times*, presided; a congratulatory telegram from President Franklin D. Roosevelt was read; a brief speech was made by H. Randolph Latimer; Migel gave a response; and the entire event was broadcast over the NBC radio network. The broadcast was recorded by the Talking Book studio and the recording placed in the time capsule sealed into the cornerstone. Among the capsule's other contents were photographs of Helen Keller, M. C. Migel, and Robert Irwin; a set of copies of the Foundation's annual reports, some issues of the *Outlook,* that day's edition of all the New York City newspapers, and a second Talking Book record, *Street Noises of New York in 1934.*

Although the Foundation staff moved into the building in late April of the following year, the formal dedication was deferred until December, when the board held its annual meeting. Among the speeches at the ceremony was one in which Migel paid tribute to his fellow trustees ("not visionaries, not maudlin sentimentalists, but sound and yet sympathetic thinkers and doers") and noted that one of them, Gustavus A. Pfeiffer, had contributed the funds for the new building's furnishings. Irwin, who accepted a key to the building from the Major, called attention to the generosity of another Foundation friend, Mrs. William A. Moore, whose gift had equipped the new building's Talking Book studios.

The conference room had been named, somewhat misleadingly, the Helen Keller Memorial Room. A symbolic key to it was presented to the living Helen by Harvey D. Gibson, treasurer of the Foundation's endowment fund, which had at that point just topped the million dollar mark. This room, furnished and decorated under the personal supervision of Mrs. Migel, was designed to hold some of Helen's memorabilia. Among its features was a panel inscribed with a motto from Helen's pen:

> "While they were saying among themselves, 'It cannot be done,' it was done."

Not one of Helen's more distinguished literary efforts, this sentence was one of nine she had drafted, at Migel's request, as possible motifs for the room. The Major had conducted an informal poll by asking several people for their preferences and then, typically enough, proceeded to ignore the opinions of the others and select the one whose idea appealed to him most strongly. But Helen had an opportunity to be as flowery as she liked when she was presented the key. After lauding Migel's "royal generosity" and terming him "the one friend of the blind who dared back their dream," she said that the new building would be one "on whose hearth the flashing wings of Hope shall fan a new flame of life for those who travel the dark way."

The original Helen Keller Room later became the office of the Foundation's executive director, but was connected by fold-back doors with an adjoining room whose walls were lined with photographs of Helen and some of the many notables she met during her long life and extensive travels, among them Alexander Graham Bell, Rabindranath Tagore, Luther Burbank, King Alexander of Yugoslavia, and Oliver Wendell Holmes. A fraction of the Foundation's collection of Keller memorabilia, the photographs on display constituted almost a pictorial biography, beginning with Helen's early childhood in Tuscumbia. Along three walls were glass-windowed cabinets displaying some of the artifacts, medals, diplomas, citations, and other mementos presented to her. One item was an autographed photograph of Mark Twain, inscribed in 1909 to Anne Sullivan Macy, "with warm regard and with limitless admiration of the wonders she has performed as a miracle worker."

From an architectural rendering of the Foundation's first building, it appears that the original design called for a four-story structure. Economy probably limited the building to three, but the change also reflected Migel's conviction that three stories provided ample space for anything the Foundation might ever need. It may have been the architects who persuaded him to top the building with a reinforced roof and a balustrade that could eventually make possible the addition of a fourth story. It was never built; when, only five years after the building opened, it was already so overcrowded that some departments were being housed in rented quarters, the need for additional space was more than could be provided by a single extra story.

A neighboring building, 11 West 16 Street, was available for purchase from the estate of its former owner and early in 1942 the Foundation bought it, together with an abutting rear structure at 18 West 17 Street, for $29,000. Both buildings were nearly a century old. The one on 17th Street was ultimately torn down and the cleared ground became a loading area for the shipping department. The one on 16th Street was a stately mansion, the former home of a New York society woman, Emily Meredith Read Spencer. It was usable with some renovation, and its architectural features, including the sweeping oval staircase that rose from the parlor floor and the panelled walls, decorated with imported wood carvings, of what had formerly been the dining room, remained for a dozen years one of the sights relished by visitors to this first annex.

As had been true in relation to the Foundation's first building and was to be the case with all subsequent property purchases, no building fund campaign was conducted. A few large gifts from trustees and, in later years, the arrival of substantial bequests, made it unnecessary. All the money received from annual contributors continued to be used exclusively for program activities.

By 1945 the immediate needs and anticipated postwar requirements of National Industries for the Blind (NIB), which had been housed by the Foundation from its inception, demanded greatly enlarged quarters. Two lots were available on West 17th Street, adjoining the rear of the Foundation's building; these were bought for $19,000 in 1945 and the existing structures torn down. A $200,000 four-story building was completed in the fall of 1947. NIB contributed $75,000 toward the cost, a sum it recovered when it moved to a new location in 1962.

By 1953 the century-old Spencer mansion was beset by so many structural defects it was no longer safe to use. It succumbed to the wrecker's ball and a new three-story structure was erected in its place. Construction of the new building, faced with red brick to match the adjoining 15 West 16 Street, and alterations to the latter to connect the two, cost close to $300,000.

At this point, the Foundation's buildings occupied three and one-half sides of a rectangle stretching through the block from 16th to 17th Street. A 12-story loft at 20 West 17 Street interrupted the fourth side. By 1960 a need for additional space prompted purchase of the loft and the creation of a corridor to connect it with the other three buildings. Initially, only 6 of the 12 floors were needed by the Foundation and the remaining floors were rented out to other nonprofit organizations, but as of 1972, only 2½ floors were occupied by others.

The loft purchase ended the acquisition of land, but not the rearrangement of space to meet changing conditions. One such rearrangement created a good-sized ground floor conference area which was named the Polly Thomson Room. Helen Keller's devoted companion had died in 1960, and the suggestion to honor her came from Nella Braddy Henney, the biographer of Anne Sullivan Macy, who had been an intimate of the Keller household since the mid-Twenties. To furnish the Polly Thomson Room, Mrs. Henney turned over the $10,000 fee she had received as a consultant in the production of the motion picture of William Gibson's *The Miracle Worker*. The balance of the funds to equip the panelled and carpeted auditorium, which was opened in 1964, came from Foundation resources.

As of 1972 the Foundation and its sister agency, American Foundation for Overseas Blind, occupied 67,300 square feet of space in four buildings whose value was carried on its balance sheet at cost, $2,043,472. That same year, however, found members of the board's Business Advisory Committee recommending that 5,000 square feet of additional space be rented to permit expansion and further automation of the Talking Book manufacturing plant.

If all of this was a far cry from the original two-room office of 1923, so was the financial picture shown in the 1971–72 annual report, which revealed total assets of $19,311,211, of which endowed funds constituted over $17 million. The Migel-Irwin-Keller trio who had striven so mightily to achieve what at times seemed an unreachable endowment goal of $2 million all lived to see it attained in 1948, but only Helen Keller survived long enough to see capital reserves go into eight figures and the yearly income from contributors hover around the million dollar mark.

Just as 1945, the year M. C. Migel gave up the presidency of the Foundation, signalled important changes in its leadership, so 1958, the year he died, also brought a new command to the fore. William Ziegler, Jr., who died March 3, 1958, at the age of sixty-seven, was replaced as president by Jansen Noyes, Jr. Elected to succeed the late Major as chairman of the board was Eustace Seligman, who had been board secretary since 1950. The new secretary was Richard H. Migel. The treasurer's post vacated by Noyes was filled by John P. Morgan II. The only title without a new name opposite it was vice-president. George F. Meyer continued in that post, which he had held since 1952.

More was involved than a change of chairs. The group now heading the Foundation were not retired philanthropists but persons active in their respective professions and, in four out of five cases, men with heavy experience in fiscal management. Noyes was a partner in the investment banking firm of Hemphill, Noyes and Company. (In 1965, as the result of a merger, the firm became Hornblower and Weeks—Hemphill, Noyes. In 1972, Jansen Noyes, Jr., was its president and chief executive officer.) Seligman was a partner in the law firm of Sullivan and Cromwell, Morgan an officer of the Morgan Guaranty Trust Company, and Migel an officer of a firm of securities dealers (he later joined a large printing firm as its financial vice-president). The sole exception to this Wall Street-oriented alignment was Meyer, who was executive director of the New Jersey Commission for the Blind.

Jansen Noyes, Jr., tall, rangy, blond-haired, with strong Nordic facial features, was forty years old when he became the Foundation's third president. Born in Montclair, New Jersey, he attended the Lawrenceville School, then went on to Cornell University where he took a degree in mechanical engineering. He was pursuing advanced study at the Harvard Graduate School of Business when the

United States entered World War II. A member of the Naval Reserve, he entered his country's service, spent the war years on active duty in the Atlantic, and was discharged in 1945 with the rank of lieutenant commander.

It was not long after his return to civilian life as a general partner in the Wall Street firm of which his father was co-founder that the youthful veteran received a telephone call from M. C. Migel. Noyes would surely be devoting some of his time to civic affairs, the Major said; how would he like to use that time for the benefit of blind people?

Noyes was interested. He knew something about M. C. Migel from the latter's son, Richard, who was with Hemphill, Noyes at the time. And while he knew nothing about blindness—up to that point he had never even met a blind person—he considered serving as a trustee of the Foundation a more stimulating activity than ringing doorbells to raise funds for local charities. Election to the Foundation board took place in June 1946; and a few months later Noyes took over the treasurer's post. He soon found himself also overseeing the financial affairs of two related organizations, National Industries for the Blind and the newly incorporated American Foundation for Overseas Blind. In similar fashion, when he became Foundation president in 1958, he simultaneously acquired the presidencies of NFB and AFOB.

Noyes' real education in the affairs of the Foundation came about when he conducted a penetrating study of its budgeting and accounting processes in 1949. He found that the long-established system of maintaining separate revolving funds for different activities failed to yield a true budgetary picture of the scope and depth of operations and financial commitments, because only net results, with income offset against expenditures, were shown. In the revised procedures adopted under Noyes' direction, gross figures were given for both expenditures and income, and the trustees evaluating budgets were able to gain a more detailed grasp of just what was happening. Analyzing the workings of these separately administered funds also brought to light the existence of overlapping responsibilities in various departments, and precipitated the administrative changes instituted by Barnett during his early years as executive director.

It was fortunate that the new president needed little or no briefing when he took over in 1958. At that point the Foundation was undergoing some crucial changes of direction. These had a number of aspects, but all centered in one way or another on the question of professionalization.

The movement toward professionalizing work for the blind began in the educational area during the late Thirties. In 1940 AAIB introduced a national certification service for teachers of blind children, and the following year AAWB launched a similar program for home teachers of blind adults. Progress, halted during the war years, resumed momentum in the early Fifties. In 1952 AAWB appointed a committee to delineate "the ideal agency for the blind," but the committee sensibly decided that "ideal" meant "such perfection as to be practically unobtainable" and devoted itself instead to considering the question of criteria and standards. Reporting the committee's position to the next year's convention, M. Roberta Townsend, its chairman, spoke candidly. Work for the blind, she said, had "been guilty in some instances of coasting comfortably on past achievements, complacent in the assurance that privileges and preferences guaranteed sound service to its clientele." However:

> A lack of standardization of services as well as an equal lack of unanimity of thinking has fostered many sporadic programs. Some continue to duplicate those already in existence, some hide behind a long list of high sounding services, no one of which is actually available to the client.

She then went on to identify a number of specific weaknesses in existing services, to suggest as a "test or model" the "best in the total programming of health and welfare in society as a whole," and to make clear the obstacles in the way of such an effort.

What the AAWB did, after hearing this forthright analysis, was to adopt a resolution asking that "a manual of useful criteria and standards for the guidance of agencies" be devised and that it be done by the American Foundation for the Blind.

At the same 1953 convention, the AAWB received and acted on a report from a committee dealing with another problem: fund-raising and public relations practices. This second group, chaired by M. Robert Barnett, was as blunt as the Townsend committee. Without naming names, its report asserted that there were

> so-called agencies for the blind which have absolutely no basis for existence in terms of necessary services to blind people, whose administrative bases are just as weak as their service, and yet who overtly seek public support for the agency and its empty program in a manner which implies to their supporters that they do have essential and substantial worth.

The report also noted that some six hundred agencies in the field of work for the blind were making that number of separate approaches to the public, with resulting public confusion and, often, sufficient irritation to cause rejection of the entire field. It criticized some prevailing practices, such as publicizing client names and photographs without prior consent and using exaggerated emotionalism and appeals to pity in fund-raising literature. Its heaviest fire was directed at "coercive types of fund-raising techniques," specifically the mailing of unordered merchandise to prospective contributors, and the use of "gimmicks" which "tend to perpetuate public notions of the stereotype of blindness, such as white canes, dark glasses, miniature mops and brooms, canisters which are strongly reminiscent of the tin cup."

What action could AAWB take to correct these abuses? The committee's recommendation was that it adopt a code of ethics and that it award an official "Seal of Good Practice" to agencies demonstrating their adherence to such a code.

Aware that in several states legislative investigations of charity rackets had uncovered deception and fraud in many organizations, including some ostensibly engaged in work for the blind, the delegates saw the value of the committee's idea. The code of ethics was adopted July 14, 1953, and covered desirable elements of agency structure and program as well as specific prohibitions against such practices as claiming falsely that products were blind-made, paying commissions to fund-raisers, and mailing of unordered merchandise.

A standing committee was empowered to issue the "Seal of Good Practice" to agencies voluntarily submitting evidence that they adhered to the code. But no great rush to acquire the seal developed; two years later, AAWB's secretary-general voiced a public reproach over the slow rate of acceptance. Only 68 agencies had applied for the seal. In succeeding years the code did pick up some speed, but it was eventually abandoned when a far more comprehensive set of standards, and a permanent structure for their implementation, made their appearance.

As it began to explore the dimensions of the arduous AAWB assignment, the Foundation discovered that before standards could be formulated for services to blind persons, some basic factual data would have to be assembled about the personnel who delivered those services. Who were they? What were their responsibilities? What qualifications of education and experience did they have? Did they earn commensurate salaries?

The aid of the federal Bureau of Labor Statistics was enlisted and a survey conducted of all agencies serving blind persons and their several thousand professional, technical, and administrative staff members. Financed in part by an OVR research grant, this produced a number of useful findings, among them the not unexpected discovery that jobs in the field of blindness were generally underpaid. There was outright discrimination in state agencies, where employees in the division for the blind often earned less than persons with the identical titles in other divisions. Equally serious was a chaotic lack of uniformity in job descriptions and in the qualifications of persons holding jobs with the same or similar titles. The day-to-day field experience of the regional consultants confirmed this, and also highlighted the difficulty of local and state agencies in recruiting qualified personnel to meet the demands of rapidly expanding programs.

Toward the end of 1959 the Foundation established a national personnel referral service to help overcome the last-named problem. It listed both job openings and available candidates all over the country and became a resource for agencies seeking executives, administrators, and practitioners, and for personnel ready for career advancement. Among the agencies, some needed help in developing appropriate job descriptions and sound personnel practices so as to attract the calibre of worker they wanted; among the job-seekers, many were encouraged to acquire the additional education or training that would qualify them for higher categories. An active promotional campaign was conducted to bring new personnel into work for the blind.

All of these efforts had a single goal, M. Robert Barnett told the AAWB in 1959: "to make sure that blind persons benefit from the social revolution that is currently taking place in this country." He was referring to the impact of the 1954 VRA amendments, which had stimulated sizable spurts in all types of rehabilitation services. The next ten years, he predicted, would show even more dramatic advances.

To achieve these advances, it grew increasingly clear, would require a structured process that embodied both standards and a method of implementing standards to serve as instruments of change. In a word, accreditation. In 1961 Noyes told his board of trustees that the time had come to move in that direction. "It is not our intention," he said,

> that the American Foundation for the Blind will itself conduct a policing program, but rather that it would arrange to expedite a service program of evaluation and accreditation which would find its authority in a democratic representation of all legitimate interests in this field. . . . [There is] enough misunderstanding, misrepresentation, and probably ineffectual activity which the public is being asked to support, that we all should join together in a pioneering effort to reduce these confusions to the greatest possible extent.

Had there been any hesitation in the board's thinking, it would have been removed by the appearance in 1961 of the influential and widely read "Hamlin Report," so designated after the name of its study director, Robert H. Hamlin. (The formal title was *Voluntary Health and Welfare Agencies in the United States—an Exploratory Study by an Ad Hoc Citizens Committee.*) Sponsored by the Rockefeller Foundation, it presented the conclusions of a group of 21 distinguished citizens after they had assessed the degree to which all types of voluntary agencies were meeting their duty of public accountability. A major conclusion was that the public "must have more objective information about agency purposes, program content, administration, physical facilities, board structure and function, personnel, financing and budgeting and relations with other agencies and the community."

The implications of the Hamlin Report were one more evidence of a swelling popular demand for some form of assurance that the nation's thousands of voluntary health and welfare agencies, supported by many millions of contributed dollars, were operating responsibly. In the professions, and in higher education, such assurance had long been provided through accreditation systems. Now accreditation had begun to come into force in secondary education, library services, the hospital field, and nursing homes, and was under development for rehabilitation centers and sheltered workshops.

By what method could a comparable system be established in work for the blind? Guidance was sought from persons outside the field as well as from those who understood its unique nature and problems. An Ad Hoc Advisory Committee on Accreditation was appointed by the Foundation in 1962; its recommendation, submitted in April 1963, was for an autonomous commission that would be responsible for both the formulation of standards and the creation of a permanent accrediting body.

Thus was born the independent organism known as COMSTAC: the Commission on Standards and Accreditation of Services for the Blind. In creating the 22-member commission, the Foundation agreed to grant it absolute autonomy of policy and procedure while accepting responsibility for financing its work. Some exploratory approaches to philanthropic foundations had already been made. Originally estimated at $350,000 over a four-year period, the final costs were

$438,000, of which the Foundation supplied $300,000 in cash and staff services and the remainder came from the Irene Heinz Given and John LaPorte Given Foundation, the Gustavus and Louise Pfeiffer Research Foundation, the Rockefeller Brothers Fund, and the Vocational Rehabilitation Administration.

The commission membership comprised a great many diverse elements. It balanced lay leadership with professional expertise, governmental services with voluntary agencies, blind persons with sighted persons, business interests with labor representation, specialized work for the blind with general community services. It embraced the major professional disciplines and drew on all geographical sections of the United States. Chosen as chairman was a man knowledgeable about accreditation but in a position of absolute neutrality where work for the blind was concerned: Arthur L. Brandon, retired vice-president for university relations at New York University.

To serve as full-time executive director of COMSTAC, Alexander F. Handel was detached from the Foundation staff. Eight other staff members were released part-time for service with the commission, and six professional persons with other affiliations were also engaged to staff the committees charged with developing standards.

COMSTAC got under way in February 1964. It selected 12 areas for development of standards, of which 5 were basic aspects of administration common to all operating agencies, and 7 were specific types of service programs in work for the blind. Technical study committees were appointed for each of these 12 subjects; the committees, whose membership ranged between 7 and 14, were selected with the same attention to balance as the commission itself. They were given a set of guidelines designed to avoid blue-sky thinking at one extreme and unduly lax criteria at the other. The key clauses were these:

> Standards should be formulated so as to set a level of acceptable performance below which no agency should fall, while simultaneously constituting a challenge to the better agencies to continue striving for improvement. Standards should be practicable. They should be based primarily on existing knowledge which has been tested in practice, leaving to future revisions whatever modifications might be called for in the light of new knowledge produced by research or experience.

As the committees went about their assignments, correspondence was conducted with specialists all over the country and progress reports were made at appropriate professional meetings. By December 1965 the standards had been drafted in sufficiently final form to warrant intensive review at a three-day national conference that was attended by some four hundred lay and professional persons. Each set of standards was analyzed and debated, line by line and page by page, in workshop sessions. Following a process of revision and clarification, based on the reactions and suggestions of the conferees, the standards were published in 1966 under the title *The COMSTAC Report: Standards for Strengthened Services*.

The national conference also served as the stage for the first public presentation of the plan for establishing the National Accreditation Council for Agencies

Serving the Blind and Visually Handicapped. NAC, as it came to be known, began on January 1, 1967, with Brandon as president and Handel as executive director. Its founders projected a ten-year plan for gradual self-support through membership dues to be paid by agencies admitted to accreditation. To help underwrite the initial years, the Foundation committed $300,000 over a five-year period and persuaded the Vocational Rehabilitation Administration and other groups to underwrite an equal sum.

By the end of 1972 NAC had accredited 47 agencies and schools for the blind; approximately the same number were in one or another phase of the self-study process that precedes accreditation. The pace was slower than had been hoped for, and additional financial help was needed from and granted by the Foundation and other sources. It was clear by then that self-support was not likely to be attained by the original target date of 1977.

Not everyone agreed with the statement by one enthusiast that accreditation would be "the most significant advance in work for the blind since the advent of the Talking Book." In some quarters the prospect of standards stipulating professional qualifications for various positions was regarded as threatening the security of blind personnel holding such jobs in public and voluntary agencies and as limiting future access to such jobs by blind persons. These same groups also regarded as inimical to the interests of blind persons employed in sheltered workshops the absence of standards calling for minimum wages, collective bargaining and other labor protections.

The principal vehicle for opposition on these and similar grounds was the National Federation of the Blind, whose militant and outspoken president, Kenneth Jernigan, conducted a vehement crusade, first against COMSTAC and then against NAC. Under the banner of consumerism, Jernigan used his organization's annual conventions, and its monthly newsletter, the *Braille Monitor,* to mount a vendetta against NAC, designed, as he put it, "to reform it or destroy it." His tactics were viewed by more conservative elements as an outright struggle for power characterized by extremist accusations of a kind that had not been seen or heard in work for the blind since the Congressional hearings on the Pratt-Smoot bill forty years earlier.

These more conservative elements continued to assert their faith in the accreditation process as an instrument for constructive progress. In 1971 the United States Office of Education awarded NAC the status of a recognized accrediting agency; it was the first such recognition in the field of special education. The Social and Rehabilitation Service continued to make annual budgetary grants. The Council of State Administrators of Vocational Rehabilitation voted in late 1972 to adopt a policy under which, by mid-1974, all rehabilitation facilities under their jurisdiction would be required to apply for accreditation, either to NAC or to a comparable body, the Commission on Accreditation of Rehabilitation Facilities. The Association for Education of the Visually Handicapped (formerly American Association of Instructors of the Blind) reacted to NFB's anti-NAC propaganda by writing the Secretary of Health, Education and Welfare: "We decry the efforts of one particular organization to impair or destroy the single organization completely dedicated to improving and maintaining high standards of service to the visually disabled in our country."

The American Foundation for the Blind remained unwaveringly convinced that accreditation was an essential ingredient in the development of quality services for America's blind citizens and reaffirmed its stand in a policy statement issued in October 1968. As further evidence of its conviction, the Foundation awarded its 1969 Migel Medal for lay leadership to Arthur Brandon, citing his leadership of both COMSTAC and NAC. No comment was made during the award ceremonies over the ironic twist which saw the same year's Migel Medal for professional achievement go to John F. Nagle, the blind attorney who was chief of the Washington office of the National Federation of the Blind.

The Foundation's policy statement on accreditation was one of a series of such statements developed by its Service Advisory Committee. The use of committees made up of trustees and others came increasingly into play during the Noyes presidency as part of a base-broadening philosophy which simultaneously brought board members into more intimate contact with program activities while giving practitioners in work for the blind greater participation in shaping Foundation policy. From its inception in 1965 through the end of 1972, the Service Advisory Committee formulated policy statements on a score of issues, among them employment, housing, income maintenance, education, peripatology, and services for the aged.

Not all of these statements accorded with popular thinking. A policy declaration on fragrance gardens, for example, asserted that these were not "in the best interests of visually impaired persons" because they fostered needless segregation and perpetuated a stereotype. A later statement applied the same negative judgment to brailled nature trails and touch museums for the blind.

Another advisory group which exerted policy-shaping influence was the Scientific Advisory Committee. A Business Advisory Committee gave its attention to questions concerning the manufacture of Talking Books and the procurement and sale of other products of importance to blind users. A Public Relations Advisory Committee was appointed in 1970 and a Publications Committee in 1971 to guide the work of the Foundation's information staff.

A dozen years after assuming the Foundation presidency, Jansen Noyes, Jr., moved into the post of board chairman, succeeding Eustace Seligman, who became a trustee emeritus. The 1970 alignment of officers brought John S. Crowley to the presidency and Mitchell Brock, a partner in Sullivan and Cromwell, to the secretaryship. Richard H. Migel, who had served as secretary since 1958, was elected to the just-created office of vice-chairman of the board. J.P. Morgan II remained as treasurer and J.M. Woolly, superintendent of the Arkansas School for the Blind, continued in the post of vice-president to which he had been elected in 1967.

John S. Crowley, forty-seven years old when he became the Foundation's fourth president, brought a fresh orientation to the office. As senior partner and director of McKinsey and Company, an international management consulting firm, he was in a position to contribute professional thinking to internal management practices and extramural relationships. A trustee since 1963, he had served on the executive and finance committees and had headed a committee on personnel to update staff salary guidelines.

Crowley's early training paralleled that of Jansen Noyes, Jr. He, too, held a degree in engineering (in his case, from the University of Rochester) and had taken graduate work at the Harvard Graduate School of Business, where he received a master's degree in business administration. He had also seen Navy service during World War II. Thereafter, however, the careers of the two men diverged, Crowley having spent most of his business life in marketing and management.

Dark-haired, dark-eyed, incisive in speech and manner, Crowley spearheaded a marketing program to bring the sensory aids developed by science and technology into greater usefulness for the nation's blind population. At the fiftieth anniversary observance, held in October 1971, he announced that the Foundation would assume responsibility for "the full entrepreneurial role" in bridging the commercial gap between drawing board and consumer—a gap which had long kept sensory and other devices from reaching their potential markets.

After analyzing the four necessary steps—making an inventory of products in various stages of development all over the world, developing a mechanism to evaluate them, defining the market potential of each, and finding manufacturers who would produce and distribute the finished products—Crowley said that, if need be, the Foundation would commit itself

> to the tasks of securing the required funding from whatever combination of sources, negotiating with various contractors for producing and marketing the products, and, finally, managing and monitoring the contractors as necessary.

The first stage of the new venture got under way soon thereafter under the direction of a marketing specialist. After analyzing the various statistical studies of blindness made in the preceding decade, his initial conclusion was that the prevalence of severe visual impairment in the United States had been greatly underestimated. The implication was that there existed a largely undiscovered market for a variety of products, ranging from sophisticated sensory aids to simple appliances, that could be useful in the lives of visually impaired people. How to pinpoint the appropriate segments of this market so as to disseminate knowledge of, and stimulate demand for, what was actually or potentially available was the next challenge to be overcome.

21

Little Things That Make a Big Difference

Short of some miraculous visual prosthesis that can produce artificial sight, what blind people have traditionally sought (and, as often as not, invented for themselves) were devices that could enhance their ability to function in personal and vocational pursuits. Whether a self-threading needle, a carpenter's level equipped with an audible signal, a notched slide rule, or brailled playing cards, each such device has represented one more step toward equalization with the sighted.

If sales figures are any indication, there exists a genuine demand for all sorts of tools, homemaking equipment, medical instruments, timepieces, games, writing and drawing aids designed or adapted for use by blind persons. The 1972 aids and appliances catalog of the American Foundation for the Blind, which listed some 300 separate items, produced $564,000 worth of orders for 124,000 pieces of merchandise. Processing of this steadily burgeoning business, about 90 percent of it in the form of mail orders, has required the employment of as many as 18 staff members; it has also meant sizable annual deficit appropriations.

The origins of this unique accommodation service flowed out of the convergence of two separate streams. One was the sale and distribution of radios and braille watches and the processing of one-fare transportation applications—three forms of direct service for blind individuals begun in the Twenties. The second was the establishment, also in the Twenties, of the Foundation's experimental shop "for the improvement and elaboration of mechanical appliances for the blind," although this shop did not initially concentrate on homely appliances for individuals but on the heavy machinery that revolutionized braille printing and writing methods. The subsequent development of Talking Book records and playback machines preempted all of the Foundation's technical and engineering resources during the Twenties.

To cope with the demand for simpler devices during this period, the Foundation imported from England's National Institute for the Blind a full line of appliances, games and canes. That the Foundation should itself work on products of this kind was not lost sight of, but the machinery manufacturing projects did not level off until the early Forties, at which point wartime shortages of manpower and raw materials for consumer goods made for further delay.

At the same time, however, the war inspired intriguing vistas of wonders to come. "It is expected," the Foundation's 1942 annual report said, "that many of the inventions which have been made to advance the war effort will, when the conflict is over, be adaptable to the use of the blind in overcoming their handicaps."

Just how would such adaptations be accomplished? The annual report for the following year raised the hope that a research laboratory would be established to study possible uses for "wartime inventions now held secret . . . as soon as they are made public." As will be seen, most of the military secrets—radar, sonar, guided missiles, and the like—yielded few immediate practical results for blind people. What did open some prompt new opportunities were technologies related to the stepped-up industrial output of the war years. A blind woman in Buffalo was credited with the idea for a device that attached to a scale and produced an audible signal when the desired weight was reached. It was taken up by a commercial firm and found immediate application, not only in industrial plants employing blind people but in the Foundation itself, which used the audio scale to speed up the packaging of twenty million Talking Book needles. A blind Canadian invented a paper currency detector whose electric eye "read" denominations by means of buzzes. While this was apparently never produced commercially, the electric-eye idea was employed by the Foundation's engineers to devise a safety attachment for sewing machines used in workshops for the blind. The attachment brought the machine to an instant stop when an operator's hand moved too close to the needle; it also had a two-tone buzzer that alerted the operator when thread was broken or ran out.

By the beginning of 1945, enough of a start had been made on a $100,000 campaign to raise funds for a technical research laboratory to set up a "model shop" and assign two men to it. It was one of these men who soon grew into a role he seemed born to fill—that of "Mr. Fixit" for America's blind people. He was Charles G. ("Chick") Ritter, who made up for the absence of formal academic qualifications by a quick intelligence, a high degree of mechanical aptitude, a wide-ranging curiosity, and a set of deep-rooted convictions about the capacity of blind people to overcome their visual handicap.

Sandy-haired, open-faced, sturdily built, just approaching middle age, Ritter was not an ivory-tower type; he left theoretical speculations to others and devoted himself to tangible solutions that would prove of immediate use. He did not have far to look for his first blind clients. They were colleagues on the Foundation staff, they were friends and friends of friends, they were visitors who came to the Foundation office and blinded veterans Ritter went to see at Valley Forge and Old Farms. The first thing one of these people asked about was a slide rule; Ritter worked out an embossed version that enabled a blind engineer to hold on to his job. Someone else needed a tactile micrometer; it materialized in due course. For the men in the military hospitals, a spill-proof, magnetized checker set was designed. Some of the most useful devices were the simplest, such as a tape measure employing ordinary wire staples to mark off inches.

Ritter's "one problem at a time" approach led him to listen attentively to the housewife who wanted a meat roasting thermometer she could read with her fingers, to the gas station attendant who needed a tire pressure gauge he could follow by touch, to the physician who could check the blood pressure of his patients with a tactile sphygmomanometer. Most of these objects required relatively simple adaptations of commercial products and the making of such adaptations became the chief task of the model shop.

But not everything needed to be adapted. Once tuned in to the specific problems of blind people, Ritter began to seek out commercial products peculiarly suited to their use. Early models of the pressure cooker had visual gauges, but so many accidents occurred that one company switched to an audible signal. Ritter saw immediately that here was a brand that could be used safely by blind persons. He located a magnetized knife rack that eliminated the danger to fingers of fumbling through cutlery drawers and a new kind of egg beater that did away with messy splashing. There were other gadgets of this kind: a safety jar opener, a flameless cigarette lighter, a whole range of interval timers that anyone could mark with dots of glue for finger-reading.

How could the nation's blind people be informed of these useful aids to daily living? And how could they obtain them? A monthly column, "The Suggestion Box," began appearing in the *Outlook* in May 1946 and was soon regularly reprinted in the *Ziegler Magazine* and a number of local periodicals for blind readers. The matter of supply was handled through the same Foundation mail order service which had long dealt in watches and radios and now went on to secure these newer items from manufacturers at wholesale prices and resell them at cost. Bit by bit, blind people were acquiring a greatly expanded discount shopping service through which they could buy the things they needed at price savings.

By the end of its first year of operation the Technical Research Department was stocking and selling 45 items; a year later, the number had increased to 84, and a year after that, to 122. The initial mimeographed price list was now too bulky to handle, and an illustrated printed catalog was produced in 1948. Copies were sent on inquiry and were also distributed through displays at meetings of blind people and workers for the blind. It was not until some years later that a mailing list was built for the annual catalog; in 1972 the computerized list comprised close to 100,000 names for the inkprint edition and 5,000 for a separate braille edition.

One of the factors in Ritter's surehandedness in identifying objects that blind people could put to practical use grew out of an informal group he called the Technical Research Council. Blind people, he was convinced, were the only true experts on what would work for them, particularly with respect to devices in professional or technical specialties. Beginning with a core of blind engineers, teachers, and other professional people in the New York area who met informally at Foundation headquarters every Thursday evening, Ritter eventually developed a list of some five hundred technical specialists all over the country he could call on for consultation. Many of these had worked out devices or methodologies to solve problems in their own work, and such solutions proved useful to others struggling with comparable problems.

Although Ritter's frequent public appearances, in person and in print, gave him national prominence, he was not alone in developing the aids and appliances service. In the early days, Michael Gregory and Martin Sheridan, who ran the model shop, along with men like J.O. Kleber, John Breuel, and Manuel Powers, also contributed ideas for adaptations and new devices. At Ritter's right hand in expediting sales and demonstrations were two attractive blind women, Ruth Wartenberg and Helen Scherer, who also doubled as photographic models in illustrating the use of some of the devices.

For all his talents, Ritter was not a trained scientist and the Foundation still cherished hopes for major technological breakthroughs in the sensory realm. Out of the circle of Ritter's unofficial consultants emerged Clifford Martin Witcher, Ph.D., who joined the staff as a research engineer in November 1947. Witcher, a native of Atlanta, held a doctorate in physics from Columbia University, a B.S. from Georgia Institute of Technology, and a master's degree from Emory University.

Blind since the age of two, Cliff Witcher had attended regular elementary and high schools, a fact he credited for his proficiency in science. Schools for the blind, in those days, did not provide laboratory work for their students. Neither, for the most part, did public high schools, which routinely excused blind students from lab courses, but Witcher was allowed to take the same science classes as his fellow students. In his high school chemistry class he developed an auditory technique for measuring acids by setting up a group of "pitch pipes"—test tubes containing measured amounts of water, each of which gave off a different sound when blown across. When a particular quantity of acid was needed for an experiment, he would add it, drop by drop, to an empty test tube until the sound from blowing across the tube matched the sound from the "pitch pipe" with the desired amount.

At Columbia, Witcher worked under the Nobel laureate physicist, I. I. Rabi; his performance there resulted in a permanent open door for blind students in Columbia's science laboratories. This was by no means a common practice; one of the earliest accomplishments of the Technical Research Council was persuading other universities to admit blind students to laboratory work.

Witcher was familiar with some of the wartime devices which were thought to hold the key to sensory aids for the blind. He had worked on radar at Bell Telephone Laboratories and on sonic and supersonic guidance devices at Haskins Laboratories. There was a pleasing irony in his coming to work for the Foundation in a research capacity; years earlier the Foundation had turned him down for a scholarship on the grounds that scientific research was an unrealistic career objective for a blind person.

Much of Witcher's early work had to do with the mechanical problems which confronted blind people in earning a living. Some of his solutions, such as a collapsible cane manufactured out of the legs of a photographer's tripod, were of use to large numbers; more than 1,200 of the then novel collapsibles were sold in a short period. Others were unique solutions to unique problems. A blind woman who operated a small dairy business in New England wrote to ask how she could make sure that all milk bottles were uniformly filled to the proper height without having to put her finger in the milk. Witcher adapted a dental aspirator which would be mounted above the bottle in such a way it would produce a distinct sound when the milk reached the desired level; it was also rigged to carry off any excess milk into the next bottle.

While such projects were useful and often challenging, they were not the kind of research Witcher had been employed to do. In early 1949, at his insistence, his responsibilities were narrowed; he would work on electronic guidance devices to the exclusion of all else. A small appropriation for equipment was allotted, but it soon became evident that the substantial sums required for such fundamental research were well beyond the resources of a voluntary agency.

Witcher had been trying to interest the Veterans Administration in picking up where military research had left off. A detailed letter he wrote to the head of the VA's Prosthetic and Sensory Aid Services in late 1948, and another that he drafted for Robert Irwin's signature in 1949, had, in fact, brought him the offer of a job with the VA to direct a research project on sensory aids. The Foundation had agreed to give him a one-year leave of absence for this purpose, but for unrecorded reasons, the plan failed to materialize (the research assignment, as will be seen, went to Thomas Benham) and the decision to have Witcher concentrate on guidance devices represented a compromise solution arranged during a period of major organizational upheaval. Irwin was retiring, a successor had not yet been found, and the trustees were trying to keep a temporarily captainless ship afloat with a minimum of disturbance.

Under the staff reorganization that followed Barnett's appointment, Witcher spent increasing amounts of time as a consultant to the university laboratories which were then beginning to tackle research on sensory problems. What interested him most was the work on cybernetics being conducted by Norbert Wiener and Jerome Wiesner at Massachusetts Institute of Technology. This body of theory concerning the information-processing and communication methods common to man and machine was opening an entirely new line of thinking, Witcher reported in mid-1950.

> We have at last come to understand that our chief difficulty lies in discovering a channel other than sight by which information can be carried to the brain fast enough and accurately enough to meet the needs connected with independent travel and the reading of printed material.

In the same report, he mentioned he had been asked to serve as an informal consultant to MIT's electronic research laboratory. Thus was forged the first link in the ever closer collaboration that was to develop between the Foundation and MIT in the ensuing decades.

Witcher resigned from the Foundation in September 1950; following a year of teaching in Chicago, he joined the MIT staff, where he developed a number of electronic devices, including an optical probe that was promising enough to reach the stage of pilot production. He was on the verge of further achievements along these lines when, at the age of forty-two, he died of a heart attack in October 1956.

By the time Witcher died, sizable amounts of money and brain power had begun to be invested in research on sensory problems. Almost all of the money came from the federal treasury, much of it channeled through the VA. The brain power was concentrated in a handful of industrial and university laboratories working under federal contract. The prime objectives were to find substitutes for sight in two major areas, reading of print and independent travel, and the origins of much of the work were to be found in the efforts of a historic wartime enterprise, the Committee on Sensory Devices of the Office of Scientific Research and Development.

Toward the closing days of the war, President Franklin D. Roosevelt addressed a letter to Dr. Vannevar Bush, director of the military research unit which had coordinated the work of the nation's scientists in weapons technology, asking how these same resources could be employed in the postwar world. Among other points raised was the question: "What can the Government do now and in the future to aid research activities by public and private organizations?"

Robert Irwin's usually fertile imagination failed him when this letter appeared in the press on November 21, 1944. Instead of perceiving the larger implications, he addressed a trivial request to Dr. Bush, asking the Office of Scientific Research and Development to help the Foundation "get a high preference rating for $3,000 to $4,000 worth of machine tools," so that it could begin work on developing appliances to overcome the handicap of blindness. So hush-hush had been the work of the Office of Scientific Research and Development that Irwin was apparently unaware that a special group within it, the Committee on Sensory Devices, had already launched basic research into the question of blindness.

The CSD was headed by Dr. George W. Corner, chairman of the Department of Embryology of the Carnegie Institution. Its other members consisted of two physiologists, a biologist, a specialist in otological research, and a physicist. There were also three consultants attached to the committee, only one of whom, the director of the Institute of Optics of the University of Rochester, had any technical knowledge of visual problems.

The committee's initial mission was to focus on the needs of blinded veterans but, as Dr. Corner later wrote, the problems of this group were "not separable from those of blindness in general."

At its first meeting in January 1944, the CSD decided to focus on two objectives: devices for reading ordinary print, and guidance devices for ranging and obstacle finding. Haskins Laboratories, an independent research organization then located in New York City, was assigned to be the coordinator. Haskins, in turn, selected contractors to design various types of apparatus: four were to work on guidance devices constructed on differing approaches to a radar principle, and one was to concentrate on a reading device that would scan printed matter and translate light impulses into some form of audible code. At a later stage, CSD adopted two additional research objectives: optical aids for the partially sighted, and perfection of a device to produce enlarged embossed images of printed matter.

Although Vannevar Bush's organization was disbanded at war's end in 1945, the work of the Committee on Sensory Devices was taken over by the National Research Council of the National Academy of Sciences with continuing financial support from the VA and the Army Surgeon General's office. CSD's appropriations came to an end in 1947; the final funds were spent on a report published in 1950, *Blindness: Modern Approaches to the Unseen Environment*, which included not only detailed accounts of the CSD-financed projects but chapters by outside specialists on major phases of work for the blind.

The Committee on Sensory Devices itself remained in existence until 1954 as a subcommittee of the National Research Council's Division of Anthropology and Psychology. Ten years later, at the request of the Veterans Administration, the Council established a new advisory group, a Subcommittee on Sensory Aids, under its Committee on Prosthetics Research and Development. Professor Robert W. Mann of MIT was the subcommittee's first chairman.

Viewed from an engineering standpoint, all the projects sponsored by the original CSD were successful in the sense that, as Dr. Corner wrote, each produced "an instrument which is able to do something not previously accomplished." But, he added candidly:

> In each case . . . we come up against the question of the ability of the human user to make practical use of the sense-stimulation afforded by these instruments. . . . Whatever missteps the Committee made arose chiefly from insufficient realization of this fact or from disregard of it.

Even in the disciplined ranks of science, the lessons learned by one generation must apparently be relearned by the next. Despite Dr. Corner's warning, sensory research during succeeding decades was dotted with engineering triumphs that worked perfectly in the laboratory and failed at the critical point of consumer use.

In the 25 years following termination of the CSD's projects, the Veterans Administration, which had contributed more than $400,000 between 1945 and 1947, invested approximately $3,500,000 more in the effort to develop reading machines and electronic guidance devices for the blind. Large sums also came from several units of the Department of Health, Education, and Welfare—the Social and Rehabilitation Service, the Office of Education, and the National Institutes of Health—and, in a few instances, from the Defense Department. Because some of these grants were shown under other labels, it is not possible to assign a definitive figure to the overall total. An estimate was made in 1968 that federal investment in blindness technology during the preceding 20 years had approximated $8 million.

There exists a voluminous body of literature tracing the history of the several dozen painstaking projects which attempted, for the most part in vain, to find viable substitutes for sight in reading and mobility. As of 1972, a handful of these projects were still current, with some already at the testing stage and one just beginning to seek a market. To describe a few of these is to convey both the immensity of the problems and the lengths to which technology went in the effort to solve them.

Since the only two sensory channels that could be employed as partial substitutes for vision were hearing and touch, all work on print-reading and guidance devices for the blind centered on converting light into sound, taction or both.

The grandfather of the family of devices that transformed a beam of light into aural output was born before World War I when a British physicist, Dr. E. E. Fournier d'Albe, made use of a phenomenon discovered 40 years earlier, the light-sensitive properties of the chemical element selenium, to construct a machine that translated light impulses into sound. He described his instrument, which he named the optophone, in a 1913 issue of a British technical journal and five years later demonstrated it, using a live blind model, Mary Jameson, before the British Scientific Products Exhibit at King's College in London.

The thought that there was any way in which she could have direct access to the printed word fascinated eighteen-year-old Mary; she was undismayed by the complexity of the system involved. As she later described it, the original "white" version of the instrument built in the inventor's laboratory

> had one selenium cell which received light reflected from the printed page being read. White paper emitted a full musical chord; the reading was done by the tones blotted out by the black print as the scanner passed along the line.
>
> In a word, reading was effected by what one didn't hear. This was not easy and the frail construction of the instrument added to one's difficulties. The focusing arrangements would slip out of place if anyone walked heavily across the room. However, by August 1918 I could manage a speed of about a word a minute, sufficient to show that print reading was possible.

It was this one-word-a-minute skill that she demonstrated at King's College, and her performance was sufficiently impressive to interest an optical manufacturing firm, Barr and Stroud, Ltd., of Glasgow, to produce a "black" version of the optophone which reversed the reading process so that the sound symbols came from the black print and not from the white paper.

The optophone used six musical notes—GCDEFG—to denote the height and shape of printed letters. Each letter of the alphabet could be identified through the unique combination of notes which signified its vertical, horizontal, or diagonal contours. Mary Jameson was one of the few people in the world who not only mastered this extraordinary code but learned to enjoy doing it. In 1972 she was still using a modernized version of the six-tone optophone at speeds of up to 60 words a minute.

Although the British machine was patented in the United States in 1920 and demonstrated to American leaders in work for the blind two years later, it failed to arouse interest as a practical reading medium and was never produced in this country. However, its polyphonic reading principle was one of those reexamined under the Committee on Sensory Devices. A basic dilemma facing the engineers who approached this assignment was described by Dr. Franklin S. Cooper of Haskins Laboratories as illustrating "the perversity of natural phenomena, that the system which offers most promise of yielding easily intelligible sounds somewhat like English should also be the system which requires the greatest instrumental complexity." Conversely, systems like the optophone that involved simpler instrumentation had the disadvantage of psychological complexity, with the major translation burden falling on the user.

Under CSD a contract was awarded to the Radio Corporation of America to see what could be developed in the way of polyphonic instruments. One of its two inventions was a machine called the "reading pencil" which used photoelectric cells and magnetic tapes to produce a chirping, canary-like sound to characterize each letter of the alphabet. Twenty-five working models of this apparatus were produced and tested, with but marginal results.

In 1954, shortly after the CSD had formally gone out of existence, the VA sponsored a technical conference on reading machines (the first of six that would be held in the next dozen years), at which sufficient enthusiasm was expressed to warrant a new start. Accordingly the VA contracted with two midwestern research organizations, Battelle Memorial Institute and Mauch Laboratories, to do further work on polyphonic reading devices.

After 13 years Battelle's efforts, as reported in 1970 by Howard Freiberger, electronics engineer of the VA's Prosthetic and Sensory Aids Research and Development Division, "culminated in the production of 10 copies of a quite rugged, fairly reliable, portable Model D Optophone fitted into a standard piece of luggage, a ladies' train case." Also evolved was a 200-hour training course in the use of the Battelle optophone, which employed nine tones instead of the six in the original version and used transistors in place of Fournier d'Albe's selenium cell.

Mauch Laboratories, which also began work in 1957, produced a series of devices. One, the Visotoner, was similar to the Battelle machine, but miniaturized. Its scanner weighed only ten ounces; with its batteries and accessories, including a tracking aid called the Colineator, the Visotoner set could fit into an attache case. A tactile variation, called the Visotactor, used vibrators on four finger-rests instead of an auditory output. Both machines were designed to be "medium cost reading devices."

Dr. Michael P. Beddoes, a Canadian engineer who independently developed a polyphonic reading machine called the Lexiphone (his instrument used hisses and clicks in addition to musical tones), observed in 1968 that such machines "can inspire tremendous and lasting affection from a very few peculiarly gifted people." One such, America's equivalent of Mary Jameson, was Harvey L. Lauer. Braille therapist at VA's Hines rehabilitation center for the blind, Lauer began the 200-hour Battelle training course in 1964. Two years later he reported he had found five "categories of efficient uses" for the instrument—proofreading his own typing, identifying currency, reading correspondence, checking bills and bank statements, identifying packaged goods—and expected soon to be able to look up material in dictionaries and reference books. His speed was slow—5 to 25 words a minute. Still, as he said at the time, "The pace is slow, the mileage is improving, but the payload is terrific."

When the first Visotoners and Visotactors were delivered, Lauer mastered both instruments, then taught the Visotoner to Margaret Butow of the Hadley School for the Blind, who proceeded to develop a 25-lesson tape-recorded screening course which the school, under contract from the VA, used as a method of locating candidates who could learn to use this reading machine. Lauer also taught the

Visotoner to a number of blinded veterans at the Hines center; they were reading print at speeds of up to 15 words a minute, he reported in 1969.

Clearly, there could never be a mass market for what some irreverent wags called the "optophone follies." An admittedly optimistic estimate made by Freiberger in 1970 projected a maximum of five hundred blind persons as the target population for the Visotoner; he thought that perhaps an equal number, who were tactually rather than aurally oriented, might be found for the Visotactor. He went on to identify the obstacles in locating these target groups, in recruiting teachers and preparing instructional materials, and in procuring machines. In 1967, when the VA bought 30 Visotoners and 10 Visotactors, the unit cost per set was $1,875. Freiberger estimated that the cost per set in a serial production run of 500 machines might come to $1,500, or a total of $750,000. On the assumption that, in a two-year period, 11 instructors could teach the skill to five hundred people, he put the cost of teacher preparation and student instruction over this period at an additional $500,000.

Clearly, few members of the target group could be expected to pay so much themselves; in virtually every case the money would have to come from federal, state, or voluntary agencies, or perhaps from corporations employing a number of blind persons. Nevertheless, it was reasoned, even this large an expenditure would prove worthwhile if it enhanced the ability of some blind persons to achieve or retain vocational independence. On this theory, in 1971 a California group began marketing an entirely different tactual reading machine called the Optacon.

The Optacon did not originate in abstract theorizing; it was prompted by a very human desire, a father's wish to ease the plight of his blind daughter. That the father happened to be an accomplished scientist was the first of two coincidences that propelled the machine from concept to serial production in less than a decade.

Candace ("Candy") Linvill was an infant when retinoblastoma, cancer of the eye, necessitated bilateral enucleation. When she reached school age her parents, who lived in a suburb, decided they would have her attend the small village school rather than be bussed to nearby San Francisco where special classes for blind children were available. The village school accepted the little girl on condition that her mother braille all of her books. Candy was already a fourth-grader when her father, Professor John Linvill of Stanford University's School of Engineering, came upon the idea that could lighten his wife's brailling chores and advance his daughter's education.

On a visit to an IBM research center in Germany, Linvill saw a high speed computer which used vibrating pins as hammers to produce its printout. "If you could print with vibratory pins, you could surely feel them" was his first thought. He went on to develop the vibratory pin notion, using piezoelectric reeds as vibrators, to the point where he could patent it.

The second coincidence took place when Linvill discovered that a colleague at Stanford Research Institute, Dr. James C. Bliss, was also working on tactual reading. An electrical engineer who had done his doctoral work at MIT as part of Professor Samuel J. Mason's group studying sensory aids and communications, Bliss was continuing sensory research at Stanford with the help of major grants from the National Aeronautics and Space Administration (NASA) and the United

States Air Force. At the point that he and Linvill met, Bliss had evolved a computer-controlled device that presented letter shapes by a series of air jets. Using Linvill's vibrating reeds in place of Bliss' air jets, the two men joined forces to evolve the basic design of the Optacon. The question then arose: could a blind person identify letter shapes presented in tactual vibration form? Candy Linvill became the first experimental subject, and it was her success at mastering what was essentially an electronic version of line type finger-reading that encouraged the inventors to go on.

As it finally emerged, the Optacon used a transistorized miniature camera, about the size of a pocket knife, to scan inkprint. What the scanner "saw" activated a set of 144 tiny vibrating reeds on a fingertip-sized tactile screen. Placed on this screen, the reader's finger felt the image produced by the vibrating reeds, an image which replicated the shape of the letter the scanner focused on. The entire unit—camera, battery-operated converter, and tactile screen—was contained in a book-sized, 3½-pound package.

Development of the Optacon was largely financed by the Bureau of Education for the Handicapped of the U.S. Office of Education, which over a four-year period made grants totalling more than $1,300,000 to perfect the instrumentation, test prototype models, and produce a pilot run of 50 machines for more extensive testing. The results were sufficiently encouraging—reading speeds of 50 words a minute were achieved after practice by a number of others besides Candy Linvill—so that, on expiration of the federal grants, Linvill and Bliss formed a commercial venture in 1971 to produce and market the Optacon.

The initial handcrafted instruments were priced at $5,000; by the end of 1972, serial production made possible a reduction to $3,450. Along with the Optacon proper, a number of accessories were developed whose price, along with the tuition for a training course, brought the total package close to $5,000. There was sufficient interest, both domestically and abroad, to engender hopes for larger-scale production at lower cost in the near future.

An approach to presenting a wider field of tactile images was developed in the late Sixties by two other California scientists, Paul Bach-y-Rita and Carter C. Collins of the University of the Pacific's Smith-Kettlewell Institute of Visual Sciences. Their invention, the Tactile Vision Substitution System (TVSS), used as a receiver a much larger expanse of body skin than the narrow compass of a forefinger. In its initial form, TVSS employed a chair with 400 plastic vibrators embedded in its back. These were linked to a small, hand-held TV camera which scanned images and reflected their shape in the vibrators, much as the Optacon did. The user leaned back in the chair to feel the pattern vibrated against his back. In a subsequent version the vibrators were moved from the back of a chair to a panel attached to a desk so that the user leaned forward to receive the image on chest and abdomen. Later still, the number of vibrators was increased and packaged in a cummerbund-shaped pad worn around the user's body. Another change was to place the formerly hand-held scanner in a pair of eyeglass frames. Teachers in the schools for blind children that tested these instruments used them to familiarize students with geometric shapes and other visual concepts.

Whatever the stage of development of the Visotoner, the Visotactor, the

Optacon, or TVSS, there was no thought in the minds of their inventors or their sponsors that they represented more than interim solutions to the reading machine problem. Far more sophisticated devices were simultaneously in process of exploration. Among the most elaborate were the VA-sponsored experiments at Haskins Laboratories to generate spoken speech from printed text. One involved six separate processes in which words "recognized" by an electronic character reader were recorded in phonemic form by means of a computer "dictionary" storing 150,000 words, were then "punctuated" by means of stress and intonation instructions also stored in the computer, then transformed by another computer program into a synthetic speech output recorded on tape for the blind user to hear.

This multimillion-dollar mechanism, obviously out of reach as a personal reading device, was designed for use in library centers; the principal argument in its favor was that it was capable of producing, at rates of 150 words per minute, intelligible synthetic speech which relieved the user of the need to master an artificial code.

Less complex were the "spelled speech" mechanisms explored in several quarters; these scanned print, letter by letter, and by means of tape reproduced the computer-stored recorded sounds that identified each letter name. The advantage of spelled speech over the optophone was that the user was spared the task of mentally translating a particular combination of tones into the letter "h"—he would instead hear a tape-recorded human voice pronounce "aitch" out of the machine's stored vocabulary. The simpler the user's task, however, the more complex (and more expensive) the machine's. An early spelled-speech machine had been developed for the Committee on Sensory Devices by the Radio Corporation of America. Built before the era of electronic miniaturization, the RCA Recognition Machine had 250 vacuum tubes; the single prototype produced was never considered a practical solution.

Also in process while these auditory translation efforts were under way were projects designed to employ the code many blind people already knew and used—braille. As has been noted, an early version of automated composition of braille textbooks using an IBM computer began at the American Printing House for the Blind in the early Sixties. Subsequent work at MIT developed a system for translating Grade 2 braille into a code compatible with any size or type of computer, and thus capable of time-sharing connection to computers employed for other purposes. In 1970 the Atlanta public school system began using this program to produce virtually instantaneous brailled lessons for its blind students.

The system, which MIT's Sensory Aids Evaluation and Development Center built with support from the Hartford Foundation, consisted of two elements, a standard Teletypewriter and a high-speed braille printer called Braillemboss. Both were linked by ordinary telephone circuit to a commercial IBM computer on a time-sharing basis. Text typed on the Teletypewriter emerged in braille from the Braillemboss at a speed of 10 characters per second. As of 1972, the 20 models of Braillemboss built by MIT were in use not only in school systems but at MIT itself for the benefit of blind scientists, and in several commercial companies employing blind computer programmers.

Professor Robert W. Mann, head of the MIT sensory aids unit, predicted in 1970 that there would be other uses, "including even broadcast stations so that blind radio announcers can get the wire service news in braille directly from the Teletype." Another potential use could be the production of brailled books from the same computer tapes used by publishers in the composition of inkprint books and periodicals. If and when technology developed to the point, often predicted by scientists, where a computer terminal was a standard feature of every home, blind people could have access to home-delivered daily newspapers in braille.

A totally different approach to making braille more accessible was simultaneously under research at the Atomic Energy Commission's Argonne National Laboratory under contract to the University of Chicago in a project supported by the U.S. Office of Education. The Argonne braille machine was designed to do away with bulky braille volumes by storing reading matter, in coded symbols, on an endless belt of magnetic tape which translated the symbols into raised braille characters. The user would feel the dots under his fingertips as the belt moved under them at whatever speed he wished; as the belt returned to the tape cartridge, the dots would be flattened out and the tape would be ready to receive impulses for the formation of new braille characters.

Invention of this device was spurred by the same motivation that had prompted John Linvill to conceive of the Optacon. The inventor, Dr. Arnold P. Grunwald, a physicist on the Argonne staff, had a young son blind from infancy. As of the end of 1972 sources of support were being sought for construction of 30 copies of the mechanism for testing.

Lack of access to printed words was not the only problem of blind readers. For students, scientists and many others, the need for drawings, diagrams, maps and other graphic material was also of importance. It was a group of blind engineers and technicians who induced the Committee on Sensory Devices to adopt, as one of its projects, the modernization of a long-existing device, the Visagraph, which could produce mechanically embossed copies of graphic material and take the place of the handmade raised line drawings that then represented the only other available method.

What gave birth to the Visagraph was a wealthy man's humanitarian impulse. In 1926 Robert E. Naumburg attended an entertainment sponsored by the Boston Committee for the Blind. The blind people in the audience, he said,

> made a more lasting impression on me than the performance. So impressed was I by their character, their philosophy, their keenness to get all they could out of life, that when I left them that evening I could think of nothing else. The next morning I began work on the Visagraph.

Naumburg's first apparatus combined sound and touch; he later eliminated the auditory element and developed a version, the Printing Visagraph, that depended on touch alone. This produced, on a thin sheet of aluminum foil, a magnified raised image of a printed page. The desk-sized machine consisted of a scanning section and a recording section that were geared together so the recording mechanism produced a relief image of the printed material scanned by a selenium cell.

Demonstrated at the 1931 World Conference on Work for the Blind, the Visagraph aroused curiosity but little practical interest. Educators, convinced that braille was a superior system for finger-reading, rejected as a throwback the idea of teaching blind people to read linear type. Despite the negative reception, Naumburg continued his work over the years, although the machine never emerged beyond the laboratory stage.

The Visagraph may have been unusable as a machine for reading text, but its ability to reproduce graphic images had practical possibilities. Under contract from CSD, and with Naumburg acting as a consultant, an independent laboratory was assigned to produce an improved version. This instrument, the Faximile Visagraph, yielded enlarged copy on heavy metal foil at the rate of about three minutes per page. It was never produced commercially, partly because there simultaneously became available a simpler copying apparatus which used a special resin that could be baked into raised form, and partly because experience showed that embossed illustrations which faithfully reproduced every detail of the inkprint original were confusing to the finger. Raised diagrams, it was found, needed editorial judgment as to what to include and what to omit.

This was particularly evident in map-making, a subject of continuous study by both educators and mobility specialists. Blind persons could be helped to extend their travel skills if provided with tactual maps of unfamiliar locations. Extensive experimentation was under way in the Sixties and early Seventies on how to evolve a set of uniform symbols that would identify such features as steps, building entrances, mailboxes, bus stops, and such differing terrains as grass, paved roads, wooded areas, and bodies of water. The problem was not merely designating symbols but how to place them on embossed maps so as to provide guidance without clutter.

Maps would undoubtedly continue to be needed, even when electronic mobility aids reached higher performance levels than was the case in 1972. As with reading machines, the effort to construct guidance devices had entailed heavy expenditures since World War II. At least two dozen separate attacks on the problem were made over a 25-year period; of these, three were still being actively pursued in 1972: the VA-Bionic Laser Cane, the Pathsounder and the Kay Binaural Sensor.

CSD, which authorized four contractors to work on guidance devices in 1944, saw the problem in two parts: short-range obstacle detectors that would safeguard the blind walker by informing him of fixed or moving obstructions in his path, and recognition devices that would provide clues for a mental construct of the environment. The initial question was which of the possible energy bands to utilize: sound, supersonic energy, visible light, ultraviolet light. For the most part, the CSD-supported projects concentrated on ultrasonic devices. All of them fell short, either because the information they provided did not yield a sufficient margin of safety, or because their signals were not clear enough to be genuinely useful.

One, however, employed a principle that held some promise. It was a wartime invention of the Army Signal Corps: a portable box resembling a battery lamp which used a narrow beam of visible light to determine range by means of optical triangulation. The light beam registered the presence of reflected obstacles through vibrations in the device's handle. Under CSD contract, 25 experimental units of this sensory aid were constructed by the Radio Corporation of America for testing. It proved to have some serious flaws, principally that it had no capability to warn the user of stepdowns or deep holes in his path. Another aspect that users found objectionable was that the vibrating handle emitted a continuous signal; a change in the signal registered the presence of an obstacle. "It was like having a continuously ringing telephone which you answered only when the ring changed," was the way this feature was described by Dr. Eugene F. Murphy, chief of the Research and Development Division of the VA's Prosthetic and Sensory Aids Service.

Nevertheless, when the VA activated a research program to pick up where CSD had left off, the decision was made to evaluate the device in field trials. The evaluation assignment was placed in the hands of a talented blind scientist, Thomas A. Benham.

Benham was, in many ways, a counterpart of Cliff Witcher. They were the same age (both born in 1914). Both had been blind since early childhood and both had pursued careers in science with no concession to their lack of sight. Following graduation from Haverford College in Pennsylvania, Benham got a job as a junior engineer in RCA's development laboratories; working on quartz crystal experiments, he devised the special techniques and instruments he needed to do his full share of the work, among them a brailled micrometer, a voltammeter which registered readings through both sound and touch, a calculator adapted for braille operation.

In full agreement with the belief that blind people could pursue satisfying careers in technical fields if expertise could be shared, Benham later launched a non-profit organization, Science for the Blind, which began by tape-recording and distributing technical literature and went on to produce a series of special instruments for blind scientists. With the help of several organizations and foundations, Science for the Blind was carrying out in 1972 a facet of the work begun by Chick Ritter's Technical Research Council a quarter-century earlier.

All of this was still in the future when, in 1950, Benham accepted the VA assignment. After trying out the Signal Corps guidance device with 67 blind persons, he reported in 1952 that about one out of five could benefit from its use; he also detailed the changes needed in design and performance that could make it more useful and efficient. The following year VA contracted with Haverford College to work out Benham's recommendations and Haverford subcontracted the engineering development to a nearby electronics firm which, after several changes of name, came to be known as Bionic Industries. In the course of a dozen years Bionic built a series of models, beginning with portable "lunchbox" carriers and moving on to smaller, flashlight-shaped machines until the development of integrated electronic circuitry made it possible to compress instrumentation into a cane handle.

This was regarded as an important breakthrough; since no obstacle detector was as yet capable of totally replacing the cane, a guidance device in the cane itself meant that the blind traveler could have one hand free. The several cane models developed in the mid-Sixties also featured something new. Previous devices had contained two detectors, one aimed at obstacles straight ahead and a second focused downward to warn of major dropoffs. Now a third channel was added, aimed upward to reflect overhanging signs or tree branches that might collide with the user's head.

Soon thereafter came development of the laser, a powerful beam of light emanating from a tiny space. In 1966 this made possible the first laser cane. Four years later, after preliminary testing and redesign, ten copies of the VA-Bionic Laser Cane were produced for use in field evaluations with blinded veterans. The instrument emitted both audible and tactile signals. The middle, or forward-looking, beam provided a tactile signal, a pin vibrating against the index finger of the hand holding the cane. The other two signals were given by tones (high-pitched for overhead obstacles, low-pitched for major dropoffs) from a small loudspeaker in the cane handle's crook.

A careful protocol for evaluation of these canes in actual use was developed by a panel of engineers and mobility therapists. Performance under varying traffic conditions would be filmed and compared with the same subject's performance using a conventional long cane. Out of twenty years of experience with guidance devices, years marked by alternating hopes and disappointments, the VA adopted this testing procedure because, as Eugene Murphy pointed out in late 1971:

> It is not enough to say that the cane is accepted or rejected by certain percentages of users. Rather it is necessary to discover the types of users for whom it is most appropriate. . . . one needs an armamentarium of devices from which selection can be made.

Any such armamentarium might have a place for the ultrasonic mobility aid invented by a New Zealand engineer, developed under British financial sponsorship and tested in more than twenty countries—a device which, in 1972, had reached about the same stage of readiness as the laser cane.

This device, the Kay binaural sensor, went through a series of engineering refinements comparable to those undergone by the laser cane as technological advances made it possible to pack electronic circuits into ever-smaller spaces. It reached the production engineering stage in 1965, a half-dozen years after Dr. Leslie Kay, then a visiting lecturer at Birmingham University (and later head of the Department of Electric Engineering of New Zealand's University of Canterbury), conceived the idea for an echolocation instrument and enlisted the support of St. Dunstan's and Britain's National Research Development Corporation in developing it.

Originally contained in a hand-held instrument about the size and shape of an ordinary flashlight, the Kay device was later redesigned to incorporate its sensor and receiver in an eyeglass frame whose earpieces were equipped with tiny loudspeakers. The power supply and control instrumentation were lodged in a small pack that could be clipped to the belt or worn elsewhere on the body.

In their 1972 version the Kay spectacles contained three tiny transducers mounted above the nosepiece between the lenses. The center transducer emitted a high-frequency sonic pulse which, when it struck an object, produced vibrations in the other two. These were converted by the control pack into sound the user heard through the minute speakers, similar to hearing aids, mounted over the earpieces of the spectacles. The volume of sound was an index of distance; the nearer the object, the louder the sound. The binaural effect—the signal reaching one ear might differ in pitch from the signal reaching the other—enabled the user to gain more precise information about the location of the obstacle.

Following testing in Europe—one British experimenter reported that over a nine-month period he walked 1,250 miles with the help of the device—a yearlong series of evaluations was conducted in the United States by Kay and a team of associates from the University of Canterbury in 1971–72. Working with mobility teachers who first trained under blindfold in the use of the device and then taught it to an aggregate of some one hundred blind users, the team found a high level of acceptance in both groups. But more work remained to be done in engineering redesign and in improving the training program, Kay reported after analyzing the test results.

One of his conclusions represented a surprising turn of the wheel. "It would appear," he wrote, "that some of the blind users could play an important role in future training programs." Acknowledging that this reversed the contemporary practice, in both cane and dog guide mobility programs, of utilizing only sighted instructors, he nevertheless found that some of the blind persons who tested his guidance device "better understood the language of the [sensory] aid and the perception of the environment which it makes possible."

A third object which had the potential of fitting into an armamentarium of mobility aids was also a pulsed ultrasonic unit, one developed at MIT by Lindsay Russell with financial support from a philanthropic foundation. Known as the Pathsounder, this lightweight device was designed specifically to detect obstacles at above-waistline level as a supplement to cane-probing at ground level. Hung on a strap worn around the neck, it was tested in the early Seventies by the VA, whose findings turned up an unexpected bonus. The device was an effective clear-path indicator for blinded veterans confined to wheelchairs.

Impressive as were the technological accomplishments represented by these three guidance devices, what emerged most clearly from a review of their performances was that all three were supplements to, and not replacements for, the more familiar mobility aids: the long cane and the dog guide. Whether engineering genius might one day conjure up a total replacement for cane or dog remained, in 1972, as problematic as whether medical technology might one day find a way of inserting TV cameras in empty eye sockets or devising some other prosthesis that could produce artificial vision. Some work on such a prosthesis had already been attempted: in England, where electrically stimulated probes inserted in the occipital cortex of a blind nurse produced images of ricegrain-sized points of light called phosphenes; in the United States, where several medical research teams were working on the concept of combining electrodes inserted in the brain with eyeglass-mounted TV cameras; in the Soviet Union, where experiments with artificial vision were conducted on dogs.

Given the impressive sums and high-powered engineering talent invested in sensory aids research over a 25-year period, what useful role could be played by a non-governmental body? This was the question repeatedly confronting the American Foundation for the Blind once government-financed efforts gained momentum in the Fifties.

Soon after M. Robert Barnett took office, he convened a series of conferences which brought together Foundation officers and technical staff members with a group of outside scientists. With few variations, the basic themes at these early meetings would be echoed time and again in the decades to follow. They were essentially these:

The Foundation should employ a small number of personnel professionally qualified to understand and evaluate the research under way in various laboratories, to maintain close liaison with the scientists conducting these projects, and to serve as consultants to them on the needs and capabilities of blind persons. It should restrict its own research efforts to those for which its staff and facilities were equipped and not venture into new and untried fields. It should take responsibility for keeping the field of work for the blind continuously informed on the progress of technical research. It should have the benefit of policy guidance from an advisory committee of leading scientific and technological specialists.

The first such committee, appointed in 1952, was small but choice: Dr. Thorton C. Fry of Bell Telephone Laboratories; Dr. William C. Geer, head of his own consulting laboratory in Ithaca, New York; and Dr. Jerome B. Wiesner of MIT. In later years, others of equal prominence served for varying lengths of time, among them Sherman M. Fairchild of the electronics firm that bore his name, Peter Goldmark of CBS Laboratories, Edwin H. Land of the Polaroid Corporation.

As of 1972, the Foundation's Research Advisory Committee was headed by the sociologist Dr. John W. Riley, Jr., a vice-president of the Equitable Life Assurance Society. Its members included Dr. Edward E. David, Jr., formerly of Bell Telephone Laboratories, and, in 1972, director of the Office of Science and Technology in the White House; Dr. Heinz E. Kallman, consulting physicist; Professor Herbert Hyman of Wesleyan University's Department of Sociology; Dr. Stephen A. Richardson, visiting professor at the Albert Einstein College of Medicine; and Dr. Wiesner, who had by then become president of Massachusetts Institute of Technology. Wiesner, who was also a Foundation trustee, had served as an advisory committee member continuously since 1952, maintaining his interest even when he was White House science advisor during the Kennedy administration.

The technical resources available to the Foundation were augmented, beginning in 1967, by the practice of appointing part-time consultants to the research staff in the areas of social science, physical science and statistics. An added technical resource, informal but intimate, was the continuous link with MIT, initiated through Clifford Witcher and subsequently brought to a more intensive level through John Kenneth Dupress, who did as much as anyone to influence the changing course of Foundation research. To see his role in perspective, it is necessary to go back to the period when Ritter and Witcher were the leading spirits in promoting the development of aids and appliances.

For a year or so after Witcher's resignation in 1950, the Foundation was without a technical research chief. The post was filled in 1952 by Charles P. Tolman, an engineer whose background included considerable experience in prevention of blindness work. He had developed a widely used tonometer—an eyeball-pressure measuring instrument which made possible early diagnosis of glaucoma. Already semi-retired when he joined the staff, Tolman remained less than three years but left some significant legacies. One was that he taught the endlessly curious Chick Ritter a great deal about low-vision aids—knowledge Ritter was to put to use in starting a service for partially sighted persons.

John Dupress was hired in late 1958, one of several new staff members in the reorganized administrative structure which consolidated social, behavioral, and technological research. The reorganized unit operated under the newly reaffirmed policy that emphasis would be put on "stimulating and motivating universities, laboratories, government agencies and direct-service rehabilitation agencies to plan and carry through research relating to blindness."

It would have been hard to find a more accomplished hand at "stimulating and motivating" than John Dupress. Many people, including his admirers, used more pungent words—gadfly, needler, prod—to describe his impact. His admirers were ardent but not particularly numerous. Dupress, who tended to be caustic, hyper-critical, and assertive in pursuit of his aims, neither sought nor attained broad popularity.

The wellsprings of this prickly personality were easily discernible. Orphaned at an early age and raised by a foster mother in his native Massachusetts, Dupress was to endure an even more traumatic young manhood. He enlisted in the Army at age nineteen, achieving such high test scores that he was assigned to an advanced communications training program at Lehigh University. Despite this specialized education, he was shipped overseas with an infantry unit in 1944. He saw action at Omaha Beach and then in the Battle of the Bulge where, in December 1944, an exploding hand grenade pierced his face and body in 26 places, including his eyes, and he was captured behind German lines.

His experience as a prisoner of war embittered him for life. The camp to which he was assigned, he claimed, carried out brutal psychological experiments on prisoners. He lost not only his eyes but his left hand, which was severed at the wrist. What remained intact was his fighting spirit.

Surgery gave him a cosmetic hand prosthesis and a pair of plastic eyes, and he went on to Old Farms for rehabilitation, and then to Princeton University, where he rolled up a good academic record, operated a small recording company, and founded an electronics club. Although his major was psychology, he was increasingly intrigued with electronic gadgetry, using a wire recorder to take down lectures, then a dictaphone to record his notes on small plastic discs. After graduation he continued to be enamored of sound recording systems. The stereophonic system in the listening room at the heart of the Connecticut home he later designed and had built was a marvel of high fidelity.

A complex, proud, and reserved individual, Dupress had no desire to be associated with other blind people, still less to make a career of work for the blind. He took the job at the Foundation because of the challenge it offered in terms of technological and human engineering. The problems entailed in harnessing science for the benefit of blind persons would never be solved, he believed, "by isolated research for the blind." Nor would those capable of solving the problems be motivated purely by altruism. "The best research minds can be obtained by presenting our problems as complex and stimulating ones rather than as charity items."

What attracted him was the opportunity to be associated with the "best research minds." And once he became a member of the Foundation staff, he lost little time in seeking them out. One of his earliest official reports read: "The Director of this Bureau [Dupress] happily announces that he has secured the interest of three additional major research facilities" whose work he would coordinate with the relevant research conducted at Massachusetts Institute of Technology. At MIT, 16 students were working on designing machines that could feed information into human sensory channels, while in two affiliated laboratories work was going forward on aspects of auditory research. Dupress himself was lecturing in the man-machine systems design course and serving as a consultant in the auditory research projects.

Despite the lack of a science degree, Dupress could and did make contributions to complex technological thinking, but where he really excelled was in seeking out sources of large-scale research grants. Among the many beneficiaries of this skill was James Bliss of Stanford, who credited Dupress with introducing him to the right people in Washington when he needed support for an early sensory aids project. However, it was this very skill at grantsmanship that eventually led to Dupress' departure from the Foundation at the end of 1963 to head a newly established unit at MIT, the Sensory Aids Evaluation and Development Center. He had been the prime mover in arranging the necessary $98,000 grant from the Vocational Rehabilitation Administration.

As director of this center, whose primary purpose was field-testing the sensory hardware evolved in MIT's laboratories, Dupress kept in constant touch with his former colleagues on the Foundation's research staff and with others in work for the blind. When, in December 1967, a heart attack ended his life at the age of forty-five, the loss was keenly felt, even by those who had never developed much personal rapport with him.

In 1960, as an initial step toward its changed role in research, the Foundation secured an $80,000 matching grant from the Office of Vocational Rehabilitation to assess the status of worldwide technology in relation to aids for the blind. The survey culminated in the first International Congress on Technology and Blindness, convened in New York in June 1962, at which papers were given by scientists and technologists from England, France, Denmark, Poland, Sweden, the Netherlands, Austria, Israel, West Germany, Canada, and the Soviet Union, as well as the United States. This first conference, whose proceedings were detailed in four volumes published the following year, was succeeded by several other international conclaves: one in Rotterdam in 1964, one in London in 1966 under the sponsorship of St. Dunstan's, and one in 1971 in New York as part of the Foundation's 50th anniversary observance. These were interspersed with a number of other research conferences held in the United States. There were many useful by-products of these meetings, not least of which was that they brought about face-to-face contacts between the technologists and the practitioners expected to make use of their work.

The necessity for continuous dissemination of information on the thrust and progress of research was one of the major themes of the 1962 international congress. To satisfy this need the International Research Information Service (IRIS) was created in 1964. Launched with the help of a federal grant and then maintained out of Foundation funds, IRIS set up a sophisticated document-handling system for the collection and indexing of research material from all over the world. The information gathered was issued in a variety of forms: bibliographies, state-of-the-art reports, monographs, conference proceedings, and a series of research bulletins which had reached 25 in number by 1972. Toward the end of that year, an updated international catalog of aids and appliances for the blind was being readied for publication. The first such catalog had been issued ten years earlier as one of the four volumes to emerge from the first technology congress.

Throughout the period that some members of the Foundation's research staff were working to help shape the electronic future, other staffers marched steadily onward with the adaptation, production, and distribution of the less sophisticated devices that could be made immediately available. Until he left the Foundation in 1959 to move to Denver for a position with the Colorado state agency for the blind, Charles Ritter continued to be the pivot of a steadily growing aids and appliances service.

One of the devices listed in the Foundation's very first catalog was a simple magnifying glass. The sales response sharpened Ritter's awareness of how many legally blind people had fragments of residual vision which the right kind of optical aid could enhance. A number of ophthalmologists responded helpfully to his quest for more information, and Ritter gradually grew highly knowledgeable about the world of optical goods: microscopic lenses for close work, telescopic lenses for distance, projection readers of various strengths and types, devices to concentrate light or to diffuse it.

The use of magnification to enlarge the image registered on the retina of the human eye was nothing new. Eyeglasses had been worn for centuries; Nero was said to have used a polished gem as a magnifier. There were, however, some new elements that led to an upsurge of interest in optical aids following World War II. One was the disintegration of the long-held belief that vision was a consumable item that had to be conserved. Ophthalmologists discovered that the use of residual vision did no permanent harm to weak eyes; the effects of eyestrain could be readily overcome by a period of rest. The other factor had to do with advances in optical technology that made possible the production of cosmetically acceptable high-strength compound lenses.

In 1924 some heartening results through the use of telescopic spectacles had been announced at a meeting of the American Medical Association in a paper given by a pair of Chicago ophthalmologists, one of whom, Jules C. Stein, went on to achieve renown in a totally different field as head of the giant Music Corporation of America. The Illinois Society for the Prevention of Blindness, some of whose clients had been included in the patient group, called the telescopic lenses to the attention of Anne Sullivan Macy at a time when she was suffering one of her periodic bouts with eye trouble. Fitted with a pair, she wrote Marion A. Campbell, secretary of the Illinois Society; "You may be as enthusiastic as you please for me in endorsing the telescopic lenses—I never knew there was so much in the world to see."

Presumably Mrs. Macy wore these glasses in the privacy of her home. They were hardly ornamental. Robert Irwin described them as "a sort of miniature pair of opera glasses attached to spectacle holders about one inch from front to back, rather heavy, and of course very conspicuous. Few people would want to be seen on the street with them."

In the years after World War II manufacturing techniques using plastic in place of glass made high-magnification spectacles lighter in weight and more acceptable. At the same time, optical firms began to produce a greatly widened range of microscopic and telescopic devices and a few forward-looking agencies for the blind began experimenting with optical aids for clients who had some residual vision. One of the pioneers was the Industrial Home for the Blind in Brooklyn, which instituted a low-vision clinic in 1953 and reported, in a follow-up study of its first five hundred clients, that optical aids had enabled a sizable number to get or keep jobs or, in the case of students, to manage academic studies more successfully. The study made clear, however, that there was little magic in any such program. Not all eye conditions could be helped, and among those that did respond, a key factor was client motivation.

At the same time one of the problems of all groups rendering low-vision services concerned the professional tensions and rivalries between ophthalmologists (medical doctors who treat eye diseases) and optometrists (non-medical specialists in refraction and correction of visual defects). Most of the former, oriented to medical or surgical treatment of eye problems, found it economically unfeasible to invest time in fitting special lenses and training patients in their use. Nor were they, in many instances, as knowledgeable about the potentialities of such optical aids as optometrists. Harry J. Spar, then assistant director of IHB, who served as a consultant on blinded veterans, summed up the situation when, in 1953, he wrote the VA's chief of physical medicine and rehabilitation that IHB's low vision clinic had

> found a number of instances in which ophthalmologists have indicated that lenses could not be helpful and in which spectacular help has resulted from the work of the optometrist. If the fitting of lenses to blinded veterans is left to the judgment of the ophthalmologist, I am afraid that many of them will not receive the help that may be available to them through the use of special lenses. I am afraid, too, that if the employment of an optometrist is left to the discretion of medical personnel, it is not likely to materialize.

One of the minor projects undertaken by the Committee on Sensory Devices before it wound up was a small optical aids survey conducted by the Dartmouth Eye Institute. The survey's major conclusion, Dr. Corner reported, was "that the possibility of designing better reading glasses of relatively high power, and projection magnifiers which throw images of print upon a screen for convenient reading should be seriously investigated." Four prototype projection magnifiers were subsequently built under CSD contract and sent to the Perkins School for the Blind for testing. "There is no doubt that the projection magnifier will be useful," Dr. Corner said after the tests were completed.

One such device, the Megascope, was designed by the Foundation's technical staff in 1953 and built to its specifications under a $21,000 appropriation for tooling and the manufacture of 100 units. The machine, a table-top unit, consisted of a tray on which reading matter was placed face down. Magnified 12 to 25 times, the print was projected on a lighted screen facing the viewer, who used an adjustable frame to move the material to be read from side to side and front to back. The first model sold out the year it came out; later models featured various operating improvements and lower prices.

The Megascope was one of several dozen optical aids—hand-held, stationary and illuminated magnifiers, pocket telescopes, monoculars, lenses of all types, light-occluding devices, etc.—that the Foundation displayed at an international congress of ophthalmologists in 1954. It was the first time such a collection had been put on view for the medical eye specialists, and it had a considerable impact. Ritter, who organized and managed the display, reported that a number of ophthalmologists

> insisted on ordering an assortment of magnifiers on the spot. Others expressed the determination to persuade agencies for the blind in their home communities to set up "seeing aid centers" where the hand magnifiers could be tried out. Still others told of plans to establish full-blown low vision clinics to work intensively on the problems.

This swelling wave of interest, together with the reports emerging from the local agencies which had begun low-vision services, led the Foundation in 1954 to embark on a three-year project of clinical investigation and evaluation of optical aids. A committee of ophthalmologists, optometrists and optical research specialists was organized with Dr. Richard E. Hoover as coordinator. Their aim was to gather data for a manual detailing principles and procedures for the treatment of low-vision disabilities. This would be accomplished, the Foundation's annual report for 1953–54 explained, "by stimulating the formation of low vision clinics in some medical schools and hospitals where uniform levels of treatment and methods of collecting data may be employed." The hope was not for "sight restoration in the ordinary sense" but to "find the best methods of using residual sight up to its maximum."

A year later the Foundation reported that it had been invited to exhibit optical aids before numerous medical groups, and that 3,000 copies of a pamphlet on the subject had been distributed. Indeed, said the 1954–55 annual report, such was the pace and degree of interest shown that the original three-year program might be completed in half that time.

The promise implicit in this optimistic start was never fully realized. Problems, perhaps not adequately anticipated, arose over sponsorship and control of low-vision clinics. Ophthalmologists wanted them located in hospital outpatient departments; this, as Spar had predicted, tended to exclude or downgrade the participation of the non-medical optometrist. On the other side, agencies for the blind had difficulty enlisting the cooperation of the medical eye specialist because of his preference for hospital settings. There were also disputes over the people to be served by the clinics.

Some of these vexing issues were reflected in a policy statement the Optical Aids Research Committee issued in December 1957. It said that a low-vision service "should be available to all age groups of blind persons—not just those who seem to be employable" and that such a service "should not be so closely identified with charity that persons who can pay . . . will not use it; neither should it be so prohibitive in price that its services cannot be purchased for the benefit of those less able to pay for it." On the last point, the statement added:

> Because optical aids are associated with rehabilitation of "blind" persons, there is an assumption that all such persons are dependent upon and entitled to a free service provided by the community. This is not always true. . . . it is hoped and believed that in the future the majority of persons with severely defective vision will receive proper fitting and follow-up services through their private practitioners.

The same walking-on-eggs approach was reflected in the carefully worded handling of the question of auspices. After naming four possible locations for optical aids services—hospital, medical arts center, agency for the blind or "any other publicly or privately maintained clinical setting where community professional resources are assembled"—the statement said that the Foundation "implies no arbitary preference for any of the foregoing settings. . . . The decision regarding sponsorship and physical location of an optical aids service and all that it entails calls for community consensus and action."

It was just about the time of this statement that optical aids clinics were approved by the federal government as components of the overall vocational rehabilitation program, and about 30 such clinics were rapidly established all over the country. With this development, the Foundation felt its pilot task had been concluded; what remained was primarily a job of medical education and stimulation. On this basis, an agreement was reached in 1960 with the National Society for the Prevention of Blindness; they would take over the national program in low-vision services, including the evaluation and distribution of optical aids. However, Barnett assured his trustees, the Foundation's interest in optical aids would "always remain high. Its function as a catalytic agent has served the nation well; its role in the future will be one of constant vigilance."

A dozen years later, that vigilance brought the question of low-vision services back onto the Foundation's priority lists. Many of the clinics were functioning at a low level; some existed in name only, while others were only open for brief hours at long intervals. Toward the end of 1972 negotiations were going on toward the possibility of a tripartite effort, under which the National Society for the Prevention of Blindness would continue to promote knowledge and use of optical aids in the medical and health professions, the National Accreditation Council would evolve an up-to-date set of standards for low-vision services, and the Foundation would set about stimulating a nationwide network of delivery systems that would embrace both the fitting of optical aids and the accompanying training and follow-up services which experience had shown to be essential elements in vision rehabilitation.

Coincidental, but aptly symbolic of the Foundation's reentry into the field of low-vision activity, was the fact that its 1972–73 aids and appliances catalog featured a new optical aid, a successor to the Megascope. The Optiscope was a portable illuminated optical enlarger that produced four-power magnification in color or black and white on a polarizing screen at a price of $295. Other projection magnifiers were also on the market, including closed circuit television setups, but they were far more expensive.

If enlargement of type by means of an optical device could make printed matter accessible to some legally blind persons, could not the same results be achieved by pre-enlarging the print?

So far as children were concerned, an affirmative answer had been found as early as 1915 when Robert Irwin, then supervisor of classes for blind children attending Cleveland public schools, organized a non-profit firm to publish textbooks in half-inch-high type. He moved the enterprise to his home in New Jersey when he came east to work for the Foundation. Never a large-scale operation (Irwin told people he conducted it as a sort of hobby), it had a catalog of some 70 titles for first grade through junior high and sales of about $10,000 a year when Irwin retired and the firm was liquidated.

A logical source for large type textbooks was the American Printing House for the Blind, because of its receipt of annual federal subsidies for the production of educational materials for blind children. The Printing House began regular publication of such books when its plant facilities were expanded in 1947; in the 1972 fiscal year it produced some 45,000 copies of close to 500 titles for use in residential schools and day classes for visually impaired children.

The hope long entertained by educators that commercial publishers would find it economically feasible to enter the field of large-type publishing began to be realized in the late Forties when a Pittsburgh firm, Stanwix House, published a few children's titles. However, it was not until the mid-Sixties, when photoenlarging and offset printing techniques brought production costs within reach, that large-type books for adult readers made their appearance. The first, John F. Kennedy's *Profiles in Courage*, was produced in an 18-point edition by Keith Jennison Books in 1965. By 1970 there were 1,500 adult and children's titles listed in *Books in Print*, and a Library of Congress reference circular listed more than 40 producers of large-type reading matter. Slightly less than half of these were trade book publishers; the balance were non-profit agencies, religious publishing houses, photoenlarging and microfilm services, and some periodicals. *The New York Times*, which began issuance of its *Large Type Weekly* in 1967, claimed 14,500 readers in 1972. A large-type edition of selected articles from the monthly *Reader's Digest* had a 1972 circulation of 5,000.

One of the findings of a 1966 study made by the New York Public Library under a grant from the United States Office of Education was that books in large print attracted not only legally blind persons but many others with "tired eyes," particularly the aging. The initial study, which placed 75 different book titles in three major branch libraries, evoked so much reader response that the federal grant was renewed for a second year to increase the number of titles and extend the service to additional branches. Large-type books were included in the National Accreditation Council's *Standards for Production of Reading Materials for the Blind and Visually Handicapped* issued in 1970, with criteria listed for typography, design, binding, paper, etc.

"Sometimes it seems no limit is in sight for the uses of large print books," Robert S. Bray of the Library of Congress wrote in 1971. He did not have in mind, he added, the particular use reputedly made by a certain Mr. Twichell. This man was a felon who, according to an anecdote related by Bray in an article in the *Large Print Journal,*

> complained to prison authorities that the print in his Bible was too small, and asked that a druggist friend be allowed to bring him another in larger type. The friend saturated the pages with corrosive sublimate which Mr. Twichell rolled into balls, and with the aid of water, swallowed them. Unfortunately, Mr. Twichell had no further need of any kind of reading material after that.

The economic factors—high unit cost and marketing difficulties—which kept optical aids and large-type books from reaching potential users among the great proportion of legally blind persons who had some degree of residual vision were even more evident when it came to the smallest sector of the blind population: those who were also deaf. When the Foundation announced in 1971 that it would mount a major effort to close the gap between producers and consumers of aids for the blind, there was no thought that there could ever be a commercially sustainable market for appliances designed specifically for the deaf-blind. As of 1972 there were only a few, one of which had been in regular production for 20 years: the Tellatouch.

Its history was an interesting example of retrograde progression. As will be seen in a later chapter, the Foundation's major efforts on behalf of the deaf-blind got under way in the mid-Forties after a number of abortive starts. When, at about the same time, the decision was made to launch a research laboratory, one of the projects listed for exploration was "an electric conversation board . . . a device which would make possible the carrying on of a conversation with the deaf-blind." The concept was a relatively simple one. A sighted person would sit facing a typewriter-like keyboard on which he would type his message, and the machine would translate the message electrically, letter by letter, into braille symbols which would surface on a plate at the back of the machine where a deaf-blind person could feel them with a fingertip.

A prototype was worked out by Kleber and later modified by Witcher. In field testing, however, this model, known as the Electro-braille Communicator, had a number of operating flaws and it was withdrawn from the market in 1952. Both Kleber and Witcher were gone from the Foundation by then, but Tolman tackled the problem and finally solved it by changing the construction principle from electrical to mechanical. Since the "electro" element was gone, a new name was needed. Rechristened the Tellatouch, the device helped end social isolation for hundreds of deaf-blind children and adults.

In the version distributed in 1972 the Tellatouch had a four-bank keyboard. The top three banks held the inkprint alphabet and numerals; the bottom bank, consisting of six braille keys arranged as in a braillewriter, made it possible for a blind person to send messages through the machine to one who was deaf-blind.

The Tellatouch and other Foundation-made appliances were sold at the cost of materials and direct labor. The initial practice of pricing aids and appliances below overall cost—i.e., without taking into account salaries, handling charges or overhead—began to be modified in 1959 when a budget review showed a deficit of $80,000 on gross annual sales of $160,000. Although the trustees formally reaffirmed at that time that "whatever the cost to the agency, this service activity should be continued as a vital and needed service to the blind," mounting sales and correspondingly climbing deficits in the ensuing years prompted a decision, in 1964, not to go on providing discounts on convenience sales of unadapted commercial items but to charge the regular retail price, to add a 20 percent charge to the wholesale cost of adapted items provided this surcharge did not bring the price up over the retail price of the same item in unadapted form, and to add a 20 percent markup for packaging, postage, and overhead to the production cost of Foundation-manufactured devices which had no commercial equivalent.

This move helped, but did not solve, the deficit problem, which came to $400,000 in the decade of the Sixties. Beginning in 1967, an effort was made to restrict sales to mail orders and discontinue the over-the-counter retail operation which, while representing less than 10 percent of the sales volume, was costly in terms of wages and overhead. Local agencies for the blind were offered attractive discounts on catalog items, but the offer failed to gain sufficient response and in 1970 Richard H. Migel, chairman of the Business Advisory Committee, reported that the upshot of explorations to establish suitable retail outlets elsewhere was that the "new location is beside our front door." Moving the over-the-counter salesroom from an upper floor to the Robert B. Irwin Room on the ground floor also mitigated one of the earlier difficulties, that of ushering blind customers through the maze of buildings that made up the Foundation complex.

Although break-even status for aids and appliances was not yet in sight in 1972, annual deficits had been reduced to some extent and the Foundation board remained convinced that the importance of this service to blind people outweighed the prospect of continuing losses. One factor in the smaller deficits was Congressional passage, in 1967, of new postal regulations which expanded the free mailing privileges long in existence for reading matter for the blind to include special devices and equipment sold at or below cost.

The 1972–73 catalog of aids and appliances, with its more than 300 items ranging in price from a wire loop needle threader (10 cents) to a diamond-dial self-winding gold braille watch complete with 14-karat Florentine finish gold bracelet ($352.95), was expected to produce sales in excess of $500,000. Computerized mailing lists and inventory controls helped keep down the costs of handling the high volume of business. Although the *Outlook,* now a professional journal, had long since discontinued "The Suggestion Box" as a monthly feature, the *Ziegler*

Magazine and other periodicals continued to inform their blind readers of the availability of new or different items through a column regularly supplied by the manager of the Foundation's Aids and Appliances Division. Following Ritter's departure, this position was occupied until 1966 by Arthur Keller; in 1972 the post was held by Ira Kaplan, who had taken it on in 1968.

The future course of the aids and appliance service will be influenced by the thrust toward moving the products of biomedical technology into the market place and the publication, some time in 1973, of the IRIS international catalog, which will list and describe some 1,100 devices of all types actually in production in 18 countries. Some of these have long been the objects of international exchange, with the Foundation both importing and exporting items from and to foreign organizations for the blind. The exchange process also embraced ideas and technology. For example the Foundation's research staff kept in steady touch with James C. Swail, a blind scientist associated with the National Research Council of Canada, who in 25 years produced or adapted close to a hundred instruments and devices, including his own version of an ultrasonic obstacle detector, Milton Graham and Leslie Clark reported in 1972 that in Western Europe research projects dealing with visual impairment had tripled in five years; in England alone, 34 such programs were under way.

There are those who believe that development of a workable visual prosthesis is only ten or twenty years away. Others are less sanguine. Still, as one psychologist put it: "The door is opening wider, no doubt, but we remain on the doorstep, full of hope."

22

One World

As the *R.M.S. Lusitania* neared the coast of Ireland en route from New York to Southampton in May 1915, a single torpedo from a German submarine made a perfect hit. In 18 minutes the liner sank; with her went 1,200 human beings, passengers and crew. Another 800 managed to keep afloat in the icy waters until rescue vessels arrived. Among these was George Alexander Kessler, an American businessman, who clung to an oar for seven hours.

During his long vigil, the fifty-one-year-old Kessler made a bargain with fate. Should he survive, he would devote his energies and his wealth to helping the victims of war. He had nothing specific in mind at the time, but during his convalescent stay in London, he heard of the work Arthur Pearson had begun at St. Dunstan's for the British war blind and made up his mind that this was the cause he would adopt for the people of all the countries fighting the Kaiser.

A less likely candidate for the role of philanthropic savior could hardly be imagined. Had the term "international jet set" existed during those years, George Kessler would have been one of its conspicuous members. He was known on both sides of the Atlantic as "the champagne king" and "the prince of the wine agents"—royal sobriquets he had earned during a flamboyant and spectacularly successful career as international distributor for the French winery, Moet & Chandon. "He had the world's greatest flair for publicity," a journalist was to say in reviewing Kessler's colorful career. His instinct for marketing was equally keen. He concentrated his efforts on the logical customers for champagne, entertaining high society at spectacular dinner parties that were designed to set tongues wagging. At one such event a Venetian theme was created by flooding a hotel ballroom to create an artificial lagoon stocked with live swans, ducks and salmon trout. A hundred white doves fluttered overhead as the twenty-four guests were conveyed by gondola to a floating platform where they dined while listening to arias by Enrico Caruso and two other opera singers.

Kessler was also an extraordinarily lucky man. He was in San Francisco at the time of that city's disastrous earthquake in 1906 and escaped death by walking out of a business conference shortly before the building it was in collapsed. In Chicago, on another occasion, he left a hotel minutes before it went up in flames. The *Lusitania* experience was his third narrow escape.

Kessler's society connections stood him in excellent stead as he went about making good on his vow. The likeliest place to raise money for the Allied war blind was in the United States, which, not yet a combatant, was prospering mightily from the sale of munitions and other goods. Six months after the *Lusitania* episode, Kessler and his wife, the former Cora Parsons, organized the B.F.B. (British, French, Belgian) Permanent Blind Relief War Fund and braved another Atlantic crossing to open a campaign. They seeded the drive with $50,000 of their own funds; Mrs. Kessler, it was reported, sold Tiffany and Company one of her jewels, a piece cut from the Cullinan diamond, to start the drive.

The names of those Kessler enlisted to form the American committee for the Fund were testimony to his social and business connections. They included Mrs. John Astor, Mrs. Cooper Hewitt, August Belmont, Dr. Nicholas Murray Butler, William H. Crocker of the San Francisco family, Myron T. Herrick, Otto H. Kahn, Frank A. Munsey, Elihu Root, E. S. Stotesbury of the Philadelphia family, and William K. Vanderbilt.

Similarly, eminent committees were established in England, France, and Belgium, both to raise funds and supervise their distribution. Royal patronage was accorded the committees in Britain and Belgium; in France the President of the Republic granted his seal of approval. After the United States entered the war in 1917, President Woodrow Wilson accepted the honorary presidency of the Fund's American section.

A variety of campaign techniques—mail appeals, benefit performances, collection boxes, subscription books—were employed to capture American dollars for the cause. Leading artists were persuaded to contribute dramatic illustrations for brochures and posters. To step up the pace Kessler arranged for one of St. Dunstan's earliest graduates, Sergeant-Major Robert Middlemiss, to tour the United States and address audiences at the benefit entertainments. A mustachioed veteran of 17 years of service in the British Army who had been blinded in battle at Gallipoli, Middlemiss personified the confident self-reliance rehabilitation could produce in a blinded soldier.

By early 1917, when more than $400,000 had been collected, the United States declared war on Germany and the Fund's already lengthy name became the A.B.F.B. Permanent Blind Relief War Fund, the first initial standing for "American." At this point it also found itself engaged in a distasteful squabble with a competitive drive, the Committee for Men Blinded in Battle. This other group had been organized by Winifred Holt, the dynamic and resourceful woman who, with her sister Edith, had taken up the cause of blind people soon after the turn of the century.

In 1906 the Holt sisters had founded the Lighthouse (the New York Association for the Blind) in New York City and encouraged the formation of similar local service agencies throughout the United States. Soon after the outbreak of the war,

Winifred Holt went to France to work for the French soldiers blinded at the front. She established the *Phare* (Lighthouse) *de France* in Paris and helped reorganize an existing agency in Bordeaux into a *Phare* as well. To raise funds for these rehabilitation units, the Committee for Men Blinded in Battle was established in the United States at about the same time as Kessler's group. Its sponsors were no less distinguished than the others; the daughter of publisher Henry Holt was not lacking in influential friends.

Since the two groups operated in different ways, they could have coexisted without rancor were it not for some imperious assertions made by Winifred during an American campaign tour for her committee in the winter of 1916–1917—assertions that were at once played up, and probably somewhat exaggerated, in press reports. The technical grain of truth in her quoted remarks was that the *Phare de France* was the only American organization giving direct service to the French war blind. This was so; Kessler's organization did not, at that time, conduct programs under its own name, but worked through locally-operated agencies in France, Belgium, and England.

In rebuttal to the Holt charges, the A.B.F.B. Fund listed the seven French agencies and schools for the blind to which it had already remitted $60,000. Allocation of these grants was under the direction of the French committee appointed by the president of France. The committee was headed by the playwright Eugene Brieux, a member of the French Academy, and its membership was made up of a former foreign minister of France, the president of the Paris Chamber of Commerce, the head of a leading French bank, the owner of the giant Creusot steel works, the grand chancellor of the Legion of Honor, and other impeccable dignitaries. In Britain, the allocation committee under the patronage of Queen Alexandra was chaired by Arthur Pearson, with St. Dunstan's the major beneficiary. (At a later point, the American end of the program shared in the $2 million ultimately collected by the Fund; substantial sums were given to the Red Cross for its work at Evergreen, and grants were also made to the United States Blind Veterans of World War I.)

With the signing of the Armistice in November 1918, many of the American war relief organizations considered their jobs done. But the A.B.F.B. Fund took the word "Permanent" in its title seriously. Need among Europe's war-blinded had not disappeared. Instead of liquidating, the Fund was incorporated in New York under a slightly different name with George A. Kessler as president. On the list of directors of the new corporation appeared a name new in work for the blind: William Nelson Cromwell.

Co-founder of a prestigious law firm, Cromwell had earned an international reputation for financial and legal wizardry in corporate reorganization; one journalist dubbed him "the physician of Wall Street." His most spectacular legal feat involved the prolonged and complex negotiations that resulted in the construction of the Panama Canal. Representing the French owners of the franchise to the selected route, which they sold to the United States for $40 million in 1902, Cromwell devoted almost eight years of his life to what Arthur H. Dean, his biographer, called a "case that was all but lost." The successful outcome brought Cromwell additional French clients and he began to spend more and more time in

France. During most of World War I he remained in his Paris home, lending his skills and much of his wealth to war relief efforts and, following the Armistice, to reconstruction measures for hard-hit sections of the French economy.

A born romantic, he was particularly proud of the Lafayette Escadrille, the volunteer corps of American aviators who flew for France before General John J. Pershing arrived with the American Expeditionary Force. He was a prime mover in the erection of the white marble temple in Paris where the 67 members of the Escadrille lost in combat are buried, and he personally endowed a fund for the memorial's maintenance in perpetuity.

William Nelson Cromwell, who left an estate of some $20 million when he died in 1948, was not born to wealth. Orphaned at an early age when his father was killed in the Civil War, he grew up in Brooklyn, New York, where his mother brought up her children "in Spartan living under extreme financial difficulties." On graduation from high school, he found a job as an accountant in a railroad office. Three years later he went to work for a law firm whose senior partner, Algernon Sydney Sullivan, encouraged him to attend Columbia Law School. He was admitted to the New York Bar in 1876. In 1879 the old firm was dissolved and Cromwell, only twenty-five years old, joined the much older Sullivan in a new legal partnership whose gross income, that first year, was $22,500. It was a modest beginning for Sullivan and Cromwell, which grew to be one of the world's largest law firms.

Cromwell never forgot the poverty of his youth. According to his biographer: "To the end of his life he carefully picked up paper clips or rubber bands on the floor, turned out electric lights and was saving and frugal in his habits." On the other hand, his personal life style was opulent. He spent little time in his office, conducting his business for the most part from a Manhattan mansion whose rooms, crowded with tapestries, paintings, and sculpture, were virtually museums of mid-Victoriana, or from an equally luxurious home in Paris. His appearance was also distinctive. John Foster Dulles, one of his law partners, described him as "an impressive figure with his shaggy white locks, his florid complexion and sparkling eyes."

It was this singular personality who succeeded to the presidency of the Permanent Blind Relief War Fund following the death of George Kessler on September 13, 1920, and it was he who directed a fundamental change in the Fund's program soon thereafter. Kessler's idea had been that the Fund would function in France and other parts of the Continent somewhat along the lines of St. Dunstan's in England, providing vocational training and education, supplementing inadequate government pensions, buying homes for those who had been taught hand crafts and establishing central purchasing and marketing facilities for their output.

Cromwell thought along different lines. Such rehabilitation programs, he believed, should be maintained by the governments and philanthropies of the respective countries; American funds should be reserved for those services no single agency could manage. Among the activities begun by the Fund while hostilities were still under way was braille printing. This, Cromwell felt, was the sort of service that could benefit all of Europe's war-blinded. But he encountered considerable initial resistance to the proposal that the Fund's resources be used for the production of braille literature and music. Opponents pointed out that few of the war-blinded could read braille or were interested in mastering it. That, replied Cromwell, might be true at the moment, but it would change. Supply would create demand.

The next year was spent in transforming a 64-room rented mansion near the Arc de Triomphe into what became one of the largest, best-equipped, and most up-to-date braille printing houses of its day. Cromwell personally contributed $30,000 to renovate the premises at 74 rue Lauriston and by early 1923 the plant was ready and its 45 employees, two-thirds of them blind, began production. Two years later some 5 million pages of braille had been printed, five periodicals were being issued in three languages (French, English, and Serbian), and a large quantity of braille music was coming off the presses.

One fact soon emerged: distribution of the plant's output need not and should not be limited to those blinded in the hostilities. Once the printing plates had been prepared, additional impressions could be made. With this recognition, the scope of what had been a war relief organization was enlarged to embrace blind people all over the world. The broadened purposes were reflected in a change of name: American Braille Press for War and Civilian Blind, Inc.

Under its amended certificate of incorporation, the Paris printing house enlarged its publishing program to issue periodicals and books in three more languages (Italian, Roumanian, and Polish) and branched out into collateral fields: manufacturing maps, diagrams and games, working on improved braillewriting machines, researching and testing various other educational and practical devices for blind users. In these respects, it was the European counterpart of the American Foundation for the Blind, and the two organizations cooperated closely.

One of its most substantial contributions was leadership in convening the international conference that established a worldwide braille music code in 1929. Two years later the theme of international cooperation was reinforced when American Braille Press joined the American Foundation for the Blind in co-sponsoring the World Conference on Work for the Blind, the first such event ever held on American soil.

Before World War I there had been several triennial international conferences of workers for the blind, the last of these in England in 1914. Once past the initial phase of postwar reconstruction, European leaders began to think of another such conclave. Robert Irwin was made aware of this desire when he went abroad in 1925 and, in his capacity as president of the AAWB at the time, he mentioned the subject at that year's convention. At the next biennial AAWB meeting, he brought up the question again. A committee was appointed to look into it, and conferred with a parallel committee named by the AAIB, which endorsed the idea when it met in 1928. In December of that year a letter went out to leading workers for the blind all over the world, asking whether they would be interested in an international conference to be held in New York in the spring of 1931.

Reporting to the AAWB when it next met in the summer of 1929, Irwin said that many favorable replies had been received although "there was a strong feeling in most quarters that the high cost of traveling would be a serious obstacle."

However, he informed the delegates, he had "taken up this matter with certain persons interested not only in the blind, but also in movements to bring about greater international good will," with the result that "sufficient funds were pledged to the American Foundation for the Blind to warrant it in undertaking to meet the expenses of this project." He had gone even further. Foundation president Migel had arranged with Senator George H. Moses of the Foreign Relations Committee to introduce a joint Congressional resolution authorizing President Hoover to call a world conference on work for the blind. The invitation would be extended through diplomatic channels: "It is hoped that in this way many countries will be induced to send official delegates at governmental expense."

A budget of $30,000 had been projected for the United States' share of the conference costs; the "certain persons" promising financial support were John D. Rockefeller, Jr., who pledged $10,000, and M.C. Migel, $5,000. The Foundation had budgeted an additional $10,000 of its own funds. Later, smaller sums came from others, including a personal contribution from Herbert Hoover. As is often the case with budgets, the anticipated cost underestimated the actual need, the final expense totalling $46,000. William Nelson Cromwell, who was also among the early contributors, responded to a last-minute S.O.S. for deficit financing by sending a messenger with a $2,500 check a few days before the conference was scheduled to begin.

The Congressional resolution was finally voted in February 1930 and the following month saw invitations go out from the United States Government to 50 foreign governments. Acceptances were received from 39 nations, although 7 later dropped out. The final number of delegates from outside the United States came to 109; they were accompanied by 36 others: wives, escorts, or guests. It proved to be the most broadly representative gathering of specialists in work for the blind that had yet been held.

The conference program was planned to cover an 18-day period, opening with a reception on the evening of April 13, 1931. There would then be four days of meetings in New York City, following which the overseas delegates would set out on a ten-day tour of various schools, institutions, and agencies for the blind in the eastern part of the United States. At the tour's conclusion the delegates would reassemble in New York for two days of summary and final action.

This elaborate plan had been worked out by a multinational program committee which met in Hamburg in May 1930. One of its decisions was to extend a number of additional invitations to supplement the delegations named by the respective governments, concentrating on people who could contribute the fruits of practical experience in work for the blind. The committee was chaired by an able Frenchman, Georges Raverat, secretary-general of the American Braille Press, who was already a prominent figure in work for the blind and was destined to play a heroic role in the years to come.

Raverat had been George Kessler's secretary before World War I. A soldier in the French Army, he was in a military hospital recovering from a wound when news came of the sinking of the *Lusitania* and his former employer's survival. Invalided out of military service, Raverat was reemployed by Kessler, this time to supervise the European operation of the Permanent Blind Relief War Fund. In the course of the Fund's development and subsequent emergence as the American Braille Press, Raverat came to acquire an intimate knowledge of all European work for the blind. An urbane and handsome figure, he was a well-organized executive endowed with tact and adroitness in human relations.

The logistics of the conference plan were not simple. Many of the overseas delegates were blind; some had little or no command of English. Their American hosts had to cope with innumerable details in arranging for the visitors to tour Boston, Philadelphia, Washington, Pittsburgh, and Cleveland with a sufficient number of American delegates to act as escorts but not so many as to overshadow the foreigners or tax the hospitality of the organizations and institutions they were to visit.

It all went off brilliantly. There was even room for the added amenity of a White House reception, arranged by Helen Keller through an exchange of correspondence with Mrs. Herbert Hoover. The language barrier at the conference sessions was overcome by means of a newly invented simultaneous translation system, the Filene-Finlay Translator, which made its American debut on this occasion.

The 558-page volume of *Proceedings of the World Conference on Work for the Blind,* published by the Foundation in 1932, still makes absorbing reading. To review the texts of the formal presentations and the transcripts of the ensuing discussions is to pinpoint both the gratifying progress achieved since 1931 and the problems that remain as grievous in 1972 as they were four decades earlier. There is poignancy, too, in noting how much of what was good and promising in 1931 lay shattered after World War II, some of it never to be restored.

Almost every European country made a substantive contribution to the conference content. The director of Vienna's Israelitisches Blindeninstitut gave a scholarly paper on "Psychological Problems of the Pre-School Blind Child." Questions of sensory perception were dealt with by the chairman of the Norwegian Federation of the Blind. The head of a school in Bordeaux presented his views on the education of young blind children. Vocational training principles to guard against older students' becoming "strangers to life" were set forth by the director of a Westphalian institution in a paper that provoked a heated debate on the ever-touchy subject of institutional education. Another German educator took on the subject of education for the professions. Italy's methods of preparing teachers of the blind were outlined by the director of Rome's teacher training school.

The employment section heard descriptions of Sweden's services for blind home workers, of how workshop programs were managed in Birmingham and in Glasgow, and of Canada's experience in placing blind workers in open industry. The president of the Italian Association of the Blind praised Benito Mussolini's government for requiring that certain government orders be assigned to workshops for the blind. Professor Pierre Villey, the influential secretary-general of the Valentin Haüy Association in Paris, described his country's decades of success in developing jobs for blind people in musical occupations but noted worriedly that "the sudden and extraordinary development of mechanical music and the radio" now constituted a serious threat to live musicians.

The only section in which American speakers predominated was that dealing with technical aids and resources. Papers were given by Edward E. Allen of Perkins on museums for the blind, Frank C. Bryan of Howe Memorial Press on braille printing methods, and Lucille Goldthwaite on library services. The beginnings made in Latin America to produce braille literature in Spanish were described by the executive of a Mexican agency. A Polish psychologist traced the history of the inventions and devices that enabled blind people to gain an education and earn a livelihood.

A separate session was devoted to conditions in the Orient. The unique, centuries-old status of blind people in Japan was depicted by Umaji Akiba, the director of the Tokyo School for the Blind. He detailed the up-to-date programs offered by his school to prepare children for the occupations traditionally followed by the Japanese blind but noted that the ancient custom of training through apprenticeship to private masters continued simultaneously. Delegates listening to Akiba's talk felt as though the pages of history were being rolled back when he said:

> Massage, shampooing, acupuncture and moxibustion are also taught by private masters who take apprentices. . . . The years of apprenticeship range from three to seven, according to age and attainment. The apprentices receive no education but, on the other hand, get plenty of work to do, and their condition is no better than that of a day laborer. In the country, these poor apprentices, even today, are sent out each evening by their masters to herald their presence by shouting or blowing on a small whistle in the streets for patients. It is heartrending, indeed, to hear their melancholy cries in the dead of night, particularly of a cold winter night.

Of equally exotic interest was the report given by George B. Fryer, superintendent of Shanghai's Institution for the Chinese Blind, who outlined the situation not only in China but in other, more primitive countries of the Far East. "The civilization of these countries, coming as it does out of hoary antiquity, is unique in itself and it is almost impossible to understand the customs, manner[s], religions and modes of thought of the people, even after long years of residence," he began. Religion and superstition

> play an important part in the lives of these peoples. A person is blind or deformed because the gods will it so—a sort of retribution for the sins of past generations—and any help or assistance that would tend to ease his punishment is quite contrary to practice, beyond a few cents with which to keep the body alive and so prolong his suffering. For this reason, the blind are looked upon with pity, but ostracized from society and forced to become pariahs and parasites upon the community in which they live. Being fatalists to a certain extent, they make the best of it and suffer in solitary silence, dragging out their darkened, weary lives, a burden to themselves and to all around.

No prevention of blindness programs existed in these countries, although much of the visual loss in their populations was readily preventable through simple sanitation and treatment measures. In China, political turmoil added to the complications. In an emotional peroration, Fryer expressed the hope that measures to alleviate these "pitiable and unenviable conditions" would one day come into being despite "the lack of funds, the lack of trained teachers and helpers, the ignorance of the masses and even the nonchalance of the governments themselves."

The theme of prevention was the subject of two other papers. "The first right of a blind person is not to be blind," declared the Spanish physician who headed an agency in Malaga where, he said, 77 percent of those without sight need not be so. Winifred Hathaway, associate director of the National Society for the Prevention of Blindness, described the special provisions that enabled partially sighted children to be educated in American day schools.

The liveliest controversy of the conference arose when Captain Ian Fraser of St. Dunstan's and Paul Guinot, secretary-general of the French National Federation of Civilian Blind, gave back-to-back papers expounding their respective views on the role of the state in relation to its blind citizens.

Fraser took the position that a basically sound system was provided by the British Blind Persons Act of 1920, which combined national pension grants with shared national and local financing of service programs conducted under local administration, often in partnership with voluntary philanthropy. Guinot denounced private philanthropy as a failure which had led to "incoherence, confusion, disorder—fruits of incompetence or ignorance" in work for the blind. Government, he said, had a legal and moral obligation to insure the welfare of its blind citizens. This obligation would be met only if blind people organized as a pressure group to secure their social rights. He proposed the formation of an international federation of associations of the blind who could "unite simultaneously and ask for the recognition of their own sacred rights" in a worldwide activist program.

Examined in detail, the specific measures urged by Guinot were not unreasonable, merely ahead of their time. He asked for compulsory free education of blind children under state-approved standards; vocational training, placement services and employment priorities for blinded adults; a system of disability pensions; tax exemptions; health services and other forms of social protection. Most of the delegates agreed, in principle, with the justice of these proposals, many of which were ultimately implemented in France and elsewhere. What aroused irritation was Guinot's hostile tone and his passionate insistence at every opportunity that blind people, and only blind people, "claim the right to organize the new work which will lead them to ultimate liberty."

When the delegates reassembled in New York following their ten-day tour they debated the proposal that a permanent body be formed to further future international cooperation. A tentative outline for such a body was submitted and adopted with minor modifications. The new organization was to be called the World Council for the Blind and would be headquartered in Paris. Its membership would begin with one representative from each of the 33 nations whose delegates had attended the conference. There would be an 11-member executive committee, headed by the Council's president and vice-president. William Nelson Cromwell and M.C. Migel were nominated for these respective offices; they were the only Americans on the executive committee, whose nine other members consisted of eight Europeans and one Japanese. Paul Guinot was elected a member, not as a representative of France but as spokesman for the several national associations of blind people.

To get the World Council under way, Cromwell and Migel agreed to underwrite its budget for the first three years at a rate of $15,000 to $20,000 a year. Thereafter, it was hoped, the member nations would be able to finance the work through dues.

Early in the discussions one suggestion had been that the World Council should be under the wing of the American Braille Press. Cromwell vetoed the idea, thinking it better for the new body to be wholly independent. The decision was a prudent one, for this first effort to create a permanent international body in work for the blind never actually took hold.

One reason was the worldwide depression of the Thirties, complicated by the political tensions that brought war at the decade's end. Another reason, at least as compelling, was the issue that had been raised by Guinot. In his authorized biography, Canada's Edwin A. Baker, who had been a delegate and a member of Raverat's program committee, had this comment to make:

> Half of the gathering in New York in 1931 had insisted that the proposed organization could function successfully only if its membership consisted entirely of blind persons. The others believed even more strongly that success depended on the combined efforts of the blind themselves and sighted workers for the blind. It had been on this divergence of philosophy, as well as on the economic situation, that the [World Council] foundered.

It was not until 1949 that postwar conditions settled down sufficiently to make possible the holding of another international assembly of workers for the blind. The Oxford Conference gave birth to a new body that did succeed in achieving permanence, the World Council for the Welfare of the Blind. Many of the people who came to the 1949 meeting were the same ones who had met in New York in 1931, and some of the basic issues they considered were the same. But almost everything else had changed: the geographic and political structures of Europe, Africa and Asia, the plight of their blind people, and the resources available to ameliorate that plight.

One of the effects of the 1931 conference was a major policy change adopted by the American Braille Press that same December. "It is not enough to talk cooperation," the Press said in announcing that it would gradually give up its role as the principal overseas braille publisher and begin, instead, to provide various countries with the equipment they needed to operate their own braille presses. According to an official history of the organization:

> By spring of 1935 the American Braille Press had founded or equipped two printing plants in France, two in Belgium and one each in Poland, Portugal, Yugoslavia, Colombia and Brazil. Periodicals formerly published by the Press were appearing from these printing plants, with financial assistance furnished by the Press. The printing of books had also been taken over by the individual plants, although the publication of music in braille continued at the printing house in Paris as well as the manufacture of stereotyping machines and appliances, games and braille writers.

It was at this time, too, that braille's major competitor, the Talking Book, emerged in the United States. American Braille Press initiated its own research on how recorded literature could fit into the European picture and in 1937 began producing its own Talking Books on flexible aluminum-base discs. But with the Nazi invasion of France in early 1940, these activities were forced underground.

One of the first ordinances passed by the German occupation authorities was that all alien property had to be declared. After the war, Georges Raverat described what he had done:

> I had to comply with it; and, in due time, I filed the necessary reports. It took ten months of the most trying negotiations to get it O.K.'d and at times I must say I didn't feel so very good! I purposely omitted to declare the fifty or more long tons of embossed zinc plates and Talking Book pure copper master discs stored in the basement, although I knew already that the Germans were strenuously endeavoring to obtain this very metal. I realized I was taking chances, but it finally turned out all right, except for many sleepless nights.

Raverat also successfully maneuvered, by means of delicate negotiations with high-placed French officials, to keep the Press offices and equipment intact, despite two Nazi efforts to requisition the premises and a separate attempt to have its braille embossing machinery shipped to Germany. The machinery remained in France, where it was used by the French Union of the War Blind.

Nine months after Paris was liberated in August 1944, war in Europe ended. The devastation left behind was almost unimaginable. In many ways, Europe's blind people were far worse off than other segments of the population. Reports reaching American agencies told of how schools for blind children had been knocked down by bombs, their braille books torn up and used for fuel, their writing slates melted down for metal, their workshop equipment looted or smashed. Blind adults were homeless, penniless; their residences and workshops had been wrecked, the raw materials out of which they had once made salable products were gone and there were none to be had, even with money.

William Nelson Cromwell, ninety one years old at war's end, was no longer in a position to supply the dynamic leadership to get postwar reconstruction under way. At his suggestion, two of his law partners, John Foster Dulles and Eustace Seligman, both of whom were trustees of the American Braille Press, opened negotiations with the American Foundation for the Blind over the possibility of taking over the Press. A member of the Foundation board since 1931, Cromwell felt its experience would be eminently useful in rebuilding the work in Europe.

In September 1945 Migel told the executive committee about the talks that had been held with Dulles and Seligman. The proposed affiliation would not be a drain on the Foundation's funds, he explained, because the Press had sufficient assets to take care of immediate needs.

In short order an affiliation agreement calling for interlocking boards of directors was worked out, and a new name decided upon. American Braille Press was reborn as American Foundation for Overseas Blind, with Cromwell as board chairman, Migel as president, Dulles as first vice-president, Seligman as secretary,

Richard L. Morris as treasurer, and Irwin as executive director. Raverat continued as European director until his retirement in 1953; he died in 1969 at the age of eighty-one.

(Subsequent changes in AFOB officership paralleled changes in the Foundation. Migel resigned the two presidencies in 1946 and was succeeded in both posts by William Ziegler, Jr., who was in turn followed by Jansen Noyes, Jr., and then by John F. Crowley. Cromwell remained as chairman of the board until his death in 1948; the post was subsequently filled by Eustace Seligman. In 1972 it was occupied by Noyes, who held the same office at the Foundation. Dulles remained an AFOB vice-president until his appointment as United States Secretary of State in 1953. Robert Irwin was replaced as executive director of both agencies by M. Robert Barnett. AFOB's other officers in 1972 were Richard H. Migel, vice-chairman of the board; Peter J. Salmon, vice-president; Alexander M. Laughlin, treasurer; and Mitchell Brock, secretary.)

Although the directors in office at the time AFOB was incorporated resolved as a matter of policy that its funds would be used for long-range programs, they recognized that initial priority would have to be given to such basic needs as food, clothing and housing for the hardest-hit segments of Europe's blind communities. True, American and international relief bodies were dispensing relief supplies on a vast scale, but limited mobility made it hard for blind people to get to the distribution centers, and when they did get there, they were often last in line and went away empty-handed. Nor did they command the resources to cope with the black markets that quickly arose for hard-to-get commodities.

Raverat, who visited most of the war areas soon after the end of hostilities, reported that warm clothing for the coming winter was the most urgent need. AFOB's first public appeal, therefore, was in the form of a clothing drive, with numerous American agencies for the blind serving as collection points for new and used garments. Before the end of 1946, some 60,000 pounds of clothing and 100,000 cakes of soap had been shipped to agencies for the blind in France, Belgium, Holland, and Norway.

The haste with which these postwar relief supplies were assembled created certain problems for the European agencies which distributed them. Eric T. Boulter, who was then serving in Greece as director of blind welfare for the UNRRA-affiliated Near East Foundation, recalled:

> We got massive sacks packed with used and repaired shoes; they were supposed to have been tied together in pairs, but most of the time they weren't. You can imagine what it was like to open one of these sacks and find 2,000 shoes, unmatched, all jumbled together. . . . That wasn't our only problem: we needed great powers of persuasion when a Greek peasant woman with feet eight inches wide from years of barefoot work in the fields insisted she could squeeze her feet into four-inch wide shoes because they had gilt ornaments.

Boulter was an Englishman blinded early in the war who had joined the London staff of the Royal National Institute for the Blind following his discharge from St. Dunstan's. Soon after the liberation of Greece he was sent to survey the situation of blind people there and to develop a master plan for education, rehabilitation and training in a nation where there had formerly been few services for the blind. In the three years he spent implementing that plan, he met Helen Keller during her first postwar overseas trip for AFOB. She was so impressed by the competence, integrity, and charm of the young Englishman that she commended him to the attention of Robert Irwin, who made his own postwar survey of Europe's blind in the company of Georges Raverat in the summer of 1947. These two concurred in Helen's high opinion, with the result that, the following year, Boulter joined the European staff of AFOB as Raverat's assistant. He was named field director in 1950, promoted to associate director in 1961, and retired from AFOB service in 1970. In his 22 years with the agency he had traveled nearly half a million miles and visited 60 countries. Retirement saw him returning to his native land, where he became director general of the Royal National Institute for the Blind.

The postwar survey findings provided essential guidelines for AFOB's initial reconstruction efforts. In many places the institutions and facilities that had formerly served blind people were all but gone. Immense quantities of supplies were needed, along with working capital to reinstate local programs. Of perhaps equal importance was the need to rekindle a spirit of hope among agencies for the blind. Not surprisingly, the common hardships of the war years had effected a degree of brotherhood previously absent. In an extensive report, "The Blind of Europe in 1947," Irwin observed:

> The blind are trying to help themselves in France. Among other self-help projects is the National Federation of the Blind. This Federation has 6,000 or more members, has established eight workshops, a convalescent home, a large cooperative, a school of massage, and is now trying to get money for a rehabilitation center. I found the president of the National Federation of the Blind, M. Paul Guinot, one of the most energetic people I have ever worked with. When I first knew him sixteen years ago he was a severe critic of everything being done for the blind in France. Today he has assumed responsibility for helping to make the work for the blind of France more effective and realistic.

Building on this base, AFOB organized a Central Committee for Blind Workers made up of representatives of France's major agencies for the blind, with Guinot at the head. With the help of an initial $10,000 grant, matched by funds raised locally, the committee organized a central purchasing and sales organization for the output of the 3,000 men and women employed in France's workshops for the blind.

The disruption of services in France was more or less duplicated in Belgium, Czechoslovakia, Poland and Austria. One of the saddest losses was the destruction by fire-bombing of the world-famous library of "blindiana" at the Vienna Institute for the Blind. Begun early in the nineteenth century, the library collection had been the repository for thousands of rare volumes and manuscripts. The sole stroke of good fortune was that many of these were duplicated in the library of America's Perkins School for the Blind under an exchange arrangement dating back several decades.

A special set of problems existed in Italy, where a closely knit nationwide system of services for the blind had been built under the Fascist regime. As in other countries, supplies and funds were needed to restore schools and workshops; raging inflation had reduced many formerly self-sustaining blind people to street beggary. A painful dilemma confronted the Italian schools for blind children. They had to comply with the orders of the postwar republican government to destroy textbooks regarded as tainted with Fascist ideology, but the government made no provision to supply the schools with the paper or metal with which approved texts could be produced in braille. AFOB undertook to furnish the needed equipment.

Possibly the most tragic situation of all prevailed in Greece. The sole school for the blind, located in Athens, had a capacity of merely 120. Some of the blind children were also missing one hand or both, the consequence of picking up unexploded grenades or land mines with which the retreating Germans had sown the fields and beaches. The only braille books in Greece were hand-transcribed. Irwin reported that when he visited the Athens school during the summer vacation he found a dozen children in residence:

> These were from Macedonia where guerrilla activities made it dangerous for the pupils to return to their homes. In one room I found four children gathered around a table where a little girl with only one hand was reading aloud from a hand-transcribed volume while the other three blind children were writing with their braille slates from her dictation, making extra copies of the book for use when school opened.

AFOB undertook to assist Eric Boulter in the Near East Foundation's effort to implement a comprehensive plan for the welfare of blind children and adults. It established a braille printing plant in Athens to supply press-made schoolbooks and helped to equip a new school in Salonika for 125 children.

By 1949 many of Europe's essential services for blind people had gained at least a start toward reconstruction, and AFOB began to look at the needs on other continents. The Oxford Conference underscored both the global problems of blindness and the necessity of enlisting the active support of the newly established intergovernmental bodies: the United Nations and its affiliates, UNESCO and UNICEF, the International Labor Organization (ILO), the World Health Organization (WHO). An official consultative relationship was established between these groups and the newly constituted World Council for the Welfare of the Blind, and Boulter, who became secretary-general of the Council when it was incorporated in 1951, was active in establishing contacts with them and their constituent nations. It was at the invitation of such governments that AFOB began the practice of assigning on-the-spot consultants to countries in all parts of the world to help establish services for their blind populations.

One of the first such enterprises was a Middle East pilot demonstration project set up in Cairo, jointly financed and operated by the UN, the Egyptian government, and several non-governmental agencies. The project embraced a comprehensive range: schooling for the young blind, training centers and workshops for adults, a braille printing facility, library and recreational activities, social services and facilities for training professional workers from other Arab countries.

In other parts of the Middle East vocational training centers were established in Jordan and Iran, support was given to schools in Iran, Iraq, Kuwait and Lebanon, a teacher training project was launched in Turkey, home teaching and rehabilitation services were begun in Syria, help was given in opening Israel's first rehabilitation center and in equipping a braille printing plant in Jerusalem. So extensive was the work in this part of the world that, in 1962, AFOB established a regional office in Beirut.

It was the fourth such overseas outpost for the New York-based organization. In addition to the office in Paris, which served Europe and the Near East, a regional headquarters for Latin America was opened in 1957, initially in Chile and later moved to Argentina. The same year saw one established for the Far East, first in Manila and later in Malaysia.

In 1952, work in the Orient was spurred when the Association for the Chinese Blind was merged into AFOB. Founded in 1938 by an American missionary, Edgar H. Rue, the Association had been unable to continue its work on mainland China once the United States refused to recognize the People's Republic after the defeat of the Nationalist Chinese forces. It had transferred its work to Formosa and to South Korea, concentrating on blindness prevention services. When Rue, who had directed its program from the beginning, died in late 1951, the Association's board asked AFOB to take it over.

Toward the end of the Korean war AFOB sent a full-time mission to South Korea, whose blind population was estimated at 70,000. The decision to make available a team of experts to develop a program of education and vocational training in cooperation with the Korean government, the United Nations, and other agencies followed a survey by Boulter, who also proposed that a Far East conference on work for the blind be convened. It was this meeting, held in Tokyo in May 1955, that led to the decision to establish a regional office for the Orient. A second Asian conference was held in Malaya in 1963, this time co-sponsored by the Royal Commonwealth Society for the Blind, a British agency which conducted programs similar to AFOB's in the territories comprising the British Commonwealth.

Latin America presented a different set of problems. For one thing, there was no uniform braille code in the Spanish language. The partnership evolved between the World Council on Work for the Blind and intergovernmental bodies helped bring on an explosive period of progress. The matter of a braille code that could be read in all Spanish-speaking lands was settled at a conference held in Montevideo under UNESCO auspices in December 1951. The way was then open for all blind people in Latin America to share in the educational and vocational advances achieved in other parts of the world. An immediate consequence was the 1953 agreement of AFOB and the Kellogg Foundation to jointly finance establishment of a modern braille printing plant in Mexico City whose output could serve the needs of the Central American republics.

It was only a beginning. In June of the following year AFOB joined in sponsoring the first Pan-American conference on blindness. Held in São Paulo, Brazil, it served as the launching pad for a newly invigorated effort to help the blind people—their number estimated at 400,000—of South and Central America. By the late Fifties constructive activity was under way in a dozen lands, with AFOB acting as technical consultant and, in many instances, supplying financial underpinning for newly emerging programs. The University of Chile inaugurated Latin America's first postgraduate course for teachers of the blind. A new braille printing center was established in Uruguay. A rehabilitation center in Havana expanded its work to provide vocational training and employment in seven trades. AFOB scholarships brought students from Brazil, Guatemala, and Haiti to the United States to study rehabilitation theory and techniques. Equipment for duplicating braille books was supplied to schools for blind children in Bolivia, Chile, Guatemala, Costa Rica. New schools were opened in the Dominican Republic and in Colombia.

The potential support of intergovernmental agencies was never overlooked. At the Pan-American conference, Brazilian leaders of work for the blind were advised on how to secure United Nations help in developing rehabilitation and employment programs. In due course the International Labor Office agreed that this would be appropriate to its function of encouraging utilization of untapped labor supplies. A vocational specialist was needed to advise the Brazilian government on how to go about training this labor supply; at ILO's request, J. Albert Asenjo of the Foundation staff was given a year's leave of absence in 1957 to undertake the assignment. It was one of several instances where needed expertise was transferred from work for the American blind to the international scene.

A new dimension was added to overseas work when, in 1961, the United States Government began the practice of allowing "counterpart funds" to be spent for research and demonstration projects under the direction of the Department of Health, Education, and Welfare. These funds derived from the sale of American agricultural commodities to developing countries, which were permitted to pay for them in local currencies instead of dollars. Countries where the supply of such American-owned currencies exceeded the United States' requirements for local expenditures were designated "excess currency countries." Under a law passed in 1961, such excess currencies were permitted to be used for purposes that could benefit mankind as a whole.

Between 1961 and 1971 the equivalent of $28 million in seven different countries was spent on 21 projects relating to blindness. The projects covered a wide range: blindness prevention and sight restoration in Pakistan, vocational training in Israel, industrial training methods in India and Pakistan, studies of vocational aptitudes in Yugoslavia, training of the rural blind in agricultural occupations in Egypt, Syria, and India. Many of these efforts were stimulated or expedited by AFOB, which was also called upon to assist in review, development and monitoring of the projects.

At the time AFOB was incorporated to absorb the American Braille Press, the intention had been to phase it out once the remaining assets had been used up in financing initial postwar relief and reconstruction activities. However, such widespread public interest had been generated by the 1946 clothing campaign that the trustees of the American Foundation for the Blind agreed to allow its own contributors' list to be used for a one-time fund-raising effort on behalf of the overseas blind. The response was sufficiently generous to cancel the original plan of winding up the affairs of the overseas agency. From this beginning, AFOB built its own list of supporters, and annual mail appeals became the method through which its funds were raised.

During the Fifties, contributions ranged between $300,000 and $375,000 a year. In 1959, when Helen Keller was nearing her 80th birthday and had made the last of the nine globe-circling tours which had taken her to 34 countries all over the world, AFOB's annual campaign was renamed the Helen Keller World Crusade for the Blind. Contributions from the public increased, topping $500,000 in 1962 when the appeal was given the added prestige of a National Crusade Committee headed by Helen's devoted friend, Katharine Cornell, a trustee of both AFOB and AFB. Toward the end of that decade, however, the state of the American economy and other factors caused a drop in giver income, resulting in annual operating deficits in six figures. Although the yield from $3 million in endowment funds helped, it was not enough to close the gap between income and expenditure.

Part of the endowment fund came from legacies. A not unexpected bequest was the $180,000 left by William Nelson Cromwell. Another large bequest, approximating $200,000, came from the estate of a man whose small annual contributions to the Association for Chinese Blind had given no hint that he would make so generous a provision in his will.

A more sizable proportion of the endowment fund came about through a kind of sweet irony. When World War I ended, Winifred Holt's *Phare de France,* housed in what had once been the Paris residence of the Vatican delegate to France, became a home and rehabilitation center for war-blinded French servicemen. The 44-room mansion, with its two gardens, coach house, and stables, had originally been leased at a nominal rental; the lease was supposed to terminate six months after the end of the war. It was extended until mid-1922, at which point the Vatican authorities, seeking to dispose of the property, gave the *Phare* the option of buying or vacating.

By this time, Winifred Holt was living in Rome, where she had organized another Lighthouse, *Il Faro d'Italia,* and had managed to raise the funds to buy a building for it. The necessity of immediately going after additional funds to buy the Paris *Phare* was more than the remnants of the Committee for Men Blinded in Battle could undertake. But Winifred Holt never lacked either daring or imagination. In Rome the fifty-two-year-old spinster had met an American art historian, Dr. Rufus Graves Mather, who proposed marriage. She decided to use her wedding to launch a campaign for $500,000 on behalf of both the French and Italian Lighthouses.

"Blind Poilus' Beacon Saved by Bridal Gifts to Miss Holt," read the headline in the *New York Evening Mail* of November 14, 1922. The article explained that the betrothed pair had asked well-wishers to refrain from giving them personal wedding gifts but to contribute cash, instead, to the campaign "needed to save the French veterans from ejection." Stories in other newspapers detailed the arrangements for the wedding ceremony, to be performed at the New York Lighthouse, noting that four of the eight bridesmaids would be blind women "attired in costumes of blue crepe de chine with blue and gold headdresses."

There is no record of how much cash actually was received, but the hoped-for half-million-dollar figure was never even approached. Enough was raised, however, to buy the Paris *Phare*, and in late 1924 it was dedicated by Marshal Foch at formal ceremonies attended by the Mathers. Not long thereafter, the couple set out on a series of world tours in which they visited schools and organizations for the blind in Europe, the Near East, Asia, and Latin America. Wherever they went they gave lectures and started movements for the welfare of blind people, founding additional Lighthouses in places like India, Peking, and Osaka. Their travels ended in 1937; Winifred Holt Mather died in 1945.

The Paris *Phare,* following its purchase and dedication, was maintained by a Franco-American committee which raised funds for its upkeep. Soon after World War II, during which the building at 14 rue Daru was used as a shelter for all types of refugees, the committee decided not to reconstitute a home for blinded veterans but to merge its efforts with the work in France of the newly formed AFOB. The *Phare*'s sole remaining asset at the time consisted of the now dilapidated mansion. A merger was duly effected and in 1950 AFOB spent $100,000 in repairs and renovations so that the property could serve as its own European headquarters.

Fifteen years later, real estate values in the heart of Paris had risen so sharply that AFOB was able to sell the land on which the property stood for $1,837,000 in cash plus other considerations valued at $500,000. The sale proceeds were augmented the following year by a demolition grant of $58,000 from the French Government. In 1972 AFOB's Paris office address was still 14 rue Daru, but it was quartered in the modern office building erected on the site of the old mansion and derived some income from subletting part of the space allotted it under terms of the sale. In the end, Winifred Holt Mather succeeded in endowing the cause of the overseas blind far more generously than even she had dreamed.

The American Foundation for Overseas Blind never pretended it could even begin to cope with all of the problems of a world blind population whose numbers were estimated at anywhere between 14 million and 22 million. Its principal thrusts were keyed to self-help: making trained specialists available to supply guidance and technical knowledge in establishing programs to assist the blind, providing seed money to get programs started, upgrading the level of professional training of those operating the programs.

The year 1968 saw adoption of a fourth objective: active promotion of blindness prevention programs in areas of the world showing the highest blindness rates, such as Africa, Asia and parts of Latin America. One aspect of the plan was cooperating with governments and international bodies in the administration of massive doses of Vitamin A to preschool children in areas of dire poverty. This simple measure, it was demonstrated in scientific tests, was an important element in preventing xerophthalmia, an eye disease caused by vitamin deficiencies in the diet of growing children. An advisory committee made up of specialists in eye care, pediatrics, nutrition, and public health was named in 1972 to guide development of these preventive activities, which were expected to assume steadily greater prominence in AFOB's work.

The early Seventies also saw changes in personnel and administration. Alex H.

Townsend, who had succeeded Eric Boulter as associate director in 1970, stepped down from the post because of ill health in 1972. The associate directorship was assigned to Harold G. Roberts, alongside his role as an associate director of the American Foundation for the Blind. R. Roy Rusk, who had been director of the latter agency's program planning department since 1967, moved to the Overseas Foundation in a similar capacity. AFOB's regional offices, originally staffed by American or British personnel, had been placed in the hands of indigenous or other persons intimately familiar with the cultural values and customs of the areas they served. This arrangement also meant less dislocation when, as conditions changed, the need for full-scale operations in particular regional offices diminished.

The element of responsive flexibility also characterized the World Council for the Welfare of the Blind in its role as a bridge between the efforts of local, national and international agencies and the network of human services financed through the United Nations family of intergovernmental bodies.

Following its incorporation in 1951, the Council adopted the practice of meeting in general assembly every five years, with interim actions in the hands of an executive committee. Its purposes remained guided by the nine-point "bill of rights for the blind" adopted at the 1949 Oxford Conference as a statement of every nation's minimal obligation toward its blind citizens:

> 1) Registration of all who fall within a standard definition of visual disability; 2) assumption by the national government of responsibility for the basic welfare of such citizens; 3) the right of blind people to rehabilitation and training for participation in the nation's economic, social and civic life; 4) provision of employment opportunities, both open and sheltered; 5) a standard of subsistence that makes allowances for the special costs of blindness; 6) visiting and teaching services for blind persons who are homebound; 7) group homes for aged or multihandicapped blind people, operated on acceptable standards; 8) provision at little or no cost of such aids, appliances and services as mitigate the handicap of blindness; 9) education of all blind children "according to their interests and aptitudes [and at a level] at least equal to that which they would have received if they had not been blind."

Membership in both the World Council's general assembly and its executive committee was based on proportional representation according to population. Under this formula, the United States held six seats in the assembly and three in the executive committee. The World Council's first president was Colonel Edwin A. Baker of Canada, who served three consecutive terms. He was succeeded in 1964 by Eric Boulter; when Boulter's five-year term expired in 1969, Charles Hedkvist of Stockholm became president, to serve until the next general assembly scheduled for Brazil in 1974.

In 1960 Colonel Baker's skillful leadership of the Council was honored by AFOB with the first Helen Keller International Award, a bronze statuette by the American sculptor Doris Caesar. The award's second recipient was Georges Raverat in 1968; the third, in 1970, was John F. Wilson, director of the Royal Commonwealth Society for the Blind. The statuette, "The Spirit of Helen Keller," went to another Briton, Lord Fraser of Lonsdale, in 1971. Plans were under way, at the end of 1972, to award it next to an American, James S. Adams. An industrialist and investment banker, Adams was to be honored both for his long years of service as a trustee of AFB and AFOB, and for his more than four decades of support for medical research to prevent blindness. That support had culminated in his role as a founder and, later, president of Research to Prevent Blindness, a voluntary organization established in 1960.

Not only did George Alexander Kessler keep the promise to God that he made during the seven desperate hours he clung to an oar in the Atlantic Ocean, he started a chain of events that bound others to the same selfless purpose. By 1972 the activities of the American Foundation for Overseas Blind had extended to 103 nations. Not even the vaulting imagination of "the champagne king" could have visualized an outcome of such dimensions.

23

The Birthright of Every Child

One of the principal social ideals resulting from the advent of democratic forms of government was the concept that made education the birthright of every child instead of maintaining it, in Toynbee's phrase, as "the monopoly of a privileged minority." However, it was not until the era of Jacksonian democracy that universal free education really took root in the United States. In earlier years, primary education had been supplied for the well-off by private academies, for the poor by church-supported and charity free schools and, in some parts of the country, particularly New England, by public schools supported through local property taxes.

The beginnings of American education for blind children also found their impetus in the Jacksonian surge toward freedom and equality. Within a single twelve-month span, 1832–33, schools were opened in New York, Boston, and Philadelphia. Founded and financed by philanthropists, they were thought of as charitable asylums rather than educational instruments, and their original names reflected this. What became the Perkins School for the Blind was incorporated as the New England Asylum for the Blind. The New York Institute for the Education of the Blind was the New-York Institution for the Blind. In Philadelphia the Overbrook School for the Blind was originally the Pennsylvania Institution for the Instruction of the Blind.

By the Civil War, 18 additional residential schools had been opened for blind children. Unlike the first three, all but one of these (the exception was Maryland) were state-operated, not as schools but as charitable institutions under the supervision of the state's welfare authorities. Many began as multipurpose asylums for the care and education of "defective children"—the blind, the deaf and, in some instances, the feeble-minded.

Much of this growth of educational opportunity was attributable to the crusading zeal of a handful of men, among whom the most conspicuous was Samuel Gridley Howe, M.D. History has played a cruel trick on Howe. His was an extraordinary and varied career, yet his name is hardly recognized while his wife, Julia Ward Howe, who wrote new words to an old tune while accompanying her husband to a Civil War battleground, is known to every schoolchild who sings "The Battle Hymn of the Republic."

In the special world of work for the blind, however, Howe was a man of legendary stature. He was born in Boston, November 10, 1801, graduated from Brown University, took up the study of medicine and had barely begun to practice when he enlisted in the Greek war of independence, a romantic struggle against tyranny begun in 1821. Howe, like others, was said to have been inspired by the example of the English poet Byron, who lost his life in the war to free Greece from the Ottoman Empire. It was said, too, that a disappointment in love acted as a further spur to Howe's hasty decision to set out for Greece in 1824. In any event he spent six years fighting and doctoring there, and an additional year traveling through other parts of Europe, before returning to Boston in 1831. Differing explanations were given for his return: that he contracted swamp fever in Greece and had to recover his health; that he came back to Boston to collect funds for the Greek cause. Both may have been true.

Whatever the reason, shortly after his return a chance encounter changed his plans and the future direction of his life. Two years earlier Dr. John D. Fisher had induced the Massachusetts legislature to incorporate "an institution for the blind of New England" in the form of a quasi-public school authorized to collect and expend funds under the direction of a board of trustees. Fisher and his fellow trustees had not yet found the right person to organize such a school when, as the story goes, they ran into Howe on Boylston Street and Fisher exclaimed, "Here is Howe—the very man we have been looking for all the time!"

Howe's daughter, Laura E. Richards, called the encounter on Boylston Street "a meeting of flint with steel." But the striking of a spark is not enough to ignite a flame unless it is applied to the right timber. Howe was that. As an earlier historian observed, "Howe was without a preliminary training for his task, yet he so combined poetic insight, the fiery zeal of the prophet, sound scholarship and business acumen, that any philanthropic enterprise was bound to prosper in his hands."

The enterprise that engaged Howe's interest that day did indeed prosper at his hands during a 44-year tenure, and so did many others. Although the school for the blind became his permanent base of operations, he also enlisted in many other social and political causes. He was active in the abolitionist movement, worked with Dorothea Dix in the crusade for humane treatment of the insane, founded and for 25 years directed the "school for idiots" that later became Massachusetts' Walter E. Fernald State School, helped Horace Mann in the campaign for universal free education, took an active role in establishing what became the Clarke School for the Deaf, served for a time as chairman of the Massachusetts State Board of Charities, spent one or more terms in the state legislature where he led a movement to reform prison conditions, and, during the Civil War, accepted an assignment to survey the sanitary conditions of the Massachusetts troops in the battlefields.

Despite this staggeringly wide range of interests, Howe was no dilettante, nor was he a mere figurehead. During Perkins' formative years he took an intimate interest in its daily operations, personally sought out and enrolled many of the early pupils, and, in the case of Laura Bridgman, devised what none before him had ever succeeded in achieving—a systematic method for communicating with a young girl who could neither see nor hear.

The idea that New England should have a school for blind children had come to John Fisher when, as a medical student in Paris, he visited the world's first such school, *l'Institution Nationale des Jeunes Aveugles*. Then four decades old, it had been founded a few years before the French Revolution by Valentin Haüy, a young intellectual fired by the humanitarian philosophies of Rousseau and Voltaire and intrigued by the metaphysical speculations of such earlier encyclopedists as Diderot. In Haüy's case, philosophy and metaphysics were transmuted into activism by his horror over a scene he witnessed during St. Ovid's Fair in Paris one day in 1771, an incident that became as familiar a story in the annals of blindness as did Paul Revere's ride in the history of the American Revolution.

Seated on a high platform outside a cafe in what is now the Place Vendôme were a handful of blind men scraping away discordantly at an assortment of musical instruments. On their noses hung huge empty pasteboard spectacles; to emphasize their blindness, the inscribed sides of the candlelit music scores faced away from them. As though this were not ridicule enough, the men were costumed in grotesque robes and crowned with dunce caps adorned with asses' ears. An advertising poster caricatured the scene to attract customers to the *Café des Aveugles* (Café of the Blind).

As he gazed at this crude carnival and heard the jeers of the crowds, twenty-six-year-old Valentin Haüy was seized with "a profound sorrow" and "an exalted enthusiasm" to do away with such an "outrage to humanity." "I will substitute the truth for this mocking parody," he told himself. "I will make the blind to read! I will put in their hands volumes printed by themselves. They will trace the true characters and will read their own writing, and they shall be enabled to execute harmonious concerts."

It was a bold and generous resolve, but Haüy took more than a decade to put it into practice. What finally spurred him to action was a concert appearance in Paris by the blind Austrian pianist, Maria von Paradis, whose accomplishments had attracted royal patronage throughout Europe. Haüy went to see her after the concert; she explained how she had learned to read and write by means of pinpricked letters and told him of other blind people who had also improvised ways of educating themselves. Encouraged, Haüy sought out a promising seventeen-year-old, François Lesueur, whom he began to teach with the use of hand-carved wooden letters. The lad had been a street beggar; his motivation for the novel experiment was Haüy's promise to pay him a wage equal to the proceeds of his mendicancy.

It was François who made the accidental discovery that led to the creation of an actual school. Handling some papers on Haüy's desk, his fingers felt a protuberance on a sheet of paper: the imprint of a letter on the reverse side of a freshly printed funeral notice. François asked his teacher whether what he felt was the outline of the letter "o." It was indeed, and it came to Haüy in a flash that if the fingers of a blind boy could detect a single letter that had been faintly raised through accidental pressure, those same fingers could do wonders with print deliberately raised. Haüy tested this insight by embossing sheet after sheet in italic script. François could distinguish every letter. In six months, he could both read and write.

A demonstration before members of the Royal Academy of Sciences drew their endorsement and the subsequent permission of the government for Haüy to open a school. In 1784 this finally took shape: 14 blind boys and girls, wards of a philanthropic society, were brought together in a small dwelling where, with Haüy as headmaster and François as his assistant, they began their education.

The school underwent numerous vicissitudes during the stormy years of the Revolution and its aftermath, and so did Haüy, who fell into political disfavor under the changing regimes. His accomplishments with blind children were recognized, however, and although he was never permitted to resume leadership of the school he had founded, he was invited, toward the end of his life, to create schools in Germany and in Russia. The Paris school had become a solidly grounded institution (with Louis Braille as one of its students) by the time young Dr. Fisher of Boston visited it around 1825.

By then there were more than a dozen other schools for the blind in as many European countries, and one of the first things Samuel Gridley Howe did when he agreed to start a school in Boston was to go abroad to see what he could learn from them. He found "much to admire and to copy, but much also to avoid."

One of the European practices he criticized was the custom of displaying blind pupils in public exhibitions. But he soon learned that if he was to attract popular support for his budding institution and, more important, cultivate positive public attitudes toward blind persons and their potential for employment, he would have to do the same. For many years Howe's school was thrown open every weekend so visitors could marvel at blind children reading, writing, doing mathematical calculations, and playing musical instruments. To convince skeptics that these children really could not see, a green ribbon was bound over each child's eyes.

Presumably the children wore these blindfolds when Howe took them on tour, as he soon began to do. His school was only four years old and had but a handful of pupils when a letter from a physician in Ohio prompted him to take three of his most accomplished students to give a demonstration before that state's legislature. It proved so effective that Ohio became the first state to make public provision for the education of its blind children; under a legislative appropriation a school was opened in Columbus in 1837 with Perkins' first graduate, A. W. Penniman, in charge. Within the next few years, Howe and his students made similar appearances before the governing bodies of 17 states. They rarely failed in their purpose.

By this time his own school, which had begun with the two little Carter sisters Howe took into his family home in July 1832, had reached an enrollment of 65 pupils and had outgrown its first separate quarters, a mansion donated by the wealthy Boston merchant, Colonel Thomas H. Perkins. In 1839 a large hotel in South Boston was bought with funds derived from the sale of the Perkins property, and in gratitude for the Colonel's permission to make this sale, the trustees voted for the school to bear his name. Perkins Institution and Massachusetts Asylum for the Blind became the new name; in 1877 the word "school" replaced "asylum" and in 1955 the name was shortened to Perkins School for the Blind.

In the Ivy League of schools for the blind, Perkins assumed the status of Harvard in primacy of origin, prestige, and public recognition. So eminent was Boston as the nation's cultural center, so self-assured was Howe as pundit, social reformer, and political power, that the two other pioneer schools were overshadowed for decades.

The New York school actually began operations four months before Perkins, even though the latter's legal birth and appointment of a director occurred earlier. By sheer coincidence, Howe's counterpart in New York, Dr. John Dennison Russ, had also served in the Greek war of independence as almoner (chief relief administrator) and the two men were acquainted. But Russ arrived independently at his resolve to do something for the blind boys he saw in New York City almshouses. Like Howe, he found an organization already incorporated, but not yet in operation, that was eager to do something for blind children. He joined forces with them and in a rented room on Canal Street three boys taken from the almshouse began their lessons on March 15, 1832. Boston's Colonel Perkins also had a New York counterpart in James Boorman, a prosperous merchant who in 1837 gave the school his mansion and grounds in what was then still an outlying district of Manhattan.

There, however, the resemblance ended. Russ did not have Howe's flair for attracting attention and support, and New York had yet to overtake Boston as either a commercial capital or a population center. Not until after the Civil War, when Howe was nearing the end of his life, did the New York school come to challenge Perkins' supremacy.

A brilliant and dynamic new superintendent was the reason. William Bell Wait tackled Howe on the question of embossed type, and although the system he himself had invented, New York Point, ultimately gave way to braille, he succeeded in diminishing and finally ending the use of Howe's Boston Line Type. But it was not only through the "war of the dots" that Wait became a potent force in the education of blind children; he also assumed a dominant role in shaping the academic philosophy of all schools for the blind once the heads of these schools came together in the professional association they called the American Association of Instructors of the Blind.

The Philadelphia school was born under the auspices of the Society of Friends, whose members were the social and civic leaders of the City of Brotherly Love. A Quaker emissary named Joshua Francis Fisher (no relation, so far as can be told, to Boston's Dr. John Fisher) traveled to Europe in 1830 to study schools for the blind; his return to Philadelphia coincided with the arrival of a German educator, Julius Friedlander, who had been in contact with the schools for the blind in Germany, England, and France and had come to Philadelphia with the purpose of starting one. Friedlander brought with him letters of introduction to prominent Quakers, one of whom, Robert Vaux, took the lead in organizing the Pennsylvania Institution for the Instruction of the Blind. Friedlander was appointed principal and began a class in March 1833; formal incorporation was approved the following January.

Credit for producing America's first embossed book, *The Gospel of Mark,* belongs to the Philadelphia school. Hand-embossed as a volunteer effort by a trustee, it used a tactile type that turned out to be illegible. Later, a variety of line type, different from Howe's Boston Line, was evolved at the school. Other achievements might have followed were it not for Friedlander's ill health, which caused his resignation a short time later. He died in 1838.

Although a subsequent head of the Philadelphia school, William Chapin, wielded considerable influence in the mid-nineteenth century, the school's major impact began in 1890, with the appointment of Edward E. Allen. What brought the youthful Allen into the national spotlight was not so much the educational theories he espoused as the changes he effected in the school's physical facilities. In 1899 he moved it out of a large congregate building in downtown Philadelphia to suburban Overbrook where, under his direction, a multimillion-dollar cottage school plant was constructed on spacious landscaped grounds. So dramatic was the change in atmosphere, so heightened was the morale of the school's students, and so impressive grew the placement record of its graduates that Allen, a former teacher at Perkins, was offered its directorship when Howe's successor died in 1906.

That successor had been Michael Anagnos, a Greek journalist Howe met when he once again took up the cause of Greek independence following the Cretan insurrection of 1866. As head of the Boston Greek Relief Committee, he went to Crete in 1867 to survey the islanders' needs. There he hired the thirty-year-old Anagnos as his "secretary for Cretan affairs" and brought him back to the United States. Within a short time the young Greek was helping the aging Howe with some of his many other interests; he also attracted the attention of Howe's eldest daughter, Julia, whom he married in 1871. By this time Howe was off on another political crusade, the nationalist revolution in Santo Domingo, and Anagnos took charge of the school in his father-in-law's frequent absences. He was the logical choice to head Perkins when Howe died in 1876.

Among the talents of Michael Anagnos was "a phenomenal gift of luring money out of benevolent citizens of Massachusetts," according to an account of the Perkins school written by one of its later directors, Gabriel Farrell. "So persuasive was he that proper Bostonians of his day would hardly dare face Saint Peter unless they had made provision for Perkins in their wills, a fact that greatly eased the financial problems of his successors." (It might be added that the tradition continued long after Anagnos' day; the 1972 annual report of the Perkins school showed assets of just under $45 million.)

Anagnos earned a place in history in three other respects. First, he founded the Kindergarten for Little Blind Children, the world's first school to begin the education of such children at age five when it was still customary to admit them at eight or nine. Originally established on separate premises in the Jamaica Plain section of Boston, the kindergarten eventually became Perkins' "lower school"; it was brought together with the "upper school" soon after 1910, when Perkins moved out of Boston to a spacious Watertown estate where an improved cottage-style school was built under Allen.

Second, he founded the great library and museum of "blindiana" assembled at Perkins through the exchange program with the Blindeninstitut in Vienna. But what Anagnos was probably best known for was his catalytic role in the life of Helen Keller. It was he who recommended the just-graduated Anne Sullivan as Helen's tutor, who gave Anne access to Howe's copious notes on the methods used in instructing Laura Bridgman, and who encouraged and steadied the shaky young teacher as she struggled to make contact with the eager mind of a headstrong child. Anagnos later arranged for Helen and her teacher to spend three years in residence at Perkins, not as regular members of the school but as guests. They might have remained longer were it not for a misunderstanding over a newspaper article about Helen that led to a contretemps between the school's trustees and the hot-tempered Anne. She and thirteen-year-old Helen left in 1893; they never returned except as visitors on ceremonial occasions.

According to the version of this incident given by Anne to her biographer, Nella Braddy, Anagnos was not personally involved in the controversy; he was, in fact, abroad at the time. Helen Keller's version, as related in *Midstream*, is differently shaded and carries a tinge of angry pique against the man she says she had "loved like a father." Anagnos, she wrote, tried to keep her and her teacher at Perkins in an effort to "manage" them. When they left, he "bitterly resented what he was pleased to call Miss Sullivan's ingratitude and shut us out from his heart."

It is tempting to dwell on the colorful lives and careers of the pioneer educators of the blind, both American and foreign. Romance and drama are there in abundance. To cite a single example, the motivation that led Edward Rushton to found England's first school for the blind was at least as stirring as Valentin Haüy's. Born in Liverpool in 1756, Rushton went to sea at the age of eleven, serving as an apprentice on slave-traders. On one occasion, when his ship was wrecked, he swam toward the same floating cask as a slave he had befriended during the voyage. The cask could not sustain them both, and the slave sacrificed his own life by pushing the exhausted boy onto the float.

Rushton never forgot it; a few years later, when an epidemic of malignant ophthalmia broke out in the human cargo of another such ship, Rushton—aware that the captain was systematically throwing overboard those slaves who were blinded by the disease and thus worthless as commodities—went into the hold to help tend the afflicted. This impulse to repay his debt to the African who had saved his life cost him his own sight. He contracted the malignancy and was blind at the age of nineteen.

The details of Rushton's young manhood are obscure; somehow he gained an education, became a minor poet, editor, and bookseller, and founded a literary club which, at his urging, agreed to establish an institution that would "render the blind happy in themselves and useful to society." The Liverpool School for the Blind was opened in 1790 (some sources say 1791). Rushton's own life had a happy ending.

After 33 years of blindness, an operation restored his sight. He lived another seven years before he died in 1814.

Unlike Haüy's establishment in Paris, the Liverpool school was not a residential institution. Its pupils boarded in the town and came for daily lessons, and one of its two small buildings was used as a workshop for blind adults. Educationally, it was not much, but it was a start, soon to be followed by larger and more conventionally organized schools in other parts of Britain. It also had the distinction of being the first school for the blind to be founded by a blind man.

Less melodramatic in origin, but of more enduring importance as an educational influence, was the school founded in Vienna in 1804 by Johann Wilhelm Klein. What later acquired the sonorous title of Imperial Royal Institute for the Education of the Blind began with a single blind lad, Jakob Braun, whom Klein took into his household and began to educate out of sheer affection. Klein was then a government official, a district supervisor of the poor; like Haüy, he effectively demonstrated his pupil's accomplishments before an official body, as a result of which he acquired additional pupils and began a school. Within a few years he succeeded in having it recognized and supported as a governmental institute.

Klein wrote extensively on his theories of education of blind children. Among the many ideas in which he was decades ahead of his time was his belief in the desirability of placing blind children in local schools alongside their sighted peers. The basic manual on education he wrote in 1819, the history of education of the blind he produced in 1837, the theories of teacher training and parent education he incorporated in subsequent books and monographs—these were so replete with forward-looking psychological and educational concepts that, according to Berthold Lowenfeld, who made a study of his life and work, Klein played "the most decisive role in the education of the blind among the German-speaking people of Europe."

Of all the foreign schools, the one which probably had the greatest impact on American methods was the Royal Normal College and Academy of Music for the Blind, a British institution fashioned by an American expatriate who ultimately earned a knighthood at the hands of Edward VII. This was Francis J. Campbell: born in Tennessee in 1832, blinded by an acacia thorn before his sixth birthday, educated in the newly opened Tennessee State Institution for the Blind, teacher of music there while completing his own schooling at the University of Tennessee, then for 13 years a teacher of music at Perkins until, at the age of forty, he brought into being the unique "college" over which he was to preside for the next 50 years.

Campbell's overall influence on American services for blind people extended far beyond the realm of education; he founded a family dynasty whose activities were to impinge on virtually every phase of constructive progress in those services. Even had he been childless, however, Sir Francis would have made a unique contribution through his seminal role in shaping the thinking which a number of those who taught in his school brought back to the United States.

As had been the case with Samuel G. Howe, it was chance that brought Francis Campbell face to face with opportunity. An accomplished pianist, he had spent two years in Europe under the tutelage of noted masters and was on his way back to America when, on arrival in London, he met Thomas Rhodes Armitage, the blind physician who had just succeeded in federating Britain's scattered organizations for the blind in an overall body that ultimately became the Royal National Institute for the Blind. Armitage was impressed by Campbell's account of the many music students at Perkins he had turned into successful professionals. Could Campbell achieve similar results in England? The peppery Tennessean was sure of it, provided he were given a free hand. In 1872 a conservatory for blind children opened in the Upper Norwood district of London. Later it branched out to become a teacher training institute as well.

To get his academic program under way, Campbell applied to Howe for a loan of some of Perkins' teachers. Howe agreed to grant leaves of absence to several but was not sanguine over the school's prospects. He called it "an exotic" which would require "the most skillful care and attention, by persons of pure and high motives, to make it take firm root and attain large growth in its foreign soil."

No such doubts troubled Campbell, who had firm ideas about how to reach his objectives. His choice of the term "college" rather than "school" suggested the policy of selectivity he proposed to follow. Admission was on the basis of intellectual promise; retention in the student body hinged on merit. Education was by no means confined to the classroom but took place virtually around the clock. In the British prep school tradition, teachers roomed in the same buildings as their pupils, took meals with them and participated in their daily routine from wakeup to lights out. Over the years, 44 Americans were imported by Campbell to teach for longer or shorter periods. Asked during a hearing conducted by a royal commission in 1886 why he employed so many Americans, Campbell replied that English teachers

> want far more waiting upon, and they will do far less than the American teachers. The American teacher never stops to think whether it is somebody else's business. . . . Supposing a boy comes in with dirty hands she is ready to go for soap and water and attend to him then and there. . . . Whereas if it was an English teacher I think she would be much more likely to ring for a servant. . . .

Campbell was a fervent believer in the value of physical exercise. He himself set the pace, leading the long hikes, the bicycle trips, the field games, the roller skating and swimming events for teachers and pupils alike. His wife and sons were also in the forefront of the fitness program. Campbell was proud of his own physical prowess; he regarded as one of the crowning achievements of his life his ascent of Mont Blanc when he was well into middle age.

Howe, too, believed in physical activity for blind youngsters, convinced that only through exercise could they overcome the natural fear of injury which locked so many blind people into sedentary existences. He resorted to stern methods to get his pupils out of doors; among the less salubrious memories of early Perkins graduates were the occasions when they were thrust into the frosty climate of the New England winter and the doors of the school locked against them until they had passed the requisite time in the fresh air. Anne Sullivan Macy told her biographer how the children "huddled against the wall, stamping their feet to keep warm."

Campbell regularly returned to Boston to recruit faculty, and it was on one such occasion that he met Edward Ellis Allen, who had graduated from Harvard College a year earlier and had begun the study of medicine. Allen came from a New England family of educators. His father operated a private academy where Edward's older brothers also taught. There were younger brothers as well, and at a point when the family fortunes were slim, there came the turn of one of these to go to college. Edward was asked to postpone completion of his medical studies and relieve the strain on the family budget by supporting himself for a time.

It was this factor, plus the intriguing prospect of living and working in England, that prompted him to apply for a teaching job at the Royal Normal College. He stayed at Upper Norwood three years—from 1885 to 1888—by which time he had decided against resuming his medical studies. His new resolve was not only to stay in teaching but to specialize in the education of the blind. As he neared the end of his sojourn, he received job offers from both the Philadelphia and the Boston schools; he chose the latter because it was closer to his family, and came to Perkins as head teacher of boys. Two years later, the tempting offer of a principalship brought him to Philadelphia. He was by then uniquely qualified.

His successor at Philadelphia, Olin H. Burritt, once pointed out that Allen was the only head of an American school for the blind in a position

> to pass upon the merits of the four embossed types struggling for supremacy in the American schools for the blind—Boston line letter, New York point, American braille, English braille; for as a teacher in Dr. Campbell's school he had learned and used English braille; at Perkins he had used the Boston line letter and, finding New York point in use at the Philadelphia school, he learned this type and continued its use for two years. . . . He believed braille was superior to all other systems and American braille superior to English braille. . . . [To] Mr. Allen belongs the credit of holding the country for braille as against New York point.

In addition to his influence on the architecture and resulting life styles in schools for the blind, Allen pioneered in several other directions, among them public school classes for the partly sighted. Classes for "myopes" had begun in England in 1909. Allen, who was by then back at Perkins as its director, had a special class opened in Boston in 1913; he went so far as to use funds from the Perkins treasury to pay for needed supplies for the five students.

Allen attributed many of his accomplishments to what he had learned from Francis Campbell at the Royal Normal College. Of them all, it was Campbell's success with job placement that made the strongest impact on American educators of the blind. Few of them, however, could go to Campbellian lengths. Sir Francis, who started out each school day with a clarion exhortation to his pupils to "storm the castle, capture the fort and take them all prisoners!" used similarly buccaneering tactics to find jobs for his graduates, particularly those trained for musical careers. He kept personally in touch with major European and American musical organizations and hammered at them to secure orchestral posts and concert dates for his talented students. For one of the most gifted, the pianist Alfred Hollins, Campbell arranged concert appearances with the Berlin, London, and New York

Philharmonics, the Boston Symphony, and other orchestras of equal renown. For these to engage a blind soloist had hitherto been "undreamt of," Hollins wrote many years later, and it happened only because of Campbell's "almost superhuman persistence."

America, too, had its pioneers in aggressive placement techniques, and one of them was Liborio Delfino, whose background could hardly have been more different from Campbell's. Delfino was a seventeen-year-old immigrant, newly arrived in the United States and working on a Philadelphia pick-and-shovel gang, when a quarry blast destroyed his eyesight and his right arm. Having spent an impoverished boyhood tending sheep and goats on a barren Italian mountainside, he had never learned to read or write. He knew only the most rudimentary English and was the sole member of his family to have come to America when the accident happened.

At Germantown Hospital, Delfino was befriended by an Italian-speaking visitor who persuaded him to enter Philadelphia's school for the blind. He had to begin in the primary grade with the school's smallest children, but he plugged away and reached graduation in 1900. A person of affectionate and cheerful disposition, and of great physical strength despite the loss of the arm, he won such popularity with both students and teachers that Edward Allen added him to the staff. Delfino did well at every assignment Allen gave him—teaching ungraded classes, making a survey of the school's graduates, inducing business and industrial firms to offer them jobs, persuading parents to enroll their blind children in the school. He soon became the school's official placement agent and manager of the salesroom which merchandised the products of its workshop and home workers. He remained a member of the staff until his death in 1937.

Many other men, both blind and sighted, earned a place in the pantheon of early educators. There was Joel W. Smith, who taught piano tuning at Perkins for 30 years under Anagnos and Allen. Blinded in early adulthood, Smith used his fine mechanical bent to devise many pieces of apparatus for use by the blind, including an early braillewriter constructed on the principle of the then newly invented typewriter. He was credited with introducing touch typing, a technique mastered by blind people long before sighted typists abandoned the original "hunt and peck" method. He devised the American braille code, which was taught at Perkins once Boston Line Letter was discarded, and which was subsequently adopted by a number of other schools for the blind. He was founder, editor and publisher of *The Mentor,* the first national print periodical dealing with work for the blind. Officially sponsored by the Perkins alumni association, this monthly was short-lived (from 1891 to 1894), but it set a pattern and cultivated an appetite later capitalized on by the *Outlook.*

There was Benjamin B. Huntoon, for nearly a half century superintendent of the Kentucky School for the Blind, founder and shaper of the affiliated American Printing House for the Blind, and prime mover in the early affairs of the AAIB. There was Frank H. Hall of the Illinois School, inventor of the first efficient braillewriter and braille stereotyper. There was Ambrose M. Shotwell, the bearded grandfatherly blind man who was both pacemaker and peacemaker in the establishment and development of AAWB. Shotwell was never a superintendent—he taught at the Arkansas school for a number of years and then was librarian at the Michigan school for several decades prior to his retirement in 1927—but the pressures exerted by him and other lower-level workers for the blind had much to do with changing the focus, and eventually the locus, of education for blind children.

There was also William Henry Churchman, blind from his seventeenth year, who in the pre–Civil War era launched three state schools—Tennessee, Indiana, and Wisconsin—as each one's first superintendent, and narrowly missed heading a fourth, the New York State School at Batavia. Churchman was generally credited with resuscitating the seemingly stillborn AAIB after an 18-year lapse; he served a term as president of the revived organization, 1876–78.

The early superintendents of schools for the blind were, for the most part, just what their titles implied. Educational policy was only one of their functions. Except for the few who headed philanthropically supported schools, the superintendents were public officials, in some cases political appointees, who were not only responsible for all aspects of institutional management but had to cultivate numerous legislative and bureaucratic relationships. Most of the tax-supported schools fell under a state board of charities; it would take many decades before one school after another succeeded in getting itself transferred to the jurisdiction of the state educational department.

Understandably, therefore, it was the privately endowed and financed schools—primarily Boston, Philadelphia, and New York—that took the initiative along purely educational lines. This they did for three days in August 1853, when the New-York Institution for the Blind hosted the meeting that laid the groundwork for what eventually became the American Association of Instructors of the Blind.

The 17 men present—14 superintendents and 3 teachers—found a lot to talk about even though their individual situations were so greatly dissimilar. The three pioneer schools had been in existence some twenty years; only two others (Ohio and Virginia) were backed by as much as a decade of experience; the remaining nine (Tennessee, Indiana, Wisconsin, Illinois, Missouri, Louisiana, Georgia, Iowa, and Maryland) had been founded less than ten years earlier, two of them (Iowa and Maryland) that very year.*

The substantive resolutions adopted at this first assembly reflected, as Francis M. Andrews and C. Warren Bledsoe noted in a historical chronicle of the AAIB,

> perennial items of policy, practice and concern: 1. National responsibility for producing embossed books and federal funds to provide other educational resources. 2. Demonstration of the capacities of blind children by showing their performance to public officials. 3. The approval of a standard embossed type [Boston Line] but research for an improved system. 4. The necessity

---

* It is puzzling that the official proceedings indicate that only two existing schools were unrepresented. The two missing schools are not identified but historical records show that four other schools were in existence as of 1853: Kentucky (founded 1842), North Carolina (1845), Mississippi (1848) and South Carolina (1849).

for a periodical concerned with blindness. 5. The approval of a standard system of musical notation. 6. Discipline of blind children as exacting as that applied with sighted children. 7. Responsibility for finding employment for graduates of schools. 8. The question of ideal architecture.

The convention's "immediate object," the proceedings noted, was "to make application to Congress for a donation for a permanent printing fund for the use of the blind" on the grounds that since Congress had

> appropriated large portions of the public lands for general education, from the benefits of which the blind have been and necessarily are excluded, their claim for a portion of the proceeds of these lands to aid in their education is both just and reasonable.

This argument was to be presented to the next session of the federal legislature in the form of a "memorial." It is not clear whether such an approach was made, but if it was, it did not succeed any more than earlier approaches to Congress made by Howe. Another resolution was for a second convention to be called, presumably in the near future, but this did not happen either. It was not until 1871, when William Churchman circulated a questionnaire asking whether there was interest in holding another convention, that the moribund organization was brought back to life.

Howe had been elected president of the as-yet-unnamed 1853 body, and it was unquestionably he who kept the fragile organizational bud from blossoming. There could have been any number of reasons for his lack of action, one of which may well have been, as Andrews and Bledsoe suggested, unwillingness to share or dilute his status as the nation's undisputed authority on the subject of blindness. But, as they also pointed out, "time was running out for Howe" when, in 1871, he received the Churchman questionnaire.

It was not merely that he was seventy. His Boston Line Type was being steadily challenged, and dot codes were rapidly gaining new adherents, thanks in large part to the energetic efforts of that fast-rising star in the education of the blind, William Wait. Within his own domain at Perkins, Howe had had to cope with a palace revolution of sorts in which younger members of the faculty questioned existing educational methods. He himself was disappointed in the practical results achieved at his school; its graduates had failed, by and large, to gain the hoped-for acceptance in open employment, and the school had found it necessary to open a workshop for some and to create internal jobs for others. He had also been saddened that the families of many former students took little or no responsibility for their future welfare, which meant the school was expected to continue acting in a parental role.

In the marathon address he delivered as guest speaker at the cornerstone-laying ceremony for the New York State Institution for the Blind at Batavia in 1866, Howe voiced these doubts publicly. He questioned whether the established schools for the blind were really fulfilling a useful function. Ruefully acknowledging his personal role in stimulating the growth of such schools—"I labored with more zeal than knowledge"—he went on to say:

> I accept my full share of condemnation when I say that grave errors were

incorporated into the very organic principles of our institutions for the blind, which make them already too much like asylums. . . . All great establishments in the nature of boarding schools, where the sexes must be separated; where there must be boarding in common, and sleeping in congregate dormitories; where there must be routine, and formality, and restraint, and repression of individuality; where the charms and refining influences of the true family relation cannot be had—all such institutions are unnatural, undesirable, and very liable to abuse. We should have as few of them as is possible, and those few should be kept as small as possible.

[Any] class of young persons marked by an infirmity like deafness or blindness . . . depend more than ordinary persons do for their happiness and for their support upon the ties of kindred, of friendship, and of neighborhood. . . . Beware how you needlessly sever any of those ties . . . lest you make a homeless man, a wanderer and a stranger. Especially beware how you cause him to neglect forming early relations of affection with those whose sympathy and friendship will be most important to him during life . . . and how you restrict him to such relations with persons subject to an infirmity like his own.

Undaunted by the fact that he was uttering these strictures at an occasion marking the construction of one of the very institutions whose practices he was deploring, Howe spelled out additional indictments. Schools for the blind, he said,

are generally wrong in receiving pupils too indiscriminately; being in most cases tempted to do so by the fact that they are paid according to the number they receive. They are wrong in receiving all pupils as boarders, when they should receive those only who cannot board at home, or in private families.

A better system, he declared, would be more selective. It would "reject everyone who can be taught in common schools," especially those who had some sight and could easily attend public day schools, "if special pains were taken with them, and special encouragement given . . . in the shape of books, slates, maps, etc."

Some of the other ideas Howe advanced were likewise well ahead of their time: Residential schools should act as screening and preparation centers, keeping some pupils a year or so for rudimentary instruction before sending them home to learn what they could in the common schools, where they would be aided by state-supplied books and apparatus and, if need be, a stipend for support. Which children, then, should receive their total education at a school for the blind? Only

the select pupils, say fifty in number, [who] should have every possible advantage and opportunity for improvement . . . the best masters, the best instruments. . . . They should be kept as long as may be necessary to qualify them to get their own living, as teachers of languages, as vocalists, as tuners of pianos, as organists, and the like.

In this last proposal lay the kernel of the idea that Francis Campbell, then a teacher at Perkins, was able to realize a few years later in England, but that Howe's own school, as a quasi-public body, could implement to only a limited extent. The state institutions were in even less of a position to exercise any real degree of selectivity. To keep a tax-supported school operating under capacity spelled political hot water for its superintendent.

Howe repeated some of these same reservations when he replied to the questionnaire he received from Churchman five years later. He saw no necessity to hold a convention, he wrote. "The great advantages which may flow from it, will be lessened by the fact, that it countenances the idea that there is greater difference between those who see, and those who do not see, than really exists."

The 1871 convention met without him, although Anagnos was present as "resident superintendent" of Perkins. This time the delegates made sure to adopt a constitution, give the organization a name and set a firm date for its next meeting a year later. Conventions thereafter were biennial. At the 1876 conclave, the plan for an appeal to Congress for support of books for blind students was revived and a committee appointed to see to it. Huntoon of Kentucky had already established a small printing house as an adjunct to his school; he chaired the committee, drafted a bill, persuaded his Congressman to sponsor it, and organized a campaign among the superintendents to rally their own representatives in the House and Senate in support. At the 1880 convention, he was able to announce that "An Act to Promote the Education of the Blind" had become law in March 1879 and the Printing House already had its first annual federal subsidy of $10,000 to provide schools for the blind with embossed textbooks. From this modest acorn grew the mighty forest which, in the 1972 fiscal year, commanded a federal appropriation of $1,590,000.

Despite Howe's warnings, residential schools continued to be built. By the turn of the century there were 37; another dozen were established during the next two decades. Of the 50 to 55 * residential schools in existence in 1972, only one—a special school for multiply handicapped blind children—was less than a half century old.

The post–Civil War period was one of sporadic growth as the nation expanded westward. California opened its school for the blind in 1867. The Oregon school, which began in 1873, soon had to shut down and remained closed for four years due to lack of both pupils and funds. In 1891 it reported it had had an average of seven pupils in the eight years since reopening, but now had sixteen, "most of them children," and hoped to double that number soon. "The reluctance of parents to send their blind children to school, and their lack of appreciation of the privileges offered gratuitously by the State, are deplored," the school's superintendent complained; what Oregon needed was a law like the state of Washington's, making it mandatory that "all defective youth be placed in some school for special training."

The same point was made by the Institution for the Deaf and Blind of Colorado, one of the many dual schools existing at the time. There, as elsewhere, the deaf pupils greatly outnumbered the blind; the Colorado count in 1891 was 74 deaf and

---

* Varying definitions of residential schools give rise to varying figures, but all counts put the number within this range.

34 blind pupils. New Mexico, then a territory, already had a school for the deaf "but the indifference of parents has retarded any active movement to provide advantages for blind children."

(Dual schools continue to exist; in 1972 there were ten, but although the physical facilities were shared and the administration was the same, faculties and classes were separate.)

The problem of compulsory education took a long time to solve. As late as 1930 there were still nine states which did not legally require parents of blind children to send them to school. As of 1972 this was no longer so; not only was school attendance compulsory for all children in all states, but local school authorities were mandated to provide educational facilities for all children.

All the schools established in the western states were tax-supported, but in the prosperous industrial areas of the East and the Middle West private philanthropy continued to play a significant role. Pittsburgh's Western Pennsylvania School for Blind Children came into being in 1890 thanks to a wealthy spinster's $40,000 bequest, augmented by gifts from other prominent citizens in the thriving steel center. Mrs. Mary X. Schenley donated a five-acre tract of land "located in a desirable part of the city and . . . estimated to be worth upward of *one hundred thousand dollars,"* H. B. Jacobs, the new school's superintendent, reported early the next year. Another contributor was William Thaw, whose widow became a lifelong friend and benefactress of Helen Keller; she was the mother of Harry K. Thaw, the man who in 1906 was to kill his wife's lover, the architect Stanford White, in a still-remembered scandal of that era.

The Western Pennsylvania School "was opened without ceremony and now has 21 pupils," Jacobs reported in early 1891. Ceremony was apparently reserved for acceptance of the deed to Mrs. Schenley's land; at a gala reception the donor was presented with an engrossed resolution of thanks in the form of "an album bound in Turkish morocco, with a clasp of solid silver, richly chased, and upon the cover a plate of gold fittingly inscribed."

Large or small, publicly or privately financed, handsomely housed or installed in makeshift quarters, the residential schools had many problems in common. A hardy perennial was the question of segregation of the sexes. Separate housing of boys and girls was taken for granted, as it was in all boarding schools and institutions, but schools for the blind went to extraordinary lengths to discourage even the most casual boy-girl social relations. In some, a student found openly conversing with one of the opposite sex was subject to peremptory expulsion. Even in the classroom the sexes were kept apart. At Perkins, Michael Anagnos went so far as to open and close the boys' and girls' departments on different days to prevent the two sexes from becoming acquainted on the trains.

It was not merely a matter of Victorian morality; behind these extreme measures lay a very real fear of perpetuating hereditary blindness through intermarriage. Edward Allen had such strong convictions on the issue that in 1930 he drew up charts to show that there were "more than 120 ophthalmic anomalies exhibiting a definite hereditary transmission" and that, of the causes of blindness in the 300 members of the Perkins student body, 196 were "probably hereditary." Most educators of the blind shared Allen's viewpoint; many had sets of siblings enrolled in their schools and some with long tenure had seen the pattern of blindness repeated in successive generations of the same family.

Apart from eugenics, there were practical considerations. "A house should have windows on at least one side," was a popular maxim underscoring the thought that the marriage of two blind people carried with it a needlessly large number of obstacles. The dangers of intermarriage were repeatedly impressed upon the students, but neither stern warnings nor the penalties attached to violation of school rules were wholly effective.

Although still opposed in principle to intermarriage, educators in schools for the blind in the Seventies have accepted the realities of adolescence and afford their pupils ample opportunity for supervised social contact in and out of the classroom. They have also made sex education a part of the curriculum.

Segregation by race was long a feature of the residential schools in the southern states, but it was taken for granted until relatively recent times. Some of the state institutions maintained two separate schools under the same management. As of 1931 there were ten (two were still in existence in 1972); there were also five independently administered schools for Negro children. Some of the southern states were slow to make any provision whatever for blind black children; Mississippi's first class was not instituted until 1929, when a special department for the blind was organized in the Piney Woods School for the Colored.

As was generally the case with all types of segregated schools, the educational facilities offered Negro children who were blind were inferior. A 1939 Foundation survey revealed that some of the schools for blind black children had to make do with hand-me-downs from their sister schools for blind white children, not merely in the form of worn furniture, chipped crockery, and threadbare towels, but also in classroom materials such as braille books whose dots were so worn down as to be all but indistinguishable. Even more serious was the lack of professional training in the teachers. As will be seen, one of the Foundation's notable contributions dealt constructively with this situation.

Beginning with the 1954 Supreme Court decision on school desegregation and the subsequent passage of various federal anti-discrimination laws, racial integra tion—in a few instances of the token variety—came into existence in virtually all schools for the blind.

The most fundamental change affecting the education of blind children began quietly at the turn of the century when the fast-growing city of Chicago decided to establish a separate local school instead of sending its blind children to the state school in Jacksonville at the southern end of Illinois. Frank H. Hall, who was then superintendent of the state school, urged the Chicago Board of Education not to build a separate institution. Instead, he recommended providing special classrooms in existing school buildings, and having the children take part in as many regular classes as possible. Hall's views were supported by a blind Chicago lawyer, Edward J. Nolan, who argued so persuasively before the Chicago education authorities as to overcome their belief that blind and sighted children could not be schooled together. Nolan's was not an easy task; the education board had already bought a lot and hired an architect.

Chicago's first class for blind children in a regular public school was opened in September 1900. It was supervised by John B. Curtis, a blind teacher Hall released from his own faculty to carry out what was admittedly an experimental venture. By 1907 Curtis was able to report that Chicago had 24 blind pupils in grade school and 5 in high school, and that while "teaching blind children in the same public school with seeing children has its limitation and cannot be applied universally . . . its claims for favorable consideration are strong."

John Curtis, born in 1871, attended the Illinois school for the blind after he lost his sight at the age of ten. Having graduated from Chicago's Hyde Park High School and earned both a bachelor's and a master's degree from the University of Chicago, he knew from personal experience about gaining an education alongside sighted students. Robert Irwin, who first met Curtis in 1908, described him as "a gentle, retiring man who never received his due share of credit," and it was no doubt at Irwin's instigation that some of this overdue credit came to Curtis when he was given the Migel Medal in 1945, ten years after his retirement. The pioneer educator died in 1951.

It did not take long for the Chicago formula to be tried out elsewhere. Cincinnati started a day school class for blind children in 1905, Milwaukee in 1907, and two years later four other cities followed suit: Racine, Cleveland, Boston, and New York. All began on a cautiously small scale, feeling their way and uncertain about how best to shape their programs. The influence and prestige of the long-established residential schools remained strong, and the advocates of public school education were not unaware of the special advantages the residential schools offered. Irwin, who was appointed supervisor of the Cleveland day classes when they opened in 1909, told the AAIB a year later that he expected to send his pupils to the residential school when they were old enough to begin learning a trade. By that time, he said, a youth would have "passed the period when the influence of the home is most essential to his development." Moreover, it would be "a stimulus to more lasting effort for a sightless person, about to launch out for himself, to come into contact with others preparing to face life under similar conditions."

Irwin was also conscious of other key elements absent in the early public school classes. He set about filling these deficiencies by adding a half-day to the school week. The pupils reported on Saturday mornings for special instruction in music and crafts. Their teachers, too, took on extra duties; they led the children on weekend hikes and organized a summer camp program for them. They also made home visits. "Teachers have been expected to visit in the home of at least one pupil each week. This is as much as can reasonably be asked of them," Irwin reported in 1916. But, he concluded, this did not provide enough coverage, so he arranged for the Cleveland office of the State Commission for the Blind to add to its staff a visiting teacher whose job would be "to supervise the home training of the blind children attending the public school classes." This step was needed because the "most earnest and persistent efforts" of the school's teachers were often "neutralized by the ignorance or indifference of parents." A tactful visiting teacher would encourage parents to allow the child to practice at home the self-care and homemaking skills learned at school. The person appointed to the new post, incidentally, was Mary Blanchard, who later became Mrs. Irwin.

In New York City the public school classes were born in a battle royal over tactile type between a group of ardent braille advocates led by Winifred Holt, representing the newly organized Lighthouse, and an equally vigorous group of New York Point adherents led by William B. Wait. The type question may have been the ostensible issue, but it symbolized a far deeper conflict. Wait saw a threat to philanthropic support for his school in the establishment of public school classes on its own New York City territory. The impetuous Winifred saw a threat to the future of her fledgling Lighthouse if what she called "the old order for the blind" were permitted to prevail. As noted earlier, the braille forces won, with assists from, among others, Frank H. Hall and Helen Keller.

By 1910 there were, all told, just over 200 blind pupils in the public schools of various cities, while the population of the residential schools came to 4,600. That year the AAIB took its first serious notice of the day school movement. The heart of the issue was put very plainly at the convention in Little Rock by George F. Oliphant, head of the Georgia residential school:

> It is no longer a question of whether the experiment of educating blind children in the public schools shall be made. It is already in progress. The only question for the institution to determine is our attitude toward the movement. Shall we help it, shall we fight it, or shall we sit still and see if it will run over us?

In the main, the school heads adopted the third alternative. A few more large cities initiated public school programs, but the movement soon reached a plateau. In 1949, nearly fifty years after Curtis' first experimental class in Chicago, the residential schools were still educating 90 percent of the nation's blind children.

Nine years later, that proportion had dropped to 60 percent and in some states, such as California, it was down to 25 percent. The cause of this sharp turnaround had little to do with instructional considerations; it stemmed from a wholly unexpected (and, for a dozen agonizing years, inexplicable) epidemic of infant blindness.

24

The Ever-Changing Children

Beginning around 1941 and growing steadily, year by year, the incidence of blindness in babies rose to alarming heights, and no one knew why. Before the mystery was solved, between 10,000 and 12,000 children had been added to the blind population of the United States, their lack of sight due to an eye condition that had a name but neither a cure nor a known cause. The name was retrolental fibroplasia (which means a fibrous growth behind the eye's crystalline lens). No cure was ever devised, but the story of how the causative factor was eventually pinpointed and reversed adds up to one of medicine's most suspenseful detective stories, complete with innumerable false leads and an almost Holmesian solution.

The first genuine clue was discovered by Theodore L. Terry, M.D., professor of ophthalmology at Harvard Medical School. In a single year he saw 6 blind infants with this strange membraneous growth at the back of the eyeball, heard of 8 other cases, and made the significant observation that all 14 babies had been born prematurely. It was Dr. Terry who gave this eye condition its cumbersome name (it came to be called RLF for short) and who first described it in medical literature. The Texas-born physician with the clipped moustache and the thinning shock of red hair, whose brusqueness concealed a deep sensitivity, found it emotionally devastating to have to tell one set of parents after another that their babies were blind and that neither surgery nor medicine knew any way of correcting the condition. Prematurely born at birth weights under three pounds, these infants had been saved from death by relatively new medical techniques. Did blindness have to be the price they paid for survival?

Theodore Terry was a dedicated scientist as well as a humane physician. With financial help from James Edgar Pew, a Philadelphia industrialist whose grandson had been Terry's first RLF patient, he set up an organization, the Foundation for Vision, consisting of a team of medical researchers abetted by a group of specialists in child development and family counseling. The latter would work with the parents of the blind infants, helping them adjust to their personal traumas and offering practical counsel on how to bring up blind babies. The team's base of operations was the Massachusetts Eye and Ear Infirmary in Boston, but its members also traveled for research and consultation to the other large eastern cities where RLF had begun to appear.

One of the most mystifying aspects of the disease was the way its incidence varied in different localities, even in different hospitals in the same locality. Initially, only Boston seemed to be affected, but once Dr. Terry had published his first report in a medical journal, word of similar cases came from a few other cities. As the data began to be analyzed, another puzzling fact surfaced: for the most part, cases of retrolental fibroplasia were occurring only in the biggest and most sophisticated medical centers, hospitals that boasted the best in equipment and care. Virtually no cases were reported from rural or suburban hospitals.

Other medical researchers soon joined Dr. Terry's team in the hunt for causes. Were there variations in the way different doctors or different hospitals treated "preemies"? In 1947 a statistical and epidemiological study by biochemist V. Everett Kinsey and research anatomist Leona Zacharias tabulated existing variations and reported that one of several points on which pediatric care in hospitals differed was "frequency of use and duration of exposure to oxygen." They were on the threshold of a vital discovery, but no one recognized it at the time. Much more credence was given to other theories from various quarters.

Could the cause be too-early or too-sudden exposure to light? In one hospital a medical team blindfolded 33 premature infants as soon as they were born and kept their eyes shielded from light until they had gained enough weight to be ready for discharge. It made no difference; 15 of the 33 developed some degree of RLF. Was it lack of Vitamin A in infants born before full term? Large doses were administered, but the trail led nowhere. A Baltimore husband-and-wife medical team developed a theory about Vitamin E deficiency as a cause, but this theory, too, petered out after extensive trials. A researcher in St. Louis pointed a finger at oxygen insufficiency as the culprit; others thought the trouble might stem from the shock of sudden changes in the oxygen levels of the incubators in which the premature babies were kept until they reached normal birth weight. If RLF were a kind of withdrawal symptom, a more gradual transition might prevent it.

All these theories were pursued with urgency and skill, but none halted the tide. By 1951 the RLF epidemic was reaching new heights, and the spirits of the men and women working to counteract it were sinking to new lows. In April of that year 25 of the principal researchers met in New York City, acknowledged that no one had nailed down either cause or cure and determined to organize a permanent committee for continuing investigation. Dr. Terry had died of a heart attack in 1946; his successor at the Boston project, Dr. Kinsey, was named chairman of the new committee.

Within a year, the committee had some telling clues to follow. Not long before, a young resident in ophthalmology at the District of Columbia General Hospital had begun to make a statistical correlation of the incidence of retrolental fibroplasia with the number of days the affected babies had been kept in oxygenated incubators. He and his associates found enough correspondence in the two sets of data to start them on a small controlled experiment. Some premature infants were placed in the routine high-oxygen (60 to 70 percent concentration) atmosphere for a month or longer. With others, high-oxygen administration was reserved for those occasions when cyanosis or other symptoms of breathing difficulty developed. The physician who pursued this line of inquiry, Dr. Arnall Patz, later explained:

> Cutting down on oxygen was much easier said than done. The night nurses were always turning it on again because they were so sure we were doing wrong. And it was a tough thing to sleep with, this business of keeping babies on low oxygen when all the teaching had been to give them plenty of it.

The results of this small study, which Dr. Patz published in September 1952, were strongly suggestive if not conclusive. In the high-oxygen group, 20 percent of the babies developed retrolental fibroplasia; in the low-oxygen group, the figure was less than 2 percent.

By that time similarly revealing hints were coming in from foreign sources. A pediatrician in Birmingham, England, became aware that her local hospital had never had a case of RLF until it replaced its leaky old incubators with airtight models. In Melbourne, Australia, another pediatrician made the same observation soon after her hospital installed its new, efficient "oxygen cots."

The aggregate number of cases from these diverse sources was too small to constitute real proof, but it was large enough to call for a major controlled study that might settle the issue once and for all. Such a study was begun in July 1953 under the joint sponsorship of the federal government's National Institute of Neurological Diseases and Blindness and two voluntary agencies. It called for simultaneous clinical trials in 18 cooperating hospitals. Each hospital would divide its caseload of low-weight premature infants into two randomly selected groups of uneven size. The smaller group would receive the standard high-oxygen treatment; the larger would be given oxygen only as needed. A total of 75 clinical investigators and 800 babies would participate.

Many of the cooperating doctors were dubious and uneasy, but within three months enough evidence was accumulated to show that the mortality rate among infants receiving oxygen only as needed was no higher than it was among those receiving the standard treatment. The ground rules of the clinical trials were promptly changed: all prematures would now be kept on restricted oxygen treatment.

Was this, finally, the solution? It took a while to know, since RLF often could not be diagnosed until the babies were several months old. But the proof, when it came, was overwhelming. Of the babies in the groups treated with routine high oxygen, 1 in 4 developed retrolental fibroplasia; of those in the groups given lower concentrations or intermittent treatment, the figure was 1 in 13. The mystery had been unraveled.

With the worldwide announcement of this discovery—the director of the National Institute of Neurological Diseases and Blindness called it "the most important single clinical advancement in ophthalmology during the past decade"—the epidemic tapered off sharply. But it did not quite come to a halt. Habitual routines proved hard to reverse. In many places Dr. Patz's experiences were duplicated. As one New York ophthalmologist remarked: "Everyone wanted to turn the oxygen on. . . . It was like giving a lollipop to the baby."

Faulty communications also played a part. Although hospitals, pediatricians, and medical schools were alerted, and articles appeared in major medical journals, a questionnaire sent out by the National Society for the Prevention of Blindness a year after the breakthrough discovery found 70 of 113 hospitals still routinely administering oxygen to all low-birthweight premature babies. In September 1955 the American Academy of Pediatrics issued a fact sheet beginning "The accumulated evidence definitely incriminates the excessive use of oxygen as a major factor in the cause of retrolental fibroplasia in premature infants" and recommending that oxygen, when administered, be in no higher concentration than 40 percent. Through a never-explained series of errors, the statement failed to be published in either the Academy's newsletter or its professional journal.

In areas like New York City, where public health officials took firm preventive measures, new cases of RLF showed a dramatic drop-off. Control mechanisms were introduced in the large medical centers whose airtight incubators had been responsible for the largest number of RLF cases. Most introduced such safeguards as using only tanks of premixed oxygen in concentrations no higher than 40 percent. But as the years went on and smaller hospitals in rural and suburban areas updated their pediatric equipment, sporadic new cases of RLF began to appear. The disease had become so rare, Dr. William Silverman said in 1968, "that most physicians lost interest because they saw so little of it."

What did attract medical interest at the time was infant death caused by the respiratory syndrome called hyaline membrane disease, for which the treatment was high oxygen administration. Once again doctors faced a difficult dilemma. Citing a 1967 survey which brought to light 33 new cases of retrolental fibroplasia, most of them incurred through treatment of premature infants for respiratory distress, Dr. Silverman warned that RLF, "the disease we thought had practically disappeared, is rearing its head once more." The accuracy of this warning was attested in 1972 when the parents of a four-year-old Connecticut child blinded by retrolental fibroplasia won a lawsuit for damages against the physicians who had treated the child at birth and the hospital where the oxygen overdose had been administered.

At the point where the medical profession could consider its end of the problem solved, a crisis point was being reached by those concerned with the thousands of young children already blinded by RLF. Keeping pace with the "baby boom" that followed the return of servicemen from World War II, the number of infants with retrolental fibroplasia peaked during the 1949–1953 period. New York State alone had 922 known cases in 1955; the children ranged in age from newborn to early teenage, with three out of four under six years of age.

Well before then, schools for the blind had begun to sense the upcoming demand. Residential schools in the epidemic areas initiated or expanded guidance services to parents of preschool blind children. They also began enlarging their facilities.

A "summer school" for mothers and their blind babies had been initiated in the Michigan School for the Blind in 1937 with good results, and a number of other schools decided on similar methods of parent counseling. Boston having been the hub of RLF discovery and concern, Perkins was the first to respond to the need for help. In the summer of 1945 it began a two-week institute at which the mothers of the RLF infants heard lectures by ophthalmologists, child psychiatrists, pediatricians, psychologists, and nursery school educators. They were given opportunity for individual consultations with these specialists and also observed the techniques used in a nursery school setup where their children, ranging in age from one to five years, were cared for. A collateral benefit was familiarization with the Perkins campus and facilities; many would be enrolling their children there in due course.

Overbrook, which began annual 12-day summer sessions of this type in 1949, soon found itself with a waiting list. It also prepared actively for the future by doubling its kindergarten facilities. On the West Coast, the Oregon school initiated annual summer institutes in 1949; with financial help from statewide fraternal bodies, it also started a successful program of placing blind preschool children in nursery schools with seeing children. The California school reported in 1953 that pupils under ten years of age already made up 40 percent of its population. Of greater significance was the fact that the number of blind children attending public schools in California had more than tripled in the preceding decade. Emotional support and guidance for parents were being supplied by a statewide program of visiting teachers.

Back in the east, Delaware, which had never established a state residential school, sending the majority of its blind children to public schools and the remainder to the nearby Maryland School for the Blind, coped with the emergency by setting up a special day nursery for blind infants; with virtually all of the state's RLF children concentrated in and around Wilmington, it was feasible to have them bussed to a single center. Funds to launch the nursery school were raised by public subscription in a 1950 campaign spearheaded by a parent group. Subsequent funding was taken over by the state commission for the blind.

The Connecticut School for the Blind reported in 1953 that its average enrollment had increased 50 percent in four years, and that the state had appropriated more than $500,000 to expand the school's facilities. The average entrance age, formerly nine, was now down to five; a greatly lengthened period of schooling was in view for the years ahead. A similar prospect was reported by Michigan, where the school had already had to increase its staff by three primary school teachers and two houseparents.

Most of these developments were recorded in the October 1953 issue of the *Outlook*, which printed a roundup of reports from various parts of the nation describing the impact of retrolental fibroplasia on educational facilities. Many schools had little to report. Located in areas not hit by the RLF epidemic, they were experiencing no pressure. Others were handicapped by the absence of hard data on which to base long-range planning. The latter problem was described by Robert H. Thompson of the Missouri school. How could intelligent planning take place without some accurate foreknowledge of demand? "We are torn between two dilemmas," Thompson wrote:

> One dilemma is the erecting of buildings for an anticipated enrollment which we hope medical science will prevent from materializing—in which case we could have mostly white elephants on our hands and second guessers would criticize us for our folly. The other dilemma is to wait to build until the increased enrollments have materialized and penalize those who have urgent need of our services by the delayed availability of adequate educational facilities. Either choice is distasteful.

Although RLF cases were restricted to relatively few states, the bulges in the affected schools sent up the national totals of residential school enrollment from 5,014 in 1949 to 5,324 in 1953. The public school figures showed really startling changes—from 656 blind pupils in 1949 to nearly twice that many—1,214—in 1953. In both instances the quantum jump still lay in the future, for as of 1953 the majority of RLF children were still too young for school.

Once the shift to public schools began in earnest, there was no reversing it; from year to year an increasing proportion of the nation's blind children would now be living at home and attending schools in their communities. The proportion of blind children educated in public schools, for so many years a flat 10 percent, reached 18.6 percent in 1953; five years later it was 48 percent; by 1962 it had reached 57 percent, and in 1972 it was apparently stabilized at just over 60 percent.

Several factors shared responsibility for the changed picture. One of the most dominant was a matter of social class. Mostly from the urban middle class, the families of the RLF children valued independence and self-direction and were imbued with greater confidence in their ability to cope and overcome than had been the case with the majority of families of earlier generations of blind children.

The postwar social climate also had its influence. It was an era of growing activism on the part of parents whose children had any sort of physical or mental handicap. Some of the major national health organizations dealing with specific disease entities—cerebral palsy, multiple sclerosis, muscular dystrophy, cystic fibrosis, and the like—came into being during this period, most of them parent-instigated. One consequence of the pressures exerted by parent groups was that school authorities were compelled to recognize the claims of all kinds of handicapped children to educational opportunity.

Demographic factors came into play as well. Public school systems previously without enough demand to establish educational provisions for blind children were now confronted with sufficient numbers to warrant setting them up. The postwar migration to suburbia spurred construction of innumerable new schools, and the parents of blind children made strong demands that resources be provided for their education.

The question about the public school movement raised by George Oliphant back in 1910—"shall we sit still and see if it will run over us?"—finally had an answer. But the answer, as it emerged, did not generate as much heat as might have been expected. By and large, those who still held the most passionate convictions on either side of the residential-public school debate were holdovers from an earlier generation. The newer leaders in education were no longer so concerned with it.

What were the main points that had divided the opposing camps? Public school advocates accused the residential schools of regimenting children, of weaning them away from their homes and families, of instilling unrealistic career expectations, of failing to prepare them adequately for the rebuffs of society. Defenders of the residential school denied these allegations, cited the excellent academic achievements of their graduates, and leveled their own charges: day classes in public schools were so inadequately equipped and so largely staffed with inexperienced teachers that the children attending them received inferior educations; blind children in integrated programs got lost in large public school classes where teachers could not possibly give them the individual attention they needed; public schools did not provide the physical training, musical, and manual arts programs at which residential schools excelled; the social acceptance of blind children by their sighted schoolmates was nominal rather than actual; blind children were largely excluded from the recreational and sports activities of the other students; blind children were needlessly indulged by both teachers and peers in matters of discipline and behavior.

The fair-minded among the educators recognized that most of these charges and countercharges had some validity, and sought to build bridges between the two forms of education so as to give blind children the best of both. One of the most useful forms of bridge-building was the practice, followed by the more progressive residential schools, of having their older students attend community high schools.

In earlier years such opportunities had been selectively granted to a handful of gifted students. First to adopt the practice on a general scale had been the New York State School at Batavia, the very institution whose cornerstone-laying ceremonies had been the scene of Howe's somber warnings against the evils of segregated education for blind children.

At the 1910 AAIB convention, Batavia reported success with sending its older students to a community high school. Among those who learned of the report was George F. Meyer, a sixteen-year-old boy just entering the ninth grade at the Washington State school for the blind. With the reluctant permission of the school's superintendent, he memorized the long walk to the nearest city, Vancouver, Washington, and enrolled in the local high school. But solving the travel problem was only the first step. As one of the colleagues associated with him in his later professional life told the George Meyer story:

> The janitor and one of the partially-seeing boys read assignments to him late into the evenings in a furnace room—the only place in the school with light that late at night. They took turns dictating the Latin textbooks letter by letter since neither had studied Latin. George hand-transcribed his own books. He was valedictorian of the 1914 class of some sixty or seventy pupils of the Vancouver, Washington High School and went on to receive his Phi Beta Kappa key at the University of Washington.

Understandably, Meyer turned into a strong advocate of public school education for blind children. In the early Twenties he organized the first such classes in Minneapolis and in Seattle; returning to Minneapolis, he spent 15 years as supervisor of classes for the blind before moving east to become executive director of the New Jersey State Commission for the Blind in 1937.

New Jersey was the perfect place for him. It was one of the few populous states that had never organized a residential school for the blind and was therefore among the pioneers in day school education. The first public school class opened in Newark in 1911 at the initiative of Meyer's predecessor, an energetic and imaginative blind woman named Lydia Y. Hayes. She had organized the New Jersey commission in 1909 and was largely responsible for shaping the state's policy toward education of the blind. She began the practice of having the state pay for reader service for blind students, rallied a corps of volunteers to produce brailled textbooks, and thriftily saw to it that when one student finished a textbook, it was handed on to the next. Blind children in rural areas, where there was not enough demand to organize classes, were sent to residential schools in the neighboring states of New York or Pennsylvania but were encouraged to return home for their high school work. Education, it should be noted in adding up the considerable accomplishments of Lydia Hayes, was only one of the commissioner's responsibilities; she directed all of the state's tax-supported work for the blind, children and adults alike.

Soon after George Meyer took over the job on Miss Hayes' retirement, he launched a new service, the itinerant teaching program, which made it possible for blind children to attend local schools even in small and scattered communities. This program, started in 1943 with a single traveling teacher, was so soundly conceived and developed that it served as a model for other states when the day school movement began its spurt of nationwide growth a decade later.

Meyer, who remained in office until five years before his death in late 1969, was a firm believer in public school education as a realistic introduction to adulthood. He compared this day-to-day exposure to the blunt facts of life in a normal home with the attitude frequently found in a residential school child, who thought of himself as a visitor when he returned home during school vacations and, consciously or unconsciously, made unfavorable comparisons between his family's modest living environment and the facilities afforded by a well-equipped residential school. Moreover, the child's feeling of alienation from his family and his community was all too often reciprocated.

Meyer's views represented one extreme; at the other was Merle E. Frampton who, throughout his 35-year tenure as principal of the New York Institute for the Education of the Blind, assumed a defender-of-the-faith mantle in proclaiming the superiority of residential school education. Frampton's attitude was best summed up in the title of a pamphlet he wrote in the mid-Sixties: *The Tragedy of Modern Day Education for the Blind as Practiced in the Integrated Public School Classes.*

Twenty elements of the "tragedy" were cited. Most were the traditional criticisms, but a few were new and rather far-fetched, such as his comment that urban transportation arrangements were "inadequate, erratic, costly and destructive of an optimum education program. How can a child be ready for study in any school after one to two hours of travel in the early morning? . . . The blind child on school arrival is ready for bed, not a rigorous program of education."

Unchanged from the stance of a book he co-authored in 1953, the gravamen of the Frampton position was that "there cannot be two 'bests' in a method" and that schools which segregated blind children for educational purposes "provide the best system so far conceived."

Despite its occasionally exaggerated rhetoric, the Frampton defense was temperate compared with the slashing attack leveled at residential schools many years earlier by Dr. Thomas D. Cutsforth, an instructor in psychology at the University of Kansas. After losing his sight at the age of eleven, Cutsforth himself had attended the Oregon School for the Blind from 1905 to 1912. He went on to the University of Oregon where he earned his baccalaureate and master's degrees and taught psychology before beginning his doctoral research.

In *The Blind in School and Society*, a book based on the research which earned him his doctorate in 1930, Cutsforth charged that graduates of schools for the blind were "very deficient in sensory and motor functions" and that this was due to the educational philosophy which steeped them in "the traditions and content of a visual development that runs counter to their personalities and is alien to their perceptual processes." The book, which had a strong Freudian orientation at a time when this viewpoint had not gained much ground in any but avant-garde circles, also dealt with the fantasy life of blind individuals, with sex behavior, personality development, and social adjustments.

Many of Cutsforth's points would later be recognized as sound, but his language was so immoderate and his criticism so unsparing that publication of the book met with a hail of offended reactions. Even the gentle, objective, and scholarly S.C. Swift described the work as "ferociously frank . . , scornfully cynical." Cutsforth's weakness, Swift wrote, "lies in the unsoundness of his generalizations—notwithstanding the fact that his judgments are delivered with all the assurance of infallibility." Samuel P. Hayes, who pioneered in the psychological evaluation of blind children, also questioned the author's fairness in building his arguments solely on cases of extreme maladjustment.

There is no record of any reaction by Helen Keller, whom Cutsforth repeatedly cited as a conspicuous example of how what he called "the hypocrisy of verbalism" subverted true educational aims. Imposing a "visual superstructure" on a child who has never had vision, he claimed, "robs the sensory world of a wealth of beauty and appreciation and leaves in its place empty husks of visual meaninglessness." The literary tradition underlying education of the blind "produced an optimum condition for word-mindedness."

Eventually Cutsforth's book gained enough respect as a piece of original thinking to prompt the Foundation to republish it long after it had gone out of print. A new edition, augmented by a speech Cutsforth had made on "Blindness as an Adequate Expression of Anxiety," was issued in 1951. Cutsforth himself was by then living in Los Angeles and maintaining a private practice as a clinical psychologist. He retired in 1959 and died three years later.

Cutsforth, whose book originally appeared in 1933, dealt only with the residential schools; he totally ignored the public school classes which, at that time, were educating an insignificant fraction of the nation's blind children. Twenty years later this was no longer true, and responsible leaders were asking themselves how well prepared were these public school systems to handle their mounting responsibilities.

In the early Fifties there was no universal answer. Pockets of experience existed in various places, but no one had put them together into either a philosophic or methodological framework. A landmark step was the week-long National Work Session on the Education of the Blind with the Sighted, which was held in August 1953. Sponsored by the Foundation, the Pine Brook Conference (so called because it took place at a camp of that name in the Adirondack Mountains) engaged the energies of two dozen experts in general and special education. The report of its findings, issued the following year, came to be a bible of first principles based, as the foreword noted, on "realistic thinking, actual experience, and a firm belief in the educational rights and needs of the individual blind child."

The conferees identified three main patterns of public school education of blind children—the Cooperative Plan, the Integrated Plan, and the Itinerant Teacher Plan—and pinned down the specific elements needed to make each of them work effectively.

The Cooperative Plan was the latter-day descendant of the earliest form of public school education, the "braille classes," in which blind children received all of their schooling from a special teacher trained in education of the blind. These were segregated classes, essentially similar to those in the residential schools; the main difference was that the child continued to live at home. At the beginning, the braille classes embraced both totally blind and partially sighted children. It did not take long, however, for the fallacy of this practice to be noted and separate "sight-saving" rooms were set aside for those pupils who had enough vision to use large print as their reading medium.

As time went on, practices in both the braille classes and the sight-saving classes underwent modification. Their pupils were sent to regular classrooms for some subjects, returning to their special home rooms for others and for supplemental help with the studies they were pursuing alongside sighted classmates. The home room teachers, who were specialists in education of the blind, provided whatever aids were needed: brailled or recorded texts, arithmetic boards, tactual maps and globes for the blind children, and large-type texts, optical magnifiers, bulletin typewriters and the like for the partially sighted. Each child's educational progress was planned and directed by his specialist teacher, who worked closely with the teachers of the regular classes the child attended. Hence the term "cooperative plan."

The Integrated Plan represented a step toward bringing visually handicapped children into closer context with their sighted peers. The blind or partially sighted child was no longer enrolled in a special home room but in an open class, and educational responsibility for him rested with the school's regular faculty. The specialist teacher of the blind operated out of what was called a "resource room," which was stocked with tactile and low-vision instructional equipment. The children came to the resource room as needed; also, as needed, members of the school's faculty consulted the specialist teacher on adaptations of classroom methods that enabled the visually handicapped child to keep pace with his fellows.

Under the Itinerant Teacher Plan the specialist instructor did not serve a single school but covered an entire district through periodic visits for consultation with teachers whose classes included visually handicapped children. This traveling teacher also saw to it that such children were supplied with texts and study materials in the forms they could use. The Itinerant Teacher Plan was a viable system for school districts in rural areas, or in large cities where each of many schools enrolled a few blind children. It worked particularly well in the junior high and high schools, where students needed less day-to-day guidance.

A somewhat different version of the Itinerant Teacher Plan, involving an operating partnership between a residential school and a state public school system, was already in existence at the time of the Pine Brook Conference. The "Oregon Plan" had been initiated in 1945 by the Oregon School for the Blind and the state's Division of Special Education. Here the residential school served as a kind of diagnostic and preparation center for blind children, equipping them with basic reading, writing, and other learning skills and then placing them in their local public schools under the continuing supervision of an itinerant teacher. A unique feature was the residential school's readiness to take the child back, if need be, for a shorter or longer period of additional training, or for ophthalmological treatment. In essence the Oregon Plan was not too different from what Samuel Gridley Howe had proposed at Batavia nearly a century earlier. But it also had a forward-looking aspect, for it presaged the climate of change that eventually would bring residential schools and public school systems into closer tandem.

Whatever the plan, each depended for its effectiveness on the knowledge and skills of the specialized teacher and on that teacher's ability to convey basic techniques to the much larger groups of teachers who had not been trained to work with blind children. The Pine Brook report outlined detailed orientation programs for the non-specialist teacher and comprehensive preparation programs at the graduate level for specialist teachers of the blind. Presumably the conferees recognized that what they proposed was more a prescription for the future than an instant remedy. Throughout the Fifties, as children born in the postwar population explosion began reaching school age, the nation faced a shortage of all types of teachers, but the shortage of those professionally qualified to work with blind children was particularly acute.

It was not a new phenomenon.

For the greater part of a century, teachers of the blind, whether in the residential schools or in the early public school classes, had acquired their skills through what was basically an apprenticeship. Many had no more than a high school education; motivation and adaptability were the characteristics sought by heads of schools for the blind. Many of those taken on as teachers were themselves graduates of the school. A few had gone through normal school and fewer still were college graduates. Actual teaching experience was a rarity.

Striving to have their schools recognized as educational facilities rather than institutions, the more progressive leaders in education of the blind were aware that qualified faculty was a prerequisite. In 1921 Edward Allen took an important step toward professionalization by establishing the Harvard Course on Education of the Blind. A six-month program operated in cooperation with Perkins by the Harvard Graduate School of Education, it earned its students credits toward a master's degree. Beginning in 1925, the course was supplemented by a second half-year program—the Special Method Course, in which the students underwent a residential apprenticeship at Perkins, attending lectures, observing classes and practice-teaching. Completion of this second unit, which was given under the direction of Jessica Langworth of the Perkins faculty, also earned graduate credits.

The same year that this twelve-month program began in Boston, a six-week summer course was initiated by I. S. Wampler, superintendent of the Tennessee School for the Blind, in a cooperative arrangement with George Peabody College for Teachers in Nashville. Those attending lived at the Tennessee School while taking instruction at Peabody from Wampler and the visiting faculty he assembled.

The two pioneer teacher training programs served different populations. The Harvard course attracted mainly newly graduated college or normal school students preparing for a career; the Nashville summer sessions were attended mostly by teachers already in service who were giving up part of their summer vacations. For various reasons, mainly financial, the Peabody program lapsed in 1928. It was revived for a single summer in 1931, but depression conditions made it a hardship for teachers to afford even the modest costs: $7 a week for room, board, and laundry ("a reasonable number of pieces," read the 1931 prospectus) and tuition at $4 per credit hour. The course was reinstated in 1935, with the help of a one-time grant from the American Foundation for the Blind.

During the same period that Allen and Wampler were striving to improve the skills of teachers in schools and classes for the blind, attempts were being made to introduce some orientation to blindness into general teacher preparation programs. The first such effort reportedly took place on the West Coast immediately after World War I when Dr. Richard S. French, principal of the California School for the Blind, and Dr. Newel Perry, his head teacher, served as lecturers in special education at the University of California. For several summers in the early Twenties, Robert Irwin held a similar post at Teachers College, Columbia University. In 1935 a more formal program was instituted at Columbia by Merle Frampton. It took the form of graduate scholarships, combining full-time study at the university with residence, proctorial and teaching duties at the New York Institute for the Education of the Blind. When the arrangement terminated in 1944, Teachers College asked the Foundation for help in restructuring its program and Berthold Lowenfeld accepted the post of lecturer in special education to fill the gap. The New York Institute's teacher training program was subsequently moved to Hunter College. Perkins, too, later transferred its course; it was moved from Harvard to Boston University in 1953.

As scanty as were the efforts to build a corps of professionally trained educators in all schools for blind children, the situation in the schools for Negro children was infinitely worse. Racial segregation not only kept black children in separate schools staffed by black teachers, but prevented those teachers from attending courses given at white southern colleges such as Peabody. Few earned enough to afford the expense of traveling to the non-segregated northern educational institutions which offered summer programs in special education.

One of the first assignments undertaken by Philip C. Potts when he joined the staff of the Foundation in 1937 was a survey of Negro schools for the blind, most of which were combined with schools for the deaf. His findings revealed such a need and hunger for training on the part of teachers in these schools that the Foundation moved to establish a pilot summer training program at a southern Negro college. The first such course was held in 1939 at West Virginia State College with the Foundation contributing Potts' time plus a modest grant to cover expenses for materials and to provide scholarships for some of the teachers who could not even manage the carfare from their homes to West Virginia.

The effort was so successful that the Foundation underwrote it for 14 successive summers. In 1942 the program was moved from West Virginia State to the Hampton Institute in Virginia, where completion of the eight-week session earned credits toward a graduate degree.

Practical results were seen almost immediately. In 1942 Robert Irwin wrote Mrs. Andrew Carnegie that "already in some of the southern states almost the entire staff of the school for the [Negro] blind is composed of teachers who have taken our summer school course." He did not mention, as he might have, that the project was the first and only one of its kind in the nation, and that it had already had a ripple effect that went beyond schools for blind children. With the help of credits earned through this course, one blind man who had been working in a broom shop became a professor in a southern Negro college; another obtained a teaching position in a state school; two others qualified for civil service appointments in public schools and still another obtained a Rosenwald fellowship for advanced study.

During most of the Forties Potts also directed a summer graduate course for teachers of the blind in the Department of Education of the University of Wisconsin, while Lowenfeld gave a similar course at the College of Education of the University of Washington. The same period also saw the Foundation heavily involved in sponsoring courses for home teachers at a number of colleges and universities, and, in cooperation with Perkins, giving a summer course for teachers of deaf-blind children at Michigan State Normal College.

There was one other key element in professionalizing the teaching of blind children that owed much to P. C. Potts. He headed a committee appointed by the AAIB in 1932 to consider the question of teacher qualifications; it was this committee that developed the three-level plan instituted by the Association for certification of teachers in schools and classes for the blind.

AAIB's teacher certification program was officially adopted in 1938 and the first awards made at its 1940 convention. By 1948, a total of 275 certificates had been issued. One explanation for the modesty of this figure was that even though the plan contained grandfather clauses which permitted the substitution of experience for academic credentials, many of the blind teachers working in the schools did not and could not measure up to certificate requirements.

It was Neal F. Quimby, superintendent of the New Mexico School for the

Blind, who ventured to grasp this nettle in public. In a 1949 address to the AAWB—an address he prefaced by predicting that his comments would displease many in the audience—he spelled out his charges. Too many blind teachers, he said, were apt to "trade on their handicaps as an excuse for poor work," to exhibit emotional instability in reacting to criticism, to either resist all change or, at the other extreme, entertain radical notions for change, to harbor "an exaggerated idea of their real abilities." Quimby, who had spent 14 years as principal at Overbrook before moving to the New Mexico superintendency, acknowledged the distinctive assets that blind teachers could bring to their work but decried the inbreeding resulting from the desire "to look after our own" that led many schools to recruit teachers mainly from the ranks of their graduates. He blamed this practice, plus poor vocational counseling, for clogging the schools with people better suited to other occupations.

Coming as they did when educators of the blind already knew of 6,000 newly blinded infants, Quimby's remarks were timely. A problem of unknown proportions clearly loomed ahead, and those conscientiously concerned over education of the rising generation of blind children had to get ready as best they could.

"The time is not far distant," Quimby also warned, "when we will require equal intelligence and training for those responsible for the children out of school hours as we do for those who work with them in the classroom." He was speaking primarily of the residential school houseparents. With schools accepting pupils at earlier and earlier ages, the role of these adults as friends, confidants and surrogate parents was one of steadily growing importance. Recognition of their influence led the Foundation, beginning in the mid-Fifties, to stage a series of regional institutes for houseparents, designed to effect a closer partnership between them and teachers, social workers, and other professional personnel in the residential schools.

By 1954, when the tide of newly blinded babies was finally ebbing, it became possible to make a realistic projection of future manpower needs in education. A study made that year under the joint sponsorship of the Southern Regional Education Board, Peabody College, and the Foundation recommended adoption of a regional plan for teacher preparation, covering 16 southern states. Under this plan, Peabody would establish a year-round training program for teachers of visually handicapped children. The program would be launched with sufficient financial support from the Foundation to support a full-time professorship, five graduate training fellowships a year, plus a number of summer school scholarships.

The Peabody program got under way in 1957, with Samuel C. Ashcroft, formerly director of educational research for the American Printing House for the Blind, as its director. The Foundation's commitment was for $50,000 over a three-year period; subsequent financing was to come from the 16 states represented in the Southern Regional Education Board. When these funds failed to materialize in sufficient degree, money for two additional years of support was voted by the Foundation.

The regional teacher training program at Peabody was expected to be the first of a number of such regional centers strategically located across the nation. The thinking was that they would replace the hit-or-miss system under which schools for the blind had to rely on nearby colleges or universities for summer training courses. As things worked out, the regional center plan proved needless. In October 1963 the passage of Public Law 88-164 expanded earlier provisions for federal support in the education of certain categories of handicapped children to embrace a wider range of disabilities, of which blindness was one. Under this law an appropriation of just under $500,000 became available to finance 14 training centers for teachers of the blind. Subsequent federal legislation further enlarged the depth and scope of support for the education of the handicapped. In 1972 professional undergraduate and graduate preparation programs for teachers of the visually handicapped existed in 27 colleges and universities in 17 states.

The early decades of the twentieth century were periods of lively ferment in educational theory. What was the real purpose of education? How and why did children learn? Traditional educational methods had been keyed to the idea that the purpose of schooling was to inculcate habits of mental discipline that prepared children for adult life. No, said John Dewey among others, education is not merely a pre-game warmup, it is the game itself. Children were not adults in miniature, they had their own sets of values, their own realities, and education should acknowledge and build on these by working with "the whole child." Progressive education, the term given to this new approach, encouraged children to pursue their own interests, wherever they led, rather than having them squeezed into precast courses of study. Learning by doing instead of learning by rote was seen as the highroad to sound intellectual growth.

This new thinking was not lost on educators of blind children. As early as 1918 Thomas S. McAloney, then superintendent of the Western Pennsylvania School for the Blind, devoted his presidential address at that year's AAIB convention to the "new education" and how it affected schools for the blind. Every educator knew that blind children, like all others, were distributed along the entire intelligence curve from dull to gifted. Therefore, said McAloney, "we should have different standards for different mentalities, and . . . each individual should be studied and standards set for him."

How could these different mentalities be evaluated? A teacher's classroom observations might well be subjective. A more objective tool was the newly emerging science of psychology. Even as McAloney spoke, two schools for the blind were already applying its techniques to measuring the intellectual capacities of pupils. One of these was the Philadelphia school where, in the fall of 1916, Principal Olin H. Burritt had instituted a Department of Psychological Research with four closely related aims. As detailed by the department's director, these were:

1. To develop and apply methods for testing the mentality of pupils in schools for the blind; 2. To apply the technique of experimental psychology to some of the problems in the psychology of the blind; 3. To adapt to the blind some of the standard tests of school subjects now so widely used upon the sighted, and if possible, to suggest improvements in the pedagogy of the blind; 4. To work towards a method of vocational guidance through the use of mental tests of various sorts.

Burritt's initiative introduced into work for the blind a new personality, Samuel P. Hayes, Ph.D., whose name was to become part of the working vocabulary of all educators of the blind for the next half century. Hayes, a professor of psychology at Mount Holyoke College, had been referred to Burritt by Dr. Henry H. Goddard, head of the New Jersey Training School for the Feeble Minded at Vineland. One of the several psychologists who had worked out an American version of the Binet-Simon intelligence scales, Goddard already knew something of the problems in testing blind children. As noted in an earlier chapter, Robert Irwin had spent the summer of 1914 at Vineland, working with him on a version of the IQ protocols that replaced vision-related items with tactual or oral tests. Although Irwin's efforts failed to produce usable results, his collaboration with Goddard bore fruit when Burritt asked for help in introducing psychological testing at Overbrook.

Goddard mentioned this request in a talk to a group of psychologists. Among them was the thirty-one-year-old Hayes, who had earned his doctorate in psychology at Cornell University with a dissertation on color blindness. The idea of working with real blindness intrigued him. He accepted the part-time post of directing psychological research at the Philadelphia school and took a half-year's leave of absence from Mount Holyoke to live at Overbrook and gain a firsthand knowledge of blind children and the methods of educating them. He also assigned one of the graduates of his Mount Holyoke course to work full-time at the school.

Hayes was a slightly built man whose looks and manner suggested a kindly clergyman (a career he had once considered) or an absent-minded scholar. But the impression was deceptive. He was a prodigious worker and a prolific writer who continued to teach at Mount Holyoke until he retired in 1940 at the age of sixty-five. He lived another 18 years after that, professionally active until the end.

At about the same time psychological work was begun at Overbrook, Perkins employed a Vassar College graduate to administer intelligence and achievement tests to its student body. In 1918 the two schools decided to join forces by having Hayes divide his consulting time between them. At this point Hayes engaged one of the brightest of that year's Mount Holyoke graduates, Kathryn Maxfield, to take over the work at Perkins under his supervision. He also added a second assistant at Overbrook. In describing these arrangements to the AAWB in 1919 Hayes made clear that:

> The use in schools for the blind of standardized tests of school subjects is still in its first or experimental stage.... Undoubtedly the standards will not be the same as those for sighted pupils, and it may take a considerable time before it will be safe to set standards for blind pupils.

He was to spend his entire professional life refining and revising these tests, trying them out in first a handful, and then a broad range, of schools and classes until, by the late 1940s, he was reasonably satisfied he had gone about as far as he could in working out instruments comparable to those used in measuring the intelligence or achievement of sighted children.

There were any number of obstacles, large and small, to be overcome. For one thing, the generalized IQ and achievement scales were constantly being revised and new psychological tests, such as the Wechsler-Bellevue batteries, brought into use. For another, the schools and classes for the blind contained children with a wide range of visual handicap, from total blindness to near-normal sight; tests for the partially sighted could not be the same as those for the children who could see nothing. Evaluation of test results also had to take into account the age of onset of blindness. A congenitally blind twelve-year-old boy, educated in finger-reading from the beginning, might well do better on a brailled test than a boy of the same age and mental capacity who had been blind a relatively short time and was not yet at home with braille. Oral administration of tests was one way of equalizing this.

The testing techniques themselves had to be made foolproof. For example, as Hayes once explained, in a true-false test in which the children used braille slates to record their answers, it was quickly discovered that

> we must not let pupils write *t* for true and *f* for false on their braille slates because the braille *t* requires four dots while *f* requires only three, so the slower or less capable pupils have only to listen to the clicks made by the best pupils and write the same letters themselves.

A way out was found by instructing the children to use *c* for correct and *i* for incorrect, since both were two-click letters.

Consistently validated over a period of more than two decades, Hayes' findings were essentially that, in the better schools for the blind,

> pupils test up to the seeing standards grade for grade. We cannot say that their educational achievement is equal to that of the seeing, for in most grades the blind tend to be about two years older, partly due to later entrance into school and partly as a result of the time consuming process of education through the fingers.

He also found that in the administration of verbal intelligence and school achievement tests, blind children needed more than twice as much time as the sighted because braille was a slower reading medium than inkprint. The substitution of oral examinations likewise slowed down the testing process.

Hayes made many efforts to work out ways of testing non-verbal areas, such as motor skills or manual aptitudes, but he did not get far, nor did he have much better luck with tests designed to yield personality profiles or vocational interest inventories. It remained for the next generation of psychologists to tackle these problems, with varying degrees of success.

Prominent in this second echelon was Mary K. Bauman, who developed a set of manual dexterity tests for blind persons during World War II. As director of psychometric work at Philadelphia's Trainee Acceptance Center, an organization which guided applicants for defense work into the training programs and industrial jobs they were best suited for, she discovered that no usable instrument existed that could test blind persons for manual or mechanical skills. She proceeded to develop her own adaptations of the performance tests used with sighted persons and tried them out with a group of blind volunteers. These were the first of many contributions Mrs. Bauman made to the development of non-verbal psychological evaluation instruments for visually handicapped people. Her increasing interest in the subject led to her establishing a psychological testing and vocational guidance service for blind persons. She gave this up in 1968 to become executive secretary of the Association for the Education of the Visually Handicapped (AEVH, formerly AAIB).

In a retrospective review published in 1972, Mary Bauman made it clear that much remained to be done in perfecting reliable performance tests for blind persons:

> Psychologists and educators alike recognize that ability takes both verbal and non-verbal forms and that to measure only one of these is to measure only half of the individual's potential. . . . [Most of the non-verbal tests] which have been developed are inadequately normed, poorly validated, and lack that body of interpretative data which could make them useful to the many psychologists who see only a few blind persons each year. . . . we know little more about the performance ability of blind people than we did in the 1930's.

As keen as were educators of the blind to use the tools of psychology for assessment of student potential, they were even more concerned with how this new science could help improve teaching content and methodology. Robert Irwin was among those who had firm convictions on the pressing need for research in educational methods. A year after the Foundation opened its offices he hired Samuel Hayes' protégé, Kathryn Maxfield, as the staff educational psychologist and assigned as her first project a study of braille reading and how it was taught. Three monographs by Miss Maxfield in as many years culminated in a basic teacher's manual, *The Blind Child and His Reading*, published in 1927, and in the decision to link future research more closely to actual practice. This was accomplished by means of an "experimental school" project, jointly sponsored by the Foundation and Perkins, in which the latter's primary grades served as a laboratory for testing new approaches.

With Kathryn Maxfield as overall supervisor and Dr. Frieda Kiefer (she became Mrs. Ralph Merry soon thereafter) as resident director at Perkins, the experimental school, known as the Department of Special Studies, began in the autumn of 1927. Following up on the braille reading study, one of the initial experiments tested the relative merits of teaching beginners to write braille with traditional slate and stylus as against teaching them the use of the mechanical braillewriter. Other experiments tried out the teaching of reading by the word method, differing approaches to arithmetic instruction, various classroom seating arrangements and a "project teaching" approach to nature study. In addition, some individual psychological studies were pursued. Diagnostic workups were made of children with learning or behavior problems, followed by remedial programs designed to help.

As the project's findings emerged, reports were issued for consideration by other schools for the blind. A major medium for this material was the *Teachers Forum,* a bimonthly periodical initiated by the Foundation in 1928 as a vehicle for exchange of news and experience in educational methods. Kathryn Maxfield served as its founding editor; Samuel P. Hayes was a steady contributor of articles dealing with psychological work; faculty members of various schools wrote on curriculum development and teaching techniques; and the editorial content gradually broadened its scope to cover a range of collateral issues.

The *Teachers Forum,* which was one element in the Foundation-Perkins partnership, continued for a number of years after joint sponsorship of the experimental school came to an end in 1932. "It is the intention of Perkins to turn the whole Institution into an experimental and demonstration school," read one official explanation in the *Teachers Forum* of September 1932. "To our regret this valuable work will be discontinued . . . owing to lack of funds," read another official explanation, this one in the Foundation's annual report for 1932. Neither told the whole story. A more revealing glimpse was given by President Migel in his report to the Foundation board at its 1932 annual meeting: "Recently the newly appointed director of Perkins Institution has expressed a desire to continue this work independently of the Foundation, and has employed our former Educational Psychologist to direct this and other work connected with his school."

Back of all these explanations lay an administrative upheaval at Perkins that for months on end had been the subject of agitated talk and rumors throughout the field of work for the blind.

In mid-1931, much against his will, Edward E. Allen was retired from the directorship of Perkins and replaced by the Reverend Gabriel Farrell, rector of the Protestant Episcopal Church of Rhinebeck, New York, who was a stranger to both education and work for the blind. Allen's colleagues and the large body of blind people who had been his students during his more than forty years of educational leadership were scandalized by the peremptory manner in which he was removed from office just one year before Perkins was to observe its centennial and Allen himself to complete a quarter century of directorship of the school. On less personal grounds, the protests centered around the choice of a non-educator to head the nation's most prestigious school for the blind at a time when all such schools were striving for professional recognition in the field of education.

Proper Bostonians that they were, the Perkins trustees refrained from public response to a flood of private and published scoldings. Had they cared to, they could well have made out a reasonable case for their actions. Allen was seventy years old; for well over a year he had been urged, first informally and then by official committee action, to prepare for retirement by finding and training an understudy. But he had dragged his heels, unable to settle on a candidate he considered qualified. In a scrapbook assembled by his wife, documenting the circumstances of his retirement, one may find not only the innumerable letters from admirers which, she wrote, "kept his heart from breaking during this most trying experience of his otherwise happy and unclouded life," but also some of his correspondence with the Perkins trustees. Reading between the lines makes it apparent that Allen had suffered from ill health for some years, and that this had affected his work. In a memorandum sent to the trustees in January 1931 he noted that when their committee had formally notified him in the summer of 1930 that he should get ready to retire, he was "stunned" but acquiesced. However, he added, "I did not tell them that having finally learned to overcome my insomnia I was then feeling like my old self again."

At the time he submitted this memorandum, in which he reviewed the accomplishments of his administration—"Perkins as it is now is largely my own creation"—he was pleading to be given additional time to hand over the reins to a successor. The trustees, however, wanted the new director to take full charge at once. When Allen resisted, they moved ahead without consulting him further. He was given a pension and the title of director emeritus to become effective with his formal retirement at the end of June 1931.

Once the initial shock wave receded, Edward Allen's friends turned to salvaging his ego. At the end of April he was made guest of honor at the dinner jointly given by M. C. Migel and William Nelson Cromwell to wind up the World Conference on Work for the Blind. Olin Burritt had already written Migel in February suggesting "the extreme desirability of the Foundation taking active steps immediately to invite Dr. Allen to accept an official relation to the Foundation," specifically as a regular contributor to the *Outlook* and the *Teachers Forum* on topics "on which he is probably better qualified to speak than anyone else in the United States." Thereafter Allen's byline was to be found on many feature articles in the *Outlook* and in every issue of the *Teachers Forum,* where he conducted a largely reminiscent column, "Dr. Allen Says."

Other honors followed. The Perkins Alumni Association and its student body petitioned the trustees to name the school's chapel for him and there were suitable dedicatory ceremonies. When it met that summer, the AAWB adopted a laudatory resolution praising Allen's accomplishments; some years later it presented him with its Shotwell Award. Probably more meaningful to him at the time of the crisis was another resolution adopted at the AAWB's 1931 convention declaring

> that boards of trustees when appointing heads of schools and institutions for
> the education of the blind . . . should place in charge of such schools and
> institutions only professional educators, and, when possible, those who are
> trained and experienced in the special work of educating the blind, and . . .
> that failure to live up to such principles on the part of boards of trustees . . . is
> to fail seriously in the performance of their higher duties and to place other
> interests before the welfare of the blind themselves and the welfare of
> society.

To Gabriel Farrell, who met his future colleagues for the first time at that very meeting, the adoption of the resolution hardly constituted a cordial welcome. But wiser heads among the confraternity recognized the futility of fighting a *fait accompli;* it was reportedly John F. Bledsoe of the Maryland School who led the way in breaking what amounted to a silent boycott and helping the newcomer feel at home.

Within a few years, Farrell made it on his own. During the two decades he was the Perkins director, he instituted many important administrative and program changes that won the respect of his fellow school heads. He was also astute enough not to repeat Allen's mistake of failing to groom a successor. When he retired in 1951, the directorship went to Edward J. Waterhouse, who had been with the school for 14 years, first as a teacher and then as head of the school's manufacturing affiliate, Howe Press. Waterhouse, too, was careful to train an understudy; when his turn came to retire in 1971, there was a smooth transition to Benjamin F. Smith. Smith, Perkins' sixth director and the first blind man to occupy the post, had started as dean of boys 20 years earlier and had been promoted successively to principal and assistant director before moving into the top spot.

Edward Allen's heart did not break after all. He remained active for a good number of years following his retirement, continuing to direct the teacher-training Harvard Course until 1949, when it was taken over by Farrell. (Under Waterhouse's administration the course was transferred to Boston University.)

Allen lived to be eighty-nine years old; his wife, the former Katherine Gibbs, whom he had married in 1891 when they were both teachers at Perkins, died in 1952, two years after him. Gabriel Farrell also lived to a ripe age; he was eighty-two when he died in 1968. Ironically, it was Farrell, the erstwhile stranger, who managed to accomplish during his retirement what Allen had long intended but never quite got around to doing. Farrell wrote a book, *The Story of Blindness*, capsulizing the history of work for the blind up through the middle of the twentieth century.

The depression years saw relative quiescence in curriculum development, although some of the residential schools managed to utilize depression manpower to enrich their supply of teaching materials. With the help of Works Progress Administration workers, the Ohio school constructed a large number of scale models for use in object teaching. In 1941 the Foundation organized a traveling collection of these models, which fitted in well with the Talking Book Education Project. Children who listened to a recorded biography of George Washington, for example, could deepen their understanding through tactual examination of a model of Mount Vernon or one of the Revolutionary War battlefields.

This same era saw the initiation of still another approach to expanding children's learning opportunities. The Dramatic Arts Project was an idea that captured the imagination of M.C. Migel. He had somehow met the actress and dramatic coach Ruth Vivian, a featured player in the Broadway hit *The Man Who Came to Dinner*, and in the spring of 1939 told the executive committee that he had personally engaged her to demonstrate at three schools for the blind how dramatics could enhance the development of poise and self-confidence.

These trial runs at the Ohio, Maryland and Minnesota schools went so well that the following summer the Major arranged, again at his own expense, to have Miss Vivian and two other coaches conduct a six-week summer course in the techniques of play production. Attended by 16 teachers from as many schools, the course was given at Rest Haven, the vacation home for blind women then still privately financed by the Migel family. Twelve blind students formed the experimental acting company for demonstration purposes.

The course's unmistakable effectiveness in training teachers to conduct dramatics programs in their schools led the Foundation to turn to the Rockefeller Foundation for a two-year grant of $30,000. The application was backed by the results of a questionnaire which established that 37 schools for the blind were keenly interested in adding dramatics to their curriculums but lacked both the financial resources and the expertise to do so. The requested funds would make it possible for three coaches to train faculty members in all of these interested schools, spending five or six weeks in each.

Grant approved, the project got under way in the summer of 1941 with a budget that provided not only the coaches' salaries but the necessary support materials: props, costumes, prompt-books and individual brailled scripts for each part in 24 separate plays. Reduced royalty rates were negotiated with the copyright holders of the selected plays, which ranged from simple one-acters for younger children to more sophisticated full-length comedies such as Sidney Howard's *The Late Christopher Bean* and Kaufman and Connelly's *Dulcy*.

The Dramatic Arts venture proved immensely popular with faculty and students alike. During its two-year span more than 200 teachers in 30-odd schools were trained in play production and direction and close to 1,000 blind boys and girls were exposed to their first taste of stage fever. Measures were also taken to correlate dramatics with the basic school curriculum. To enrich classroom work in such subjects as history, English, and social studies, a series of 13 one-act plays, "Dramatic Hours in American History," was produced on Talking Books along with corresponding sets of brailled scripts and prompt-books.

For the first year after Kathryn Maxfield's departure from the Foundation to become director of personnel and research at Perkins, she continued to function as editor of the *Teachers Forum,* sharing responsibility with Eber L. Palmer, who had just come on staff as Foundation assistant director. Palmer took over as sole editor in September 1933 and remained in charge until he left in 1937 to head the New York State School for the Blind at Batavia, at which time editorship was transferred to his successor as assistant director, P. C. Potts. The *Teachers Forum* continued as an independent publication until the end of 1941, after which it was merged with the *Outlook.*

Miss Maxfield remained at Perkins less than two years before moving to a new job where she could pursue what had become her major interest: the psychological study of preschool blind children. In early 1934 she became director of the Arthur Sunshine Home and Kindergarten for Blind Babies in Summit, New Jersey.

Founded in 1909, this was an institution with a complex and not altogether praiseworthy history, that had just undergone a thorough internal reorganization. The new director was employed to give the organization a fresh start. The Home, which had formerly provided primarily custodial care for a mixed population of blind babies and older, mentally retarded blind children, would now adopt a two-pronged service program: as a laboratory where the needs of preschool blind children might be studied, and as a training center for counselors who would visit blind babies in their own homes and extend guidance to their parents.

While still on the Foundation staff Kathryn Maxfield had made a preliminary survey seeking "productive avenues of approach to the problems of the preschool blind child." Case records of 110 such children under the care of nine agencies were analyzed, but the results were foggy and the only conclusion to be drawn was that "the gate to the proper field of knowledge eludes discovery."

Some of the fog was dispelled by what Miss Maxfield accomplished at the Arthur Home before lack of funds forced it to close its residential unit in 1938, and by the studies she conducted during later stages of a long professional career. Her work laid some solid foundations for the major changes that took place in pre-school services during the Fifties.

That work with blind children had to begin at an early age had long been recognized. Every teacher had seen children report for school who had not yet learned to use a knife and fork or to tie their shoelaces; some were physically underdeveloped and lacking in basic motor skills; some were excessively timid; some were addicted to such "blindisms" as eye-rubbing, facial contortions, rocking and swaying of the body or other forms of self-stimulation; some were so totally self-absorbed as to be unable to relate to others.

Such developmental lags were less apt to denote intellectual deficiency than inadequate upbringing during the formative years. In the early days of education of blind children, most schools bemoaned this situation but accepted as inevitable that each newly admitted child's first year of education would have to focus as much on overcoming poor parental training as on introducing cognitive learning. Here and there, however, special nursery schools were set up on behalf of blind babies, notably those born to desperately poor families or those maltreated by ignorant or indifferent parents.

The nation's first came into being in Connecticut in the late nineteenth century when Emily Welles Foster, a wealthy and devout churchwoman of the Lady Bountiful era, literally stumbled over a small boy sprawled on the floor of a dimly lit hallway in a Hartford tenement, where she had gone in search of one of her Sunday School pupils. After she had picked him up and assured herself he was not hurt, she learned that he was "blind Tony," aged seven, who spent most of his days lying in the hallway and drumming his feet against the wall.

Seeking out the boy's parents, Mrs. Foster found they were non-English-speaking Italian immigrants whose provincial dialect was so different that they could not understand the phrases she studiously mastered in standard Italian. This dialect was the only language little Tony knew, but somewhat like Anne Sullivan, who at that very time, 1888, was in the early stages of her work with Helen Keller, Mrs. Foster determined to find a way to communicate with him. As she herself was to say, she felt that "language was the key by which the door of his shut-in mind might be opened to our world."

Within a few months she had learned enough of Tony's dialect to begin to teach him the equivalent English words. When, to give him a taste of fresh air and sunshine, she occasionally took the boy to her suburban home for a day or two, she became aware of how much more rapidly he responded to teaching in surroundings where there were fields and trees and birds to provide him with new sensory experiences. Tony's parents could also see the difference, and soon agreed to surrender their son to Mrs. Foster's care. He was joined at her home by another blind child taken from the Hartford almshouse.

Emily Foster's initial objective was to prepare these little boys for schooling; at the time, the state of Connecticut had an arrangement under which it could send 20 pupils a year to Perkins. She accomplished this, but her aims soon broadened to embrace a more general interest in the welfare of all blind people. Among those she encountered while organizing a social club for adult blind residents of Hartford was an attorney, Frank Cleaveland, who in 1893 helped her persuade the Connecticut legislature to enact a bill establishing a Board of Education for the Blind separate from the state's department of charities. It was the first such autonomous agency in the nation, and ironically, its primacy nearly led to its untimely demise. In 1899 the legislature debated a resolution to abolish it "because no other state had one." (A few years later this was no longer a fact; in 1907 Massachusetts established an independent state commission for the blind.)

Under the Connecticut statute, which provided that any visually impaired resident who could not be educated in the common school "is entitled to be educated in such a way and for such a time" as the newly created board decided, the nation's first nursery for neglected blind babies was established in Hartford in 1893 with the help of funds raised by Emily Foster and others she recruited. It was later moved to Farmington, where it remained in operation until the premises were destroyed by fire in 1934. By then social conditions had changed. The ophthalmia neonatorum responsible, in Mrs. Foster's day, for the blindness of so many newborn infants had been largely eradicated, and no one could have anticipated retrolental fibroplasia. Connecticut's nursery was never rebuilt; in its place, the Board of Education for the Blind engaged a "mother's counselor" to serve blind infants through home visits.

The straight-backed, blue-eyed Emily Welles Foster, whose portrait hangs in the offices of the present-day Connecticut education board, served as one of its members by appointment of the governor until her death in 1918. Long before then she had the satisfaction of seeing her first protégé, Antonio Martello, become the self-supporting and respected newsvendor at Hartford's railroad station.

Second in seniority of service for preschool blind children was the Boston Nursery for Blind Babies. It was founded in 1901 by Isabel Greeley who, as a teacher in the Perkins kindergarten, came to realize that the five- and six-year-old children enrolled there would have benefited by much earlier care and training. Her ideas attracted the support of Boston society and the nursery, which started in a private house with three or four small children in residence, soon moved to larger quarters with room for 25. In 1934 a day nursery program was added which, according to an account published at the time, served all preschool children with impaired vision "whether they have no sight or only slightly defective sight" but not "children of low mental capacity." This nursery was still in existence in 1972, although its name had changed to Boston Center for Blind Children and the basic emphasis of its services had been reversed to focus on diagnostic service and residential treatment for emotionally disturbed children who had visual disabilities.

A handful of other residential nurseries subsequently came into being, but by World War II most of these had either closed their doors, changed their programs or been absorbed into general service agencies. For the most part, the nurseries were supported by voluntary contributions; the Los Angeles Nursery School for Visually Handicapped Children, for example, was established in 1938 by Delta Gamma, a sorority group. There was little governmental support for such programs; an item in the *Teachers Forum* in May 1930 noted that, as of that date, only 13 states were financing services for blind babies.

When the retrolental fibroplasia epidemic struck, many parents turned for guidance to community agencies—child care and family service organizations—

whose social work staffs tended to focus less on the day-by-day training of the blind child than on the emotional and psychological impact of blindness on overall family structure and relationships. These social workers knew relatively little about practical training techniques; what they did know, and dealt with, were ways of helping parents come to terms with their feelings about having a blind child.

A 1944 psychological research study analyzing the influence of parental attitudes on the personality development of a blind child divided these attitudes into five fairly distinct but occasionally overlapping categories: acceptance of the child and his handicap, denial of the effects of the handicap, overprotectiveness, disguised rejection, and open rejection. The adjustment mechanisms produced in the children by these differing parental attitudes were also grouped into five classifications: compensatory behavior, denial, defensive behavior, withdrawal, and non-adjustive behavior. While these two sets could not be shown to have a one-to-one correspondence, the general conclusion of the author, Dr. Vita Stein Sommers, was that

> blind individuals tended to make a wholesome personal and social adjustment whenever their early life afforded them a reasonable amount of economic, physical and emotional security, whenever they were fully accepted by the members of their family, and the parents were able to face their handicap in an objective way.

None of the later in-depth studies of the blind children—or, for that matter, the general child development studies conducted by authorities such as Erikson— differed materially from this postulation.

In an effort to crystallize and disseminate such insights the Foundation convened a three-day National Conference on the Blind Preschool Child in early 1947. The extent to which interest in this subject had moved out of the restricted circle of agencies for the blind into broader professional areas was evident from the roster of speakers, among them Dr. Lauretta Bender, senior psychiatrist of New York's Bellevue Hospital, Dr. Arnold Gesell, director of Yale Medical School's Clinic of Child Development, and Anna W. M. Wolf of the Child Study Association of America.

Included in the recommendations in the published conference proceedings were two that promptly drew fire from the residential school heads. One was that "the accent should be on leaving the child in his family and providing the family, particularly the mother, with guidance and, if necessary, case work help" from social workers in general casework agencies. Such social workers, though not specifically experienced in the problems of blindness, could nevertheless make use of "sound child-psychological and psychotherapeutic principles." Day nursery services could be a resource for children while their parents were receiving this guidance.

The other was a statement by Robert Irwin that, for the sake of overall unification, responsibility for service to preschool children should be assumed by state commissions for the blind.

At the opening of the next AAIB convention, William E. Allen of the Texas School for the Blind devoted much of his presidential address to an attack on these recommendations. Under optimum conditions, he said, keeping children at home and sending them to day nurseries might be all right in large metropolitan cities, but it was no solution in states like his, where pupils in the school for the blind were drawn from 95 counties scattered over a wide territory. As for state commissions, they dealt primarily with blind adults. Work for the preschool child was

> clearly within the field of the residential school for it bears no resemblance to vocational training and placement of the adult blind. Training of the pre-school blind child is a forerunner of the primary work done in residential schools. Can you picture a nursery school for the seeing under the control of a United States Employment Bureau?

What Allen was really driving at was the threat that what he termed "social work thinking" would undermine residential school education. Joseph G. Cauffman of Overbrook reinforced that point in his speech. He acknowledged that the social worker had much to contribute "but the program in my estimation should be controlled by educators."

The fears that underlay these protests were real enough. The residential school heads were speaking at a time when a powerful anti-institutional trend dominated child welfare services. All over the country orphanages were being disbanded and their wards placed in foster homes. Child development studies dwelt strongly on the damaging effects of maternal deprivation and the need for the very young child to have a one-to-one relationship with a mothering figure, something not even the best-run congregate institution could supply.

But the fears were also premature. In 1948 the retrolental wave had not yet reached its peak; in a state like Texas, the first case of an RLF-blinded child had yet to appear. During the next two decades sheer numbers would provide enough "business" to tax the facilities of all types of educational programs for blind children. But the suspicion and bitterness touched off by the Foundation-sponsored conference remained and festered for a considerable time. The Foundation, some educators alleged, was out to denigrate and destroy the residential schools.

True, Robert Irwin had never made a secret of his bias in favor of public school education. One of the first challenges faced by Barnett when he succeeded Irwin was to persuade the educators that both his personal attitude and the Foundation's official policy were even-handed. An early staff appointment lent credence to this avowal. As consultant in education Barnett appointed Georgie Lee Abel, whose entire professional experience had been in residential schools: Tennessee and Idaho, where she taught, Iowa where she served for eight years as principal, Overbrook where she held an administrative post. Soon after taking office in August 1950, she addressed an open letter to educators to declare that her office would serve "as a sort of clearing house for outstanding contributions to the education of blind children" from all sources, and that "in all things of an educational nature we hope to develop a sane and sympathetic philosophy which we can share and explain."

A study of programs for preschool blind children, which was Miss Abel's first major undertaking, revealed the paucity and uneven quality of existing services and led to a second national meeting on the subject. Unlike the 1947 conference, which had been opened to a large general audience, the 1951 event was a concentrated four-day work session for 35 selected participants representing education and such collateral disciplines as ophthalmology, psychiatry, psychology and social work. The conference report contained nothing to upset anyone. Its most tangible result was the Foundation's employment, the following year, of a consultant in preschool education, Pauline Moor, whose professional experience in parent guidance included six years on the RLF research team organized by Dr. Theodore Terry.

As the retrolental wave subsided and the incidence of blind infants diminished, the problem of preschool training grew less acute. By the end of the Fifties many of the special services that had sprung up to meet the RLF emergency had been phased out. Within a few short years, however, the nation saw a new crop of blind babies, smaller in total number but in far worse shape. These were the infants born to mothers who, early in pregnancy, contracted rubella (German measles) during the 1963–65 epidemic.

The effects of maternal rubella on the children such mothers bore were seldom limited to a single anomaly. Deafness, cardiac impairment, motor handicaps, and mental deficiency, singly or in combination, were the principal conditions found in these babies; where blindness was added to one or more of these anomalies, the resulting problem was severe.

No exact figure was ever obtained as to the number of multiply handicapped blind children born during this epidemic; one of the more authoritative sources estimated that eye defects were found in 15 to 20 percent of the 30,000 cases. The absence in many states of laws requiring compulsory reporting of blindness (and the lack of enforcement in some states which did have such laws on the books) frustrated efforts to arrive at national counts of either the prevalence or incidence of blindness from any cause. That a blind rubella child also had an additional handicap which was regarded as his major disability meant that many such children were assigned to institutions where agencies for the blind were either unaware of their presence or unable to help them. Although a number of special services were established for multiply impaired blind preschool children, and some schools for the blind organized special educational programs as these children began to reach school age, it could not be claimed, as of 1972, that these efforts represented a comprehensive solution.

Concern with preschool blind children in the Seventies centers on improving delivery of services. The lower incidence and scattered distribution of blindness in babies have eliminated the need for the kind of crash programs that coped with the RLF problem, but these same factors have left parents of blind infants with less ready access to needed help. Recognition of this problem led the Foundation to adopt, as one of its newest priorities, a continuing program of advocacy to help insure delivery of comprehensive services—from parental counseling to special education to vocational guidance and prevocational training—for every blind child. A National Task Force on Early Child Development was organized in early 1972. Under its guidance a number of national and regional seminars were conducted, intensive field surveys were made and two pilot projects were initiated to explore improvement of delivery systems in urban and rural areas respectively. The task force also took note of an increase in the incidence of anophthalmia—the absence of eyes—in newborn infants and at its behest the Foundation began building a national roster of children with this condition. An effort was simultaneously under way to enlist the interest of the National Institutes of Health in undertaking medical research into the cause of anophthalmia, whose etiology is unknown.

"In theory, none of us admits the feeble-minded; in practice, we all have them." When he made this statement to his fellow educators at the AAIB convention in 1916, Olin H. Burritt was spotlighting a long-standing dilemma of schools for blind children. It was this very dilemma that led him to initiate psychological testing at Overbrook, in an effort to identify those children who frustrated the goal of demonstrating that blind children were as capable of academic achievement as the sighted.

That goal was valid enough for the great majority of pupils in schools for the blind. What was also true, however, was that some cases of blindness resulting from hereditary or prenatal causes were accompanied by severe mental retardation, emotional instability or both. And a third truth was that society had made no provision for such children other than placing them in mental hospitals or state schools for the retarded that had no educational services for them.

Borderline cases usually found their way into the residential schools or into the early public school classes for blind children. Robert Irwin reported in 1915 that a study of the sixty blind pupils enrolled in Cleveland's public school classes showed "four feeble-minded children and two suspicious cases who will probably prove within two or three years to be feeble-minded." That same year Cincinnati opened a special public school class for blind children of low mental development. "I do not feel that this is an ideal plan, but I think it is the best that can be provided by a day school," Irwin commented.

What *was* the ideal plan? Irwin didn't know, and neither did anyone else, either then or fifteen years later, during the 1930 White House Conference on Child Health and Protection, when a spirited colloquy took place between the heads of institutions for retardates and a spokesman for schools for the blind. Two of the former, including Vineland's famous Dr. Goddard, came out flatly in favor of institutional placement. In a statement which rings strangely in modern ears, he said: "The feeble-minded, whether deaf, blind, seeing or hearing, have a right to be happy and they are happy in a well-managed institution. . . . The Vineland inmates are the happiest group of people I have ever seen."

The superintendents of three other state schools offered a less Pollyannaish view. For the most severely retarded blind children, they said, there was really no alternative to institutional care. However, borderline cases—one superintendent identified these as having an IQ between 40 and 80—"should first be given an opportunity in the school for the blind, and be permitted to remain there as long as the child is making progress." Not only might such a child do better in the company of other blind children, his presence in a group of sighted retardates was a disturbing influence. The solution, said Dr. E. R. Johnstone, who had by then succeeded Goddard at Vineland, was that the schools for the blind should develop special classes for children whose IQs were higher than 30.

Just the opposite, maintained Samuel P. Hayes, speaking for Perkins, Overbrook and schools for the blind in general. The mental institutions should set up special units. "The simple educational activities adapted to low-grade intelligence can be modified so that children with little or no vision can still succeed in them. . . ." Placing such children in schools for the blind only frustrated them and usually resulted in their being sent home. This sometimes created a moral dilemma. "In many cases these homes are highly undesirable, and the residential schools often keep quite unsuitable children on the chance of improvement rather than . . . cut off all hope." Schools and classes for the blind had to be relieved of these children, Hayes asserted, because "an undue amount of teacher time has to be given to them" and because their continued presence took up space that "might better be given to promising younger people on the waiting list."

It was clearly a stalemate, and the White House Conference recognized it as such. All the Subcommittee on the Visually Handicapped could do in its final report was recommend that a study be made "to effect some agreement as to placement of responsibility for the training and care of the blind feeble-minded."

Forty years later, the problem had yet to be definitely resolved, but circumstances had brought about both of the proposed solutions. A number of state hospitals and schools for the retarded did in fact set up special units for blind children, and a number of schools for the blind did in fact establish special units for children whose multiple disabilities made for retarded functioning. In addition, there were two private boarding schools and several public school programs exclusively devoted to serving blind children with severe learning problems.

The first such private school was organized in 1921 in a Philadelphia suburb by a forceful, incurably optimistic woman named Jessie Royer Greaves. She had been in her mid-twenties when, having just graduated from what was then called the Emerson College of Oratory in Boston, she visited Overbrook and convinced Edward E. Allen that the pupils would benefit from a course in "physical expression and declamation," which combined public speaking, dramatics, and an exercise regime to overcome awkward body mannerisms. In 1902 Miss Royer (she had not yet married the artist Harry Greaves) became a part-time faculty member; she continued to conduct her special course for 25 years, even after the event that prompted her to start a school of her own.

In 1920 Mrs. Greaves returned to Overbrook following the summer vacation and found that a number of pupils in her class had been sent home because of low IQ scores. She was indignant; from her personal knowledge she felt sure that, despite their poor intellectual ability, these children had potential which could be developed in a non-competitive learning environment. She knew, too, that only two alternatives faced those dismissed: vegetation at home or commitment to a state institution.

Early in 1921 Mrs. Greaves opened the Royer-Greaves school; its hyphenated name was a joint memorial to her late father and the young husband who had died two years earlier. Her fundamental formula, as she later described it, was "music, conversation and much love." With these as opening wedges, she devised ways of training her pupils in self-care and social behavior, of overcoming their speech defects, of building their self-confidence and spurring them to achievement.

Steadfast adherence to her goals over a 40-year span won her the Lane Bryant Award in 1961, six years before she died at ninety-two. Another school like hers—the Hope School in Springfield, Illinois—was founded in 1957 by the parents of a mentally retarded blind daughter.

By this time there had surfaced a growing national concern over the large number of deviant blind children who were either too intellectually limited or too emotionally disturbed to be eligible for schools or day classes for the blind. A 1956 survey of New York State's 2,200 blind children had shown one out of ten to have retarded mental development; it had also shown that a large number of the children in this fraction had additional disabilities, with cerebral palsy and epilepsy leading the list.

To grapple with the problem of such multiply handicapped children, national workshops were sponsored by the Foundation in four successive summers beginning in 1959, in conjunction with the special education departments of universities in different parts of the country: Northwestern, Peabody, San Francisco State and Minnesota. The objective was to enlarge the "small but growing corps of persons throughout the United States who have common interest, common concern, and some common bodies of knowledge in regard to this severe problem." The distilled thinking of the four workshops appeared in two compelling publications. *No Place to Go*, edited by Kathern F. Gruber and Pauline M. Moor and published in 1963, presented a poignant picture of the "lost children within the blind population." *No Time to Lose*, edited by Miss Moor out of material derived from a seminar the following year, provided a frightening national picture. It asserted that 25 percent of all blind children under the age of 20 were not then (1964) receiving any educational service, but that many among them could in fact be helped through patient, sensitive and skillful handling. One point made in both publications was that routine psychological evaluations of these children and their potential were often misleading due to the absence of accurate measuring instruments applicable to blind children. Case histories were cited to demonstrate that, in spite of dismaying predictions based on routine tests, many children had been helped to a gratifying level of functioning. But there was no surefire formula; methodology was necessarily exploratory and educators had to find the courage to persist with "conviction, love, patience and a creative, daring spirit."

Whether prompted by this daring spirit or by more practical considerations, it proved to be the residential schools that took up the largest share of the challenge posed by the multiply impaired blind child. Among the earliest to make the effort was the Michigan School for the Blind which, in 1962, reported that 35 of its 280 students had severe multiple handicaps and were being taught in separate classrooms and housed in a separate dormitory. This school reported in 1965 its conclusion, drawn from some years of experimentation and study, that "if special treatment and care were provided, a surprisingly large percentage of these children could be habilitated sufficiently so that they might enter either day school classes or residential schools."

The dimensions of the national problem were assessed in 1966 by the Foundation's research staff, which circulated a questionnaire among more than 1,000 schools and classes for blind children, state and local hospitals, voluntary and public agencies concerned with blindness. Admittedly incomplete, the responses produced a sample of some 8,900 multiply-impaired blind children; on the basis of the sample, a total national figure of 15,000 such children was estimated. This, wrote Milton D. Graham who compiled the survey report, posed "a national problem that can only be met by a massive national effort to provide services and training." The dollar figures associated with such an effort were also massive—a projection of $50 to $75 million a year for a five-year experimental program involving 4,000 specially trained teachers plus supporting personnel—but, as Graham pointed out, the expenditures might properly be offset against the ultimate total costs of lifelong institutionalization for the approximately 25 percent of these children receiving care at public expense in state institutions.

A possible approach to this monumental task, suggested in a 1968 Foundation policy statement, was to develop regional facilities for diagnostic, treatment, educational, and rehabilitation services so that those in need would find them within a reasonable distance from their homes and no single state would have to assume the full costs. As will be seen in the next chapter, a regional plan was then beginning for one group, the deaf-blind; as of 1972 no comparable arrangement had been established for other categories of multiply impaired blind children.

A more immediate approach, stressed at a 1968 regional institute conducted in the Southwest, was that a larger investment be made in in-service training of both teachers and other personnel in schools for the blind. Charles C. Woodcock, superintendent of the Oregon school, put the existing residential school situation in plain focus. In Oregon, he said, the public school program for the blind was so well developed that "the multiply handicapped child is the challenge that we at the residential school are facing now. These are the children we are going to serve and either we will serve them or we will go out of existence."

Addressing the same conference, in whose sponsorship the Foundation was joined by a group of Texas state agencies and by the Department of Special Education of the University of Texas, J. Max Woolly, superintendent of the Arkansas School for the Blind, supported Woodcock's observations about the demands made on staff: "Only the emotionally strong, well-prepared teacher can survive." The Arkansas school was then serving 36 multiply impaired blind children, using a separate building for this program. Woolly described some of the pupils: a six-year-old girl, not toilet trained, who until she entered the school had spent much of her time sitting on her father's lap; a seven-year-old boy who had never eaten anything except baby foods because his mother had never had the stamina to insist that he learn to chew; another child whose bizarre behavior made him appear "more like a little frightened animal than a little boy"; several children whose excessive hyperactivity could only be controlled by medication. Said the Arkansas superintendent: "The challenge of providing for these children is at times almost beyond human endurance, yet we are convinced after these few years' experience that a great many of these boys and girls can lead independent, happy, contributing lives."

As schools for the blind gradually accepted the task they had so strongly resisted in previous decades, the mental hospitals and state schools for the retarded also began to yield ground. As of the mid-Sixties, some softening of their traditionally negative attitudes toward educational service for blind inmates could be perceived. The Children's Division of the Syracuse Psychiatric Hospital (later known as the Fairmount Institute) established a unit for severely disturbed blind children in 1964 and reported, five years later, that their experience had been comparable to that of the schools for the blind: i.e., with intensive staff effort and the closest kind of interdisciplinary teamwork, these children could be helped to break out of their isolation, relate to other people, control aggressive drives, acquire basic self-care skills, and participate effectively in an educational curriculum.

In a Massachusetts institution for retardates, the Walter E. Fernald State School, a demonstration project on teaching motor development and mobility skills showed that up to 40 percent of the school's 240 blind residents were capable of responding to instruction. In Michigan the Plymouth State Home and Training School set aside a separate building for its 110 blind residents, most of whom were children, and initiated an educational program using differential teaching and motivational techniques according to each patient's age and ability. Close integration with families and community made it possible for some of these children to leave the institution.

Public school educational systems also grew less hesitant about tackling services for the blind child with additional handicaps. In a few cities special day school programs were inaugurated by multiservice agencies for the blind.

The gradual emergence of these efforts did not take place in a social vacuum. Much of the momentum was stimulated by the broader movements on behalf of all handicapped children, movements which drew ever-greater support from public opinion and were increasingly bolstered by federal financing. In this climate, the heads of schools for the blind, although understandably reluctant to abandon their long-cherished emphasis on academic excellence, came to accept the need for a changed role.

From a historical viewpoint, the metamorphosis had philosophic justification. There would never have been schools for the blind in the first place had other educational facilities for visually handicapped children existed. The residential school of the Seventies was continuing to meet the unfilled needs of its day. It was providing academically sound educational opportunities for normally endowed blind children from isolated rural areas where public school facilities could not be efficiently supplied. It was doing the same for children whose families were unable to provide suitable home environments. And increasingly it was supplying special services for children who could not benefit from the usual educational facilities.

There was one other aspect of change that differentiated the contemporary school for the blind from its pioneer antecedents. This was its role in relation to another kind of misfit, the partially sighted child who had too little vision to manage the work in a public school but too much to be taught by tactile methods.

The presence of such children in schools for the blind had always been a matter of concern. Originally they were accepted for the same reason as the totally blind children—there was simply no other place for them to go. But they were a social and educational problem. Before the era of large-print books and optical aids, they were taught touch reading, which often proved to be a self-defeating exercise. In the same 1916 speech that opened up the question of retarded pupils, Olin Burritt also talked about the partially sighted:

> We have tried for years to make them use their fingers in lieu of their eyes. In our determination to circumvent nature we have resorted to all sorts of devices from aprons to cover their hands to huge pasteboard collars about their necks which give a classroom equipped with this last device an appearance quite like a monastery.

Burritt argued that such children, if they lived in large cities, should attend their local public schools and be given supplementary assistance by a special teacher employed for that purpose. Arrangements of this kind were already in existence in Boston and Cleveland. "But what about the pupil with partial sight who comes from the sparsely settled rural community? I see no other way than that we must provide him with the necessary eye-instruction in our special schools."

It took a good many years for the eye-instruction formula to be put into effect with any degree of universality. Most schools for the blind stayed with finger-reading for all pupils. Somewhat faster progress was made in the public schools, where either the "Boston system" or the "Cleveland system" was followed. The Boston procedure—a segregated class for semi-sighted children—was initiated by Edward E. Allen in 1913; the Cleveland procedure, originated by Robert Irwin soon thereafter, was a cooperative plan in which partially sighted children took oral work with their regular grades and did their written work in a specially lit and equipped "sight-saving" room under the guidance of a special teacher.

Both systems were predicated on the then prevailing theory that vision had to be "conserved" to prevent further deterioration. It was natural, therefore, that the education of partially sighted children should become a major program element in the work of the National Society for the Prevention of Blindness, which had been organized in 1908. Edward M. Van Cleve, who in 1915 was named managing director of that organization (then known as the National Committee and not yet independently staffed) while serving simultaneously as principal of the New York Institute for the Education of the Blind, emphasized the semantic value of calling these public school classes "sight-saving" rather than "classes for children of defective sight" or "classes for the semi-blind." Their popularity was enhanced, he said, "and the willingness of parents to have their children attend them is secured, by laying emphasis upon the conservation element in their purpose."

As a logical outcome of its advocacy, the NSPB for many years exercised professional leadership in dealing with the education of partially sighted children, operating along lines parallel to the Foundation's work on behalf of children with more severe visual handicaps. This separation of function continued until 1967 when the two national organizations recognized that their respective programs, particularly in the area of teacher training, had moved so close together as to represent duplication of effort. An agreement that year consolidated the two activities under Foundation auspices.

Although a few residential schools started separate sight-saving classes during the Twenties and Thirties, the pace did not really pick up until the middle and late Forties; at the end of that decade 17 or 18 schools for the blind were maintaining specially equipped classrooms in which partially sighted children were taught by visual methods. One reason for the acceleration was that enrollment in residential schools was declining as a consequence of the postwar growth of public schools and classes. Another was a by-product of the 1943 Vocational Rehabilitation Act amendments which, although primarily aimed at services for blind adults, inspired a wave of vision testing and follow-up remedial medical and surgical procedures for visually handicapped children. A joint NSPB-Foundation study in the Maryland and Florida schools for the blind in 1943 found correctable eye defects in a substantial number of pupils who acquired enough sight, after the necessary remedial measures had been taken, to be capable of visual instruction.

The stepped-up movement of the residential schools into education of the partially sighted engendered a certain amount of protest among those who opposed any growth of institutionalization; the professional literature of the Forties featured a number of articles and speeches on both sides of the issue. There was also some backstage maneuvering in opposition to the legislative change which in 1946 authorized the American Printing House to add large-print books to the educational materials it supplied on quota allotment to the schools and public school classes for blind children. The opposition proved futile. A federal survey made in 1960 showed that more than half of the children in the public school classes for the visually handicapped read large print; in the residential schools the print readers came to a substantial 29 percent.

These proportions were more or less unchanged as of 1970, when Printing House statistics showed that of 8,411 children registered in schools for the blind, 4,722 were braille readers, 2,302 read large type, 426 read both, and 961 read neither. The same source revealed that of the 12,812 children enrolled in the public school systems, large-type readers numbered 7,626, or about 60 percent, and braille readers 3,059, or about 24 percent. Also of interest in these statistics was that 12 percent of the combined registration of 21,223 read neither braille nor large type. This last category embraced non-readers, readers of regular ink print and those who were educated primarily by means of recorded materials.

The Sixties saw a state of truce descend on the long-standing issue of residential versus public school education for blind children. Both types of program achieved record heights in enrollment and settled into a fairly steady ratio of 40 percent educated in schools for the blind and 60 percent in public school systems.

Along with the cooling of tempers there gradually developed more amicable teamwork between the professional organization of the educators and other major elements in work for the blind. The American Association of Instructors of the Blind democratized its structure under a revised constitution, adopted in 1952, which had the effect, as its then president, Neal F. Quimby, put it, of changing "from an organizational setup in which the superintendents and a few selected delegates controlled the group, to one in which every member has an equal voice." The change also involved a broadening of the membership base to include persons "affiliated with or interested in" education, guidance, vocational rehabilitation and placement work. AAIB, said Quimby, was no longer "a closed shop." Special efforts began to be made to enlist the interest of the public school educators as well as of such non-teaching personnel as the residential school houseparents. By 1956 AAIB could report a 40 percent membership increase to 1,145; by 1972 this figure had more than doubled to just under 2,500.

Along with expansion came growing pains. One of the measures adopted in tandem with the revised constitution called for AAIB to have its own professional journal. Since discontinuance of the *Teachers Forum* a decade earlier, the field of education had felt the need for a medium specializing in its own interests. To fill the gap, the *International Journal for the Education of the Blind* was founded in 1951, initially as an independent non-profit quarterly under a board of trustees headed by Josef G. Cauffman. The early financing and actual printing were supplied largely by the New York Institute for the Education of the Blind under Merle Frampton. In 1954 the *Journal* was designated as AAIB's official organ and its production moved to the American Printing House for the Blind, with Paul J. Langan, then superintendent of the Kentucky School for the Blind, as editor. As was invariably the case with professional publications of limited circulation, subscription income failed to cover costs and subsidies were needed.

A more serious financial problem was the need for a permanent office and a full-time executive to serve the expanding membership. In 1957 AAIB opened negotiations with the Foundation on "a plan of cooperative endeavor." The educators' earlier suspicions that the Foundation was biased against residential schools had been largely dissipated, partly as a result of forthright speeches made by M. Robert Barnett at the 1952 and 1954 conventions in which he brought the whispering campaigns into the open, and partly because, under Barnett's administration, the Foundation had repeatedly demonstrated its impartial interest and concern in all forms of education. A number of other steps had also brought the two organizations into closer coordination. Under the Foundation's bylaw revisions of 1951 the president of AAIB automatically became a member of the board of trustees (as did the president of AAWB).

The first fruits of AAIB's approach to the Foundation consisted of a $9,000 grant to finance three jointly sponsored institutes in 1958. The following year saw an agreement under which the Foundation undertook to supply $75,000 (in equal installments over a six-year period) as a subsidy toward AAIB's operating budget. On the basis of this assurance AAIB was able to establish office headquarters and employ an executive secretary. The incumbent, as of 1972, was Mary K. Bauman. She had become the executive in 1968, the year the organization changed its name to Association for the Education of the Visually Handicapped (AEVH).

Although profound changes have taken place in the educational provisions for blind children in the 140 years since the first schools opened their doors, the essential goals and many of the problems remain the same.

The United States never favored a closed system for blind people similar to that in some European countries, where many blind persons spent their childhood years in a residential school, their working years in a handicrafts workshop and a home for blind persons on the same premises, and their final years in a retirement home within the same compound. From the beginning, the objective in American work for the blind was integration into open society, with all this entailed in terms of physical, social, and economic mobility.

The education of blind children continues to focus on these aims. Gymnastics and sports constitute important parts of a curriculum designed to give blind children the stamina, agility, and confidence essential to moving about with ease and efficiency. Interscholastic athletic contests, aimed at developing a competitive "never say die" spirit, are encouraged, not only against other teams of blind youngsters but against sighted teams in those events (wrestling, bowling, weightlifting, swimming) where blind contestants can compete on equal terms. Much effort has been devoted in recent years to having blind children gain entree to the regular community programs of such youth organizations as Boy Scouts, Girl Scouts, 4-H Clubs, and others.

Structured orientation and mobility programs now exist in virtually all schools for the blind and in a growing number of public school programs. These are expected to expand as additional trained peripatologists become available.

The question of vocational preparation continues to be a paramount concern. As with all children, the education of blind youth has moved along two basic tracks: the academic, reserved for students preparing for college or a career in business; and the industrial, which originally specialized in the traditional "blind trades" but later opened up to train students in the mechanics of carpentry, metal, and electrical work which would qualify them for assembly line jobs in open industry.

The development of hand skills has come to be seen as an important element in the education of all blind children, as much for avocational purposes as for future employment. When the number of blind children educated in public schools equalled and then began to exceed the number in the residential schools, it became a matter of heightened national concern that, in most public schools, blind students were automatically excused from the manual training courses customarily given in the seventh and eighth grades. The problem, it was recognized, was that the public school industrial arts teachers lacked knowledge of how to bring blind children into a shop program; most did not even know they were capable of mastering the necessary skills.

In 1959, under contract with the then Office of Vocational Rehabilitation, the Foundation convened a national conference on principles and standards of industrial arts education for blind students. Those attending included vocational rehabilitation counselors, placement workers, public school principals, industrial arts teachers and supervisors in public schools, and a similar group working in schools for the blind. They spent three days hammering out a detailed plan, complete with curriculum guides, demonstration lessons, and equipment lists, which could serve as working blueprints for integration of blind students in shop classes. These were tested out in a series of summer sessions for industrial arts instructors. High hopes were entertained, but the benefits proved to be temporary and limited in extent. As of 1972 the degree of participation of blind boys in shop classes in public schools is still in need of substantial expansion. The same holds true of girls in home economics classes, and of both sexes in physical education programs.

Much also remains to be done in the preparation of blind students for productive and satisfying work lives. The acquisition of specific skills is only part of the process; realistic vocational guidance and the inculcation of good work habits and sound mental attitudes are also important elements of prevocational training. In 1972 a National Task Force on Career Education listed 24 separate measures that could be taken to increase the introduction of blind persons into the mainstream of work opportunities, retraining them as need be when former career channels closed and new ones opened. The overall thrust was that education should have as its target "placement and recycling of individuals on a lattice of open career options."

25

The Loneliest People

Helen Keller called them "the loneliest people on earth." Gabriel Farrell termed them "children of the silent night." "The muffled drums" was the name some gave themselves in England.

They were the deaf-blind, regarded by the few people who even knew of their existence as the most hopeless, the most helpless of human creatures, deserving of pity and protection but unreachable, unteachable. It was no wonder that the one such person the world did know about—the one whose life and accomplishments defied the popular stereotype—was regarded as enough of a miraculous oddity to be booked on a vaudeville circuit.

But Helen Keller was not the only person—or even the first—to be helped out of what she described as "the double dungeon of darkness and silence." There were others before her, others came later, and there will doubtless be more in the future, for it was less than thirty years ago that the world began to acknowledge the existence of this heretofore hidden layer of humanity. And with that acknowledgment came new efforts at rescue and salvage—efforts spurred on by Helen herself in the face of decades of discouragement.

As of 1972, the number of known deaf-blind persons in the United States was put at 12,000, equally divided between children and adults. Knowledgeable authorities estimated that there were at least 3,000, and perhaps as many as 8,000, additional deaf-blind persons who had not yet been located.

Of the known population, relatively few were in Helen Keller's condition, i.e., totally without sight or hearing. Although the language varied somewhat from situation to situation, the basic definition of deaf-blindness was "legal blindness plus inability to understand connected discourse through the ear, even with amplification." This meant that many deaf-blind persons had traces of vision or faint degrees of hearing, or both, but that neither sensory channel was sufficiently functional to serve by itself or as a substitute for the other. It was the absence of the substitution factor that made deaf-blindness so disabling a condition.

As with simple blindness or simple deafness, the kind and extent of handicap were governed by individual factors. Degree of loss, as well as age of onset and the order in which the disabilities occurred, all made a difference. It was the rare deaf-blind person who was born that way. At one time, childhood infections such as scarlet fever or meningitis sometimes produced simultaneous blindness and deafness, but in later years, when raging infections of this type had been largely eradicated, simultaneous onset seldom occurred. Judging by contemporary sample studies of segments of the adult deaf-blind population, deafness more often preceded blindness than vice-versa; the interval before the onset of the second disability ranged from a few years to a good many.

The person who grew up as a deaf child and then lost the use of his eyes had visual memories to draw upon but had learned to be dependent on vision to receive (and usually to give) communication by means of sign language or lip reading. The situation was reversed for the blind person who subsequently lost the hearing that had been his main source of orientation and communication. The age at which first one and then the other sensory channel was blocked was also a crucial factor in the nature and dimension of the overall problem confronting the individual. The person beset with deaf-blindness in adulthood, after he had had an education, was in a very different plight from the preschool child who still had everything to learn.

This is perhaps the point at which to dispose of the "darkness and silence" image evoked by the popular catch phrases used to describe deaf-blindness. An English business executive who lost his hearing in young adulthood and, a dozen years later, was blinded in an automobile accident, wrote a compelling account of his experiences and sensations during the first months of double disability—"a period of furious frustration"—and went on to describe the world as he perceived it:

> What is it actually like to be deaf-blind? I can only tell you what it is like for me. What it's like for a person who has never seen or heard, I do not know.
>
> First, it is neither "dark" nor "silent." If you were to go out into a London fog—one of the thick yellow variety—and then close your eyes, you would see what I see. A dull, flesh-colored opacity. So much for literal "darkness. . . ."
>
> Nor is my world "silent" (most of us wish it were so!) You have all put a shell to your ear as children and "listened to the waves." You may, at times—when dropping off to sleep perhaps—have "heard" the clang of a bell in your ear, or a sound like the shunting of railway wagons, or a shrill whistle, or the wind moaning round the eaves on Christmas Eve. All these have I perpetually. They have become part of the background. Cracklings, squeakings, rumblings—what I hear is the machinery of my being working. The blood rushing through my veins, and little cracklings of nerves and muscles as they expand and contract. In short, my hearing has "turned inwards."

This man had a bank of visual and auditory memories on which to draw. Severe as they were, his problems were less devastating than those of a person whose congenital or early deafness rendered him unfamiliar with sound and gave him an absent or imperfect command of speech, or a person whose lifelong blindness resulted in a limited, perhaps distorted, grasp of objects and spatial relationships.

All told, it was this lack of homogeneity in a sparse, widely scattered and often hidden population that for so long baffled and discouraged those who strove to release deaf-blind individuals from the bonds of personal and social isolation. It was next to impossible to devise methods of education or rehabilitation that could be universally applied.

Those same eighteenth-century philosophers whose metaphysical inquiries into the nature of intelligence led them to speculate on whether a blind person, restored to sight, could recognize visually the objects he knew intimately through touch also pondered the theoretical question of whether it was possible to educate anyone who lacked access to the two principal avenues of knowledge. The two French clergymen who were pioneers in devising an instructional system for the deaf were interested in pursuing this inquiry, but neither succeeded in locating a suitable deaf-blind subject. In the United States, the American Asylum for the Education of the Deaf and Dumb, which Thomas Hopkins Gallaudet founded in 1817 after studying the methods developed in France, did have such a subject, a young woman named Julia Brace, but little progress was made in teaching her anything but the simplest kinds of self-care. The reason may well have been that although Julia had lost sight and hearing at the age of four, she was eighteen before she became a pupil at Gallaudet's school in Hartford, Connecticut, in 1825.

Samuel Gridley Howe apparently saw Julia soon after opening his school for the blind in Boston in 1832; he wrote of "closely watching" her and concluding that the effort to penetrate the mind of such a person "should not be abandoned, though it had failed in her case as well as in all that had been recorded before."

It did not take long before Howe came upon his chance to succeed where others had failed. In 1837 he was escorted to a New Hampshire farmhouse where he met seven-year-old Laura Bridgman—deaf, blind, incapable of speech, and nearly devoid of the sense of smell, all due to a virulent bout of scarlet fever that had nearly taken her life when she was a two-year-old baby. Moved by the child's plight, and intrigued by the challenge she presented, Howe persuaded Laura's parents to entrust her to his care.

Laura was an appealing little girl—slender and fair, with delicate features—and Howe, who had yet to marry and have children of his own, had a fatherly fondness for her. But his motivation in attempting to open her mind had religious and intellectual as well as humanitarian considerations. Charles Darwin had not yet written his *Origin of Species*, but the startlingly heretical theory of man's evolution from primates was already being promulgated and Howe was among those who held that the God-given human soul was what distinguished men from beasts. His descriptions of his experiences in teaching Laura emphasized his spiritual convictions. His early efforts—taking a few common objects, attaching to them labels that spelled out their names in raised letters, and training Laura to associate the shape of each word with the object to which it was attached—these, he wrote, involved only imitation and memory. "The process had been mechanical and the success about as great as teaching a very knowing dog a variety of tricks." It was not until Laura had been taught to recognize the individual letters of the alphabet, had learned to pick out and arrange into word form the letters that she associated with particular objects, and had become aware that these letters could be used in different combinations to denote different objects that, as Howe put it,

> the truth began to flash upon her—her intellect began to work—she perceived that here was a way by which she could herself make up a sign of anything that was in her own mind and show it to another mind; and at once her countenance lighted up with a human expression: it was no longer a dog, or parrot,—it was an immortal spirit, eagerly seizing upon a new link of union with other spirits!

Years later, in his memorable Batavia address, Howe recapitulated his work with Laura and threw down an even more direct challenge to the Darwinists: "She took hold of the thread by which I would lead her out, because she had all the special attributes of a human soul. No created being devoid of these attributes could do it. Try ye, who believe that an ape or a chimpanzee differs only a degree from man!"

After the first weeks, during which Howe personally taught Laura, he assigned a special teacher to work with her under his direction. The next step was to teach her that there was a different and faster way to represent the letters of the alphabet than by laboriously picking out their shapes in cast metal. This was the manual alphabet of the deaf, in which fingers held in different positions and combinations signified the 26 letters. Laura learned how to receive and give these finger signals and thus was forged the third link in the chain of communication that freed her from isolation. Other links were added. She was taught to read books embossed in Howe's raised type, to write with a pencil using a grooved board to guide the lines, to do simple arithmetic, and to master sewing and other kinds of handwork. There was no effort to teach her the use of voice; Howe later said he regretted not having made the attempt, but too many other things were then claiming his attention, among them his marriage to Julia Ward in 1843. Laura's main communication channel remained finger-spelling, at which she became adept, and many of the blind children at Perkins (including Anne Sullivan) learned the manual alphabet so they could converse with Laura and, later, with the four other deaf-blind children taken into Perkins during Howe's lifetime.

Laura Bridgman outlived her benefactor by 13 years, remaining at Perkins until her death in 1889. After two attempts to return her to her family proved unsuccessful, Howe left a provision in his will to insure she would continue to be sheltered at the school to the end of her life. She was by no means a liability. In fact, the attention called to her by Charles Dickens in *American Notes* brought Perkins world renown. (The novelist, who visited the school in 1842, "did not deign to notice anything or anybody except Laura," one of the girl's teachers observed in her diary.)

Dickens' enthusiasm, remarkable in a man so outspokenly critical of institutions, was the fortuitous factor that opened the gates of liberation for Helen Keller. As pointed out in an earlier chapter, it was reading *American Notes* forty-plus years later that prompted Helen's parents to begin the inquiries that led to Anne Sullivan, who spent six months studying Howe's reports on the instruction of Laura Bridgman, and talking with the aging Laura herself, before heading south to Alabama in March 1887.

Anne Sullivan, whose teaching techniques were brilliantly intuitive, carried Howe's methods a long step forward when she decided to communicate with seven-year-old Helen in complete sentences rather than teach her isolated words. This insight came to her barely a month after her arrival at the Keller home. On April 10, 1887, she wrote:

> I am going to treat Helen exactly like a two-year-old child. . . . I asked myself, "How does a normal child learn language?" The answer was simple, "By imitation." The child comes into the world with the ability to learn, and he learns of himself, provided he is supplied with sufficient outward stimulus. He sees people do things, and he tries to do them. He hears others speak, and he tries to speak. But long before he utters his first word, he understands what is said to him. I have been observing Helen's little cousin lately. She is about fifteen months old, and already understands a great deal. . . . She obeys many commands like these: "Come," "Kiss," "Go to papa," "Shut the door," "Give me the biscuit." But I have not heard her try to say any of these words, although they have been repeated hundreds of times in her hearing, and it is evident that she understands them. These observations have given me a clue to the method to be followed in teaching Helen language. I shall talk into her hand as we talk into the baby's ears. I shall assume that she has the normal child's capacity of assimilation and imitation. I shall use complete sentences in talking to her. . . .

Two weeks later she was able to report:

> The new scheme works splendidly. Helen knows the meaning of more than a hundred words now, and learns new ones daily without the slightest suspicion that she is performing a most difficult feat. She learns because she can't help it, just as the bird learns to fly. . . . [W]hen I spell into her hand "Give me some bread," she hands me the bread, or if I say, "Get your hat and we will go to walk," she obeys instantly. The two words, "hat" and "walk" would have the same effect; but the whole sentence, repeated many times during the day, must in time impress itself upon the brain, and by and by she will use it herself.

It seems reasonable to conjecture that this creative concept contributed heavily to Helen Keller's masterly command of language. Her ability to express herself in graceful, often poetic, prose far outstripped the childish constructions in the journals the adult Laura Bridgman kept. It was not merely a matter of advanced education. Helen was not yet ten years old when she sent an impulsive letter to the poet John Greenleaf Whittier with sentences like these: "When I walk out in my garden I cannot see the beautiful flowers but I know that they are all around me; for is not the air sweet with their fragrance? I know too that the tiny lily-bells are whispering pretty secrets to their companions else they would not look so happy."

Her teacher may have helped Helen with this and comparable letters (indeed, it was alleged by some that she dictated them), but how, then, explain the talent for expression in the letters Helen sent Anne Sullivan during a long summer separation? Months before the letter to Whittier, Helen wrote from Tuscumbia to "Dearest Teacher":

> I am sitting on the piazza, and my little white pigeon is perched on the back of my chair, watching me write. Her little brown mate has flown away with the other birds. . . . Little Arthur is growing very fast. . . . I will take his soft chubby hand in mine and go out in the bright sunshine with him. He will pull the largest roses and chase the gayest butterflies.

It was the following winter, when Helen and her teacher were in residence at Perkins, that they heard of a deaf-blind girl in Norway, Ragnhild Kaata, who had been taught to speak. The headmaster of the school for the deaf in which Ragnhild was a pupil anticipated what is now called the vibration method by placing the six-year-old girl's hands on his lips so that she could feel and imitate their movements. Helen at once aspired to a comparable achievement and for a number of years took speech lessons, first from a private teacher, then at a school for the deaf and, later, again from private teachers as well as from Anne Sullivan. It was a milestone in her young life when, at the end of the first 11 lessons, she was able to articulate "I am not dumb now," but the enunciation was halting and garbled, and, as Anne Sullivan's biographer was to write, the aim of Helen and her teacher to have Helen achieve normal speech was

> the only one of their heroic undertakings in which they have confessed defeat. It is no secret that Helen's voice is the great disappointment of her life. . . . To those who are accustomed to it, it is easy to understand and not unpleasant to hear, rather like listening to someone with a queer foreign accent. But strangers, as a rule, do not find it easy to follow.

If there was a single repetitive theme in everything Helen Keller wrote from childhood on, it was the desire that something be done for others afflicted like herself. She instilled this desire in a number of others. Among those who befriended her during her earliest years was William Wade, a well-to-do landowner in western Pennsylvania who became the patron of every deaf-blind child and adult he could find. Wade made no effort to establish an organized channel of help but, in the manner of the times, made individual persons the objects of his private beneficence, distributing books, typewriters, sewing machines, looms, bicycles, dolls, vacation trips, and whatever else seemed calculated to bring pleasure or profit to barren lives.

It was, in fact, through one such impulsive gift that he met Helen in the first place. After reading a letter published in a children's magazine in which she described her small dog, Wade remarked to his sister, "That is not the sort of dog a blind child needs, she ought to have a mastiff." He promptly arranged to send her one, and her letter of thanks, in which she said she planned to name the dog Lioness, began a correspondence between the nine-year-old child and the fifty-year-old philanthropist that led to Helen and her teacher's spending a summer, and later a winter, as guests of the Wade family at their estate in Oakmont, Pennsylvania. Helen's account of their first meeting showed the remarkable sensitivity of her sense of smell: "He met us at the train in Pittsburgh, and I recognized him at once by the tobacco he used, the scent of which had permeated the letters he sent me."

Wade's delight in Helen and his appreciation of what could be accomplished by an eager mind despite the absence of vision and hearing was in line with his long-held interest in the question of deafness. Toward the closing years of his life (he died in 1912 at the age of seventy-five), he wrote a monograph, *The Deaf-Blind*, which was the first effort at constructing a roster of deaf-blind persons in the United States, giving an account of their education, their accomplishments, and their status. The first edition of this book, published in 1901, listed 72 such persons Wade either knew or had heard of; in a second edition, published three years later, the list came to 110 names, the majority supplied by schools for the deaf.

The huge dog Wade gave Helen also managed to play an incidental role in the history of work for the deaf-blind. A mistaken fear for the public safety caused a policeman to shoot Lioness soon after her arrival in Tuscumbia, and Helen's letter to Wade, reporting this unfortunate event, was published in a magazine at his initiative. It prompted a deluge of spontaneous public subscriptions to buy Helen another dog. But Wade had already sent her a replacement,* so she decided to divert the contributed money to a fund Michael Anagnos was then raising for the upkeep of Thomas Stringer, a four-year-old deaf-blind boy who had just been brought to Perkins from a Pennsylvania almshouse.

Stringer, who spent 20 years at Perkins, became one of the school's legendary figures. His academic accomplishments were modest, but he was extraordinarily adept with his hands and grew into a first-class craftsman in woodworking. Following his graduation from Perkins in 1913, he went to live with a guardian, his economic future secure thanks to the $1,000-a-year income from the fund Anagnos had raised, plus what he earned by constructing vegetable crates for sale to local farmers.

During Perkins' first century, 18 deaf-blind children were educated there, with varying degrees of success. A few other schools for the blind, and a large number of schools for the deaf, also contained pupils with a second disability. Among the best known of these were two educated in schools for the deaf. One was Kathryne Mary Frick, who was graduated in 1925 from the Pennsylvania Institution for the Deaf and, five years later, came to public notice through an autobiography published in the *Atlantic Monthly*. The other was Helen May Martin, who was educated at home and in her late teens entered the Kansas School for the Deaf; she was a talented pianist who learned to read music scores in New York Point, memorized them, and made frequent concert appearances throughout the Middle West during the Twenties.

An exceptional case was that of Helen Schultz, who received virtually all of her

---

* The second mastiff, named Lion, also had a short life; it was put to death by Helen's father after it had bitten Anne Sullivan in the hand.

education in the public schools of New Jersey. She was the subject of an article, "The Education of a Girl Who Cannot See or Hear," which Lydia Hayes, chief of the New Jersey Commission for the Blind, wrote for the *Outlook* in 1926, describing how Helen attended a public school in Jersey City until she was eleven, when her mother died. She spent the next year at Overbrook and then returned to her home state where, adopted by a family living in suburban Montclair, she completed her education in a local public school. Except for the year she spent at Overbrook, Helen Schultz did not have a private teacher-companion constantly at her side; she made friends with schoolmates and received whatever supplementary help she needed from them, from her teachers, or from those at home, first her mother and then her adoptive guardian. Having had hearing until she was seven, Helen had command of speech. She received communication through the manual alphabet from those who knew it, through printing in her palm from those who didn't.

What Lydia Hayes omitted to mention in her article was that she herself was the person who had adopted Helen. This was made known a few years later when Walter Holmes, editor of the *Ziegler Magazine*, wrote an article describing Helen's efficient management of the Hayes household. She could cook, sew, knit and crochet in addition to reading braille and using the typewriter. Later she married Lydia Hayes' nephew and moved to the Middle West.

Helen Schultz was exceptional because, until 1931, deaf-blind children who received any kind of formal education in a school for the blind or a school for the deaf were assigned to special teachers on a one-to-one basis. One of Gabriel Farrell's first acts as the new director of Perkins was to change that. As he later described this innovation,

> instead of employing a teacher for each pupil, a special department was opened with teachers trained in speech-building for schoolroom instruction and attendants to care for the children outside of the classroom. In making this fundamental change, it was hoped to secure more skilled teachers on a professional basis and by distributing responsibility to avoid both the loneliness of Laura Bridgman after her school work terminated and the life-long dependence of Helen Keller upon first Mrs. Macy and later Miss Thompson (sic).

The change at Perkins was not altogether self-generating; it was stimulated, at least partly, by a train of outside events that were then arousing new public interest in the problems of deaf-blindness.

In 1927 a Montreal publisher issued a book, *Hors de Sa Prison*, in which the author, Corinne Rocheleau, told the chilling story of a deaf-blind girl named Ludivine Lachance. The daughter of illiterate parents living in a remote village in Quebec, Ludivine lost sight and hearing before her third birthday; for the next 13 years she led the life of a half-tamed animal. As summarized in an English-language review of the book:

> Her body was clad in but a single garment, more like a sack than an article of clothing; her hair knew neither brush nor comb; her nails were like the talons

of the hawk. A small cell-like room was partitioned off for her use in a corner of the kitchen; it had no window and no furniture but a straw ticked bed. The prisoner of darkness would allow no other stick nor stool in her dungeon and broke chair or table if such were introduced. When air became a vital necessity, she searched out a crack in the outer wall of the house, and, putting her mouth to it, sucked in great draughts of the refreshing element. She ate like a wild animal, using her hands to convey the food to her mouth, and bolting it without perceptible mastication.

When Ludivine was sixteen, the village curé finally persuaded her parents to let her be taken to the convent school for deaf-mutes in Montreal, conducted by the Sisters of Providence. There, for the remaining seven years of her life (she died of tuberculosis in 1918), the half-crazed, half-savage Ludivine was patiently brought by devoted nuns to a semblance of human dignity. She was taught cleanliness, self-care, some rudiments of language, a few manual accomplishments, and was instructed, to the limits of her understanding, in the Catholic faith.

It is not clear whether the author of Ludivine's story, a deaf woman who was herself a graduate of the convent school, knew Ludivine, but she apparently did know the nuns who had taught her and a number of other deaf-blind girls brought up under their care. Preparing to write her book, Corinne Rocheleau sent inquiries to schools for the deaf and schools for the blind in both Canada and the United States, asking about any deaf-blind pupils they might have had. Her researches led her to a Cincinnati woman, Rebecca Mack, who had also long been interested in the welfare of the deaf-blind and had begun to keep a list of all such persons who came to her notice. The two women joined forces to compile a register of 655 names of deaf-blind children and adults; their idea was to publish these in book form, much as William Wade had done early in the century.

The field of work for the blind became aware of this project when, in September 1928, the *Outlook* published a long article by Miss Rocheleau describing her researches and pleading for joint action by organizations concerned with the blind and those concerned with the deaf. Interest in the subject was heightened when, soon thereafter, Sherman C. Swift devoted his "Book News" column in the *Outlook* to a detailed synopsis of *Hors de Sa Prison* which, having been published in French, was not widely known in the United States. That same year saw the publication of a new book, *Laura Bridgman, the Story of an Opened Door*, by Laura Richards, daughter of Samuel G. Howe. The second installment of Helen Keller's autobiography, *Midstream*, appeared around the same time.

The two professional associations in work for the blind took note of these stirrings. In 1928 the AAIB voted to appoint a committee of three "to cooperate with a like committee from the National Association of Instructors of the Deaf to consider the feasibility of a sane plan for the education of the deaf-blind." When the AAWB met the following summer, it went beyond the question of education to consider the overall dimensions of the problem. Two important points were brought out in the summary of its discussions:

No plan of education for the deaf-blind would be complete without the giving of some consideration to after care, since the plight of the adult deaf-blind is recognized to be quite as serious as his plight as a child. Over-education without means of self-realization for social adjustment was stressed as holding grave possibilities for unhappiness in the individual.

There was less agreement as to a solution. . . . A more or less centralized plan for the education of the deaf-blind might have its advantages, but whether an independent institution should be built and maintained for this purpose, or whether the work should be done in conjunction with certain schools for the deaf, the blind, or the deaf and blind already established, seemed open to question. . . .

The opinion was unanimous, however, that the question was one deserving the careful study of the American Foundation for the Blind.

The Foundation was already in the picture. It had been approached by the Volta Bureau, research arm of the American Association to Promote the Teaching of Speech to the Deaf (later known as the Alexander Graham Bell Association for the Deaf) to co-sponsor publication of the Rocheleau-Mack book and had, in fact, voted some money on condition that the published material consist only of the 55-page introductory section in which Corinne Rocheleau outlined the overall problems of deaf-blind persons and the existing provisions for help to them. The Foundation objected to publication of the 110-page "biographical section" prepared by Miss Mack on the grounds that its listing of 665 deaf-blind persons was inadequately documented.

This suggested excision was not acceptable to the authors of *Those in the Dark Silence* and in 1930 the full text appeared under the Volta Bureau imprint, with the publishing costs underwritten by Miss Mack, a woman of some means. The book was a curious piece of work. Nine out of ten listings in the "biographical section" gave only initials and the name of the state in which the subject lived, and most of these entries were meaningless: e.g., "S.S., New York. Adult. Reads embossed type. Typewrites." or "I.W., Georgia, Adult. Lives with her mother." Only 65 or so entries were identified by name; their biographical information consisted of sketches supplied by the subject, or a member of the family, or his or her teacher, or material derived from press clippings. The explanation the authors gave was that names had been used only with express permission.

Despite its grotesqueries, publication of *Those in the Dark Silence* served a purpose. Deaf-blindness was the subject of one of the round-table discussions at the 1931 World Conference on the Welfare of the Blind and a formal recommendation was made that the major organizations interested in work for the deaf and work for the blind join forces to tackle the problem. The Foundation thereupon opened negotiations with the Volta Bureau and with the American Federation of Organizations for the Hard of Hearing, and in the closing days of 1931 the three agencies announced the formation of a Joint Committee on the Deaf-Blind.

A three-pronged approach was agreed upon. The Volta Bureau would establish a national register of deaf-blind persons, using the Rocheleau-Mack lists as its nucleus. The hard-of-hearing group, which had chapters in many different cities, would verify and update the register by interviewing persons on the list to determine their situations and their needs. The Foundation's role would be to devise model laws and to campaign for state legislation to initiate or improve provisions for the education of deaf-blind children and the care of deaf-blind adults.

Two representatives of each of the three organizations made up the membership of the Joint Committee on the Deaf-Blind. The chairman was H. M. McManaway, superintendent of Virginia's dual school for the deaf and the blind and president of the Volta Bureau's parent organization. Corinne Rocheleau (she had now become Mrs. Wilfred Rouleau) was the Volta Bureau's other nominee. The American Federation of Organizations for the Hard of Hearing was represented by its executive director, Betty Wright, and another staff member. The Foundation members were Anne Sullivan Macy and Robert B. Irwin, who was named secretary of the joint committee.

It all sounded very promising, but the committee was star-crossed from the outset. None of the three constituent organizations had the money to do a real job. The Volta Bureau, which held a legal option on the contents of the Rocheleau-Mack register, had been unable to find a source of funds to get it into shape. This immobilized the hard-of-hearing group's assignment, and frustrated the Foundation, which needed accurate names and addresses of deaf-blind persons in any given state before it could launch effective action in that state's legislature. There were personality clashes, mainly between Mrs. Rouleau and Mrs. Macy, which brought in Rebecca Mack on the one side and Helen Keller on the other. These came to a head in charges and countercharges, some substantive and others petty, in an angry six-way correspondence that also involved M. C. Migel and Robert Irwin. The upshot was the Foundation's decision in early 1933 to withdraw from the joint committee and to proceed on its own to build a register of the nation's deaf-blind population, on the strength of which legislative initiatives could be pursued.

A few years later Rebecca Mack relented, largely at the urging of Helen Keller with whom she had long been acquainted. She had kept a duplicate of the register and in 1936 gave it to the Foundation, which made an effort to validate it by means of a detailed questionnaire sent to every state welfare department, school for the blind, and school for the deaf.

The results were disappointingly scanty, and resources were lacking to conduct the case-by-case field investigations that would have been productive. The Foundation, then striving to complete its own endowment fund, was unwilling to deflect attention from what it considered its primary responsibility to several hundred thousand blind people by mounting a special campaign on behalf of a much smaller number of deaf-blind persons. But it did make some sporadic attempts to obtain extra-budgetary grants; in 1931 an approach was made to the W. K. Kellogg Child Welfare Foundation and some years later, when the Will Rogers Memorial Fund for handicapped children was established in tribute to the journalist who had died in an airplane crash in Alaska, Helen Keller solicited the fund's trustees for an allocation on behalf of deaf-blind children. Neither effort brought results.

One small windfall did come about; in 1932, when Helen was chosen by *Pictorial Review* as that year's "woman who has contributed most to womanhood and humanity," the honor was accompanied by a $5,000 award. Helen turned the money over to the Foundation as an earmarked fund to be spent at her discretion for help to individual deaf-blind persons. Beyond this, and an occasional small appropriation from the Foundation treasury to supply deaf-blind individuals with such items as braillewriters, no further efforts were made on a national scale for the next ten years.

Why did this first national effort to join forces with organizations interested in the deaf turn out to be such a fiasco? Migel, who hastily took himself out of the picture, no doubt regarded the whole matter as a squabble among temperamental women. Irwin's motivations for withdrawing the Foundation from the Joint Committee for the Deaf-Blind were a little more complex, but neither man wished to become embroiled in what was essentially a long-standing animosity toward Anne Sullivan Macy by the educators of the deaf.

From early on, Helen Keller's outspoken teacher had criticized the methods used in schools for the deaf. In the two years, 1894–96, that Helen attended the newly opened Wright-Humason school for oral teaching of the deaf, Anne had written to John Hitz, the first director of the Volta Bureau, deploring the "plodding pursuit of knowledge" of the children in the school and the "stupidities" practiced by their teachers. This hardly endeared her to the teachers of the deaf, and they found equally offensive the patronizing tone in which she sought to find excuses for them: "I pity them more than I blame them. When you consider the huge doses of knowledge which they are expected to pour into the brains of their small pupils, you cannot demand of them initiative or originality." Nor did it please them to learn that Alexander Graham Bell, founder of the Volta Bureau, was "so delighted" with Anne's comments that he invited her to prepare a paper on the subject for the next convention of teachers of the deaf.

When, in 1901, William Wade published the first edition of *The Deaf-Blind*, his prefatory remarks reflected the resentment of educators of the deaf against the widely publicized statements that Anne Sullivan had wrought a miracle in bringing awareness of language to Helen Keller:

> The education of the blind-deaf is by no means the difficult task commonly believed. It may be said positively that any good teacher . . . is fully qualified to teach a blind-deaf pupil, after she learns the manual alphabet. Such a teacher has intelligence, patience and devotion, and these constitute the whole equipment required.

Wade did not spell out what he was aiming at in these remarks, but their meaning was clear to all who knew that a plan was then afoot for the creation of a special school which would serve as a training institute where Helen and Anne would instruct teachers of the deaf-blind in Anne's methods. Helen took Wade's preface to be a denigration of Anne's accomplishments; she also saw it as an effort to thwart this prospect of her gaining a secure livelihood once she graduated from Radcliffe. She was further offended by the fact that among the illustrations in this first edition was a photograph showing her with Arthur Gilman, head of the Cambridge school where she had prepared for college admission. For the sake of her future, Gilman had thought that Helen's day-and-night dependence on her teacher should be terminated, and he had, for a time, succeeded in convincing her mother of this.

Wade was among those of Helen's influential friends who agreed with Gilman (he wrote Helen that he had, in fact, originated the idea and that Gilman was merely his "agent," but Helen chose not to believe this). Others, including Helen's chief financial sponsors, disagreed, and there ensued an anguishing tug of war which ended in victory for Anne Sullivan. Helen regarded the publication of the photograph as a betrayal, and she wrote Wade a reproachful letter:

> . . . in the "Monograph," which came a few days ago, there are indications that you, my dear, kind Mr. Wade, are willing to sacrifice truth and justice to a mere prejudice, and I must utter an indignant protest, though it cost me inexpressible pain. Knowing as you did my feelings towards Mr. Gilman, was it right to ignore them and print a picture of me with him without my consent? This picture stands for something which is gone—something which he killed long ago. When it was taken, I believed that he was a good, true friend. Now I know he was my worst enemy.

In the second and final edition of his book, which appeared in 1904, Wade backed off somewhat. He used a solo photograph of Helen—one showing her capped and gowned for her Radcliffe graduation—and, in a new foreword, went to great lengths to express his admiration for Anne Sullivan's achievements. But he continued to challenge the belief that Anne's educational approach represented a new discovery. By this time, Helen Keller's *The Story of My Life* had been published and had evoked ecstatic public reactions over Anne Sullivan's role in Helen's education. This troubled Wade, and he wrote a letter to the *School Journal* insisting "there was no mystery about the education of the blind-deaf, no marvelous genius required, nor any complex intricacies to be unraveled." He reprinted the letter in the second edition of his monograph, along with articles written by other teachers of blind-deaf children describing their methods, which were essentially the same as those of Helen's teacher. He also sought to lay to rest the assertion, voiced by many, that Helen Keller was largely the creature of her teacher's genius. Helen, he said, was a prodigy and it was "dangerous nonsense" to deny it, "for it loads down other teachers of the blind-deaf with the weight of mistaken feeling, that if they could only pursue such methods as Miss Sullivan's, they would make Helen Kellers of their pupils."

Anne Sullivan agreed with him in this last statement and said so repeatedly. As she once put it:

> I have never thought that I deserve more praise than other teachers who give the best they have to their pupils. If their earnest efforts have not released an Ariel from the imprisoning oak, it is no doubt because there has not been an Ariel to release.

It was in this second edition of *The Deaf-Blind* that Wade declared openly what he had only intimated in the foreword to the first edition.

The only thing in "The Story of My Life" that I can see may be mischievous, is the proposal that Helen and Miss Sullivan should carry on a school for the blind-deaf. . . . *The one thing* the interests of the blind-deaf demand above all others, is the recognition by the public, and particularly by State boards of education, that it is the duty of the States to educate these unfortunates. If a special school, under the charge of two such distinguished personages, is required to educate the blind-deaf, good-bye to all hopes of the States undertaking it.

Wade's clear-eyed vision of the overall needs of deaf-blind children grew from his intimate knowledge of the field of education of the deaf. He was an original member of the American Association to Promote the Teaching of Speech to the Deaf and an occasional contributor to its periodicals. At the convention of the American Association of Instructors of the Deaf held in St. Louis in 1904 in connection with the Louisiana Purchase Exposition, he was awarded a gold medal for "his benefactions to deaf-blind children and for his untiring zeal in finding and providing education for such children in the United States."

So much for William Wade. But Corinne Rocheleau and Rebecca Mack regarded themselves as his ideological heirs, asserting that since his death, no one had taken an interest in the deaf-blind. Anne Sullivan Macy may also have seen the two women in this light, and she was not a person who easily forgot or forgave. "Mrs. Macy's stand on the subject of other teachers of the deaf-blind has been most unjust and a constant aggravation to said teachers, many of whom have done work that is truly remarkable," Corinne Rocheleau Rouleau wrote M. C. Migel when the work of the Joint Committee on the Deaf-Blind had reached an impasse. Helen's teacher, she said, "would be a permanent obstacle to harmonious work in the committee." She was piqued by the fact that Mrs. Macy had refused to see her or allow her access to Helen and had scornfully dismissed her as "that Frenchwoman." She could not refrain from slapping back: "I am a perfectly good American by birth and even count Yankee Colonial ancestors, which is probably more than Mrs. Macy could say for herself."

The well-meaning but sometimes maladroit Rebecca Mack also had complaints to make about the way Helen Keller's household treated her. A plaintive letter she wrote Helen brought a rebuke for persistence and a stern lecture castigating the "unfriendly spirit" in which she and Mrs. Rouleau were withholding their register.

It may all have been a tempest in a teapot, but the fact was that as the tempest raged, the teapot boiled dry. A decade passed before it was refilled.

The man who got national action simmering again was the amiable Irishman whose unique blend of idealism, persistence and personal charm had already won him a permanent niche in the annals of work for the blind. Peter J. Salmon, a hero of the workshop campaign which culminated in the Wagner-O'Day Act, played an even more seminal role in the activation of services for the deaf-blind. He did it by means of a well-timed ploy.

In observance of Helen Keller's sixty-fifth birthday in June 1945, Salmon staged a luncheon at the Industrial Home for the Blind, of which he was by then executive director. It was a rather exclusive affair; in addition to Helen, the other principal guests were 13 deaf-blind men trained for employment in the IHB workshop, which had just earned an Army-Navy "E" citation for its war production record. In a statement extensively covered by the press, Helen cited these 13 men who "have all proved their capabilities, strength and human dignity" and urged that training and employment programs similar to IHB's be established in other parts of the nation. This could be done, she suggested, through the cooperative leadership of the Foundation, the IHB, and Perkins.

Months of preparation had preceded this announcement. Still aglow over her recently completed tours of military hospitals, Helen was psychologically ready for a new challenge. The impressive wartime record rolled up by blind and handicapped workers in all types of industry had swept away some long-held prejudices and misconceptions; the climate of public opinion now seemed ripe for an advance. A small but solid body of experience had been built up, largely by IHB, to demonstrate that, given the right kind and amount of help, deaf-blind persons could become productive workers; a similar body of experience proving the educability of deaf-blind children had been developed at Perkins and a few other schools.

The original plan Helen put forward was for a quasi-autonomous body, the National Council for the Deaf-Blind, to be established as an administrative division of the Foundation but financed through a separate campaign. Together with Peter Salmon she outlined a detailed program. Migel was sympathetic. He wrote William Ziegler, Jr., who would succeed him later that year as Foundation president, that "now, in the autumn of her life, we should endeavor to aid [Helen] in this project, which would so greatly add to her happiness and be a gratifying achievement for the Foundation."

The only debatable point was launching a separate organization and a separate campaign; the Foundation decided to set up a new department for the program and to create, instead of the proposed council, an advisory body called the Helen Keller Committee on the Deaf-Blind.

The advisory committee held its first meeting in September 1945, and the new department got under way the following January with Dorothy D. Bryan as director. Mrs. Bryan, whose background included experience in special education, rehabilitation, and social work, began where the efforts of the preceding decade had left off—by initiating a nationwide drive to locate deaf-blind individuals, to ascertain their medical, social, and financial status and, by developing a complete and accurate register, to grasp the extent of the existing needs. The flaw in previous efforts to help the deaf-blind, the committee felt, had been the decision to complete a national register before beginning a service program; this time, the two processes would move ahead simultaneously.

The service program envisaged was primarily stimulation of state and local agencies to care for their deaf-blind populations. However, this proved to be so slow a process that in less than a year the Foundation found itself taking on a direct service role as well. As casefinding went along and urgent needs were uncovered which local resources were not ready or able to meet, the department began to supply hearing aids, vibrator alarm clocks, typewriters, braillewriters, and other tangible aids that could encourage or restore functioning in deaf-blind individuals.

The department's function soon grew even broader. A scholarship program was begun to enable promising deaf-blind young people to go to college. For the benefit of potentially employable adults, a series of short-term courses was financed to bring workshop supervisors from all parts of the country to Brooklyn, where they could learn IHB's tested techniques of communication, rehabilitation and vocational training. To increase educational opportunities for children, courses for teachers of the deaf-blind, cosponsored by Perkins, were conducted for three successive summers at Eastern Michigan University's school of special education.

One of Dorothy Bryan's first observations, as she crisscrossed the nation and visited scores of deaf-blind persons in their homes, was the great hunger for a medium which would help allay their feelings of isolation by providing them with news of the world and each other. In 1947 the Foundation began a monthly magazine, *Touch and Go*, produced in inkprint and braille and sent free of charge to all deaf-blind adults. In addition to news digests, it contained a variety of articles, stories and poems, many written by its readers.

The national register grew slowly at first. Beginning with fewer than 1,500 verified names, it rose to over 1,900 in 1948. The workload, however, grew fast, and in 1948 Annette Dinsmore was added to the staff as assistant director of the Department of Services to the Deaf-Blind. Two years later she succeeded Mrs. Bryan as director, in which capacity she remained until her retirement in 1971.

Annette Dinsmore was still another example of the right person in the right place at the right time. She began her career as a teacher of deaf children; following the bout of infection that left her totally blind at the age of thirty, she earned a graduate degree in social work, joined the staff of the Philadelphia Department of Public Assistance and then became supervisor of home teaching for the Pennsylvania State Council for the Blind. A tall, sturdy woman with a ready smile, a quick wit, a gift for empathy, and a large fund of common sense, she became to hundreds of deaf-blind people what Kay Gruber had become to the war-blinded: a warm personal friend who kept in touch through intimate correspondence, remembered birthdays and anniversaries, introduced people to others with like interests, and was an unfailingly dependable source of counsel and help in all sorts of situations. She and her Seeing Eye dog became welcome visitors, not only in the households of deaf-blind persons all over the country, but also in the offices of the state and local agencies she persuaded to extend services to them.

Of all the barriers that imprisoned deaf-blind persons, the greatest was difficulty in communication. One of the first steps in the new program was production of a pamphlet, *Working with Deaf-Blind Clients*, which aimed at bridging the communications gap between staff members of local social agencies and the deaf-blind persons who needed their services. The pamphlet contained a number of simple pointers and was illustrated by photographs showing the finger and knuckle positions of the most feasible communication method, the one-hand manual alphabet. The hand photographed in this pamphlet, issued in 1947, was the hand of Helen Keller.

Two years later, when a more comprehensive guide on the subject was to be issued, an embarrassing discovery was made. Several of the illustrated finger positions were wrong! It fell to Annette Dinsmore to tell Helen Keller that some new photographs would be needed, and to explain why. Annette regarded the assignment with trepidation. If the world's best known deaf-blind person was not the ultimate authority on the manual alphabet, who was? A tactful approach occurred to her en route to Helen's home. The divergences between the standard finger positions and those Helen was accustomed to using were comparable, she explained, to the differences between distinctive individual penmanship and "Palmer Method" handwriting. Amenable to this face-saving explanation, Helen was happy to pose her right hand in the conventional configurations.

The expanded handbook, *Methods of Communication with Deaf-Blind People*, was issued in 1951 (a revised edition was produced in 1959 and a prize-winning documentary film on the subject was made in 1963). It offered several choices, depending on the individual situation of the deaf-blind person. Those whose deafness had preceded blindness (and they were in the majority) were apt to know the one-hand manual alphabet; those whose disabilities occurred in the reverse order were apt to know braille. Those whose hearing and sight were both lost in middle life or later might not know either, but could nonetheless learn to use one of the simpler methods.

The one-hand manual alphabet had been used for centuries by deaf people. Along with the sign language of the deaf, it was said to have originated in Spanish monasteries whose monks were under a vow of silence. It could be learned in a fairly short time by a sighted or a blind person and had the advantage of relative speed. In the American version, the letter *B*, for example, was represented by pointing the four fingers, tightly held together, straight up, while the thumb was bent across the palm. To form the letter *I* the speaker made a fist with the thumb and first three fingers, but pointed the little finger straight up. The various finger positions (see illustration on overleaf) were formed into the cupped hand of the deaf-blind person.

The British manual alphabet was slightly different. There was also a two-hand alphabet, seldom used because it was awkward and slow.

Some deaf-blind persons received communication by means of the standard Morse Code, which had the advantage of permitting dot-dash touches on any part of the body or even through floor vibrations which could be felt across a room. Another such code, devised by a deaf-blind man named Cross, was based on a system of taps and strokes applied to the back of the hand or elsewhere on the body. It was similar to a dot-and-stroke method developed by the Austrian, Hieronymus Lorm, in the nineteenth century. The Lorm Alphabet was widely used by deaf-blind persons in central Europe.

With a person blind from childhood, it was also possible to communicate through braille hand speech, in which the speaker pointed to the dots in an imaginary braille cell in the receiver's palm, or pressed the receiver's fingertips into braillewriter combinations.

There were also some simple auxiliary aids. One of the oldest was the alphabet glove, which enabled a sighted person to spell out words by touching the letters printed on a thin glove worn by the deaf-blind person. A touch on the top of the thumb was *A*, one at the base of the ring finger was *R*, one on the second joint of

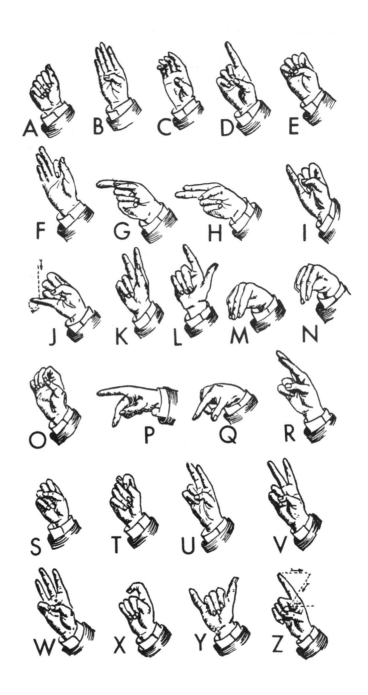

the index finger was *G*, etc. This required little effort by the sighted communicator but considerable memorization on the part of the deaf-blind receiver. Easier, but slower, was printing-in-the-palm, which spelled out messages to people who either had a visual memory of print or could be taught to recognize the shapes of printed letters. Slower still were the alphabet plate, which reproduced the print alphabet in embossed form, and the alphabet card, which was embossed with braille letters and overprinted with each letter's inkprint symbol. With these devices the speaker spelled out words by placing the blind person's finger on the correct symbols.

As noted earlier, it took several years to perfect a mechanical device for speedier communication; the problem was finally solved in 1954 by the invention of the Tellatouch, a small machine that enabled a sighted or blind person to communicate with a deaf-blind person who could read braille. Another device was a pocket-sized braillewriter whose output was on a strip of plastic tape. Annette Dinsmore usually took one of these on her field trips, along with a Tellatouch and various types of hearing amplifiers.

An early system for telephone conversations, the Tactaphone, was the product of cooperative work between the Illinois Bell Telephone Company and the Hadley School for the Blind. It required a knowledge of the Morse Code by both parties. The sender used his dial to transmit the code's dots and dashes (dialing number 1 for dot, number 4 for dash) while the deaf-blind person at the other end received the code through his fingertips by means of a vibrating disk installed in the base of his telephone. A later version, the Sensicall, was developed through cooperation of the New York Telephone Company and IHB; it did away with the dialing and permitted the code to be sent either by voice or by means of a separate button. Later still came the Tactile Speech Indicator, a portable device which did not require special installation but could be used with any telephone.

How could a deaf-blind person, alone at home, know there was someone at the door or on the phone? Some had electric fans hooked up to doorbell or phone bell so they could feel the air current activated by the ring. A more modern approach used an electronic instrument, similar to the radio pagers carried by hospital physicians; instead of "beeping," the wireless transmitter, worn in a shirt pocket, vibrated against the body. Two such devices were being tested in 1972, one developed by MIT's Sensory Aids Evaluation and Development Center and the other by Bell & Howell. Even the possibility of group communication among deaf-blind persons was being explored; an experimental European device operated on a relay system similar to that in telephone conference hookups.

Slow and patience-demanding as all of these methods might be, for the socially marooned deaf-blind person they represented a precious lifeline of interpersonal relationship which many had thought lost forever. There were cases where such surrender was needlessly premature—where the fitting of a proper hearing aid made two-way voice communication possible, or where surgical treatment restored vestiges of functional vision.

In the first five years of the Foundation's deaf-blind department, field trips by its staff covered 36 states; five years later, the remaining states had been visited and the volume and quality of local services to deaf-blind adults showed an appreciable upsurge. Field trips invariably resulted in additional casefinding; by 1970 the national register contained the names of 4,000 adults and close to 800 children.

The effort to increase job opportunities was uphill work. In 1956 a national workshop was conducted and a report subsequently published (*Vocational Training and Employment of Deaf-Blind Adults*), but it failed to have much impact on the state rehabilitation counselors who held the key to jobs. Burdened with large caseloads of less gravely handicapped people who could be trained and placed with less time, effort, and expense, the counselors almost invariably classified deaf-blind applicants as "non-feasible" for employment. It was not until 1962, when the Industrial Home for the Blind put on a full-scale regional research and demonstration program, that the first appreciable dent was made.

More than forty years of service to deaf-blind adults preceded this landmark demonstration. Not long after the youthful Peter Salmon joined the staff of IHB in 1917 as its business manager, a deaf man who had lost his sight applied for a place in the agency's broom shop. Salmon saw no reason not to take him on, and taught the shop supervisor the manual alphabet, which Salmon had picked up during his years as a student at Perkins. This first deaf-blind worker in the broom shop proved so satisfactory that opportunities were given to others as the years went by. As of 1945, a dozen deaf-blind men were employed in the IHB workshop and seven more were receiving other types of rehabilitation services from the parent agency. At this point IHB decided to establish a separate deaf-blind department, and it was the formal opening of this unit, as well as the launching of a national drive, that Helen Keller's 65th birthday luncheon celebrated.

The department's objectives went beyond employment. Almost as urgent as jobs was the need for social contacts and personal development. A program of parties and picnics, games and outings, club activities and hobbies not only enriched the lives of the participants but deepened the insights of the IHB staff into the problems and potentialities of this group.

Sensitive to their human needs, Peter Salmon assumed the role of realistic apologist. "One thing to be kept in mind always," he wrote, "is the fact that no matter how complete the rehabilitation of a deaf-blind person may seem to be, there will always be a certain amount of frustration, irritability, suspicion and restlessness, as a result of the difficult limitations imposed by the double handicap."

Salmon never played down either the difficulties or the gratifications of serving the deaf-blind. The work, he said,

> requires patience, compassion, intuition and selflessness far above and beyond that required in work for the blind. The worker must be able to accept trivial demands and childish possessiveness. He must be able to continue when no progress is evident; much of the work with this group is tedious. He must be willing and able to give time—any amount of time; work with the group is slow. And yet, work with no other group is more rewarding in terms of personal satisfaction. Let the worker with the deaf-blind follow through . . . and he will find himself sharing in the liberation of a soul, an experience granted only to the privileged few.

It was in this spirit that IHB undertook, in 1956, a comprehensive two-year study of 63 deaf-blind clients, their characteristics, limitations and potentials, and in a seven-volume report presented the evidence that intensive rehabilitation could measurably assist the vocational and social adjustment of a large percentage of deaf-blind adults. The findings of the federally financed study occupied a major session at the 1958 AAWB convention. A lead-off statement by Mary Switzer, director of the Office of Vocational Rehabilitation, emphasized that it was largely fear that had so long delayed the start of rehabilitation service for this group:

> fear among the deaf-blind that their disability placed them automatically on a fringe of society from where there was little chance of escape.... fear among rehabilitation workers ... that, because of a lack of guideposts and tools, they were inadequate to cope with the special problems inherent in deaf-blindness.

Thanks to the IHB study, she continued, guideposts were now at hand. It was OVR's hope that rehabilitation agencies in other parts of the country would now enlarge the entrances to opportunity wedged open by the study; the federal government stood ready to back the development of a number of regional rehabilitation centers for the deaf-blind.

Disappointingly, her offer found no takers. An ice-breaker was needed, and in 1962 IHB launched one as a demonstration project—the Anne Sullivan Macy Service for Deaf-Blind Persons, funded by Miss Switzer's agency. Designed to embrace the 15-state northeastern region, the project was called upon to stretch its borders as it progressed; in the end it served clients from 17 additional states, some as far away as Oregon and New Mexico.

Over a period of seven years, and at a cost of $500,000, the Anne Sullivan Macy Service worked with 171 deaf-blind men and women who underwent six-week evaluation periods that were followed, on the average, by eight months of intensive rehabilitation treatment. The results went a long way beyond the findings of IHB's earlier study by demonstrating that, on completion of such a specialized course, deaf-blind men and women could return home to their own communities, or be resettled in new communities, to function with a good deal of independence and self-direction. Optimum results necessitated continuing services from a community agency; one of the most significant effects of the demonstration was that those agencies that had referred clients for rehabilitation showed a marked increase in willingness to work with additional deaf-blind persons. However, as Peter Salmon noted in a monograph which summed up the experience and findings of the project, the real trouble was that many agencies would not take that first step and make a referral for service. "The true failure," he said, "lies in not trying."

No one would ever accuse Peter Salmon himself of not trying. The man in whose honor Helen Keller willed 25 percent of her residuary estate to IHB's deaf-blind program—because, as her last testament stated, she regarded Salmon "as a most active, disinterested champion of the deaf-blind [who] has put unremitting enthusiasm, energy and resourcefulness into the effort to break their captivity of double affliction"—this man was not content to stop with a demonstration project. Already past retirement age, he mobilized and led a five-year legislative campaign which succeeded in incorporating in the 1967 amendments to the Vocational Rehabilitation Act a provision for a federally financed National Center for Deaf-Blind Youths and Adults.

It was not yet the final hurdle. In a general appropriations cutback, the 90th Congress adjourned without approving funds for the center's first year of operations. Striving to remedy the omission as soon as possible, Salmon wrote every federal legislator that, unlike the drastic protest actions of other disadvantaged groups, there would be "no riot or sit-in" on the part of the deaf-blind: "we are dealing with silent men and women who are not only unorganized but so much isolated that they have little knowledge of what is going on. . . ."

The needed initial appropriation was approved early in the next Congressional session and June 1969 saw the execution of a contract by HEW's Social and Rehabilitation Service assigning operation of the National Center to IHB.

Obtaining funds for construction of the center's residential and treatment facilities also met with a series of frustrating delays. In the original planning, a modest facility had been envisaged at a projected cost of $2.5 million for land and construction. Then a windfall deeded the National Center 25 acres of surplus federal land in Sands Point, Long Island, and a more adequate facility became possible. Zooming construction costs had already made the original sum unrealistic; the added factor of a larger facility meant that $5 million more was needed in building funds. This sum was included in the Rehabilitation Act of 1972, passed by Congress but vetoed by the President. The following year it appeared as an earmarked item in the HEW appropriations bill for fiscal 1973, which likewise met a Presidential veto. Hope remained that the funds would be released in fiscal 1974.

In the interim, the center operated out of temporary quarters. Forced to restrict its client group to 17 or 18 persons at a time, instead of the proposed 50, it was moving ahead with other parts of its overall program: regional offices for case-finding, screening and follow-up; public education activities; and week-long training sessions for staff members of local agencies preparing to serve deaf-blind clients.

Where deaf-blind children were concerned, events followed a different course. Only 133 children—as against ten times that many adults—appeared on the list with which the Foundation's Department of Services to the Deaf-Blind began in 1945. There was every reason to believe that the actual number in both categories was at least twice as large, but whereas some types of immediate service could be offered to adults, there was little that could be done for children without adequate facilities for education.

The deaf-blind department at Perkins, begun in 1932, had been serving an average of 12 to 15 children annually; in 1940 its enrollment reached a high of 18. The New York Institute for the Education of the Blind opened a deaf-blind department at about that time, and in 1943 the California School for the Blind did likewise. An additional handful of children were receiving individual instruction in scattered schools for the deaf as well as in schools for the blind. All told, the nation was educating perhaps three or four dozen deaf-blind children; the rest were immobilized by a pair of tight bottlenecks. There was the reluctance of schools that could cope with a single handicap to take on the complex, expensive, and often frustrating challenge of educating a child with a second sensory deficiency, and there was the absence of qualified teachers who could do the job.

Although the numbers picture was dismal, the prospects for meaningful educational achievement were more hopeful than ever before. Thanks to the pioneering work of a spirited southern woman, Sophia Alcorn, the "Tadoma method" of sensing and replicating sound vibrations was bringing to many deaf-blind children the one gift Helen Keller envied more than anything else—the power of understandable speech.

It was just before World War I that Miss Alcorn, newly graduated from the normal school operated by the Clarke School for the Deaf in Massachusetts, joined the faculty of her native Kentucky's school for the deaf. Soon after her arrival the school accepted its first deaf-blind pupil, eight-year-old Oma Simpson, and assigned the child's training to the new teacher. "Miss Sophie," as she came to be called throughout a long and distinguished career, was dissatisfied with the half-measure represented by the manual alphabet; less than a year after she began with Oma, she started to teach her orally. She placed the child's sensitive fingers on her mouth, jaw and throat to feel the movement and vibrations as different sounds were formed, then had Oma place her fingers on her own face to duplicate these movements and vibrations. During the ten years Oma was in Miss Sophie's charge at the Kentucky school, she learned not only to comprehend speech by "reading" the resonances she felt in touching the speaker's face, but also how to produce speech. "She could carry on a conversation with anyone with whom she came in contact," her teacher wrote.

When the Simpson family left Kentucky, taking Oma with them, Miss Sophie moved, too. At the South Dakota School for the Deaf she met her second deaf-blind child, Tad Chapman, with whom she began oral instruction at once, deferring the manual alphabet stage. Tad was taught words by tactile methods, his fingers tracing the letters his teacher fashioned out of sandpaper. Unable to see the drawings or use the mirror by means of which deaf children learned lip positions, Tad was taught vowel sounds by touching the lip position diagrams Miss Sophie constructed out of pipe cleaners. After four years of work with Tad, Sophia Alcorn turned him over to Inis B. Hall, another teacher at the South Dakota school, whom she had trained in the method she named "Tadoma" after her two pupils.

If deaf children unable to see could learn speech with the help of their fingertips, could such tactile methods help sighted deaf children acquire more natural speech patterns than they could through visual instruction? Intrigued by this question—"I am constantly amazed at how much the fingers can convey to the brain"—Miss Sophie spent the remaining years of her professional career at the Detroit Day School for the Deaf, exploring the use of vibration techniques for teaching language and speech to sighted deaf children. It was Inis Hall who stayed with the education of the deaf-blind; when Tad Chapman was admitted to Perkins in 1931, she was asked to accompany him and to launch the school's deaf-blind department. From that day forward, all Perkins' deaf-blind pupils who were capable of learning it were taught by the vibration method, which Miss Hall modified and amplified as she gained experience in its use with different children. In 1943 she moved to the California School for the Blind to head its newly opened deaf-blind unit, remaining there until her retirement in 1952.

Inis Hall was an instructor at one of the summer graduate courses jointly sponsored by Perkins and the Foundation at Eastern Michigan University in 1949, 1950, and 1951. Although enthusiastically received, these courses, attended mainly by teachers of the deaf, failed to produce a sufficient yield of qualified instructors for doubly handicapped children, whose known numbers were steadily growing. The Foundation's register showed 190 deaf-blind boys and girls under the age of twenty in 1953; six years later the children's list held 350 names.

What was happening with these 350 children? A 1959 report gave some details. About 20 were preschoolers under the age of five, 80 were attending schools which had departments for the deaf-blind, 70 were in institutions for the mentally retarded, and 180—just over half the total—were living at home, not enrolled in any educational program whatever.

Numerically, the situation was not much different in 1962 when M. Robert Barnett delivered a detailed report on the deaf-blind to the AAWB convention. He did, however, add a significant detail. The Foundation was keeping a "watching list" of children who, though not yet classifiable as deaf-blind, were showing progressive losses in hearing, vision or both; there were 50 children known to be moving toward deaf-blindness.

Neither Barnett nor anyone else possessed the power to predict that, by the time AAWB met two years later, the nation would be in the midst of the maternal rubella epidemic that was to add not just 50 but hundreds upon hundreds of deaf-blind children to the national picture.

Disappointed by the negligible results of the summer graduate courses for teachers, in 1952 the Foundation approached the AAIB and its counterpart, the Conference of Executives of American Schools for the Deaf, asking each professional association to appoint a committee to explore the question of how deaf-blind children could be given better opportunities for education. The two associations held a conference in April 1953 at which they joined forces with the Foundation to organize the National Study Committee on Education of Deaf-Blind Children. Although the committee's roster was high-powered, and an amicably cooperative spirit prevailed in its meetings of the next few years, no more constructive results were produced than had been the case more than 20 years earlier, when the first attempt had been made at forming an operating partnership between educators of the deaf and educators of the blind.

There were, however, some useful by-products of the committee's brief existence. The Iowa School for the Deaf, which had a unit for deaf-blind children, initiated a three-year undergraduate teacher training program in 1953; although the program was later discontinued, it did yield a few more teachers. More enduring was the one-year graduate course organized in 1955 by Perkins, originally in affiliation with Boston University and later with Boston College. For more than a decade it was the sole such teacher training program, and it made possible a steady buildup in Perkins' deaf-blind unit, which grew to 79 children in 1972. The Perkins course produced about five new teachers a year, most of whom were employed by the school; there was little surplus for other parts of the country.

An effort to meet that need was made by the Foundation in 1954 when it employed Sophia Alcorn, then newly retired from the Detroit school where she had spent 23 years as principal, to serve as consultant to a western school for the blind then opening a deaf-blind unit. She subsequently visited and screened 64 deaf-blind children uncovered through a new casefinding sweep. When her one-year consultancy ended, the Foundation added two staff members to its deaf-blind department to pursue casefinding and field consultations to local agencies.

Locating deaf-blind children, training teachers to work with them, mobilizing community resources to serve them, were all hurdles; but trickiest of all was evaluating each child's developmental status to determine degree of disability, potential for learning, and the kind of preschool or educational program best calculated to meet his or her needs. A diagnostic facility was required, where individual assessments could be made and individual courses of treatment prescribed.

What may well have been the Foundation's cardinal contribution to the education of deaf-blind children was its decision in 1957 to sponsor such a diagnostic clinic at the Syracuse University Center for the Development of Blind Children.

For the next 12 years the center conducted monthly diagnostic sessions for deaf-blind children. Over this period, 75 children were brought in, each child accompanied by one or both parents and by a social worker from his home community. The costs of the services, travel, and maintenance expenses were defrayed by the Foundation when not available from other sources. Each session lasted four days, in the course of which a team of specialists examined the child, interviewed the parent or parents, and consulted with the accompanying social worker, whose role was to give psychological support and reassurance to parents under considerable emotional strain and then to take responsibility for implementing the evaluation team's recommendations.

The 36 boys and 39 girls were residents of 21 states; they ranged in age from under two to twenty-one, with about half under school age. Following evaluation, most of the children of school age were enrolled in the educational program recommended by the diagnostic team; a small number were deemed in need of institutional care. For the preschoolers, developmental programs in their home communities were prescribed.

To explore the dimensions of such developmental programs, the Syracuse team conducted and the Foundation financed two six-week treatment sessions during the summers of 1961 and 1962, working first with four and then with eight children whose problems were exceptionally severe because of one or more handicaps in addition to deaf-blindness. These sessions were designed to ascertain what was involved, professionally and administratively, in serving such multi-handicapped children. Hindsight shows this pilot effort to have been prescient; the rubella epidemic was yet to come.

A vexing problem which arose repeatedly throughout the Fifties concerned the deaf-blind children who were ready for schooling but whose states neither maintained schools that could serve them nor provided funds to pay for their education in out-of-state schools. Such children could hardly be kept in deep-freeze while the necessary laws and appropriations were enacted; the Foundation met the situation by paying out-of-state tuition fees for a total of 44 of these youngsters, while simultaneously striving to have the deficiencies in state laws remedied.

By the early Sixties, all states were in a position to accept financial responsibility for the education of their handicapped children and the tuition subsidy program was discontinued. At this time, too, the Foundation modified its policy of supplying free tangible aids to deaf-blind adults; it determined in future to pay only half the cost, leaving the respective local communities to find the remainder. The new policy had the desired salutory effect; local responsibility for the needs of deaf-blind residents soon grew to a point where this subsidy program could be terminated as well.

As was the case with help to deaf-blind adults, it took action on the part of the federal government to swell services for deaf-blind children from a trickle to a more adequate flow. Teacher training took an upturn in 1966 when federal funds for special education of the handicapped became available. The first two schools to offer graduate programs for teachers of the deaf-blind (in addition to the ongoing Perkins–Boston College program) were Peabody College for Teachers and San Francisco State College. At about the same time Michigan State University organized a similar course on an undergraduate level. As of the end of 1972 these schools had expanded their services to offer both graduate and undergraduate programs, and five additional colleges had been added to the teacher-preparation roster.

The major breakthrough in education came with the passage in 1968 of Public Law 90-247 which authorized operational grants for a limited number of "model centers" for schooling of deaf-blind children and also called for establishment under federal auspices of ten regional centers. The latter were not schools but coordinating bodies, each serving five to seven states, whose responsibilities embraced casefinding, referrals, development of consultation and training programs for parents and teachers, and promotion of new services. As the result of intensive investigations conducted by teams of professionals in each region, 3,600 deaf-blind children had already been located as of early 1972. The federal coordinator of these regional centers reported at that time that 1,200 of the 3,600 had been placed in a variety of educational and training programs and about 800 were in state institutions for the mentally retarded. With 1,600 remaining at home and receiving no services, it was clear there was still a long way to go. Some new programs had been initiated, however, among them "crisis care centers" which were short-term residential treatment facilities for the deaf-blind child and his parents. These performed essentially along the lines originally tested at Syracuse, involving diagnostic evaluation of the child, parent counseling, and follow-up services in the home community.

To insure continuity from infancy to adulthood, liaison was established between the regional centers for children (which were administered by HEW's Office of Education) and the National Center for Deaf-Blind Youths and Adults (which was administered by HEW's Social and Rehabilitation Service). The plan was that once the National Center came into full operation, deaf-blind children in their middle or late teens for whom advanced education was not feasible would be referred to the adult facility for vocational rehabilitation and training.

With the creation of these federal facilities, the Foundation phased out its direct service programs on behalf of the deaf-blind. It turned over its registers to the appropriate new bodies and discontinued its staff work to coincide with Annette Dinsmore's retirement in 1971. But it continued to maintain a watching brief over the national picture, prepared to intervene, if need be, in the future.

Will the new generation of deaf-blind children produce a Helen Keller? Leaving aside the question of personality and the unique circumstances of Helen's life, there is no reason why other deaf-blind persons should not match or exceed her achievements.

For nearly half a century Helen Keller stood alone as the only person lacking sight and hearing to have acquired a college education, but in 1950 Robert Smithdas was graduated from St. John's University in New York; in 1954 Richard Kinney received his baccalaureate summa cum laude from Mount Union College in Ohio; in 1959 Jackie Coker took a degree from California's College of the Pacific; and before the Sixties ended, four other deaf-blind men and women had earned caps and gowns. All seven were helped by $1,000-a-year Helen Keller Scholarships; this was the one scholarship program still continued by the Foundation as of 1972.

Smithdas, Kinney, and Miss Coker were among the eight outstanding deaf-blind persons awarded gold medals at the 1966 Anne Sullivan Centennial Commemoration, a year-long event jointly sponsored by Perkins and IHB and culminating in a memorial service attended by 3,000 persons at the Washington National Cathedral.

Bob Smithdas, who went on to earn a master's degree in rehabilitation and was subsequently awarded honorary doctorates by Gallaudet College and Western Michigan University, was professionally employed in 1972 as director of community education of the National Center for Deaf-Blind Youths and Adults, a logical outgrowth of his long-time affiliation, in a similar capacity, with IHB. Dick Kinney in 1972 was the new executive director of the Hadley School for the Blind, following a number of years as its assistant director. Both men were published poets. Jackie Coker in 1972 was continuing her work as a rehabilitation teacher for the blind employed by the State of California.

As for what the future may produce by way of singular personalities and signal accomplishments, much depends not only on the inherent talents of the individual but on his good fortune in encountering the person or persons who can ignite the spark. As the sociologist Herbert Rusalem once said about Anne Sullivan: "Perhaps the real miracle was a statistical one. Of all the possible teachers who could have been assigned to Helen Keller, the task fell to the one teacher in a million who was equal to the task."

26

Open Channels

Long before work for the blind proliferated to a network comprising hundreds of local, state, and national organizations, its leaders recognized that open channels of communication were essential if blind people as a group were to improve their lot.

It was in this belief that one of the responsibilities stipulated in the American Foundation for the Blind's articles of incorporation was to "assemble, systematize and disseminate all available data in any way relating to work for the blind." Among the items in Article VII of the 1921 bylaws was that the newborn organization was to issue an inkprint and an embossed magazine devoted to work for the blind, "or avail itself of the services of such periodicals already in existence."

The founders did not name the existing periodicals they had in mind, but everyone knew which were meant. The inkprint vehicle was the *Outlook for the Blind;* the embossed periodical was the *Matilda Ziegler Magazine for the Blind.* By coincidence, both had been started the same year although under separate auspices and in sharply differing circumstances.

The *Ziegler* had a slight head start, its first issue appearing in March 1907; the *Outlook* made its debut the following month. The events that began the former might have made the plot of a Horatio Alger story.

In 1906 a shy, middle-aged bachelor named Walter G. Holmes made one of his periodic business trips to New York from Memphis, Tennessee, where he was business manager of that city's *Commercial Appeal.* Leafing through the *Herald,* then New York's largest daily newspaper, he came across an item describing a legacy which bequeathed $25,000 each to organizations for the deaf, for the crippled, for orphans, and for several other charitable purposes. Impulsively, Holmes dashed off a short note to the editor. Why, his letter asked, had the blind been overlooked in this sweeping generosity? Blind people were greatly in need of benefactors; a great deal of good, for example, would result from a fund to finance the production of tactual reading material which cost far more than the average blind person could afford. He illustrated his point by noting that a book like *Ben Hur*, which sold for $1 in inkprint, cost $30 to $40 in embossed type.

Within 24 hours, Holmes' letter evoked a reply: "I saw your communication today and as I am interested in doing something for the blind along the printing line I would like to communicate with you. (Signed) E.M. Ziegler."

Holmes may have recognized the surname; it had been in the news just a few years earlier, when William Ziegler sponsored two unsuccessful Arctic expeditions to discover the North Pole. What did not occur to him was that E.M. Ziegler was a woman and, in fact, the widow of the millionaire industrialist who had financed the polar explorations.

This, and more, he discovered at his first interview with the delicate-featured, sixty-five-year-old Electa Matilda Ziegler. He learned that their mutual concern over the plight of blind people stemmed from similar causes: Mrs. Ziegler had a blind son, Holmes had a blind brother. As Holmes later recounted: "Mrs. Ziegler said that she had always wanted to do something for the blind and that if I would take charge of a magazine for the blind, as I already had some knowledge of printing as well as editorial work, she would finance it."

Throughout his nearly forty years of editorship of the *Matilda Ziegler Magazine for the Blind*, Holmes produced a periodical that admirably answered the needs of its readers. Thousands of letters came to "Uncle Walter"—letters seeking intimate advice as well as practical information, letters responding to the heart-to-heart personal opinions he voiced in his "Publisher's Chat" column, letters expressing gratitude for the magazine that, for many, was their major link with the world at large. A single word from the avuncular editor had fantastic motive power. When his column suggested that readers observe the 20th anniversary of the magazine's founding in 1927 by sending Christmas greetings to Mrs. Ziegler, more than 1,200 letters arrived, most of them bearing the postscript, "I typed this myself." The way Holmes' readers felt about him had come vividly to light earlier that same year when Robert Irwin, then president of the AAWB, conceived the idea of commemorating the magazine's milestone by a surprise tribute to the editor. Without Holmes' knowledge, Irwin sent a letter to the *Ziegler* readers asking them to donate from ten cents to a maximum of one dollar for the purchase of a gold watch to be presented to Holmes at the AAWB convention. The response was so overwhelming that, even though all gifts in excess of a dollar were returned to the senders, enough money came in to buy not only the watch but an automobile.

The presentation was made by Helen Keller in a warm and graceful speech in which she told Holmes, "you have a chimney corner all to yourself in our hearts." It was the perfect metaphor for the self-effacing man who had resolved, from the outset, to aim his magazine not at the gifted and the brilliant but at people of modest intellect and attainments. What Holmes produced was a monthly that paid little attention to blindness per se—"we know enough of that from experience," Helen had written in endorsing this approach—but whose contents came as close as possible to those of an inkprint magazine of general interest. His editorial formula consisted of fiction, non-fiction, and poetry reprinted from a wide variety of sources, a résumé of the major news of the month and, in almost every issue, a letter or article by a blind person describing how he or she had worked out the problem of earning a living, managing a household or achieving some other practical goal.

The *Ziegler*'s news résumés were a wondrous miscellany. The May 1937 issue, for example, contained a series of short paragraphs dealing with the passage of the Wagner Labor Act, easy divorces in Arkansas, the coronation of George VI of England, the status of the Loyalist war in Spain, sit-down strikes, a Suwannee River memorial to Stephen Foster, a fire in an Illinois church, the illness of Pope Pius, a new way of preventing colds, the drought in China, the accidental electrocution of a researcher in a cancer laboratory, the diary of two young men frozen to death in a snowstorm, an explosion in a Texas school house, the mysterious "curse" associated with those who had opened the tomb of Tutankhamen, the wedding of Franklin D. Roosevelt, Jr., to Ethel DuPont—a veritable smorgasbord of news tidbits interspersed with a few jokes to freshen the mental palate.

In this same issue the "Publisher's Chat" dealt with Holmes' idea for a "friendship league," a plan by which mobile people, sighted or blind, would act as big brothers or sisters to visit, read to, escort, and render other friendly services for homebound blind persons. It was one of the rare instances in which Holmes, who usually avoided the role of crusader, attempted to stir up social action. He subsequently presented the idea at an AAWB convention, carefully pointing out that he was not advocating a new national organization but hoped for spontaneous local groups. The convention took no official stand on his proposal, but the idea did materialize in a number of communities.

Holmes' determination not to get involved in controversial issues was manifest from the beginning. The *Ziegler*'s early years coincided with the period when the "war of the dots" was reaching fever pitch. Its editor took no sides. The magazine was issued in both braille and New York Point, the two type styles having approximately equal readership at the time. Although schools for the blind stopped teaching New York Point after 1917, the *Ziegler Magazine* continued to put out a Point edition until 1963 for the benefit of the ever smaller number of readers whose fingers knew only this style of tactile print. In 1934 a Moon type edition was added, in recognition that many elderly readers no longer had enough fingertip sensitivity to distinguish dot cells but could manage the larger and simpler linear outlines. It was kept going until 1965. As of the end of 1972 the *Ziegler Magazine* was appearing only in braille, but a recorded edition was under consideration.

Electa Matilda Ziegler lived long enough to see the 25th anniversary of the magazine in March 1932; she died six months later at the age of ninety-one. Well before her death she established a fund to ensure continued financing of the publication to which she had reluctantly given her name. The original plan had been to name it simply "Ziegler," but, as Holmes noted in the first issue: "To impress on the world that this great gift is from a woman, the friends of Mrs. Ziegler have prevailed on her to call it the *Matilda Ziegler Magazine for the Blind.*"

Although braille readers were steadily declining in number, the *Ziegler Magazine*, which at one time had a subscription list of more than 12,000, was still reaching 7,000 subscribers in 1972; its actual readership was estimated at more than twice that number since many copies were shared. In 65 years of existence, the magazine had only three editors: Holmes until 1946, Howard M. Liechty for the next 23 years and, beginning in 1967, Arthur S. Keller.

Walter G. Holmes died February 7, 1946, in a fall from the window of his New York hotel room. The mystery surrounding the circumstances of his death was never cleared up; there was nothing in the nature of the cheerful, even-tempered, eighty-four-year-old man to suggest suicide, and although he occasionally had spells of vertigo, an accidental fall through a window opened wide in New York's winter climate seemed unlikely. Some of his intimates were convinced, although police investigation failed to confirm, that the frail octogenarian had been pushed out of the window by a robber to whom he had trustingly opened his door. One reason for their belief was that Holmes, who normally carried a substantial amount of cash, had empty pockets when his body was found. If these suspicions were warranted, it was a sadly ironic end for a man whose life had been lived in the Lincolnesque tradition of malice toward none.

Howard M. Liechty, who had been Holmes' assistant since 1939, had a background in education and spent the first nine years of his professional career as a teacher in American supported schools in the Near East. The depression brought him back to the United States and to a job at the New York Institute for the Education of the Blind, where he acquired an interest in blindness that made him receptive to the offer of a post with the *Ziegler* when Holmes decided it was time to groom a successor.

Liechty came to play a unique role in the blindness communication network. Five years after he assumed editorship of the *Ziegler Magazine*, he accepted a second assignment as managing editor of the *Outlook for the Blind*. This dual editorship, which lasted 14 years, enabled him to bridge the interests of the rank and file of blind people who read the former, and of workers for the blind who depended on the latter as their professional journal. Liechty retired from the *Outlook* at the end of 1965 and from the *Ziegler* in mid-1967. The intervening year saw him honored by his professional colleagues with the AAWB's Alfred Allen Award for Outstanding Service to the Blind.

Arthur S. Keller, who took over from Liechty at the *Ziegler*, moved into the post from the sales managership of the Aids and Appliances Division of the American Foundation for the Blind. He had been a government administrator before joining the Foundation's technical research staff in 1959.

Holmes' two successors maintained his traditions, both in editorial approach and in intimate, service-minded relations with readers. Early in the magazine's existence, it began the practice of supplying readers with brailled watches, clocks, and other tangible aids at cost price; the braille watch service was subsequently turned over to the Foundation, but as of 1972 the *Ziegler Magazine* was continuing to offer subscribers a few bargain items, notably typewriters and alarm clocks.

The net worth of the $600,000 endowment fund left by Mrs. Ziegler for the upkeep of the magazine grew over the years to the point where its income greatly exceeded the magazine's needs. The trustees of the Ziegler Foundation adopted the policy of using this surplus income for other services to blind people. It made grants to the American Foundation for the Blind for such purposes as a survey of library services in 1955 and a comprehensive study of New York State's educational facilities for blind children in 1956. It also channeled funds for educational or research purposes to the Industrial Home for the Blind, the Perkins School, Recording for the Blind, and other direct service agencies. Among its larger beneficiaries were the Lavelle School for the Blind, a Catholic residential and day school in New York City, which used the money to add high school grades to its curriculum; and the YMCA in Darien, Connecticut, for construction of a swimming pool and initiation of a swimming program for blind children. As of the end of 1972 the Ziegler Foundation's assets aggregated some $4,750,000 and were producing an annual income of over $250,000, of which about $70,000 was spent for continuing publication of the magazine.

Until his death in 1957, William Ziegler, Jr., headed the foundation established by his mother; its 1972 officers included Matilda Ziegler's grandchildren, William Ziegler III and Helen Ziegler Steinkraus, the latter maintaining her father's interest in the American Foundation for the Blind by serving on its board of trustees.

The first thing contemporary visitors to the *Ziegler Magazine* offices see as they step off the elevator is a large oil portrait of an elderly gentleman dressed in a conservative business suit. Radiating from the kindly face is the avuncular benevolence that led thousands of blind people who had never seen Walter Holmes or touched his hand to think of him as a treasured friend.

A pair of portrait busts flank the elevator in the main entryway to the American Foundation for the Blind's building complex. One is of Helen Keller; the other is of Electa Matilda Ziegler, to whom a blind physician once wrote, "I would rather do what you are doing for the blind than be President of the United States or the King of England."

Neither oil portrait nor statue of Charles Francis Faulkner Campbell is on view in any public place, possibly because the volatile founder of the *Outlook for the Blind* never sat still long enough to pose. Unlike Walter Holmes, who held the same job for 39 years, Campbell occupied seven different positions between April 1907, when the first issue of the *Outlook* appeared, and May 1923, when he turned the magazine over to the American Foundation for the Blind. The *Outlook* was the one constant thread in his life during this period, and its editorial desk moved with him from Massachusetts to Pennsylvania to Ohio to Maryland to Michigan.

There was no Electa Matilda Ziegler in Campbell's life to underwrite 100 percent of the cost of an inkprint magazine devoted to furthering the interests of blind people. Producing the *Outlook* was not only an unpaid moonlighting operation, but one which involved the editor in a constant scramble for funds.

As different as were the situations and the personalities of the two men who began publishing ventures within a month of each other, they had one essential quality in common: an unshakable faith in the capacity of blind people to live dignified and useful lives. Both had been brought up in the presence of blindness —Holmes with his older brother, Campbell not only with a blind father but in daily association with the blind children who attended the school his father headed, England's Royal Normal College.

Charles ("Charlie" to almost everyone) Campbell was born February 19, 1876, to Francis (later Sir Francis) Campbell and his second wife, the former Sophia E. Faulkner, whom he married in 1875 soon after the death of his first wife. Sophia had been among her husband's fellow teachers at Perkins; she was one of the first Perkins staff members released by Samuel G. Howe to help get the Royal Normal College started. Their son spent the first 16 years of his life within the walls of the college, an enthusiastic participant in its many sports activities. In 1892 he was sent to the United States for his secondary school education. He lived with an aunt while attending high school in Concord, Mass., and then entered the Massachusetts Institute of Technology, from which he graduated in 1901.

Apparently Charlie was never tempted to diverge from the field his parents were engaged in. Planning to become a teacher of blind children, he spent the next year in Leipzig studying educational methods, particularly in music. Then he joined the faculty of his father's school. A year there, part of which he devoted to making a collection of lantern slides and filming a "cinematograph" showing blind people at work and at play, led him to conclude that he needed a more rapid road to achievement. Even were he to wait for his father's retirement, still a decade away, his older half brother, Guy, who had been on the school's staff for more than twenty years, had precedence. In the United States Charlie could serve as a missionary for his father's distinctive ideas on how blind children should be prepared for life.

There was also a more personal fascination tugging at him from across the Atlantic. During his stay in Boston he had fallen in love with the attractive and accomplished art teacher Wilhelmina Dranga. That her suitor was a few years her junior did not keep Wilhelmina from responding to the lithe and wiry young man whose deep-set dark eyes under bushy brows, firm chin, and neatly-trimmed military moustache surmounting a wide, mobile mouth conveyed an aura of optimistic self-assurance. They were married soon after his arrival in 1903.

Armed with his newest slides, Charlie began immediately to seek audiences for the "cinematograph and lantern lecture" he called "Seeing by Touch; the Practical Training of the Blind." Innate qualities of humor, enthusiasm, and genuine conviction, along with a natural flair for salesmanship, made him a winning public speaker who could evoke a response from every kind of group. One of his first lectures, given before the Twentieth Century Club and Women's Educational Industrial Union of Boston, yielded immediate results. It brought about a new organization, the Massachusetts Association for Promoting the Interests of the Adult Blind, and with it, a job for Charles Campbell as field agent and executive officer.

The newborn organization became the platform from which he exerted leverage to open new opportunities for blind adults. It was under its auspices that in 1904 he launched an "Experiment Station for the Trade Training of the Blind," one of the nation's first industrial training and placement ventures to look beyond the traditional "blind trades." So effective was it in demonstrating that blind workers could be guided to produce salable articles of practical and artistic merit, and that capable blind persons could even be placed in open industry that, when the Association's next goal was achieved—that of having Massachusetts establish a permanent state commission for the blind—one of the commission's first acts was to take over the training station and name Campbell as its superintendent.

Never at a loss for ideas, Charlie then proposed that the Massachusetts Association pioneer in a new direction by sponsoring a magazine to provide a continuous communication link among workers for the blind all over the country. He was keenly aware of the need for such a medium by dint of his personal role in activating the American Association of Workers for the Blind in 1905 and his acceptance of its secretaryship. If those engaged in serving blind people were ever to become a potent force, they needed a more regular mode of interchange than a biennial convention.

Thus was born the *Outlook for the Blind*, a quarterly whose purpose was clearly stated in the opening editorial of Volume I, Number 1, April 1907. It was to be "a forum for the free and open discussion of all topics connected with work for the blind. . . . We have no theories of our own to advocate, no projects to exploit. Our only desire is to be of service to the great cause of helpfulness to the blind."

It was not literally true that Campbell had no theories of his own to advocate. He harbored fervent convictions on many subjects, particularly on the educational methods used in schools for the blind, but with scrupulous self-discipline he kept the pages of the *Outlook* impartial, giving space to all sides of all questions. Considering that the periodical made its appearance during a period when the "war of the dots" was racing toward a climax, he succeeded admirably in maintaining an unbiased editorial stance. The *Outlook*, wrote the California educator Richard French, was an "active synthesizing agent, . . . a place for discussion away from the heat of personal conflict," with "the very impersonality of paper and ink becoming essential factors contributing to a final solution."

The first issue of the *Outlook* was a creditable effort for a man with no previous publishing experience; Charlie's sole helper was Wilhelmina, who designed the layout and placement of illustrations. Among the contents was a roundup of recent news, a report on the work of the newly formed New York City Lighthouse along with the text of the speech given by Helen Keller in its behalf, a historical survey by Dr. Robert C. Moon of the work of the Pennsylvania Home Teaching Society, an announcement of the forthcoming convention of the AAWB, and an extended survey of the principal European institutions for the blind.

Most of this material was reprinted from other sources, a pattern that was to characterize the *Outlook* throughout Campbell's editorship. In the absence of any sort of reportorial staff, the dearth of original material was unavoidable. But it was by no means a total liability. By culling the best and most relevant from a variety of sources, Campbell gave his readers an overview of information and opinion to which the average workers for the blind had scant access. He filled his pages with documents of lasting importance, sometimes stretching the lengthier ones over several issues. Nowhere else could the contemporary reader or the later historian find the full texts of the two public hearings before the New York City Board of Education in 1909, in which the arguments for braille and the arguments for New York Point were expounded and disputed. The *Outlook* devoted 46 pages in two successive issues to this material, and another page to reporting the Board's crucial decision in favor of braille.

Were it not for the *Outlook,* which published in installments the proceedings of the 1907 and 1909 conventions of the AAWB and held the type for later binding in pamphlet form, there might have been no record of what was said and done at those seminal conclaves. Nationwide distribution of the information was undoubtedly a factor in the doubling of attendance at each succeeding convention of the fledgling organization.

To the *Outlook,* too, belonged a share of the credit for the successful campaign against ophthalmia neonatorum and the formation of the National Society for the Prevention of Blindness to carry the fight against needless loss of sight to all parts of the country. Issue after issue carried bound-in reprints of documents put out by medical journals, hospitals, and social agencies stressing the need for state laws and community action to ensure the simple prophylactic measures that would halt the incidence of "babies' sore eyes."

To familiarize potential readers with the new magazine, copies were sent to every school and agency for the blind, to all members of both the AAIB and the AAWB, to the civic organizations Campbell had addressed during his wide-ranging lecture tours, and to everyone else he could think of who might be willing to invest 50 cents a year for a subscription. (By the fourth issue the price was raised to $1.) More substantial support came from a few sources—grants of $50 a year from each of the four largest schools for the blind, and donations from a few well-to-do private individuals. The first year's costs were fully underwritten by the Massachusetts Association for the Blind, and for the next few years the Massachusetts Association met the deficit between income and outgo in amounts averaging $1,000 to $1,200 annually. After nearly four years, a flyleaf printed in red ink was inserted in the Summer 1910 issue, warning readers that the Massachusetts Association was not committed to financing the magazine indefinitely and that unless other agencies found the publication sufficiently useful to support it through bulk subscriptions or annual grants, the *Outlook* would perish.

Campbell felt the magazine would have a firmer base, financially and in terms of prestige, if it had the official endorsement of the two professional associations in work for the blind. The question was taken up by the AAIB at its 1912 convention. Following a somewhat fence-straddling report by Olin Burritt, Eben Morford, then president of the AAWB, rose to declare: "You people here, the Instructors of the blind, have got first chance, and if you don't do it, the Workers will. The *Outlook for the Blind* has got to continue, it is going to continue, a way out is going to be found."

Both associations agreed to lend their names as sponsors, but it was not the "way out" because the sponsorship was purely nominal. The AAIB had little by way of funds, the AAWB had even less. However, some of the individual members did try to raise or contribute a little money. It was never enough; during the 16 years that the *Outlook* appeared under Campbell's editorship, its pages were punctuated with pleas for support laced with threats of collapse. In point of fact, Charlie never dreamed of giving up. The *Outlook* would continue, he wrote Edward Allen in 1912, "even if the magazine is reduced to a four-sheet pamphlet produced by some mimeographed process."

What genuinely distressed Campbell was the lack of realism in education of blind children that left the great majority of residential school graduates totally unprepared to earn a livelihood. "After Graduation—What?" was a key question he posed in publishing a survey of schools for the blind in the October 1908 issue. It was a question that went unanswered by most of the respondents. Few schools followed up their graduates, and fewer still were ready to face the implications of their failure to follow up. Campbell put his own thoughts on the subject in the letter to Allen: "The Outlook at least can bring forward some of the facts as shown by the pitiable condition of *hundreds of graduates* of schools for the blind throughout this country."

It is a foolhardy man who expects to be liked for forcing others to confront unpalatable truths. Charlie Campbell was no fool; he knew he was making enemies when he dwelt on the shortcomings of the schools. But, he told Allen, he and Wilhelmina had "long ago agreed that we would make any reasonable sacrifice in an effort to bring about a change."

Much the same motivation led Campbell to accept any job that seemed to hold the possibility of effecting progress. In 1910 the Pittsburgh Association for the Blind was organized and Campbell was offered its directorship. He moved himself, his family, and the *Outlook* to the steel center in June of that year, expecting to launch a comprehensive statewide program of help for blind adults. To emphasize the statewide compass, his first move was to get the agency's name changed to the Pennsylvania Association for the Blind. However, the realities of the assignment proved so much narrower than his expectations that when, a year or so later, he was offered the job of organizing the work of the newly established Ohio Commission for the Blind, he was off to Columbus. Approaching the new task with characteristic energy, he initiated so broad a spectrum of programs that the commission's budget tripled in five years.

Columbus was also the site of the Ohio State School for the Blind, of which Edward Van Cleve was superintendent. When Van Cleve left to become principal of the New York Institute, Campbell applied for the vacated position. He was appointed in 1916 and had barely started on what he regarded as a mission of educational rejuvenation when the United States entered World War I and he was irresistibly captivated by the plans for the Red Cross Institute at Evergreen. Leaving his wife, who held the title of assistant superintendent, to finish out the school semester, Campbell took off for Baltimore.

At this point Charlie's wife was not Wilhelmina Dranga Campbell but her younger sister, Mary. Wilhelmina had died of pneumonia in late 1911, leaving three small children ranging in age from three to seven, and their aunt had come to the bereaved household to care for them. She and Charlie were married the following year. "Aunt Mary" admirably filled her sister's shoes in all respects but one: marital love. That this second marriage was not a happy one may well have been a major factor in propelling Campbell to Evergreen in 1918, there to remain for more than three years until the Red Cross closed out its program, Evergreen was taken over by the Veterans Bureau, and Mary had secured a divorce.

Financially the *Outlook* had suffered even more than usual during the war years; it also suffered from the pressures on its editor during the immediate postwar period, when Campbell was putting it out from Baltimore simultaneously with the

Evergreen Review. To give the latter national distribution he bound the two publications together in a manner confusing to the reader and even more bewildering to later researchers. There must have been many moments when he was tempted to let the *Outlook* lapse, but he held on in the hope that the Red Cross Institute would become a permanent body and the *Outlook* its official organ. No sooner had this particular dream been extinguished than another was kindled—that some kind of national organization would soon materialize, although different in compass from what had been visualized for the Institute. By the time Campbell accepted a new job in Detroit, the American Foundation for the Blind was a corporate reality; from then on, it was merely a question of keeping the magazine going another year or so until the Foundation opened for business in 1923.

In 1922 Charles Campbell married his former secretary, Zelma Leath, and became executive director of the Detroit League for the Handicapped, a vocational agency whose program embraced workshops, home industries, and social services for all types of physically handicapped persons including, but not restricted to, the blind. As noted earlier, he had hoped to be head of Evergreen but was passed over for the top job. He had probably hoped, too, to be named to the staff of the Foundation, but this did not happen either. As responsible as anything else for these near misses was the gossip surrounding his marital situation. The feelings he had ruffled in entrenched circles of power by his persistent attempts to reform work for the blind now found a convenient outlet in whispered moral outrage. For public consumption, Campbell's forced retreat from work for the blind was attributed to his frequent job changes. Latimer put it as diplomatically as he could when he wrote: "Essentially a promoter, restless by nature and restive under restraint, this intrepid leader was swept on irresistibly by visions of things worth doing, so rapidly from one environment to another as to thwart the complete fulfilment of any one of his noble ambitions."

If Charlie was wounded by rejection, he did not show it. It was not in his nature to nurse resentments. Irrepressibly optimistic, he plunged into his new assignment with vigor and imagination. Helen Keller was to say of him that "wherever he went, he started things moving; he always knew what to do, and before the sun of his spirit obstacles melted away."

It must have been a particular source of satisfaction to Campbell that in Detroit, under the aegis of a generalized agency, he was able to accomplish a project he had repeatedly and unsuccessfully advocated during his two decades in work for the blind. This was a residential training program in domestic science for blind girls. With the support of the Detroit Junior League, late 1930 saw the opening of a rented house, the hiring of a housemother, and the movement into the residence of seven blind children, ranging in age from nine to thirteen and selected from pupils in Detroit's public school classes for the blind. They were to have a year of continuous residence in the League house, while attending public school classes and spending weekends and holidays at home so as not to lose contact with their families. The children included boys as well as girls; younger children would be trained in activities of daily living, while the older girls got actual homemaking experience.

Campbell saw this program as a bridge between residential school and day

488   *The Unseen Minority*

school education, one which skirted the pitfalls of institutionalization on the one hand and the inability of families to provide practical instruction on the other. The idea was sound, but the timing unfortunate. The depression soon choked off financial support for League activities, and in late 1933 Campbell moved over to the Detroit Community Fund's public education department. He died on December 28, 1935, a few weeks short of his sixtieth birthday, "worn out but not rusted out," as Edward Allen put it in the six-page obituary article which led off the Campbell memorial issue of the *Outlook* in February 1936.

Complicating the production of this tribute to the magazine's founder was an incident that was a revealing postscript to Charles Campbell's life. When Campbell left work for the blind and went to Detroit in 1922, he regarded the move as the opening of a clean new page. Whether it was his wish, or the wish of his bride, the impression was allowed to grow that Zelma was his second wife and not his third. So far as his new associates were concerned, "Aunt Mary" had never been anything but that. As soon as word reached Zelma Campbell that preparations were in progress for a memorial issue of the *Outlook*, she wrote Robert Irwin an anguished letter, pleading that any biography of her late husband omit reference to his marriage to Mary. At least, she begged, no such reference should appear in those copies of the magazine that went to subscribers in Detroit. She would be willing to meet the costs of printing an expurgated edition for circulation there.

This request landed Irwin in an awkward spot. The issue then in preparation was scheduled to contain two major biographical articles—one the lengthy obituary by Allen, and the other a piece by Latimer (actually a chapter from his forthcoming book of memoirs) which dealt with all seven members of the Campbell family who had been of significant service to blind people. By no means the least of these seven was Mary Dranga Campbell who, after her divorce from Charles, had gone on to build an independent, nationally known, and highly respected career in work for the blind.

Irwin had no trouble persuading Allen to incorporate the information about Charlie's marriage to Mary in a single paragraph that could be dropped out without breaking the article's continuity. The piece by Latimer, however, could not be handled so simply. Irwin wrote explaining the situation and asking if, as a last favor to Charlie, Latimer would be willing to condense his article to deal "only with the Campbells who had passed on": Sir Francis and his second wife; his elder son, Guy, who had succeeded him as head of the Royal Normal College; Charlie; and Charlie's first wife, Wilhelmina. The two survivors to be omitted would be Mary and Guy's wife, Louie Bealby Campbell, who had held the principalship of the college for five years after her husband's death.

Latimer did not take kindly to the proposition, answering that he preferred to withdraw his article altogether. Now it was Irwin's turn to demur. He and Evelyn McKay, who was then editing the *Outlook*, devised another solution. The Latimer piece was printed in the memorial issue as an unpaged insert, not listed in the table of contents and slipped out of the expurgated copies sent to Detroit. Latimer was not told of this in advance; by the time he saw the issue, it was too late to do anything except send a dignified protest to Irwin, who responded with a not-quite-truthful explanation:

The photographs in your article needed to go on smooth paper, and as we needed additional reprints of it, it was decided to run the entire article on shiny paper and put it in the center of the *Outlook*. . . . It was for the sake of economy in making additional reprints that the pages were not numbered.

That same day he wrote Charlie's son, Francis, who had been an uncomfortable intermediary in the conspiracy of kindness: "I hope I never again get mixed up between two women in a similar situation."

It was the only time in the *Outlook*'s history that its pages were used in any but the most straightforward way, and it is difficult to think of anyone other than Charles Campbell for whose sake any kind of deception, however well meant, would have been entertained for a moment.

Survivorship was the principal characteristic of the periodical turned over to the Foundation early in 1923. The personal and professional stresses which preoccupied Campbell's last years of editorship were reflected in the magazine's paucity of content and irregularity of appearance. Some of the final issues held little more than the *Evergreen Review* sandwiched between a few pages of scattered news notes.

The fledgling Foundation was not much better prepared to do a professional job of magazine production. The first issue under its auspices appeared in May 1923 as Number 1 of Volume 17. It employed a larger type face and used illustrations more lavishly than Campbell had been able to afford, but it was amateurishly written and edited. It was not until Charles Hayes, for whom putting out the magazine was only one of many responsibilities, hired a former newspaperwoman as assistant that the *Outlook* began to assume distinctive shape and tone. These differed noticeably from the past. Campbell's *Outlook* had perforce been a journal of news and record, its target audience those professionally engaged in work for the blind. The Foundation saw the periodical as a medium for reaching beyond this limited circle; its purpose, the agency's first annual report declared, should be broadened to include material "which would also be of interest to friends of the Blind who have no professional connection with the work."

Following this guideline, Hayes used the magazine as a tool in the Foundation's campaign of public education, emphasizing themes of hope and encouragement. He filled its pages with success stories about blind people making good, not merely in such traditional professions as law and music but in widely varied occupations: ice and coal delivery, poultry raising, manufacture of bird houses, invention, journalism, advertising, the performing arts. So carried away was he by this accent on the affirmative, he even reported the "success story of a blind dog" which had been the subject of a feature article in a popular magazine.

Distribution of the *Outlook* during these years reflected its expanded purpose. Campbell had never succeeded in lifting the paid circulation to more than 1,000, although his press run went to a few hundred extra copies for promotional use. By 1927 the print order had risen to 9,000, the subscription list having been swelled by inclusion of the magazine as a perquisite of a $10 membership in the Foundation. The need to economize during the depression years led to discontinuance of this practice, and circulation never again came close to the 9,000 figure. Even during the dozen or so years, beginning in the early Fifties, when a subscription at a nominal fee was included in the membership dues of, first, the AAWB and later the AAIB as well, the total paid circulation never went much beyond 4,000. As of 1972, when these arrangements were no longer in force, the paid list for the inkprint edition was just over 3,000. A braille edition, initiated in 1931, and a recorded edition, begun in 1959, added fewer than 1,000 subscribers to the total.

Once the *Outlook* had dropped its Foundation membership subscription category, it altered its focus to concentrate on the bread-and-butter concerns of service to blind people. When it began publication of the *Teachers Forum* in 1928, the Foundation had discovered that there was a genuine hunger for substantive professional material among educators. A comparable hunger was becoming manifest in other phases of work for the blind and the *Outlook* now set out to satisfy it. In so doing it could hardly overlook the fact that the activities of the Foundation itself were among the most fertile breeding grounds of professional progress. Considerable space was given to reporting the Foundation-sponsored conferences, workshops, legislative initiatives, books and reports on subjects of professional concern.

During World War II the *Outlook* added a monthly feature, "News and Views of the AAWB." Since travel restrictions precluded the holding of conventions, it was useful to have a major channel for communication with the scattered members of the organization. Once the war was ended, *News and Views* became AAWB's independently issued house organ.

Editorial policy was one of the matters which came under scrutiny when M. Robert Barnett became the Foundation's director. As part of his strategy of cultivating teamwork with the two professional associations, both the AAIB and the AAWB were asked to appoint official correspondents for the magazine. A group of advisors summoned to a conference on editorial policy recommended that news of Foundation activities be deemphasized and more space be devoted to articles by practitioners with ideas or experiences to share.

To underscore the changed direction, the word "New" was added to the magazine's title as of 1951 and a sprightlier format was introduced under the aegis of a new editor who, in the January 1952 issue, described his policy:

> The *New Outlook for the Blind* shall be a vehicle for the dissemination of information and knowledge, for the free expression of findings and experiences, of valid theories identified as such, and of opinions, all within the limitations of courtesy and good taste, high professional standards, and respect for other opinions.

Repeated invitations were issued over the years for articles that fit into this formula, but the field of work for the blind was slow to accept the thought that the magazine was something more than a Foundation house organ. Surgical removal of all Foundation news was recommended by the Service Advisory Committee in 1965 and a new quarterly vehicle for the excised material, the *AFB Newsletter*, was launched the following year, leaving to the *New Outlook* the single role of professional journal. A completely revised format emphasized the change.

The austerely professional *New Outlook* of 1972 was no longer the all-purpose medium Charles Campbell had envisioned 65 years earlier, and even less the cheerful messenger of high hopes and glad tidings that it became under Charles Hayes. Most of its contents were of a technical nature, often research-oriented and couched in the kind of esoteric professionalese that rejoices the heart of the doctoral candidate but glazes the eye of the general reader. Because it devoted minimum space to news per se, it no longer served as a running chronicle of changes in professional personnel, program developments in individual agencies, retirements and deaths of old-timers. News of legislation was now consolidated in the Foundation's quarterly *Washington Report.* Major papers given at professional conventions could be found in proceedings or collections of selected papers published by the respective organizations. The subject matter formerly covered by a "Research in Review" column was issued in greatly expanded form in the Foundation's *Research Bulletin* series. Those in search of news of people in the field had to turn to the house organs of the professional associations and their subgroups.

Such fragmentation was not unique; the same splintering characterized communications in other fields of human service in which the growth of professionalism produced ever-narrower specialization.

One reason, perhaps, why the *Matilda Ziegler Magazine for the Blind* remained unaltered in content, format, and purpose during the same 65 years that the *Outlook* underwent repeated changes was that the *Ziegler* had long continuity of editorship. Such was not the case with the *Outlook.*

Following the first 16 years under Campbell, the editor was Charles B. Hayes from 1923 until his death in 1936. As of April 1931 the name of Evelyn C. McKay appeared in the masthead as associate editor. She kept this title even during the five years following Hayes' death, when she was in sole charge. At the end of 1941, when the *Outlook* absorbed the *Teachers Forum,* the *Forum's* editor, P. C. Potts, also became an associate editor of the merged publication. Simultaneously there appeared a managing editor, Lucille (Lucy) Goldthwaite, a retired librarian who had long edited the *Braille Book Review.* It was during her brief editorship (she resigned in June 1944) that the magazine became a monthly, appearing ten times a year (it wasn't published during July and August), a schedule maintained ever since. Originally a quarterly, it had been stepped up to five issues a year in 1933.

Evelyn McKay's name disappeared from the masthead with the issue of May 1943; she was replaced by Enid Griffis, formerly a member of the fund-raising staff, who was given the official title of associate editor in tandem with Potts. The two carried on without benefit of a top editor until November 1946 when Miss Griffis left and Warren Bledsoe was named editor. His tenure was the shortest on record; after putting out nine issues he took a leave of absence to work with the Veterans Administration in rehabilitation of the war-blinded and then decided to stay on in federal service. Potts was left alone to put out the magazine until October 1951 when Howard M. Liechty, already managing editor of the *Ziegler Magazine,* was given the same title for what had by then been christened the *New Outlook.* Liechty stayed on until his retirement in 1965; at the beginning of the following year the managing editorship was transferred to Patricia Scherf Smith, who was continuing in the post as of 1972.

As of February 1955, the name of M. Robert Barnett began to appear in the masthead as editor-in-chief. It was more than a titular honor; Barnett reviewed all the magazine's contents and wrote many of its editorials, in addition to contributing his signed column of personal opinion, "Hindsight," from October 1956 to January 1964.

Change of editorship was often accompanied by change of format. Campbell's *Outlook* was booksize (6×9 inches); its cover was a typographical arrangement featuring a list of the issue's major contents. This remained the basic design until the Foundation became publisher. For the next dozen years the cover of the *Outlook* was a four-color illustration, "Lifting the Veil of Darkness," which depicted an angelic-faced woman unshrouding the head of a bare-throated young man, his mouth open in eager anticipation of the pile of books on the table before him. Contributed by Percy Van Eman Ivory, a pupil of the famous illustrator Howard Pyle, the painting was typical of the art nouveau style of magazine and calendar illustrations of the period.

Discontinuing inspirational content in favor of professional material made this sentimental cover inappropriate, so the magazine reverted to a starkly simple typographic arrangement in 1935. In 1951, along with the change in title to *New Outlook,* the cover typography was revised. Further changes were made in 1955, but the most drastic format alteration came in January 1964 when the page size was enlarged to 8½ × 11 inches. Three years later saw the introduction of an entirely new look, inside and out, featuring abstract two-color cover designs and a different, more modern style of page layout, marked by liberal use of white space.

The subscription fee also underwent change over the years. Campbell's price of $1 a year remained in effect until 1920, when it went up to $1.50. When the Foundation took over three years later it raised the rate to $2 and kept it at that level for more than thirty years. In May 1956 the price went to $3, where it remained until the beginning of 1968. At that point, following a cost analysis which showed that publication of the inkprint edition was costing the Foundation more than $10 per subscription, a total price structure revision was introduced. The braille edition had long been offered at $1.50 a year, the recorded edition at $5. Under the new structure, all three editions were priced at $6 each. These rates did not make it possible to break even on costs, but they did effect a lowering of the annual subsidy.

Advertising income, which had been important in balancing Campbell's books, was inconsequential to the Foundation when it took over; an early decision was to eliminate the kind of ads that had filled as many as fifty pages of an issue in Campbell's time. These were largely from the Boston area and offered men's furnishings, ostrich feathers, bakery products, undertaking and embalming, Turkish baths, dry-cleaning, and other local goods and services. There was also a sprinkling of patent medicine ads: "Camphorated Saponaceous Dentifrice"; "Geneva Water" for stomach, liver, and kidney troubles; "Dr. Green's Nervura"; and the like. Campbell had nothing to do with soliciting the ads; they were totally within the province of C. Bradford Mudge, a blind Bostonian who earned a living from commissions on the advertising he secured for the *Outlook,* and possibly for other periodicals as well. No doubt Campbell knew the advertisers were making more of a philanthropic gesture than an investment in merchandising, but he may well have rationalized that the ends—a source of livelihood for a blind man and a needed financial prop for the magazine—justified the means.

The 1923 resolve of the Foundation executive committee that "advertising be limited to that specifically helpful to the blind" was still in effect as of 1972.

Charles Campbell left one other enduring legacy to work for the blind: the useful compendium that eventually became the biennial *Directory of Agencies Serving the Visually Handicapped in the United States.* Its 18th edition was being readied for publication at the end of 1972. The directory originally came into being because no sooner had Campbell begun publishing the *Outlook* than he was besieged with questions about facilities for blind people. His first editorial surveys, printed in the form of fold-out tables, were the fruits of fact-finding questionnaires he sent out in 1908. "Industrial Establishments for the Blind in the United States," which appeared in the July 1908 issue, listed data on 16 workshops in 12 states: date of founding, amount of floor space, kinds of goods made, annual sales, number of blind wage earners, average weekly wage, whether or not a boarding home was maintained for the workers, etc. The next issue saw a comparable table on schools for the blind, detailing the number of students and teachers, subjects taught, reading system or systems used, library contents, physical training facilities, and follow up programs in respect to graduates.

The enthusiasm with which this hitherto unavailable information was received led to the idea of compiling a comprehensive directory. In 1916 Charles and Mary Campbell published *Institutions for the Blind in America*, with plans for periodic updating, but complications in their personal and professional lives kept the latter idea from materializing.

Production of an updated directory was one of the early goals the Foundation set for itself. It came off the press in 1926. The second edition was issued in 1931 and the third in 1938. A biennial publication schedule was subsequently adopted and maintained.

The directory was the first book of substance published under the Foundation imprint. Two others appeared in a 1929 publication list—*The Blind Child and His Reading* by Kathryn Maxfield, and *Blind Relief Laws—Their Theory and Practice* by Robert Irwin and Evelyn McKay—along with seven staff-written monographs on aspects of education, vocations, and legislation.

A major publishing venture was the *Proceedings of the World Conference on Work for the Blind*, which appeared in 1932. That same year saw publication by the Foundation of its first book written by a non-staff member, *From Homer to Helen Keller—a Social and Educational Study of the Blind* by Richard S. French, principal of the California School for the Blind. Five years later came H. Randolph Latimer's memoirs, *The Conquest of Blindness*.

What of the Blind?, a symposium by a score of authors on various aspects of blindness and services for blind people, appeared in 1938; a supplementary volume was issued in 1941. Both were edited by Helga Lende, who during the same period compiled *Books About the Blind*, an annotated bibliographical guide published in 1940 under a grant from the Carnegie Corporation. A revised and updated edition, issued in 1953, listed 4,200 entries, many in the form of unpublished masters' and doctoral theses in the Foundation library collection.

As work for the blind moved toward greater professionalization, publications grew increasingly technical in nature. Most of the material issued during the Fifties consisted of conference proceedings or staff-edited material drawn from them. Beginning near the end of that decade and continuing into the Seventies, an increasing number of research studies dotted the publication list. As of 1972, a total of 26 volumes in the research series had been issued. Other books and monographs in the catalog of 70 Foundation publications then in print dealt with psychological studies, education, multihandicapped children, rehabilitation problems, attitudes among and toward blind persons, vocations, and social work services.

Listed in the same catalog were more than forty pamphlets and fliers available free of charge as public education materials. They covered a wide range of subject matter: *Facts About Blindness, Blindness and Diabetes, Dog Guides for the Blind,* brief biographies of Louis Braille and Helen Keller, *Careers in Work for the Blind, Why Not Hire a Blind Person?, Toilet Habits, Suggestions for Training a Blind Child.*

These materials, along with the six periodicals then being issued under Foundation editorship *(New Outlook for the Blind, AFB Newsletter, Washington Report, Research Bulletin, Talking Book Topics, Braille Book Review)* were produced by the agency's information department with a staff of 14 professionals. Of all Foundation units, this one had seen the largest proportional growth in the 50 years since the entire information staff consisted of Charles Hayes (who also doubled as director of field services) and a single assistant. Incorporated in the 1972 information department were the public education division, the publications division, the records center, and the Migel Memorial Library.

A circulating reference library that would make material on blindness readily available to professional workers had been one of Robert Irwin's early priorities. During his graduate years at Harvard, he had made extensive use of the "blind-iana" collection at Perkins. However, few people were in a position to travel to Massachusetts for research purposes; what was needed was a system that could bring books to people. As early as 1925 Irwin voiced the hope that the Foundation could be instrumental in this. The following year he succeeded in persuading the trustees to appropriate $1,000 to begin a book collection, and by 1928 the Foundation was able to report that its library already comprised 800 bound volumes plus a sizable number of pamphlets, records, and manuscripts.

There were some antiquarian prizes in this early collection; the oldest was a two-part work published in London in 1684, Richard Standfast's *The Blind Man's Meditations* and *A Dialogue Between a Blind Man and Death.* Of less interest to the bibliophile, but far more useful for practitioners, were the materials donated by people like Ambrose Shotwell, who forwarded his 50-year collection of pamphlets, reports, and periodicals on work for the blind. Numerous other individuals and agencies also responded to the plea that they clear out dusty shelves and attic boxes and donate their contents to the new repository. The pioneer schools and agencies helped by supplying bound sets of their annual reports as well as quantities of duplicate materials from their own library collections.

So rapidly did the collection grow that a full-time librarian was needed, and in March 1929 Irwin hired Helga Lende, a recent graduate of what later became the Columbia University School of Library Science. She was a real find—a Norwegian, with a degree from the University of Oslo, who had a reading knowledge of German, French, and Spanish in addition to the Scandinavian languages. But, as Irwin confided in a private letter to Latimer, dated October 22, 1929, her English was "not all that could be desired." Furthermore, "Mr. Migel was not present at the meeting at which Miss Lende was elected and he has never quite approved of her." It would be up to those trustees who, as professionals, recognized the importance of a library, "to save Miss Lende's salary from elimination from the budget."

Latimer cooperated, Migel relented, and Miss Lende's English improved to the point where she became one of the Foundation's most prolific writers and editors as well as its librarian. In 1963 she savored the delicate irony of seeing the handsome new Migel Memorial Library wing dedicated in honor of the man who had perceived so little use for a library in the first place.

By the time Helga Lende retired in 1964, the Foundation library held close to 25,000 items in many languages: books and periodicals about blindness and work for the blind, books by or about blind persons, novels featuring blind characters, sociological and psychological works bearing on aspects of blindness. As of 1972 the collection stood at over 30,000.

The circulating function of the library, which enabled teachers, students, and researchers all over the country to borrow books by mail, was soon enlarged to include preparation of reading lists on specific subjects. As of 1972 some fifty different reading lists were available and readers' advisory services, rendered by the three professional librarians on staff, were averaging 3,000 requests a year.

In the late Thirties command of the publications division also fell to Miss Lende, when, following the death of Charles Hayes, stopgap measures were employed to cover his varied responsibilities. It was under her direction that, in 1951, a publications series was begun in nine categories which saw 56 titles issued—largely monographs and edited proceedings on aspects of legislation, vocational problems, preschool services, education, community planning, technical and social research. These were in addition to some major books published during the Fifties and early Sixties: Louis Cholden's *A Psychiatrist Works with Blindness*, a revised and expanded edition of Thomas Cutsforth's *The Blind in School and Society*, and Robert Irwin's *As I Saw It*.

One book that eluded publication despite years of effort was a biography of Sir Francis Campbell. Irwin, who had his heart set on having such a book written under Foundation sponsorship, opened negotiations with Edward Allen in the early Thirties, but nothing came of them. Even earlier, Charles Campbell had urged his mother to do the job, but Lady Campbell was diffident about her writing ability. Charlie himself should probably have done it, but he, too, had reservations about his literary skill.

After Charlie's death, his son Francis sent the Foundation for safekeeping a 100-lb. box of correspondence, reports, photographs, and other data—more than 10,000 items in all—pertaining to his grandparents. Charlie had accumulated these materials for use by a future biographer. The documents were stored until Irwin's retirement, when he took them to Puget Sound, no doubt planning to use them in the history he was compiling. Somehow he failed to identify the box as being on loan from the Foundation, with the result that, on his death, it was considered part of his estate. Irwin's sister, Mrs. Edna Irwin Davis, decided to donate the Campbell papers to the Library of Congress, where they have remained on file in the Manuscript Division since 1953, awaiting the creative touch of a writer who could do justice to the man who, his son said, "absolutely did not know the meaning of the word 'impossible.' "

The 1963 internal reorganization of the Foundation consolidated the publications division, the library, the public education division, the legislative office, and the central files into a single information department headed by Helga Lende until her retirement the following year. This administrative structure was still in effect as of 1972 except for the legislative unit, which had been moved to the office of the executive director.

The central files were included in this setup in recognition of their archival value. The classification and organization of the files had begun a dozen years earlier in what proved to be a fitting coda to the notable career of Mary Dranga Campbell. She was seventy-five years old when she took on the assignment of sorting, screening, and putting in order the thousands upon thousands of yellowed letters and documents stored in the basements and attics of the Foundation buildings. Undismayed by the accumulated grime of more than three decades, and drawing on her early library training as well as on a half-century of intimate knowledge of work for the blind, she salvaged vast quantities of source material bearing on past projects, legislative activities, and research efforts. She completed the task in three years and lived another three in retirement before death claimed her in 1957.

Taken all in all, Mary Dranga Campbell's contributions to work for the blind were not unworthy of either the man she had once married or the man who was briefly her father-in-law. Even before she became Charles Campbell's wife, she had begun to roll up a respectable professional record. After taking library training at Stanford University, she spent six years as cataloguer of the Indiana University Library, then entered the Chicago School of Civics and Philanthropy (later called the School of Social Service Administration of the University of Chicago) and did some research in eugenics as part of her field training. During her marriage to her widowed brother-in-law she was assistant editor of the *Outlook* and assistant superintendent of the Ohio School for the Blind. At the end of World War I, when her marriage dissolved, she spent three years abroad in charge of child welfare work in Serbia and another three years lecturing in the United States on the social welfare problems of the battered Balkan states.

In 1926, she came back to work for the blind, beginning as executive director of the newly created Council for the Blind in the Pennsylvania Department of Welfare. Three years later she was named executive secretary of the Missouri Commission for the Blind; after three years there, she became director of work for the handicapped in the Brooklyn Bureau of Charities. Toward the end of 1934 she resigned to take on what proved to be her longest job, as head of the social service division of the Seeing Eye. There she remained for 11 years, until retirement shortly before her seventieth birthday.

A photograph taken when she completed her Foundation assignment in 1954 projected much the same image as one that had appeared in the *Outlook* 40 years earlier: a substantially built woman whose square-cut features, firm chin, and piercing eyes bespoke intelligence, determination, and large reserves of inner strength. "She was not an easy person," was the comment of a man who knew her in her prime. "She could be extremely critical of others, often to the point of intolerance, but no one could question her dedication or the high standards of discipline and duty she set for herself." Age softened her—those who came to know her in later years commented on a graciousness of manner and a youthful viewpoint that constantly enlarged the circle of people who fondly addressed this indomitable descendant of the Vikings as "Aunt Mary." Her professional accomplishments were twice recognized by her colleagues, once in 1950 when the AAWB gave her its Shotwell Award, and again in 1955 when the Foundation honored her with the Migel Medal.

The spadework done on the Foundation files served as the nucleus for the present-day records center, whose scope was enlarged when it became the repository for Helen Keller's private papers following her death on June 1, 1968. Bequeathed under Helen's will, which also made the Foundation residuary legatee of her literary rights and royalties, the collection consisted initially of some 32,000 items of private correspondence, manuscript texts, notes, legal documents, photographs, and press clippings, plus 36,000 pieces of fan mail. Cataloging of the Keller collection and its preservation was assigned to Marguerite Levine, supervisor of the records center. In 1972 an acquisition program was begun to fill gaps in the collection, notably those created when Helen's Connecticut home was destroyed by fire in 1946. Plans were also under way for microfilming the papers.

Important as it was to build communication and information resources that could strengthen services for blind people, it was at least as essential to enhance public understanding of those services and what they accomplished. The "weeks for the blind" conducted in the Twenties were early measures toward this end; so were the well-advertised public appearances of Helen Keller. But because so many of these efforts, whether national or local, were tied to appeals for contributions or legislative benefits, they tended to be counterproductive in their net effect on public opinion. Placement agents seeking industrial work opportunities for blind people repeatedly found employers readier to give checks than jobs.

The paradoxical effects of publicizing the needs of blind people had an impact on the beneficiaries as well. Hector Chevigny, who had strong feelings on the subject, declared that pity "is the luxury of the giver and the destroyer of the recipient." No one disagreed, nor was there any lack of insight into causes. Repeated studies pinpointed the origins of the stereotypes and the hidden hostilities aroused by the very thought of blindness. Understanding the problem, however, was only the first small step toward solving it.

Public relations had just begun to emerge as a professional discipline with its

own set of ethics and structured procedures when, in the early Twenties, the
Foundation approached the task of influencing public opinion. For the first two
decades or so, the public relations function was regarded primarily as a handmaiden
to fund-raising. In the mid-Thirties, in one of her periodic bursts of irritation at the
Foundation, Helen Keller wrote Walter Holmes:

> I doubt if any organization in America of the importance of the Foundation
> has such an ineffective, uninspired publicity department. Its endeavors are
> positively pitiful, and have the effect of confusing the public. It seems very
> strange that with all the able business people connected with our work
> nobody should point out that stupidity and cheapness usually go hand in hand
> . . . publicity of a high order demands brains, experience and ingenuity, and
> all these cost money.

Helen was reacting, in part, to the Foundation's refusal to go along with her and
her teacher's scheme for manufacturing and merchandising a "Helen Keller Doll."
As envisaged by Helen, the doll would have had a tiny booklet attached to its arm,

> telling the wonderful Fairy Tale of how the Lady with the Golden Key had
> unlocked the dungeon of King Dark, released the little deaf-blind Princess
> and led her forth into the beauty and joy of the sun-warm world. Then there
> was to be a tender appeal to the children of the nation to help the grown-up
> Helen Keller to open all doors and shuttered windows in the lives of blind
> people everywhere. . . .

When the Foundation rejected the idea as impracticable, Helen and Anne considered carrying it out as a private money-making effort but were persuaded to
abandon it as undignified commercialism.

The Foundation was probably right about the questionable taste of the doll
proposition, but Helen was right, too, in her criticism of the Foundation's public
education efforts at the time. Publicity specialists were hired for temporary periods
(three or six months) and then released, a system which saved money but precluded continuity of planning. A more stable arrangement was effected in the
Forties, when a full-time man was employed, but it was not until late 1952, with
the advent of Gregor Ziemer, that a sustained public education effort got under
way.

In April of that year Winthrop K. Howe, Jr., a blind man from Rochester, New
York, who was a Foundation trustee and a member of the New York State
Commission for the Blind, raised the issue of improving public education at an
executive committee meeting. "All members present generally agreed that the
need was evident but that the method for meeting it was not clear," the minutes of
the meeting reported. Actually, the method was simple enough: hire a competent
person, supply him with an adequate budget, and give him his head in exploring
avenues of influence.

Ziemer filled the bill. He had behind him a long and colorful career as author,
educator, foreign correspondent, and lecturer. Energetic, imaginative, and su-
premely self-confident, he was not in the least fazed by the scope of his assignment:

"correcting and readjusting the misunderstanding of blindness in the mind of the sighted world." In the dozen years he spent as director of public education before retiring in 1964, he opened numerous new channels of communication in campaigns which twice won top awards from the American Public Relations Association. Under his direction there emerged a steady stream of press kits, spot announcements, taped radio and TV programs, and a variety of other informational materials for use by schools, service clubs, police departments, and many other outlets.

Aware that attitudes are more apt to be shaped indirectly than through outright propaganda, Ziemer prepared and distributed to the media, to writers and lecturers and other opinion molders, a list of "32 misconceptions about blindness." Sample items:

> Blind people can eat without having to be fed.... Blind people don't feel people's faces to get acquainted with them.... Not all blind people can read braille.... Blind people are not all musical geniuses.... They can't foretell the future any more than any one of us.... Not all blind people become paragons of patience and resignation when they become blind.

Another insight was that constructive national educational campaigns could readily be undermined by poorly conducted local efforts. Much of the Foundation-produced material was therefore sent out to agencies for the blind for local adaptation and distribution. Supplying content was only half the job; the other half was to equip these agencies, few of which had public relations staffs, with knowledge of basic techniques. In 1957 the Foundation held the first of seven annual public relations workshops for local agencies. Following Ziemer's retirement, the idea lapsed for several years, but it was partially revived in 1971 when members of the Foundation's information staff addressed AAWB group sessions concerned with public relations.

During Ziemer's tenure an elaborate new dual format emerged for the Foundation's annual report. One version, with extensive text and pictures, was designed for the professional audience and major contributors; a shorter and more modest version keyed to fund-raising went to 250,000 annual contributors. After four years a simpler, less expensive, single edition served both audiences, but a hallmark of every Ziemer-produced annual report was that even the briefest managed to include a photograph of him. The backstage role customarily played by public relations people was one he airily rejected.

The Foundation's director of information in 1972 was Patricia Scherf Smith, who had joined the staff in 1965 as director of the publications division following ten years of experience as an editor and public relations specialist in the medical and hospital field. Under Mrs. Smith, who became head of the information department in 1968, a vigorous policy of public education was resumed, with special emphasis on the audio-visual field.

That decades of high-level effort had yet to succeed in shaping favorable public opinion was emphasized in 1971 when the Foundation's 50th anniversary symposium devoted major sessions to the subject of "Attitudes toward Blindness."

These became the springboard for renewed attempts "to find rational ways of dealing with an irrational problem." The following year saw the holding of six regional meetings on attitudes, at some of which participants were blindfolded at luncheon so they could experience sightlessness for themselves. The goal of these and comparable projects was to create realistic knowledge that could loosen, and eventually replace, age-old prejudices born of ignorance.

27

The Road Ahead

As it was a hundred years ago, a thousand years ago, five thousand years ago, the key that will unlock the final gate to freedom for blind people lies not within their own grasp but in the hands of the rest of society.

The twentieth century has seen giant strides toward integration in education, in the economic sphere, in the social and communal aspects of life. Yet pockets of prejudice linger. The frontal attack—exhorting the public to abandon its fears and misconceptions—has thus far made little headway. Far more has been accomplished by subtler, if slower, forms of persuasion: by the ever more common spectacle of blind people matter-of-factly going to school or working at jobs, traveling unescorted on the streets and public conveyances, maintaining households, participating with neighbors in social and recreational pursuits, fulfilling their roles as citizens in communal and political movements.

The thought, persistence, and devotion—not to mention the uncounted millions of dollars—invested in achieving such gains have been documented in preceding chapters. As the last quarter of the twentieth century approaches, the field of work for the blind, evaluating its unfinished business and sorting its priorities, ponders a series of urgent questions. How are these gains to be safeguarded? Where do they need to be shored up? In what directions should new advances be attempted?

Indispensable to any kind of planning is the need to know the dimensions of the overall blindness problem. Estimates of the visually handicapped population in the United States that range from under 500,000, according to some authorities, to as many as 1,700,000, hardly constitute a sound base for realistic deployment of resources. More than 40 years of effort to arrive at a uniform definition of blindness which would take into account functional factors other than mere visual acuity, of attempts to develop uniform diagnostic techniques and to secure nationwide regulations for compulsory reporting of visual impairment, have not brought satisfactory results. The job remains to be done.

Allied with the demographic dilemma is the need to know and do more about the causes of blindness and the measures that can prevent or mitigate them. Many people continue to suffer needlessly from visual limitations that can be overcome, partially or even totally, through medical intervention or through proper prescription and use of low-vision aids. This is true even in cases where loss of vision is caused by the degenerative diseases of advancing age. New impetus is needed for extending medical and low-vision services to all population groups, for training professional and paraprofessional practitioners in these services, for expanding the operations of existing low-vision clinics and establishing new ones, for publicizing their availability and encouraging use of their facilities.

Renewed vigilance is needed, too, to head off future epidemics of blindness among children. Public health authorities are currently expressing concern over the failure of many low-income families to observe infant inoculation precautions. Reliable vaccines to shield children from measles, polio, rubella, scarlet fever, and other disabling diseases are readily available, but alarming numbers of young parents are neglecting to provide their infants with these protections. The rising incidence of venereal disease among all groups in the population is another potential cause of blindness that cannot be ignored.

As of 1972 the children severely damaged by the rubella epidemic of the mid-Sixties had reached school age. For at least the next decade or two, they will constitute a continuing challenge. Some will need extended, perhaps lifelong, custodial care. For others, existing programs of education, rehabilitation, and vocational preparation are largely inadequate. New thinking, new resources, and new techniques will have to be created. It is an open question (but one not yet universally faced) whether the residential schools for the blind will gradually phase out their traditional programs of academic and vocational education and serve exclusively as treatment centers for children with additional impairments.

Fresh thinking is also needed for the benefit of children whose sole impairment is blindness. Although six out of ten are already being educated in the public schools, and the proportion seems likely to increase, the quality of instruction is uneven and, in many places, leaves much to be desired. Too many teachers, never indoctrinated in how to cope with the special needs of blind pupils, handle the problem ineptly, showing overindulgence at one extreme or neglect at the other. Intensified efforts to achieve more enlightened teacher preparation remain high on the priority list. Equally urgent is the need for a new surge in parent guidance so that preschool blind children will be more adequately prepared for functioning in educational programs.

Even in many of the better public schools, blind students are not getting the benefits of a rounded education when they are automatically excluded from physical education classes, shop work, or home economics courses. Questions are beginning to be raised in educational circles about resource rooms. Is over-reliance on them becoming an expedient way of ghettoizing blind children?

More serious yet is the paucity of realistic vocational preparation and guidance services for teenagers. In 1972 the Foundation established a Task Force on Career Education to seek new solutions, both in the school systems and in the state vocational rehabilitation agencies, whose sometimes stultified thinking about career options for blind persons constricts the range of guidance and placement services offered young people. Questions are being raised about the unusually high proportion of visually handicapped youth enrolled in college programs. Does this represent sound planning for future careers, or is it merely a postponement of reality?

The basic thrust of vocational rehabilitation is also in need of reshaping. The product of wartime conditions, when the nation's consciousness was focused on manpower needs, the amended Vocational Rehabilitation Act of 1943 has been administered to accentuate the vocational rather than the rehabilitative aspect of its mandate. Today, thirty years later, technology has altered the need for manpower, and there are legitimate reasons for questioning whether emphasis should not be shifted to rehabilitation per se, so that the Act's provisions may also encompass persons outside the labor market, such as the elderly or the severely impaired, for whom improved functioning can result in less social and economic dependency.

Increasing attention to older Americans has been a dominant theme in the overall socio-political thinking of the Sixties and Seventies. At the beginning of the century, only 4 percent of the United States population was sixty-five or older. By 1960, increased longevity had raised this proportion to nearly 10 percent, and elderly men and women, better educated and more aware of their rights as human beings and their power as voters, began to make themselves felt as a significant force. A profusion of organizations, voluntary and governmental, arose to deal with the needs and demands of the aging.

In contrast to the one-in-ten ratio of the elderly in the general population, more than half of America's blind persons are in the over-sixty-five bracket. But at best, according to some sources, only 9 percent of the total resources for help to blind persons is directed to the needs of the elderly. The reasons are complex but stem from the same basic factor that accounts for the neglect of all aging persons: America's emphasis on a youth- and achievement-oriented culture. On top of this is the inertia induced by traditional patterns of social service delivery and the absence of any strong incentive to alter them.

In an effort to supply such incentive the Foundation, in 1968, assigned a program priority to the cause of the aging and appointed a Task Force on Geriatric Blindness to assess the dimensions of the problem and initiate steps to deal with it. In its four-year tenure the task force moved out in a number of directions. To ascertain whether blind persons could be assimilated into the programs of "golden age" centers and the like, it sponsored pilot projects in which five different cities in New York State tried out a variety of approaches. The results were uneven, but the overall experience indicated that, given enough time, motivation, and funds for such special services as transportation, this kind of integration with sighted peers could help overcome the major burden of social isolation among the elderly blind.

Another step took the form of a grant to the Community Service Society of New York to test the feasibility of including blind persons in that agency's Project SERVE (Serve and Enrich Retirement by Volunteer Experience), in which elderly men and women worked as volunteers in mental hospitals. Here, too, results were promising.

On a national scale the task force established links with other organizations concerned with aging, among them the American Geriatrics Society, a body of physicians specializing in treatment of the elderly. It participated in the effort to gain Congressional passage of the bill introduced in the Senate in 1971 by Jennings Randolph under which elderly blind persons would become eligible for rehabilitation services through the Vocational Rehabilitation Act. The effort failed because of a Presidential veto, but undoubtedly it will be renewed in the future.

The task force also contributed ideas toward the documentation of blind persons' needs in the deliberations of the 1971 White House Conference on Aging. It stimulated the convening of six regional symposia on the problems of the aging blind and the production in 1972 of an illustrated handbook, *An Introduction to Working with the Aging Person Who Is Visually Handicapped*, designed to serve as a practical guide for families and for those whose jobs bring them into daily contact with the elderly blind. The task force was replaced in mid-1972 by a standing Advisory Committee on Aging to ensure continuing advocacy on a national scale in this area.

Inevitably, lacunae exist between advocacy and action. How well geared are the providers of service to reorganize their programs or realign their priorities? How convinced are these agencies of the necessity or validity of making fundamental changes? In the late Sixties, two severe jolts to complacency seemed to have only transitory effects. One, the publication in 1969 of Professor Robert A. Scott's *The Making of Blind Men*, accused the agencies making up the "blindness system" of concentrating on only a small and select portion of the nation's blind people—the young, the employable, and the educable—and of holding these persons in captive dependency for needlessly long periods. By squeezing clients into a kind of Procrustean mold that fit their own concepts of attitudes and behavior patterns of blind people, the agencies were shaping those they served into "a learned social role." Moreover, Scott charged, agencies competed with one another for preferred types of clients and were unwilling to surrender any of their prerogatives, even in the face of unmistakable duplication of services.

Scott's accusations were reiterated in an even more sweeping body of criticism incorporated in a document prepared by the Organization for Social and Technical Innovation (OSTI) for the Subcommittee on Rehabilitation of the National Institute of Neurological Diseases and Blindness. Based on a one-year study of "blindness, its prevention and management, including rehabilitation," the OSTI report echoed and elaborated Scott's theme.

Not unexpectedly, many of the Scott and OSTI assumptions, as well as much of their data, met with indignant rebuttals. But however faulty the data, or exaggerated the implications, the basic philosophic issues reflect valid problems to be faced in the years to come. The "blindness system" assailed by these documents is a literary fiction; the "system" concept implies a degree of structure and an agreement on common goals and standards that has yet to exist. If an overall strategy for change is ever to develop, it will have to be preceded by a virtual revolution in social thinking—a revolution that discards the "cost-benefit" yardstick, which measures service costs against return on dollar investment, in favor of the human-benefit criterion that the function of society is to serve its members. In the American political and economic climate of the early Seventies, such a turnaround in values seems a long way off.

This is not to say, however, that the need for change is being ignored. The accreditation process, though advancing more slowly than was hoped, is producing critical self-examination and reevaluation of programs among the more progressive agencies and schools for the blind. As the base of accredited organizations broadens, pressure will inevitably be exerted on the weaker agencies to upgrade their practices. Liquidation or merger is the prospect faced by organizations whose programs, however useful they may once have been, no longer warrant continuation.

Accreditation, while serving to improve the performance of individual agencies, cannot supply the complete answer. There remains the problem of autonomous, sometimes superfluous services for particular religious or ethnic segments of the blind population, for special occupational groups, for different sexes and age groups. How to coordinate the activities of these free-standing organizations, how to end program duplications at the one end and bridge gaps in service at the other, will be a complex and long drawn-out piece of business, and the need for it is as yet barely acknowledged.

A logical source of strength in tackling such problems might seem to be blind persons themselves, who have to shuttle from one agency to another for an array of services. Most large cities have loosely organized groups of blind persons affiliated with one of two national associations, but their energies are more often focused on broad global concerns than on specific local issues. The larger and older national group, the National Federation of the Blind (NFB), currently centers its efforts on strident but largely unproductive attacks against long-established agencies and organizations in work for the blind. The younger and more moderate association, the American Council for the Blind (ACB), concentrates on a variety of self-help projects, both independently and in concert with national and local agencies.

The one arena in which both organizations have ever realized any real degree of their potential is that concerned with federal legislation, where their numbers could make an impact. Here, however, even the dissident NFB has been able to make itself felt only when it joined forces with the very groups it might be simultaneously attacking on other grounds—the American Foundation for the Blind, the American Association of Workers for the Blind, the Association for the Education of the Visually Handicapped, the Blinded Veterans Association, and the National Council of State Agencies for the Blind. Over the years, the NFB has made a number of efforts to go it alone in legislative campaigns, but it has yet to achieve a single-handed victory.

The most conspicuous experience of this kind took place beginning in 1957 in relation to a legislative proposal the NFB persuaded then Senator John F. Kennedy to introduce: "A Bill to Protect the Rights of the Blind to Self-Expression through Organizations of the Blind." This innocuously-titled measure, ostensibly designed to safeguard blind employees and clients of agencies benefiting from federal funds, contained a sleeper provision proposing that "the Secretary of Health, Education, and Welfare shall to the fullest extent practicable consult and advise with authorized representatives of organizations of the blind" and that policies and procedures should be formulated to "encourage" state agencies to do likewise.

As NFB's president rightly said, that last provision would give his organization "tremendous leverage," a fact which caused the principal spokesmen in work for the blind to voice strenuous objection to the bill. Their added reservations were on the broader philosophic grounds that such a law, by strengthening separatism, would impede the more desirable goal of integrating blind persons into general society. A resolution adopted by the AAWB at its 1957 convention charged that the bill "embodies a completely unsound and retrogressive concept of the responsibilities and privileges of blind persons as citizens."

The Kennedy bill, and its companion House measure introduced by Nevada Congressman Walter S. Baring, were the subject of extensive hearings conducted by the Subcommittee on Special Education of the House Committee on Education and Labor in March 1959. The hearings also took testimony on several collateral bills calling for the appointment of a Presidential study commission to examine the nation's services for blind persons. About half of the 50 witnesses who testified over a five-day period were NFB representatives urging adoption of the "right to organize" measure, while most of the remaining witnesses, representing the major organizations in work for the blind, testified in opposition to the Kennedy-Baring bill and in favor of a Presidential study commission.

A solo position was taken by one witness, Dr. Merle E. Frampton, whose testimony skirted the "right to organize" issue and centered on opposition to the study bills. That Frampton had a hidden agenda in so doing became clear two months later when the House subcommittee decided that instead of recommending any of the bills discussed at the hearings, it would set up its own staff study with Frampton as director. Virtually the sole accomplishment of this two-year exercise was to deflect the naming of a Presidential body and arrest the momentum of the "right to organize" bill. The latter could easily have been reintroduced by the NFB, were it not for an internal upheaval which saw the resignation of its founder and president, Jacobus ten Broek, and the split-off of some of its member groups into the separate American Council of the Blind. By the time the intramural squabbles had been settled and ten Broek resumed the NFB presidency after a five-year hiatus, his organization was zeroing in on new targets.

A brilliant legal scholar, impressive in appearance and commanding in manner, Jacobus ten Broek was graduated from the California School for the Blind and went on to secure a law doctorate, a graduate degree in political science, and a post as instructor at the University of California. He gained stature in California welfare circles through his appointment, in 1950, to that state's Social Welfare Board and his ascent to its chairmanship ten years later. He was an authority on constitutional law as well as on welfare legislation, and a prolific writer on these subjects.

Ten Broek first tasted the satisfactions of group action when he participated in the formation of the California Council of the Blind in the mid-Thirties. In 1940 the council joined with six other state organizations of blind people to form the National Federation of the Blind as a protest against what ten Broek called "the oppression of the social worker and the arrogance of the governmental administrator." (This was during that early period of the Social Security Act when blind people harbored legitimate grievances against the arbitrary manner in which Title X, Aid to the Blind, was being administered by many public welfare bureaus.) The NFB grew rapidly; by 1960 it could claim affiliates in 47 states and attract 900 delegates to its 20th anniversary convention.

Ten Broek's initial goals were not in conflict with those of others in leadership positions. In 1948 he said that all he asked was that qualified blind people "be given an equal chance with the sighted." The early activities of Federation members were concentrated on demolishing what they regarded as the barriers to this goal. Working with other groups, they played helpful roles in the struggle to force civil service commissions to end discrimination against employment of physically handicapped persons, in the campaign to open more vending stand opportunities for the blind in public buildings, and in the drive to gain more equitable treatment for blind persons in state vocational rehabilitation programs.

The real rift between the Federation and its erstwhile partners began in 1953, when the AAWB adopted its Code of Ethics and labeled as unacceptable the practice of raising funds through the mailing of unordered merchandise. This hit NFB squarely in the pocketbook, since its principal means of support came through the mailing of remit-or-return boxes of greeting cards. In 1957 the United States Post Office's Fraud Division issued a complaint against the NFB, charging that the letters accompanying the greeting card mailings falsely implied that all or most of the $1.25 asked for the merchandise would be used to assist the blind, whereas in fact the NFB's yield from each sale was only 15 cents. The complaint was dropped when the NFB agreed to amend its future literature to specify the exact amount accrued from each sale.

This incident, and the fact that it was fully reported in both the nation's press and in the major communication channels of work for the blind, gave the Federation the sense of being embattled; its list of "enemies" grew to embrace virtually the entire field of work for the blind. Such extremism gave way, in turn, to insurrection among some of its state affiliates; NFB conventions in the late Fifties and early Sixties saw bitter floor fights on motions to censure, suspend, or expel state chapters that objected to the autocratic structure which centered all organizational and fiscal power in the person of President ten Broek.

A report in the September 1958 issue of the *New Outlook,* describing the heated atmosphere of that year's NFB convention in Boston, drew a furious attack against the Foundation for publishing it and the Foundation promptly rose to the top of NFB's enemy list. However, the factional rivalry disclosed in the report was real enough. It came to a head in 1961 when ten Broek resigned as NFB president, blaming "internal strife and chaos." He returned to the presidency in 1966, and held the post until his death from cancer two years later at the age of fifty-six . He was succeeded by Kenneth Jernigan, a graduate of and former teacher at the Tennessee School for the Blind, who had moved ahead professionally to become director of the Iowa State Commission for the Blind.

Under Jernigan, the NFB entered a heightened phase of militancy, targeting its opposition first at the Commission on Standards and Accreditation of Agencies for the Blind (COMSTAC) and then at COMSTAC's successor, the National Accreditation Council (NAC). Against the latter it employed many of the same tactics used by other "rights" groups during the Sixties—mass picketing staged for maximum media coverage, along with a mail campaign addressed to senators and congressmen demanding that the federal funds which helped support NAC's budget be withheld because the council had inadequate consumer representation. This was accompanied by an unremitting barrage in NFB's house organ, the *Braille Monitor,* demanding that half of the accreditation council's board of directors be appointed by, and subject to the control of, the Federation. None of these devices had achieved their aim as of the end of 1972.

Paradoxically, at the same time as this warfare was being waged against the youngest (and presumably the most vulnerable) national body in work for the blind, NFB's Washington office continued for the most part to work in harmony with the established agencies on legislation affecting blind persons. In 1970 an informal group, consisting of the heads of the seven major organizations for and of the blind, began a series of semi-annual meetings to seek common ground in policy matters. One of the seven was the NFB, represented by Jernigan; another was the American Council of the Blind, represented by its then president, Judge Reese H. Robrahn of Topeka, Kansas. The ACB had 34 affiliates in 1971. Like the NFB, it had a blind lawyer as its Washington representative. Durward K. McDaniel worked in close cooperation with both NFB's John F. Nagle and Irvin Schloss, the Foundation's Washington man; the trio constituted the principal spokesmen for blind persons in the nation's capital.

The future course of these organizations of blind persons is difficult to predict. If they follow the developmental sequence of other dissident groups which emerged in the Sixties, they may sooner or later conclude that the surer, if slower, road to reform lies in working within the system rather than through attempts to tear it down, and in joining forces with the sighted community rather than marching under separatist banners.

For their part, most agencies for the blind have been slow to recognize legitimate demands for consumer representation in their policy-making bodies, but this, too, may well see change in the years ahead as collateral community organizations give way to pressures for a broader base. A true and equal partnership between blind and sighted persons in work for the blind remains a milestone yet to be reached.

At the same time there is no dearth of intramural problems. To cite just a handful:

The merest beginning has been made in affording orientation and mobility training to all who can benefit by it. There is an ever more pressing need to redefine the role of the workshop as a therapeutic agency or as a place of terminal employment for those unable to function in competitive jobs. There is an equally urgent need for vigorous action to end exploitative workshop practices where they exist. The impasse on vending stands in federal and state buildings must somehow be broken, and new opportunities actively pursued in factories and commercial buildings. Psychological tests truly applicable to the rehabilitation needs of blind people must be devised, and a more effective counseling role found for the psychologist. Agencies for the blind must be helped to end their isolation, build two-way working relationships with other community service organizations, and expedite the integration of blind persons into programs serving the sighted. Similarly, there needs to be a much greater degree of interdisciplinary exchange and cooperation, so that staff members who provide social, educational, recreational, and health services in these general agencies are better geared to work comfortably and constructively with blind persons. The technologically sophisticated sensory aids already available must be made more accessible, and there must be encouragement for continuing research on simpler, better, and lower-priced devices to mitigate the handicaps of blindness.

In the closing decades of the twentieth century, these and comparable challenges require at least as much creativity and clear-eyed leadership as those with which the century began. The cardinal difference is that there now exist tested and tempered agents of change which can mobilize the needed resources of brains, boldness and financial investment.

> We in the United States . . . are today at the beginning of a movement which will not rest until all preventable blindness has been prevented, until the competent blind have found a recognized place of usefulness in the community, and until the condition of the rest, the aged and otherwise handicapped, has been truly ameliorated.

A worker for the blind in Massachusets sounded this call to action in 1908. It echoes still.

Chapter Notes

Key to Abbreviations

PERSONS

MRB—M. Robert Barnett
CFFC—Charles F. F. Campbell
RBI—Robert B. Irwin
HK—Helen Keller
HRL—H. Randolph Latimer
ASM—Anne Sullivan Macy
MCM—M. C. Migel
PJS—Peter J. Salmon

ORGANIZATIONS

AAIB—American Association of Instructors of the Blind
AAWB—American Association of Workers for the Blind
AFB—American Foundation for the Blind
BVA—Blinded Veterans of America
LC—Library of Congress
NFB—National Federation of the Blind
Perkins—Perkins School for the Blind, formerly Perkins Institution and Massachusetts
    Asylum for the Blind

PERIODICALS

Outlook—Outlook for the Blind, 1907–1950; *New Outlook for the Blind,* 1951
TBT—Talking Book Topics
TF—Teachers Forum

Unless otherwise indicated, all correspondence, minutes, and memos referred to are in AFB files.
Books identified by author's name or title only are listed in the Bibliography.

1. MYTHS, TABOOS AND STEREOTYPES

2 "in Wagria and other Wendish lands": French, 34
2 "Ox liver, roasted and pounded": Ross, 12

3 "Now blind": Lines 563-568

3 "to have to tell a person that he is blind": Cholden, 18

3 –Other psychiatrists have equated: Otto Fenichel, "Scotophilic Instinct and Identification," *International Journal of Psychoanalysis,* 1937, cited in "Attitudes toward Blindness", 6

4 "a mediaeval ignorance": *Mainstream,* 79

4 "To suppose there can be": 1848 annual report, Perkins, 37

4 "Dark night": Act III, Scene II, lines 177-180

4 –Working with paired blind and sighted subjects: Michael Supa, Milton Cotzin and Karl M. Dallenbach, " 'Facial Vision': the Perceptions of Obstacles by the Blind," *American Journal of Psychology,* April 1944, 133-183.

4 –The same conclusion had been reached: Griffin, 57-64

5–As reported in the *Official Bulletin of the Chicago Medical Society:* Vol. 21, p. 29

5 "Miss Huggins gave": *JAMA,* June 17, 1922, 1891

5 –In the same issue: 1892

6 –A follow-up study: Robert H. Gault, "An Unusual Case of Olfactory and Tactile Sensitivity," *Journal of Abnormal Psychology and Social Psychology,* 1922-3, 395–401

6 –A statement by her: *Christian Science Sentinel.* January 26, 1929, 436

6 –Willetta later changed her name: telephone conversation with author, November 2, 1970

6 –the Italian criminologist: cited in Edwards, 63

6 –Their opinion was shared: Tom W. Gerber, "Call Blind Claim Hoax," *Boston Traveler,* September 11, 1957

6–Soviet scientists who examined Rosa: Stanley Krippner and Richard Davison, "Parapsychology in the U.S.S.R.," *Saturday Review,* March 18, 1972, 57

7 –American interest in the subject: R. P. Youtz, "Can Fingers See Color?," *Psychology Today,* February 1968, 36-41

7 "to be able to blow your own nose": Lloyd W. Greenwood, "Return to Manhood," *BVA Bulletin,* December 1947

7 "that Louis, moved probably by the misery": French, 47

8 "Unquestionably the most worthy": Mrs. George S. Kessler quoted in *Boston Sunday Herald,* November 12, 1916

8 –In 1918 an estimated $31 million: Best, 96

10 "an age of rose-colored nightmares": Snowman, 11

11 ". . . the oldest form of tax-supported": Robert S. Lynd and Helen Merrell Lynd, *Middletown,* Harcourt, Brace & World, 1929, 467

11 "extends ready sympathy": ibid.

2. Five Days at Vinton

14 "In 1895, at St. Louis": Norman Yoder, "American Association of Workers for the Blind, 1895–1964," *Blindness* 1964, 151–175

15 "We ask that blind persons": ibid.

18 "Though I was as blind as a chicken": *Outlook,* Spring 1914, 30

19 "The Executive Committee": *Outlook,* Fall 1920, 46

20 "We were neither reckless": *Outlook,* Summer 1921, 89-90

21 "The work being done for the blind": *Evergreen Review,* July 1920

22 "late of Purdue University": *Outlook,* Spring 1919, 1

22 "Resolved, that this Association": *Outlook,* April 1920, 31

23 "a properly constituted organization": *Outlook,* Summer 1921, 91

3. TALENT HUNT

26 "a competent sighted man": letter, HRL to Charles B. Hayes, December 28, 1921

26 "This man need not necessarily be": letter, MCM to Leo B. Durstine, August 2, 1922

27 "We have come to the conclusion": letter, MCM to RBI, October 31, 1922

29 "There is a more or less ill defined fear": *Outlook,* Summer 1922, 42–44

30 "the receipts of the sale": *Outlook,* June 1924, 6–7

31 "He has a genius for harmonizing": letter, ASM to MCM, June 25, 1925

31 "Olympia, the nearest city": *Washington Alumnus,* January 1945

32 "ran a cigar stand": ibid.

34 "were, to say the least, unconventional": Latimer, 272

34 "it became Mr. Irwin's direct responsibility": ibid.

4. THE SECOND CAREER OF MAJOR MIGEL

37 "The lamentable fact": quoted in Irwin, 22-3

39 "Strangely enough": letter, RBI to Murray B. Allen, June 14, 1941

40 –The War Department was in need of silk: a detailed account of this is in Marquis James, "The Profiteer Hunt," *American Legion Weekly,* June 8, 1923, 7 ff.

42 "an anonymous friend": *Outlook,* June 1924, 5

43 –Ability to handle figures: this anecdote, as well as many other details of MCM's personal and family life, from author's interviews with Parmenia Migel Ekstrom, December 1970 and January 1971

5. THE FACTS OF BLINDNESS

46 "inadequate, unrealistic, inequitable": Richard E. Hoover, "Toward a New Definition of Blindness," *Blindness* 1966, 99–106

47 "Now we are confronted": letter, RBI to HK, December 6, 1933

47 –Senator Jennings Randolph recalled: hearings, House Select Subcommittee on Education, November 30 and December 8, 1970, 61-2

48 "from two to two-and-one-half times": *Outlook,* March 1947, 62

49 "reported 48,929 blind persons": Farrell, *Story of Blindness,* 213

49 –A much higher rate: Carl Kupfer, M.D., quoted in *The Standard-Bearer,* National Accreditation Council, Winter 1971, 3

49 "army of the aged blind": Hyman Goldstein in Proceedings of the Research Conference on Geriatric Blindness and Severe Visual Impairment, 13

50 "In practically every instance": Catherine Brannick in report, 15-16, bound in as insert in *Outlook,* Spring 1910

52 –According to the government-sponsored study: Blindness and Services to the Blind in the United States, 26

52 –A functional breakdown of the $469 million: ibid., 35

6. THE PERFECT SYMBOL

54 –While still in college: quotations are from typescript, December 7, 1903, in HK collection of AFB

55 "desire to have me educated": Teacher, 77

55 "For & in behalf": "Mark Twain's Letters," *Harper's Monthly,* October 1917, 645

56 "It is superb!": ibid.

56 "hoped that the possession of money of their own": Braddy, 178

56 "My sense of pride mutinies": *Midstream,* 209, 72

56 "all through my life": ibid., 74

56 "It required a powerful temperament": *Teacher,* 80

58 "Our present idea": letter, MCM to CFCC, November 27, 1923

58 "For years, I have felt": letter, CFCC to MCM, November 30, 1923

59 "You will be interested": letter, RBI to CFFC, January 22, 1924

60 ". . . we have been working": letter, MCM to CFFC, April 18, 1924

62 "In order to insure the perpetuity": *Outlook,* Fall 1924, 43

63 "She will not endorse": letter, Charles B. Hayes to MCM, December 8, 1924

64 "Unfortunately, a good many thoughtful givers": letter, CFFC to MCM, February 18, 1925

64 "I know that nearly everybody has heard of me": *Midstream,* 151, 152–3

65 "Try to imagine": *Outlook,* September 1925, 26

66 "map out a programme": letter, MCM to ASM, May 12, 1925

67 [Y]our treatment of Helen Keller and me": letter, ASM to MCM, n.d., probably early November 1925

68 ". . . if, in the judgment of the American Foundation for the Blind": letter, MCM to ASM, November 6, 1925

70 "that Miss Keller be placed on the staff ":letter, RBI to Herbert H. White, July 12, 1926

70 "I have not written": letter, HK to Herbert H. White, July 6, 1926

71 "unquestioning faith": Stetson B. Ryan, *Outlook,* February 1934, 35

71 "It is my recollection": letter, Herbert B. White to HK, August 6, 1926

72 "the money difficulty remains the same": letter, HK to Olin H. Burritt, October 22, 1926

72 "The truth is": letter, HK to Burritt, February 24, 1927

73 "But I am going to make a further request": letter, ASM to MCM, May 18, 1927

73 "I regret deeply": letter, ASM to MCM, July 4, 1927

74 "Also, please send me a memorandum": letter, MCM to HK and ASM, June 19, 1929

74 "It is most dear of you": letter, HK to MCM, June 24, 1929

74 "It's time to say how much I thank you": letter, ASM to MCM, October 1, 1929

74 "Helen is a slow, painstaking worker": letter, ASM to MCM, January 18, 1930

75 "There is no disguising the fact": letter, HK to MCM, January 18, 1930

75 "As to being impatient with you": letter, MCM to HK, January 29, 1930

75 –At the next executive committee meeting: minutes, January 22, 1930

75 –She cited Victor Hugo's parable: letter, HK to MCM, February 4, 1930

76 –When Anne was convalescing: letter, MCM to Robert Moses, May 29, 1935

76 "I am not gifted": letter, HK to Burritt, October 22, 1926

77 "Your letter goes right to the heart": letter, Gustavus A. Pfeiffer to HK, November 25, 1929

7. "Action Is Our Watchword"

80 "Action is our watchword": *Outlook,* May 1923, 24

80 "There is no endowment": letter, MCM to President Warren G. Harding, November 8, 1922

81 "I recommend that $100,000 be added": letter, C. R. Forbes to Senator Francis Warren, January 11, 1923

81 "If the Foundation did not do another stroke": letter, MCM to Olin H. Burritt, January 17, 1923

81 "is in no position to justify": letter, Frank T. Hines to RBI, February 7, 1927

82 "The truth is our Veteran readers": letter, RBI to General David C. Shanks, April 6, 1925

85 "more than $21,000 has been saved": *Outlook,* October 1933, 155

85 –As early as 1907: Newel Perry, "New York's Provision for the Higher Education of the Blind," *Outlook,* April 1908, 47

86 –A Committee on Scholarship Awards: *Outlook,* June 1925, 5

86 –successfully functioning as teachers of the sighted: *Outlook,* September 1929, 16

86 –the overall number of recipients exceeded 300: Director's Report of Activities, AFB, first quarter, 1961-2

87 "The Foundation furnished the director": Annual Report of Director of Research, AFB, October 20, 1924, 1–2

88 –Expectations had been given an invigorating boost: letter, Thomas B. Appleget to MCM, January 29, 1927

88 –Rockefeller promptly made good: letter, Appleget to MCM, June 11, 1928

88 "to establish the following rule": letter, MCM to Charles B. Hayes and RBI, November 18, 1925

88 "I do not see how we could function": letter, RBI to MCM, November 19, 1925

89 –At its next meeting: minutes, AFB executive committee, January 27, 1926

89 "He says that he will continue": letter, RBI to HRL, June 29, 1927

89 "it makes little difference": letter, RBI to HRL, July 7, 1927

89 "In my opinion": letter, HRL to MCM and AFB executive committee, May 5, 1928

8. THE LANGUAGE OF THE FINGERS

94 –the skeleton of his right hand: Farrell (Story of Blindness), 98

96 –The school's music teacher was the first to yield: S. Pollak, "My Autobiography and Reminiscences," *St. Louis Medical Review,* 1904

96 "The world is at last in accordance": *Outlook,* December 1929, 13

97 "Many still living": Irwin, 47

98 "I really believe": letter, RBI to MCM, June 29, 1929

98 "It is my belief that a little common sense": Lende et al., 17

99 "were almost dumbfounded": Edward E. Allen in *Frank H. Hall,* memorial brochure, quoted in Hendrickson, 10

100 "At first I thought of making": *Outlook,* Summer 1909, 43-4

101 "The work is done by the electric motor": ibid.

103 "Bob Atkinson was blinded": *Outlook,* April 1964, 132; also *The Seer,* December 1943, 7

103 –In actual fact": Westrate, 110

105 "an original fellow": letter, RBI to Dr. Frederick B. Keppel, July 12, 1927

105 "interpointing, while it saves about one-third": letter, Barr to MCM, June 17, 1926

105 "The work we have received from the Foundation": letter, Atkinson to MCM, March 9, 1929

106 "A little friendly competition": letter, RBI to Franklin F. Hopper, October 25, 1927

106 "I do not think it wise:" letter, Atkinson to MCM, March 9, 1929

108 "has everything one could want": quoted in *Outlook,* February 1934, 18

113 "I should like nothing better": quoted in Gertrude T. Rider, "Annual Report on Braille Transcribing," *Outlook,* March 1925, 19

9. BOOKS FOR THE BLIND

116 "The library departments for the blind": Irwin, 70

116 "disgruntled by the loss": Lende et al., 210

118 "We have what we believe": quoted in letter, RBI to HK, December 13, 1932

119 "Would you contemplate": hearing, House Committee on the Library, March 27, 1930, 10

119 "would save himself a lot of grief ": ibid.

120 "Books are the eyes of the blind": ibid., 21-22. The text as printed in the hearing record gives the word "consummation" in the last line of the second paragraph. The speech draft in the Helen Keller archives shows the word to be "consolation."

120 "a complete monopoly": ibid., 32

121 "a certain tendency": ibid., 34

121-2-Dialogue, Schafer and Crail, 7-8

122 -Barr testimony, ibid., 14-23

122 "I am very glad we have had this chance": ibid., 26

122 "We do not come here to split or destroy": ibid., 28

123 -Crail then introduced a new letter: text of letter, ibid., 29-39

124 "Fully 90 percent": Atkinson testimony, ibid., 40-47

124 "Leaving aside the question": Irwin testimony, ibid., 47-50

124 "They are self-constituted bulwarks": ibid., 53

125 "this is not a criminal", ibid., 55

125 -Atkinson then resumed his testimony: ibid., 57-71

125 "has for the past two years": second hearing, 120-122

127 "would be vicious": *Congressional Record,* February 28, 1931, 6568

127 "I did most of the cross-examining": ibid., 6570

128 "If we, after the hearings": ibid., 6572

128 "because no service would be rendered": ibid., 6575

128 "which is as much if not more": letter, Atkinson to MCM, October 22, 1931

10. THE TALKING BOOK

130 "a coincidence not without irony": Lucy A. Goldthwaite in Lende (ed.), Vol. 1, 179

131 "a scheme simmering": letter, RBI to George F. Meyer, April 23, 1924

131 "If we do not die too young": letter, RBI to Frank C. Bryan, February 10, 1925

132 "I have always dreamed": letter, RBI to A. C. Ellis, June 13, 1941

133 "I have in my office": letter, RBI to Frederick P. Keppel, March 26, 1932

133 "could be loaned": letter, RBI to Keppel, March 29, 1932

135 "the doggondest collector": quoted in MRB, "Hindsight," *Outlook,* January 1959, 39

135 "Since the purpose of the original bill": letter, Herbert Putnam to Senator Jesse H. Metcalf, December 22, 1932

136 "When it has been made perfectly clear": letter, MCM to Metcalf, January 10, 1933

136 -In *As I Saw It:* p. 75

137 "who is absolutely disinterested": *Congressional Record,* March 3, 1933, 5726

137 "we can declare ourselves": ibid., 5732

138 "IF EXECUTIVE COMMITTEE": cable, HK to MCM, September 22, 1933

138 "The only thought which sustains me": letter, HK to MCM, September 29, 1933

139 should "include books which the rank and file": letter, RBI to H. H. B. Meyer, March 14, 1934

140 "when you list": letter, Meyer to RBI, May 7, 1934

141 "there are those who are ever eager": letter, Atkinson to MCM, April 10, 1934

141 "adhere to the system of constant turntable speech": Report of the Advisory Committee Appointed for the Consideration of Talking Machines to Be Used with Talking Books for the Blind, June 12, 1934

142 "when I told him": letter, Atkinson to MCM, July 6, 1934

142 "You must send for Alexander": Kaufman and Hennessey, 177

143 "the magician of words": letter, HK to Will Rogers, April 1, 1930

143 "Here's my little dab": letter, Rogers to HK, May 27, 1930

143 "would render practicable the transcription": letter, RBI to Keppel, January 18, 1935

143 "that you will [some day]": letter, RBI to Ellis, January 26, 1935

144 "there is some probability": letter, Ellis to RBI, February 5, 1935

144 "the machines for using these records": *Congressional Record*, May 6, 1935, 7258

145 "Please, dear Mr. Roosevelt": HK note, n.d., on back of letter from FDR dated February 7, 1929

146 "If you wish us to do so,": letter, MCM to Herbert Putnam, July 25, 1935

147 "a nice messy job": letter, RBI to HK, August 30, 1935

148 "My first impressions": reprint from *Congressional Record*, June 16, 1936

148 "I have 16 counties": "A Few Unsolicited Letters Received from Blind Persons Who Have Been Lent WPA Talking Book Machines," memo in AFB files, n.d., ca. October, 1936

149 "shall give preference to non-profit-making": Public Law 76-118, June 7, 1939

150 "would make us more independent": letter, RBI to MCM, June 12, 1937

151 –In mid-1936 a teacher: Kenneth Longsdorf, "The Talking Book in English Classes," *TF*, May 1936, 97

152 "The speed of the average braille reader": Lowenfeld, "The Talking Book Goes to School," *TBT*, March 1940, 14

152 "comprehension of narrative material": report to the W. K. Kellogg Foundation, December 1943

11. The Beloved Voices

153 "This thing of recording a book": letter, RBI to Harold T. Clark, January 20, 1933

155 "We have auditioned literally hundreds": unsigned memo in AFB files, "Personalities Who Have Recorded for the Talking Book," n.d., ca. 1943

155 "give to the works they present": Robert S. Bray, "Library Services for the Blind," *Bulletin of the Society of Military Ophthalmologists,* September 1968, 19

155 "as long as I can speak": quoted in *TBT*, September 1964, 95

156 "Fifteen years ago I lost my sight": letter, C. E. Seymour to Alexander Scourby, January 29, 1941

156 "Having heard myself on recordings": letter, Dean Acheson to Alan Hewitt, July 9, 1971

156 "Many of our patrons": letter, Martha R. Stewart to Robert S. Bray, March 23, 1966

157 "Whereas the printed play": *Outlook,* October 1940, 142

157 "Under the operations of the copyright law": David C. Mearns, "The Story Up to Now" in 1946 annual report, LC, 165

160 "prepare a general recording of talks": letter, Joseph P. Blickensderfer to RBI, September 6, 1945

161 "We were receiving requests": Alison B. Alessios, "The Case for Recording—As a Librarian Sees It," *Outlook,* December 1947, 287

162 "never gets irritated": Don Crawford, "Recordings for College Students," *Outlook,* December 1947, 284

163 "pending the time when the Library of Congress": letter, Mildred C. Skinner to Charles H. Whittington, March 20, 1951

166 "the history of cooperation": letter, Evans to RBI, December 18, 1947

174 "There was a free afternoon:" Robert Bray conversation with author, July 22, 1971

175 "We are touched that you found it possible": letter, Mamie Eisenhower to MRB, September 30, 1955

12. A Share in the General Welfare

178 "It is useless": holograph letter, MCM to RBI, February 20, 1935

178 "I was unable to find out": letter, RBI to Sinclair, July 26, 1935

180 "This assistance has improved": *Outlook,* October 1936, 151

180 "If those of us": *Outlook,* February 1937, 12

180 –Vivid illustrations of the initial affects: quotes in this section from "The Social Security Act and the Blind," *Outlook,* October 1936, 148-156

182 "If eye examinations and medical service": "Present Status of Work for the Blind in the United States," address at Reading, Pa., November 3, 1939

184 "In my travels": HK, testimony before the Kelley Committee, October 3, 1944

185 "As one of a large family": hearings, House Committee on Ways and Means, May 6-10, 1946, 1047

185 "what we are afraid of ": ibid., 1077

185 "I think you are as good a friend": ibid., 1078

187 "Peter, . . . you people can walk out": PJS conversation with author, August 31, 1970

13. The Showcase of the Blind

191 "Work shapes a day": Henry Fairlee, "The Middle Class," *McCall's,* July 1970, 102

192 "employment of the blind side by side": RBI, Report of the Director of Research and Education, 1926, 4

194 "to strongly recommend that the federal government": quoted in *Outlook,* September 1927, 20

194 "the complete control of federal buildings": Conference on the Schall Bill (S.2819), November 18, 1930

195 "blind persons to sell papers": quoted in *Outlook,* February 1934, 4

195 "is to be confined to the selling of newspapers": Treasury Department Circular Letter No. 251, June 16, 1933

195 "the use of a chair or stool": letter, MCM to L. W. Robert, Jr., June 27, 1933

196 "to be appointed by the President": H.R. 5694, introduced May 19, 1933

196 "quite a champion of street beggars": memo, RBI to MCM, April 27, 1933

197 "with the full understanding that your Department": letter, MCM to Henry Morgenthau, Jr., December 12, 1934

197 "The Federal Government is spending billions": House Report No. 1095, 74th Congress, 1936, quoted in "Vending Stand Program for Blind Persons," mimeographed, AFB, 1957, p. 57-8

198 "This legislation would allow the setting up of stands": Senate Report No. 2052, 1936, quoted in ibid., 56–7

199 "It fell to me as a young newly-blinded man": "Influence of the Randolph-Sheppard Act on the Employment of Blind Persons," in *Blindness* 1966, 140

199 "To appeal to an employer": "Placement Work as a Business," *Outlook,* June 1930, 18

200 "There is nothing in our experience": quoted in Jennings Randolph, "The Story of the Randolph-Sheppard Act," *Blindness* 1965, 5

201 "are usually better off financially": "Present Vending Stand Programs and the Outlook for the Future," AAWB proceedings, 1951, 116–122

201 "prohibit government employee welfare associations": *Outlook,* June 1951, 194

202 "The intent of Congress to give preference": Statement by Graham A. Barden at meeting on Vending Stands in Public Buildings, August 1, 1951 - transcript in AFB files

202 "as a result of the action of the Secretary of Agriculture": Statement by MRB to Subcommittee on the Rehabilitation of the Handicapped, House Committee on Education and Labor, May 1954

203 –it was also in violation of two rulings: These were the Report of the Comptroller General of the United States to the Congress, August 10, 1949, B-45101, 32 Comp. Gen. 124; and Report of the Comptroller General to the Attorney General, August 29, 1952, B-111086, 32 Comp. Gen. 124

204 –S. 2461: introduced June 20, 1969

205 "Stealing from the Blind," Marjorie Boyd, *Washington Monthly,* December 1972, 27-36

205 "The conferees are deeply concerned": quoted in AFB *Washington Report,* December 1972, 4-5

205 –An even more ominous development: "U.S. Plans a Curb on Blind Venders," *New York Times,* November 25, 1972

206 –The first instance of industrial placement: Irwin, 147–8

207 –His characteristic approach was illustrated: Herbert Yahraes, "They Are Happy Days," *Collier's,* April 22, 1950, 87

208 "Class instructors have observed": Charles R. Borchert, "Blind Trainees Succeed in Industry," *Outlook,* February 1967, 44-46

208 "husky fellow with the flashing teeth": Yahraes, op.cit., 17

14. THE WORKSHOPS

209 "In this department the blind feel perfectly independent": 1841 annual report, Perkins, 14-15

210 "In some instances those entering the institutions": Irwin, 151–2

210 –A 1908 survey of the 16 workshops: "Industrial Establishments for the Blind in the United States," *Outlook,* July 1908, unpaged insert following 102

211 –Many years later a knowledgeable observer: PJS conversation with author, August 31, 1970

212 "work in cooperation with the American Foundation for the Blind": quoted in PJS, "Sheltered Workshops Under the NRA," *Outlook,* June 1934, 112

212 "charitable institutions . . .": Administrator's Order X-9, March 3, 1934, quoted in ibid., 114

213 "I don't think that the Foundation could possibly do": letter, PJS to MCM, March 15, 1937

213 "first we would like to secure": quoted in LeFevre, 6-7

214–He alleged that workers for the blind: letter, Merle E. Frampton to Senator Burton K. Wheeler, March 11, 1938

215 –replied with a patient explanation: letter, RBI to Frampton, March 28, 1938

215 "all the economic functions": Frampton, "Socio-Economic Forces and Their Effect on the Social and Vocational Readjustments of the Visually Handicapped," AAWB proceedings, 1935, 237-248

216 "The Committee on Executive Department Expenditures": Irwin, 158

216 "Congressman Hamilton Fish," ibid., 160

217 "knew very little about the bill": ibid.

217 "–Many years later, Peter Salmon: 1970 Senate hearings, Handicapped Workers Legislation, 37

219 "an air of skepticism": LeFevre, 16

219 "the ability of blind workers to produce": ibid., 18

220 –In mid-1940 an Army order: memo, C. C. Kleber to MCM, August 12, 1940

221 –in pre-NIB days many a workshop: memo, C. C. Kleber to RBI, December 8, 1943

222 "Steps should be taken immediately": Proceedings of the Meeting of the Postwar Planning Committee, December 13, 1943, 7

222 "acceptable workshops for the blind": Office of Vocational Rehabilitation, Cooperative Relationship Memorandum No. 11, n.d., circulated with NIB Bulletin, June 22, 1945

224 –Still another change during the postwar years: "The Expanded Program of N.I.B.," *Outlook,* January 1951, 9-11

227 –the National Federation of the Blind initiated legislation: H.R. 9801; reported in "Hearings on Minimum Wage for Blind Workers," *Outlook,* October 1960, 275-279

228 –Passed in 1966 over vigorous opposition: Public Law 89-601, approved September 23, 1966

228 "more impressed with the oddity": *The Seer,* May 1937, 25

230 –Some witnesses at the Congressional hearings: Commissioner Edward Newman, Hearings, Amendments to the Wagner-O'Day Act, subcommittee of the House Committee on Government Operations, April 20-21, 1971, 25

15. THE MAGNA CHARTA OF THE BLIND

232 "[state agencies for the blind] feel that a system": AFB circular letter, "Important Legislation Affecting the Blind," September 16, 1942

233 –Companion bills to amend the Vocational Rehabilitation Act: H.R. 7484 (Barden bill) and S.2714 (LaFollette bill)

233 "It is my intention": letter, Paul V. McNutt to Senator Robert F. Wagner, February 9, 1943

234 –As a precautionary countermeasure: "Why Rehabilitation of the Blind Is a Function of a Special Agency for the Blind," enclosure to AFB circular letter, November 17, 1943 and reprinted in *Outlook,* December 1943, 275-6

234 –Five years after its enactment: Michael J. Shortley quoted in minutes of NIB General Workshop Committee, February 2, 1948, 18

235 "many people who have spent the greater part of their careers": "The Vocation Rehabilitation Act Related to the Blind," Journal of Rehabilitation, September October 1970, 29

238 "the real challenge": Mary E. Switzer and Warren Bledsoe, "U. S. Government Sponsored Research to Study Blindness," *Blindness* 1964, 2

240 –When the Act was amended once again: Public Law 90-391

240 "pressured by the need to show": Testimony on HR 15827 and 16134 before the Subcommittee on Education, House Committee on Education, April 8, 1968, 11

241 "who have unusual and difficult problems": fact sheet, National Rehabilitation Association, quoted in *Congressional Record,* June 10, 1971, 5063

241 "that an elderly blind diabetic": statement to Select Subcommittee on Education, House Committee on Education and Labor, February 1, 1972

242 "When my sight went": Pierce, 41

242 –a 1969 survey showed: elementary and secondary school figures in Ewald B. Nyquist, "The Importance of Employing Blind Teachers in the Public Schools," *Outlook,*

January 1971, 6; college and university figure estimate in letter, D. C. McFarland to author, April 26, 1972

244 –A law passed in 1948 forbade discrimination: Public Law 80-617, approved June 10, 1948

244 –The problem was solved in 1962: Public Law 87-614, approved August 29, 1962

16. THE WAR-BLINDED, WORLD WAR I

245 "I will never be a blind man": quoted in Fraser, 27

246 –When the first actuarial survey was made in 1922: ibid., 190

247 "the Aladdin of the modern world": "Address Delivered at Evergreen January 15, 1919 by Sir Arthur Pearson," *Outlook,* Spring 1919, 21-30

248 –In 1924 the United States Veterans Bureau reported: untitled memo in AFB files, n.d., ca. 1946/7, citing figures received from Veterans Bureau

248 The remainder of the 800 men": letter, S.M. Moore, Jr., to Helga Lende, October 14, 1942

249 –In two days of strenuous work: James Bordley, "Plans of the U. S. Government for Soldiers Blinded in Battle," *Outlook,* October 1917, 54-58

249 "in such subjects as reading and writing": ibid., 56

250 "that the Secretary of War was not inclined": quoted in Alan C. Woods, M.D., "The Story of the Red Cross Institute for the Blind," *American Journal of Ophthalmology,* October 1943, 1011-1024

251 –In France, for example: Harper, 22

251 –The British system also differentiated: Twersky (1947), 125

252 "A high school student sat next to a man": Alexander M. Witherspoon, "Eighteen Months at the Red Cross Institute for the Blind," *Evergreen Review,* September 1920, 78

252 –The Red Cross saw its overall function: "The Red Cross Institute for the Blind," pamphlet, n.d., reprinted in *Outlook,* July 1918, 35-41

253 "to do anything that would help": "Pointing the Way," pamphlet, n.d., 15

254 –More than half the men had had little formal education: 1920 annual report, Federal Board for Vocational Education, 394

255 "In one instance an agent of the Board": ibid., 395

255 –Smith-Fess Act: Public Law 66-236, approved June 2, 1920

256 –Vance, when he resigned: letter, Joseph E. Vance to MCM, December 7, 1922

257 "If we were to go into a war ten years from now": letter, RBI to James L. Fieser, May 13, 1925

17. THE NEW BREED

259 –A public declaration to this effect: "Federal Aid Urged for War-Blinded," *The New York Times,* September 10, 1942

260 –The plan outlined a three-stage program: letter, RBI to Frank T. Hines, January 12, 1943, enclosing memorandum, n.d., "Suggestions for the Handling of the Problems Resulting from the War"

260 "We have complications": letter, RBI to Clutha Mackenzie, May 27, 1943

261 –In July 1943 the Office of the Surgeon General: "Rehabilitation of the Blind in Army Hospitals," n.d., enclosed with letter, Lt. Col. Malcolm J. Farrell to RBI, July 16, 1943

263 "a good substitute for an obstacle course": Twersky (1947), 72

264 "the thing on which he had come to place the most confidence": "Army Service Forces

Old Farms Convalescent Hospital (Sp)," manuscript of speech, n.d., (author not given but probably Lt. William A. Jameson), 7

265 –A study made by Colonel Thorne: "A Statistical Review of 367 Blinded Service Men, World War II," *American Journal of Ophthalmology,* October 1946, reprinted in *Outlook,* May 1947, 129–136

266 "one of the greatest achievements": Colonel J. H. King, Jr., "Army Ophthalmology," *Military Surgeon,* February 1955

266 "that newly-blinded persons could learn to be blind": H. Kenneth Fitzgerald and J. Albert Asenjo, "Rehabilitation Centers—Their Growth and Development," *Blindness* 1965, 53

266 "visit our blind hospitals from time to time": letter, Lt. Col. M.E. Randolph to RBI, January 31, 1945

267 –Their offer was promptly accepted: letter, Omar Bradley to RBI, December 11, 1945

270 "Although this committee has been in existence": letter, RBI to Carl R. Gray, April 22, 1948

270 "I am only here some 100 days": letter, Carl R. Gray, Jr., to RBI, April 23, 1948

270 "straighten out this problem": letter, Gray to RBI, May 11, 1948

270 "selection of personnel": letter, RBI to Gray, May 20, 1948

271 "As an entirely civilian organization": letter, RBI to MCM, December 6, 1944

271 "I am not quite sure just what is needed": letter, RBI to Kathern Gruber, December 27, 1944

272 "the boys will need most of our services": letter, Kathern Gruber to H. V. Stirling, March 16, 1945

272 "about fifty times as much": letter, RBI to Barton, April 7, 1944

273 "hanging on to every ounce": letter, Rosalie F. Cohen to RBI, February 26, 1944

274 "It's hard work": letter, Polly Thomson to Ida Hirst-Gifford, November 28, 1944

274 "You are the most impressive": letter, W. R. Dear to HK, August 6, 1945

274 "To be permitted to kindle even one light": letter, HK to MCM, January 13, 1945

274 "gaiety carried me back to my girlhood": letter, HK to Colonel Hardaway, Bushnell General Hospital, February 5, 1945

275 –disability compensation rate for anatomical loss: 1945 figure, P.L. 182; 1954 figure, P.L. 695; 1972 figure, supplied to author by Douglas C. MacFarland

276 "should have been enough to make the most inveterate": Warren Bledsoe, "From Valley Forge to Hines: Truth Old Enough to Tell," *Blindness* 1969, 113

276 "Why all this fuss": confidential memo, PJS to RBI, August 8, 1947

276 "Carl Gray could not see": Paul B. Magnuson, *Ring the Night Bell,* Little Brown, 1960, 325-326

277 "sincere, healthy minded, emotionally balanced": quoted in John D. Malmazian, "The First 15 Years at Hines," *Blindness* 1970, 62

278 "There were numerous occasions": Malmazian, op.cit., 63

278 "an environmental therapy": "Facts About the Rehabilitation of the Blind at the Veterans Administration Hospital at Hines, Illinois," VA Fact Sheet No. 10-7, June 1950

280–Kendrick's interest in war-blinded men: Baynard Kendrick, "Autobiographical Memoirs," *Blindness* 1970, 79 ff.

281 "There is no question about Kendrick's": letter, Thayer Hobson to RBI, December 10, 1945

282 "a flying wedge": quoted in *BVA Bulletin,* October 1946, 11

282 "quietly, without general appeal": *BVA Bulletin,* October 1948, 7

284 "The group is relatively well educated": p. 12-13

285 "a month before the veteran leaves": minutes, Conference on Blinded Veterans of the Vietnam Era, April 6-7, 1972, 49

286 "Instead of the respect and acclaim": letter, Belle McLure to R. L. Robinson, February 22, 1972

18. THE THREE-WHEELED CART

287 "Our students are a most heterogenous group": Cholden, 33-34

289 "to conduct a campaign for the prevention": "The Re-Education of the Blind Adult," AAWB Proceedings, 1919, reprinted in *Outlook*, Summer 1919, 47-52

291 "it is to be doubted if any one code": "Standards of Requirements for Home Teachers," *Outlook*, April 1935, 67

293 "that professional home teaching embraces": "Home Teacher Certification Standards," *Outlook*, May 1960, 180-181

293 "misdirected many blind young people": "Home Teaching a Specialty," AAWB proceedings, 1951, 17

294 –Using a telephone console unit: *Outlook*, October 1968, 261

294 "The newly blind adult will always need someone": Juliet Bindt, "Modern Trends in the Education of the Adult Blind," *Outlook*, June 1953, 181

295 –A 1950 Foundation survey of 11 centers: *AFB Bulletin*, Social Research Series No. 1, July 1950

295 "The greatest variation in travel training": ibid., 16-17

296 "The student usually comes from a protected environment": ibid., 17-18

296 "the best and only authorities": Langerhans and Red Key, 10

297 –the amended Medical Facilities Survey and Construction Act: Public Law 83-482

298 –scrounged trucks: Henry A. Wood conversation with author, October 22, 1970

298 "It is difficult to tell a person": 664–675, reprinted in *Bulletin of the Society of Military Ophthalmologists*, September 1968

298 "the wrong kind of hope": Cholden, 25

299 –Addressing a conference of ophthalmologists: "When Prevention Fails—Then What?," address at joint conference of Pan-American Association of Ophthalmology and National Society for the Prevention of Blindness, March 27-31, 1950, reprinted in *Outlook*, June 1950, 159-164

299 "a period of mourning for his dead eyes": Cholden, 76-77

299 "learning to use the other gateways": Fraser, 95

299 "the language of the senses": *The Open Door*, 137

300 –computer-age thinking found expression: Emerson Foulke, "The Personality of the Blind: A Non-Valid Concept," *Outlook*, February 1972, 33–37

19. MOBILITY, KEY TO INDEPENDENCE

302 "The importance to every blind man": reprinted in *Outlook*, April 1949, 106-110

303 "the three great founding fathers": Berthold Lowenfeld, "Johann Wilhelm Klein: A Portrait," *Blindness* 1971, 229-231

304 "The newly blinded man taking his first steps": Chevigny, 52-53

304 "would not be caught using": letter, RBI to Robert I. Bramhall, April 6, 1928

304 "a dirty little cur": letter, RBI to Kate M. Foley, January 29, 1930

304 "the very index and essence": letter, Edward E. Allen to RBI, January 23, 1929

305 –it was estimated that close to 4,000 dogs: Dorothy Harrison Eustis, "Guide Dogs for the Blind," in Lende et al., 184

305 –French military authorities: P. Hachet-Souplet, "The Blind Soldier's Dog," *Beacon* (London), May 1918

305 –an article on the same subject: Eustis, "The Seeing Eye," *Saturday Evening Post,* November 5, 1927, 43-46

305 "overbred, overfed": Eustis, "Lead Dogs for the Blind," *Outlook,* March 1929, 16-19

306 "turn out 60 to 70 dogs": letter, Eustis to RBI, January 21, 1928

306 "As I see it": letter, RBI to Eustis, January 25, 1928

307 "If Massachusetts will undertake the job": letter, RBI to Bramhall, op. cit.

307 –the dog school in Potsdam had recently been in touch: letter, E. Liese, Ausbildungs-stelle für Blindenführerhunde, to RBI, March 6, 1928

307 "The author well remembers": Irwin, 173

307 –he took the occasion to announce: "Blind Youth Travels 5,000 Miles with Dog," *The New York Times,* June 12, 1928

308 –challenging Humphrey's ability to teach dogs: letter, Potsdam school to AFB, January 30, 1929

308 "a mind that absorbs": Hartwell, 11

308 "55 men have started on the road": "The Guide Dog Movement" in Zahl, 369-370

309 "in Germany, a nation of dog lovers": op. cit. in Lende et al., 186

309 "wiry and as full of bounding energy": Frank and Clark, 71

311 "estimated current capacity is slightly in excess": Finestone et al., 31-32

312 "be able to demonstrate by actual blindfold test": California Business and Professional Code, Chapter 915, Statutes of 1947, Chapter 1249, Paragraph 1, p. 2760

312 –He was not even convinced: letter, RBI to Harold F. Warman, April 3, 1945

314 –An outline of the apprentice training program: Koestler, 249

315 –In the wake of this accident: AFB circular letter, January 15, 1936

315 –a policy statement that more or less reversed: MRB memo, "Official AFB Attitude and Policy Regarding the White Cane and Its Ramifications," April 20, 1961

316 –As a service to its readers: "Manual for Orientors," *Outlook,* December 1947, 271-279

316 "served chiefly to whet the appetites": Donald Blasch, "Orientation and Mobility Fans Out," *Blindness* 1971, 9

316 "The war blind at the outset": letter to editor, *Outlook,* June 1954, 201-203

317 "with the sensorium": memo in AFB files, "Mobility Technician," n.d. but internally identified as developed from conference of November 4, 1952

317 "the increasing recognition of the danger": letter, Thomas J. Carroll to Kathern F. Gruber, September 26, 1953

317 "the teaching of mobility was a task": "Standards for Mobility Instructors," 3

318 –Spokesmen for long-accepted professions: e.g., Herbert Rusalem, "The Dilemma in Training Mobility Instructors," *Outlook,* March 1960, 82-87

318 "give formal recognition to those": Koestler, 225

319 "become a fetish": Carl McCoy, letter to editor, *Outlook,* May 1969, 157

320 "Within reasonable limits, travel is safe": *Outlook,* February 1947, 37-38

320 "There seems to be a great feeling of need": memo, G. L. Abel to K. Gruber, June 9, 1953

321 –A statement subsequently issued by a dozen authorities: "Dog Guides and Blind Children," 1963, text reprinted in Koestler, 247-248

321 "I would like to encourage you": Paul A. Kolers in Proceedings of the Rotterdam Mobility Research Conference, 241

322 "I walk with my head": Arnold Auch, "Blindness and Travel," *Outlook,* October 1949, 213

20. The Watershed Years

323 –The ranks of its founders: Latimer died in 1944, White in 1934, Hamilton in 1941, Morgan in 1943, Lindsay in 1939, Miss Sherwin in 1938; Mrs. Gage retired from board in 1935 and died in 1948

326 –Under the mandatory staff retirement system: minutes, AFB executive committee, April 2, 1936

326 –persuaded the trustees to let him continue: minutes, AFB executive committee, April 26, 1948

326 –the committee had never seriously considered: conversation with author, January 12, 1973. The other members of the executive search committee were Ziegler, R. H. Migel, Salmon and Farrell

327 –the official photograph: frontispiece, *Outlook,* November 1949

331 –In 1959, ten years after Barnett took over: minutes, October 22, 1959, 66

334 –he insisted upon meeting the additional $30,000 cost: letter, RBI to trustees, January 30, 1935

335 "would add greatly to its stability": letter, MCM to HK, May 16, 1933

336 –But Helen had an opportunity to be as flowery as she liked: text of HK speech printed in *Outlook,* December 1935, 195

340 "been guilty in some instances of coasting": "Criteria and Standards of Services for the Blind," AAWB proceedings, 1953, 106-109

340 "a manual of useful criteria": E. A. Baker, *Plan for the Preparation and Publication of a Manual of Useful Criteria and Standards for the Guidance of Agencies Serving the Blind,* ibid., 109-110

340 "so-called agencies for the blind": "Report of Study Committee on Principles and Standards of Public Relations and Fund Raising for Agencies for the Blind," ibid., 142-146

341 –But no great rush to acquire the seal: Alfred Allen, "The Code of Ethics: An Appraisal," *Outlook,* November 1955, 317-320

341 –There was outright discrimination: Alexander F. Handel conversation with author, January 22, 1973

341 "to make sure that blind persons benefit": text reprinted in *Outlook,* November 1959, 330-333

342 "It is not our intention": Report of the President, AFB, October 26, 1961, 3

343 "Standards should be formulated": Koestler, 9

344 "the most significant advance": PJS, quoted in *Outlook,* January 1966, 4

344 "to reform it or destroy it": *Braille Monitor,* August 1972, 387

344 "We decry the efforts of one particular organization": letter, Lee W. Jones to Caspar W. Weinberger, January 2, 1973

346 "to the tasks of securing the required funding": "Moving Bio-Medical Research into the Marketplace" in Graham (1972), 178-184

21. Little Things That Make a Big Difference

348 "wartime inventions now held secret": 1943 annual report, AFB, 14-15

350 –There was a pleasing irony: Ritter, Clifford M. Witcher, *Outlook,* November 1956, 341-342

351 –A detailed letter: Witcher to Eugene F. Murphy, November 19, 1948; "another that he drafted": RBI to Murphy, January 17, 1949

351 "We have at last come to understand": memo, C. M. Witcher to C. H. Whittington, June 16, 1950

352 "What can the Government do": quoted in "Roosevelt Urges Peace Science Plan," *New York Times,* November 21, 1944

352 "get a high preference rating": letter, RBI to Vannevar Bush, November 24, 1944

352 "not separable from those of blindness in general": Zahl, foreword, x

353 "an instrument which is able to do something": George W. Corner, "The Committee on Sensory Devices," in Zahl, 438-439

353 –In the 25 years following termination of the CSD's projects: figures through 1964 from "U. S. Veterans Administration Research Concerning Blindness" in *Blindness* 1964, 48-54; additional data through 1972 supplied to author by Howard Freiberger, March 1973

353 –An estimate was made in 1968 that federal investment: Blindness and Services to the Blind in the United States, 104

354 "had one selenium cell": "The Optophone: Its Beginning and Development," *Bulletin of Prosthetic Research,* Spring 1966, 25-28

354 "the perversity of natural phenomena": "Research on Reading Machines for the Blind" in Zahl, 521

355 "culminated in the production of 10 copies": "Reading Machines for the Blind, the Veterans Administration, and the Non-Veteran Blind," VA document R-701204, December 4, 1970, 3

355 "can inspire tremendous and lasting affection": Toward an Improved Octophone —Experiments with a Musical Code," AFB Research *Bulletin* No. 16, 1968, 42

355 "The pace is slow": "Potential Uses of the Optophone," *Bulletin of Prosthetics Research,* Spring 1966, 32–36

355 –Lauer also taught the Visotoner: Research and Development in Aids for the Blind, VA document, October 1969, 4

356 "If you could print with vibratory pins": Interview with John Linvill, *Stanford Engineering News,* January 1970

358 –Far more sophisticated devices: Franklin S. Cooper and Patrick W. Nye, Plans for the Evaluation of a High Performance Reading Machine for the Blind, National Academy of Sciences 1971, 57

358 "including even broadcast stations": "The Blind in the Age of Technology," *Outlook,* September 1970, 202

359 "made a more lasting impression": Robert E. Naumburg, "The Beginnings of the Visagraph," *Outlook,* September 1928, 22-23

361 "It was like having a continuously ringing": remarks at 1971 AAWB convention (author's notes)

362 "It is not enough to say that the cane": The VA-Bionic Laser Cane for the Blind, National Academy of Sciences 1972, 81

363 –one British experimenter reported: Walter Thornton, "The Binaural Sensor as a Mobility Aid," *Outlook,* December 1971, 324-326

363 "It would appear": "The Sonic Glasses Evaluated," *Outlook,* January 1973, 7-11

365 "stimulating and motivating universities": AAWB proceedings, 1959, 83

366 "The best research minds can be obtained": quoted in "Kay Gruber's Column," *BVA Bulletin,* May-June 1961, 10

366 "The Director of this Bureau happily announces": Director's Report of Activities, AFB, third quarter, 1959-1960, 22

366 –Among the many beneficiaries of this skill: James C. Bliss conversation with author, October 26, 1971

368 "You may be as enthusiastic as you please": quoted in "Telescopic Spectacles and Magnifiers as Aids to Poor Vision," *Outlook,* March 1926, 54

368 "a sort of miniature pair of opera glasses": letter, RBI to Ian Fraser, June 22, 1933

368 "found a number of instances in which ophthalmologists": letter, Harry J. Spar to A.B.C. Knudson, June 8, 1953

368-9 "that the possibility of designing better reading glasses": op. cit. in Zahl, 436

369 "insisted on ordering an assortment": "Optical Aids in Ophthalmology," *AFB Enlightener,* October 1954, 6

370 –On this basis, an agreement was reached in 1960: minutes, AFB executive committee, February 2, 1960, 75-6

370 "always remain high": Director's Report of Activities, AFB, first quarter, 1960/1961, 15

371 –(Irwin told people he conducted it as a sort of hobby): letter, RBI to Mary V. Hun, January 19, 1926

372 "Sometimes it seems no limit is in sight": "Some Thoughts on Large Type," *Large Print Journal,* April 1971, 3-4

372 "an electric conversation board": unsigned memo in AFB files, "Projects for Proposed Research Laboratory," n.d., ca. 1944

373 –a budget review showed a deficit: MRB, AAWB proceedings, 1960, 79

373 "whatever the cost to the agency": minutes, AFB executive committee, October 22, 1958, 61-62

373 –new postal regulations which expanded the free mailing: Public Law 90-26, December 16, 1967

374 –Graham and Clark reported in 1972: *AFB Newsletter,* Winter 1973

374 "The door is opening wider": Charles E. Hallenbeck, "Recent Research on Advanced Communications Aids for the Blind," *Blindness* 1970, 115

22. ONE WORLD

375 "He had the world's greatest flair": A. J. Liebling, "After Repeal—the Good Old Days?," *New York World-Telegram,* October 28, 1933

375 –At one such event a Venetian theme was created: Alfred Harvey, "The Gondola Dinner," *Cartons Mondains-Cir,* Paris, September 1, 1905

376 –Kessler was also an extraordinarily lucky man: Eric T. Boulter conversation with author, September 22, 1970

376 –a piece cut from the Cullinan diamond: "Who's Who Abroad," *Chicago Tribune* European edition, January 17, 1926

377 –In rebuttal to the Holt charges: minutes, B.F.B. Permanent War Relief Fund, October 10, 1916; also circular letter, idem, March 23, 1917, and "Work in France of the American-British-French-Belgian Permanent Blind Relief War Fund Described in French Official Reports," *Outlook,* January 1918, 81-86

377 "the physician of Wall Street": quoted in Dean, 113

378 –He was a prime mover: *Time,* February 15, 1932, 23-24

378 "in Spartan living": Dean, 5

378 "To the end of his life": ibid., 115

378 "an impressive figure": foreword to Dean, ii

379 "there was a strong feeling in most quarters": "Report of the Joint AAWB-AAIB Committee on a World Conference of Workers for the Blind," AAWB proceedings, 1929, 183-185

380 –responded to a last-minute S.O.S.: letter, RBI to William Nelson Cromwell, December 9, 1935

381 "the sudden and extraordinary development of mechanical music": Lende et al., 161-162

382 "Massage, shampooing, acupuncture": ibid., 261

382 "The civilization of these countries": ibid., 264-265

383 "The first right of a blind person": ibid., 275

383 "unite simultaneously and ask for the recognition": ibid., 336-345

384 "Half of the gathering in New York": Campbell, 148

384 "By spring of 1935": Lacy, 34

385 "I had to comply": "Service for Overseas Blind," *TBT*, March 1946, 3

386 –Before the end of 1946, some 60,000 pounds: 1946 annual report, AFOB, 2

386 "We got massive sacks": conversation with author, September 14, 1970

387 "The blind are trying to help themselves": multigraphed typescript, n.d., ca. 1947, in AFOB files, 2

388 "These were from Macedonia": ibid., 3

390 –Between 1961 and 1971 the equivalent of $28 million: Martin E. McCavitt and Judith E. Turner, "Special Foreign Currency Program of the Social and Rehabilitation Service," *Blindness* 1971, 183-204

391 "Blind Poilus' Beacon Saved": quoted in Bloodgood, 149

391 "attired in costumes of blue crepe de chine": *Boston Herald,* quoted in *Outlook,* Summer 1922, 40-41

393 "1)Registration of all who fall within": *New Beacon,* London, September 1949, reprinted in *Outlook,* October 1949, 223-228

23. The Birthright of Every Child

395 "the monopoly of a privileged minority": "A Study of History," abridged, Oxford University Press, 1947, 292

396 "Here is Howe": this anecdote is related in many annual reports of the Perkins School for the Blind, e.g. 1971, 61

396 "a meeting of flint with steel": Richards (1935), 71

396 "Howe was without a preliminary training": French, 115

397 "a profound sorrow": Sizeranne, 58

397 –The lad had been a street beggar: Benjamin B. Huntoon, address to AAIB convention, 1910, reproduced in *Outlook,* Autumn 1910, 107 ff.

398 "much to admire and to copy": 1971 annual report, Perkins, 61

398 –a green ribbon was bound: that the color of the ribbon was green is mentioned in Dickens "American Notes"

400 "So persuasive was he that proper Bostonians": Story of Blindness, 63

401 –According to the version of this incident given by Anne: Braddy, 154-156

401 –Helen Keller's version: Midstream, 73

402 "the most decisive role": Lowenfeld, op. cit., 229-231

403 "an exotic": 1874 annual report, Perkins, 137-138

403 "want far more waiting upon": Report of the Royal Commission on the Blind, the Deaf and Dumb, etc. of the United Kingdom, minutes of evidence given 12 May 1886, p. 371. Published London, 1889

403 "huddled against the wall": Braddy, 58-59

404 "to pass upon the merits": "Edward Ellis Allen, D. Sc., An Appreciation," *Outlook,* June 1950, 151-156

404 "storm the castle": quoted in Edward E. Allen, "The Challenge of Sir Francis Campbell," *TF*, January 1932, 54

405 "almost superhuman persistence": letter to editor, *TF*, September 1932, 11-12

406 "perennial items of policy, practice and concern": "Chronicle of the American Association of Instructors of the Blind," *Blindness* 1972, 5

407 "appropriated large portions of the public lands": proceedings of the first convention, American Instructors of the Blind, 1853, 5

407-8 "I accept my full share of condemnation": Batavia address, September 6, 1866, published by Walker, Fuller & Co., Boston, 1866, 38

409 "The great advantages which may flow from it": letter, August 7, 1871, in AAIB proceedings, 1871, 13-20

409 "The reluctance of parents": *The Mentor*, September 1891, 267

410 "but the indifference of parents": ibid., 264-266

410 "located in a desirable part of the city": *The Mentor*, April 1891, 117

410 "an album bound in Turkish morocco": *The Mentor*, August 1891, 236

410 "more than 120 ophthalmic anomalies": "Some Experiences and a Prophecy Which Seem to Prove Wise and Right the Perkins Tradition of No Coeducation of Blind Boys and Blind Girls," *TF*, January 1939, 59-60

412 –By 1907 Curtis was able to report that Chicago had: "Education of the Blind in the Chicago Public Schools," *Outlook*, July 1907, 35 37

412 "a gentle, retiring man": letter, RBI to Kathern F. Gruber, September 12, 1939

412 "passed the period when the influence of the home": "Place of the Day School in the Work of the Blind," AAIB proceedings, 1910, 40-42

412 "Teachers have been expected to visit": "Coeducation of the Blind and the Seeing," *Outlook*, Summer 1916, 54

413 "It is no longer a question": "The Education of the Young Blind in Institutions versus in Schools with the Seeing—the Advantages and Disadvantages of Each," AAIB proceedings, 1910, 31-37

24. THE EVER-CHANGING CHILDREN

416 "Cutting down on oxygen": quoted in Steven M. Spencer, "Mystery of the Blinded Babies," *Saturday Evening Post*, June 11, 1955, 19-21, 97-106

416-17 "the most important single clinical advancement": Pearce Bailey, "Clinical Success with Three Eye Conditions," *Outlook*, June 1955, 222

417 "Everyone wanted to turn the oxygen on": Dr. Loren P. Guy quoted in Spencer, op. cit., 101

417 "that most physicians lost interest": "Prematurity and Retrolental Fibroplasia," *Sight-Saving Review*, Spring 1969, 42-46

419 "One dilemma is the erecting of buildings": *Outlook*, October 1953, 229-230

420 "The janitor": Josephine L. Taylor in Abel, 44

421 "inadequate, erratic, costly and destructive": p. 14 of pamphlet

422 "very deficient in sensory": Cutsforth p. 190

422 "the traditions and content of a visual development": ibid., p. 166

422 "ferociously frank": "Book News: A Sightless Scholar's View," *Outlook*, June 1933, 141-142

422 "the hypocrisy of verbalism": Cutsforth p. 15

422 "robs the sensory world": ibid., p. 51

423 "realistic thinking, actual experience": Pine Brook Report, 8

426 "already in some of the southern states": letter, May 9, 1942

427 "trade on their handicaps as an excuse": "The Employment of Blind Teachers in Schools for the Blind," AAWB proceedings, 1949, 33-36

428 "we should have different standards for different mentalities": "The New Education and Its Relation to and Influence upon the Education of the Blind," AAIB proceedings, 1918, 5-11

428 "1. To develop and apply methods": Samuel P. Hayes, "The Work of the Department of Psychological Research at the Pennsylvania Institution for the Instruction of the Blind, Overbrook," AAWB proceedings, 1919, reprinted in *Outlook,* April 1920, 5-8, 19-20

429 "The use in schools for the blind of standardized tests": Hayes, ibid., 19-20

430 "we must not let pupils write": "A Historical Review of Achievement Tests for the Blind," *Outlook,* December 1948, 300-304

430 "pupils test up to the seeing standards": "The Needs of the Blind Child in the Field of Educational Psychology" in proceedings, International Conference of Educators of Blind Youth, Bussum, Netherlands (1952), 179

431 "Psychologists and educators alike": Mary K. Bauman, "Psychological Testing and Blindness—a Retrospect," *Blindness* 1972, 192-193

432 "kept his heart from breaking": p. 151-157 of scrapbook in the possession of AFB Migel Memorial Library

432 "I did not tell them": ibid., 161-167

433 "the extreme desirability": letter, February 20, 1931

433 "that boards of trustees": AAWB proceedings, 1931, 78

435 "productive avenues of approach": "The Pre-School Blind Child: A Preliminary Study," *TF,* March 1934, 62-65

436 –The nation's first [such organization] came into being in Connecticut: For details of the Emily Welles Foster story, see Dorothea Simpson, "Light on Dark Paths," published 1971 by the Norwich (Conn.) Free Academy

437 "whether they have no sight": Olive McVickar, "A Nursery School for Children with Impaired Vision," *TF,* September 1939, 12-16

438 "blind individuals tended to make": Sommers, 103

438 "the accent should be on leaving the child in his family": Proceedings, National Conference on the Blind Preschool Child, 144-145

439 "clearly within the field of the residential school": "President's Report," AAIB proceedings, 1948, 9-13

439 "but the program in my estimation": "Some Necessary Steps in Organizing an Institution in a Residential School for the Blind for Mothers and Blind Babies," ibid., 34-38

439 "as a sort of clearing house": "An Open Letter to Educators in Schools and Classes for Blind Children," *Outlook,* November, 1950, 254-255

440 –one of the more authoritative sources estimated: John L. Sever, M.D., "Rubella Epidemiology and Vaccines," *Sight-Saving Review,* Summer 1967, 68-72

441 "In theory, none of us admits the feeble-minded": "President Burritt's Address: The Education of the Blind a Highly Complex Problem," AAIB proceedings, 1916, 8-14

441 "four feeble-minded children": "The Recognition and Training of Blind Feeble-Minded Children," *Outlook,* Summer 1915, 29-32

441 "The feeble-minded, whether deaf, blind": quoted in "A Place for the Blind Feeble-Minded: A Symposium," *TF,* May 1931, 8-11

442 "The simple educational activities": ibid., 10

442 "to effect some agreement": ibid., 11

442 "music, conversation and much love": "Helping the Retarded Blind," *International Journal for the Education of the Blind,* April 1953, 163-164

443 –A 1956 survey of New York State's: Cruickshank and Trippe, 189, 201, 209, 214

443 "small but growing corps": Director's Report of Activities, AFB, first quarter, 1962–3, 8

443 "conviction, love, patience": No Time to Lose, p. 44-45

443 "if special treatment and care": Anna S. Elonen and Margaret Polzien, "Experimental Program for Deviant Blind Children," *Outlook,* April 1965, 122-126

444 "a national problem that can only be met": Graham (1968), 3-4, 19, 22

444 "the multiply handicapped child is the challenge": The Blind Child Who Functions on a Retarded Level, 11-18

444 "Only the emotionally strong, well-prepared teacher": ibid., 44-49

446 "We have tried for years": "President Burritt's Address, etc.," op. cit., 12

446 "and the willingness of parents": quoted in NSPB Publication 149, "Education of Partially Seeing Children," 1952, 3

447 "from an organizational setup": "The New Constitution of the American Association of Instructors of the Blind," *Outlook,* February 1953, 47-48

449 –They spent three days hammering out a detailed plan: "Industrial Arts for Blind Students"

450 "placement and recycling": Harvey E. Wolfe, position paper prepared for National Task Force on Career Education, March 16, 1972

25. THE LONELIEST PEOPLE

452 "What is it actually like": "Merlyn" (pseudonym), "Behind the Silent Facade," *New Beacon* (London), February 15, 1942, 17-20

453 "should not be abandoned": from an article by Howe in *Barnard's,* quoted in Howe and Richards, 38

454 "The process had been mechanical": 1840 annual report, Perkins, 26

454 "the truth began to flash upon her": ibid.

454 "She took hold of the thread": Howe, Batavia address, op.cit., 28

454 "did not deign to notice anything or anybody": quoted in Fish, 10

455 "I am going to treat Helen": HK, The Story of My Life, Magnum edition, 372-373

455 "The new scheme works splendidly": ibid., 373-374

455 "When I walk out in my garden": letter, November 27, 1889, ibid., 288

456 "I am sitting on the piazza": letter, August 7, 1889, ibid., 203-204

456 "the only one of their heroic undertakings": Braddy, 151

456 "That is not the sort of dog a blind child needs": quoted in "In Memoriam, William Wade," *Outlook,* Autumn 1913, 47-48

457 "He met us at the train in Pittsburgh": ibid.

458 "The Education of a Girl, etc.": *Outlook,* June 1926, 12-16

458 –This was made known a few years later: "Without Sight or Hearing," *Outlook,* December 1930, 24-26

458 "instead of employing a teacher for each pupil": Children of the Silent Night, 32

458 –In 1927 a Montreal publisher: *"Hors de Sa Prison"* (Arbour & Dupont)

458 "Her body was clad": Sherman C. Swift, "Book News," *Outlook,* December 1928, 59-62

459 –a long article by Miss Rocheleau: "The Deaf-Blind in America," *Outlook,* September 1928, 14-19

459 "to cooperate with a like committee": AAIB proceedings, 1928, 440

459-60 "No plan of education for the deaf-blind": AAWB proceedings, 1929, 159

460 –The Foundation thereupon opened negotiations: *Outlook,* March 1932, 1-2

461 –The upshot was the Foundation's decision: letter, RBI to H. M. McManaway, January 17, 1933

462 "plodding pursuit of knowledge": quoted in Braddy, 176

462 "I pity them more than I blame them": quoted in ibid., 177

462 "The education of the blind-deaf ": Wade, first edition, preface

462 –he wrote Helen that he had, in fact: letter, June 23, 1901

463 ". . . in the 'Monograph' ": letter, June 28, 1901

463 "there was no mystery": letter of February 20, 1904, reprinted in Wade, second edition, 65

463 "dangerous nonsense": Wade, second edition, 8

463 "I have never thought that I deserve": Address to Educational Institute of Scotland, September 27, 1932

464 "The only thing": Wade, second edition, 8

464 "his benefactions to deaf-blind children": *Association Review,* December 1904, 431

464 "Mrs. Macy's stand on the subject of other teachers": letter, December 2, 1931

464 "unfriendly spirit": letter, HK to Rebecca Mack, January 21, 1932

465 "have all proved their capabilities": text quoted in press release, Industrial Home for the Blind, June 27, 1945

465 "now, in the autumn of her life": letter, MCM to Ziegler, August 13, 1945

470 "One thing to be kept in mind always": PJS, "The Deaf-Blind," in Zahl, 231-232

471 "fear among the deaf-blind": AAWB proceedings, 1958, 26-28

471 "The true failure": PJS, 52

472 "no riot or sit-in": letter, PJS to Congressman Hugh L. Carey, June 12, 1968

473 "She could carry on a conversation": Sophia Alcorn, "Development of the Tadoma Method for the Deaf Blind," *Journal of Exceptional Children,* January 1945, 117-119

477 "Perhaps the real miracle": *Outlook,* April 1966, 108

26. Open Channels

479 "I saw your communication": quoted in pamphlet, "The Story of the Ziegler Magazine," adapted from 50th anniversary issue of the *Ziegler,* March 1957

479 "Mrs. Ziegler said that she had always wanted": quoted in id.

479 "you have a chimney corner": *Outlook,* September 1927, 13

479 "we know enough of that from experience": quoted by Holmes in op. cit., 53. He was paraphrasing what HK wrote Mrs. Ziegler, when the forthcoming magazine was announced: "Several of the [existing magazines for the blind] devote too much space to our afflictions, of which we already know enough by experience." November 14, 1906

482 "I would rather do what you are doing": letter from physician in Lancaster, Ohio, contained in binder of 1927 anniversary letters in the possession of the *Ziegler Magazine.*

484 "active synthesizing agent": French, 253-254

485 "You people here, the Instructors": AAIB proceedings, 1912, 33

485 "even if the magazine is reduced": letter, CFFC to Edward E. Allen, April 30, 1912

487 "Essentially a promoter": Latimer, 169-170

487 "wherever he went, he started things moving": "Memories of Charles F. F. Campbell," *Outlook,* February 1936, 7

488 "only with the Campbells who had passed on": letter, RBI to HRL, January 13, 1936

488 –Latimer did not take kindly: letter, HRL to RBI, January 14, 1936

489 "The photographs in your article": letter, RBI to HRL, March 16, 1936

489 "success story of a blind dog": *Outlook,* December 1928, 40

490 "The *New Outlook for the Blind* shall be a vehicle": p. 4

493 "advertising be limited": minutes, February 25, 1923, 84

496 "absolutely did not know": letter, CFFC to RBI, January 20, 1928, in Box 31 of Sir Francis Campbell papers in Library of Congress collection

497 "She was not an easy person": comment by PJS in conversation with author, August 31, 1970

497 "is the luxury of the giver": Chevigny, 222

498 "I doubt if any organization in America": letter, HK to W. G. Holmes, February 21, 1935

498 "All members present generally agreed": minutes, April 8, 1952, 122

27. The Road Ahead

505 "A Bill to Protect etc.": S. 2411, introduced June 27, 1957

506 "tremendous leverage": Jacobus ten Broek quoted in *Outlook,* September 1957, 321

506 "embodies a completely unsound": AAWB proceedings, 1957, 81-82

507 "the oppression of the social worker": 1940 letter, "To the Blind of the Nation," quoted in Perry Sundquist, "The First Thirty Years," *Council Bulletin,* California Council of the Blind, November/December 1970, 18-26

507 "be given an equal chance": "A Bill of Rights for the Blind," *Outlook,* December 1948, 310-314

507 "internal strife and chaos": quoted in Raymond Parsons, "NFB Convention," *Outlook,* November 1961, 307

509 "We in the United States": Lucy Wright address at Massachusetts State Conference of Charities, October 20, 1908, reprinted *Outlook,* October 1908, 118

Bibliography

In addition to the sources listed below, references to specific magazine articles, book chapters, etc. can be found in the Chapter Notes. To conserve space, the American Foundation for the Blind, publisher of much of the professional literature on blindness, is identified by its initials.

Abel, Georgie Lee, ed. *Concerning the Education of Blind Children.* AFB, 1959.

Adams, Samuel Hopkins. *A. Woollcott, His Life and His World.* Reynal & Hitchcock, 1945.

Allen, Frederick Lewis. *Only Yesterday.* Harper, 1931.

Allied Health Careers for Blind and Visually Handicapped Persons: A Workshop Report. AFB, 1972.

American Association of Instructors of the Blind. Proceedings, biennial, 1871 ff.

American Association of Workers for the Blind. Proceedings, biennial, 1907 through 1971.

American Foundation for the Blind. Annual reports, 1924 through 1972.

American Printing House for the Blind, Inc.: Its History, Purposes and Policies. 1966.

———. Annual reports, 1966 through 1972.

Attitudes Toward Blindness. AFB Social Research Series No. 1, 1951.

Bell, Donald, ed. *An Experiment in Education: the History of Worcester College for the Blind.* London: Hutchinson & Company, 1967.

Best, Harry. *The Blind.* Macmillan, 1919.

Bindt, Juliet. *A Handbook for the Blind.* Macmillan, 1952.

The Blind Child Who Functions on a Retarded Level. Proceedings of Regional Institute, Austin, Texas. AFB, 1969.

Blind Workers in U. S. Industries. Washington: National Society for the Blind, 1943.

Blindness and Services to the Blind in the United States. Cambridge, Mass.: Organization for Social and Technical Innovation, Inc. (OSTI), 1971.

Blindness. Annual, 1964 through 1972. Washington, D.C.: American Association of Workers for the Blind.

Bloodgood, Edith Holt, ed. *First Lady of the Lighthouse: A Biography of Winifred Holt Mather.* New York Association for the Blind, 1952.

Braddy, Nella. *Anne Sullivan Macy: The Story Behind Helen Keller.* Doubleday, Doran, 1933.

Campbell, Marjorie Wilkins. *No Compromise: The Story of Colonel Baker and the C.N.I.B.* Toronto: McClelland and Stewart, 1965.

Carroll, Thomas J. *Blindness: What It Is, What It Does, and How to Live with It.* Little, Brown, 1961.

Chevigny, Hector. *My Eyes Have a Cold Nose.* Yale University Press, 1946.

——— and Braverman, Sydell. *The Adjustment of the Blind.* Yale University Press, 1950.

Cholden, Louis S. *A Psychiatrist Works with Blindness.* AFB, 1958.

Clark, Leslie L., ed. *Proceedings of the International Congress on Technology and Blindness.* 4 vols. AFB, 1963.

The CNIB Story, 1918-1968. Toronto: Canadian National Institute for the Blind, 1968.

Conference of Administrators of Rehabilitation Centers for Blind Persons. AFB, 1961.

Cosgrove, Elizabeth. *Home Teachers of the Adult Blind.* Washington: American Association of Workers for the Blind, 1961.

Cruickshank, William M. and Trippe, Matthew J. *Services to Blind Children in New York State.* Syracuse University Press, 1959.

Curtis, Scott; Donlon, Edward T. and Wagner, Elizabeth, eds. *Deaf-Blind Children: A Program for Evaluating Their Multiple Handicaps.* AFB, 1970.

Cutsforth, Thomas D. *The Blind in School and Society.* Appleton, 1933. Republished, AFB, 1951.

Dean, Arthur H. *William Nelson Cromwell, 1854-1948: An American Pioneer in Corporation, Comparative and International Law.* Privately printed, 1957.

Dickman, Irving R. *Living with Blindness.* New York: Public Affairs Committee, 1972.

———, ed. *Sex Education and Family Life for Visually Handicapped Children and Youth: A Resource Guide.* New York: Sex Information and Education Council of the United States and AFB, 1972.

———. *What Can We Do About Limited Vision?* New York: Public Affairs Committee, 1973.

Dinsmore, Annette B. *History of Deaf-Blind Services at the American Foundation for the Blind.* Unpublished manuscript. AFB, 1970.

———. *Methods of Communication with Deaf-Blind People.* AFB, 1959.

Directory of Agencies Serving the Visually Handicapped in the United States. Biennial, 1965 through 1971, AFB.

Dufton, Richard, ed. *Proceedings of the International Conference on Sensory Devices for the Blind.* London: St. Dunstan's, 1966.

Edwards, Frank. *Strange People.* Lyle Stuart, 1961.

851 Blinded Veterans: A Success Story. AFB, 1968.

Farrell, Gabriel, *Children of the Silent Night.* Watertown, Mass.: Perkins School for the Blind, 1956.

———. *The Story of Blindness.* Harvard University Press, 1956.

Fifty Years of Vocational Rehabilitation in the U.S.A., 1920-1970. Washington, D.C.: United States Department of Health, Education, and Welfare, Social and Rehabilitation Service, 1970.

Finestone, Samuel, ed. *Social Casework and Blindness.* AFB, 1960.

———, Lukoff, Irving F. and Whiteman, Martin. *The Demand for Dog Guides and the Travel Adjustment of Blind Persons.* New York: Research Center, New York School of Social Work, Columbia University, 1960.

———. *Guide Dog Training for Blind Persons*. Research Center, New York School of Social Work, Columbia University, 1957.

Fish, Anna Gardner. *Perkins Institution and Its Deaf-Blind Pupils*. Watertown, Mass.: Perkins Institution, 1934.

Fitting, Edward A. *Evaluation of Adjustment to Blindness*. AFB, 1954.

Frampton, Merle E. and Kerney, Ellen. *The Residential School*. New York Institute for the Education of the Blind, 1953.

Frank, Morris and Clark, Blake. *First Lady of the Seeing Eye*. Henry Holt, 1957.

Fraser of Lonsdale, Baron. *My Story of St. Dunstan's*. London: George G. Harrap, 1961.

French, Richard Slayton. *From Homer to Helen Keller: A Social and Educational Study of the Blind*. AFB, 1932.

Frick, Kathryne Mary. "In the Dark Alone." *Atlantic Monthly,* April 1930; "Groping in the Dark," ibid., May 1930; "Light at Last," ibid., June 1930.

Goldish, Louis Harvey. *Braille in the United States: Its Production, Distribution and Use*. AFB, 1967.

Gowman, Alan G. *The War Blind in American Social Structure*. AFB, 1957.

Graham, Milton D. *The Deaf-Blind: Some Studies and Suggestions for a National Program*. AFB, 1970.

———. *Multiply Impaired Blind Children: A National Problem*. AFB, n.d., ca. 1968.

———, ed. *Science and Blindness: Retrospective and Prospective*. AFB, 1972.

Griffin, Donald R. *Listening in the Dark*. Yale University Press, 1958.

Gruber, Kathern F. and Moor, Pauline M. *No Place to Go: A Symposium*. AFB, 1963.

——— and Voorhees, Arthur L., eds. *The Grove Park Report: Principles Underlying Nonmedical Vocational and Rehabilitation Preparation Services for Blind Persons*. AFB, 1961.

Harley, Randall K., Jr., *Verbalism Among Blind Children*. AFB, 1963.

Harper, Grace S. *Vocational Re-Education for War Cripples in France*. Washington: American National Red Cross, 1918.

Hartwell, Dickson. *Dogs Against Darkness*. Dodd Mead, 1942.

Haycraft, Howard. *Books for the Blind and Physically Handicapped*. Fourth edition, revised. Washington, D.C.: Library of Congress, 1972.

Helms, Arthur. *Tape Recording Books for the Blind*. AFB, 1962.

Hendrickson, Walter B. *Frank H. Hall and His Braille Writer*. Jacksonville, Ill.: Illinois Braille and Sight Saving School, 1968.

Howe, S. G. and Richards, Laura. *Laura Bridgman*. Privately printed, Boston, 1903.

IHB Optical Aids Service Survey. Brooklyn, N.Y.: Industrial Home for the Blind, 1957.

Industrial Arts for Blind Students: Report of a Conference on Principles and Standards. AFB, 1960.

Instruction in Physical Orientation and Foot Travel for Deaf-Blind Persons. Brooklyn, N.Y.: Industrial Home for the Blind, 1966.

International Catalog, Aids and Appliances for Blind and Visually Impaired Persons. AFB, in press.

Irwin, Robert B. *As I Saw It*. AFB, 1955.

Itinerant Teaching Service for Blind Children: Proceedings of a National Work Session. AFB, 1957.

Josephson, Eric. *The Social Life of Blind People*. AFB, 1968.

Kaufman, Beatrice and Hennessey, Joseph, eds. *The Letters of Alexander Woollcott*. Viking, 1944.

Keller, Helen. *Midstream, My Later Life*. Doubleday, Doran, 1929.

———. *The Open Door.* Doubleday, 1957.

———. *The Story of My Life.* Century, 1904. Magnum Easy Eye edition, Lancer Books, 1968.

———. *Teacher: Anne Sullivan Macy: A Tribute by the Fosterchild of Her Mind.* Doubleday, 1955.

Kendrick, Baynard. *Lights Out.* Morrow, 1945.

Kerby, C. E. *Blindness in Preschool Children.* New York: National Society for the Prevention of Blindness, 1954.

Kim, Yoon Hough. *The Community of the Blind: Applying the Theory of Community Formation.* AFB, 1970.

Koestler, Frances A., ed. *The COMSTAC Report: Standard for Strengthened Services.* New York: Commission on Standards and Accreditation of Services for the Blind, 1966.

Lacy, Bernard. *An International Adventure: A Brief History of the American Foundation for Overseas Blind, 1915–1965.* New York: AFOB, 1965.

Langerhans, Clara and Redkey, Henry, eds. *Adjustment Centers for the Blind: Findings of the Spring Mill Conference.* AFB, n.d., ca. 1951.

Latimer, Henry Randolph. *The Conquest of Blindness.* AFB, 1937.

LeFevre, Robert. *The Story of the Wagner-O'Day Act.* New York: National Industries for the Blind, 1966.

Leighton, Isabel, ed. *The Aspirin Age.* Simon and Schuster, 1949.

Lende, Helga. *Books About the Blind.* AFB, 1940. Revised edition, 1953.

———. *Federal Legislation Concerning Blind Persons in the United States and Insular Possessions.* AFB, 1952.

———, ed. *What of the Blind?* AFB, Vol. 1, 1938; Vol. 2, 1941.

———, McKay, Evelyn C. and Swift, Sherman C., eds. *Proceedings of the World Conference on Work for the Blind.* AFB, 1931.

Library of Congress. Annual reports, 1934 through 1970.

Linsner, James W., ed. *Proceedings of the Mobility Research Conference.* AFB, 1962.

Lowenfeld, Berthold, ed. *The Blind Preschool Child.* AFB, 1947.

———. *Our Blind Children.* Second edition. Springfield, Ill.: Charles C. Thomas, 1964.

———, ed. *The Visually Handicapped Child in School.* John Day, 1973.

———, Abel, Georgie Lee and Hatlen, Philip H. *Blind Children Learn to Read.* Charles C. Thomas, 1969.

Lukoff, Irving Faber and Whiteman, Martin. *The Social Sources of Adjustment to Blindness.* AFB, n.d., ca. 1972.

Lydon, William T. and McGraw, M. Loretta. *Concept Development for Visually Handicapped Children.* AFB, 1973.

McAulay, John H. *Vocational Schools as Training Facilities for Blind Workers.* AFB, 1954.

McMurtrie, Douglas C., ed. *Abstract-Catalogue of Literature on the War Blinded.* Baltimore: Red Cross Institute for the Blind, 1919.

The Mentor. Monthly, 1891–1894. Alumni Association, Perkins Institution for the Blind.

The Middletown Lighthouse for the Blind: A Survey. AFB, 1957.

Monbeck, Michael E. *The Meaning of Blindness.* Indiana University Press, 1973.

Moor, Pauline M. *A Blind Child, Too, Can Go to Nursery School.* AFB, 1962.

———. *No Time to Lose.* AFB, 1968.

National Academy of Sciences, *Evaluation of Sensory Aids for the Visually Handicapped.* 1972.

———. *Sensory Aids for the Blind.* 1968.

National Accreditation Council for Agencies Serving the Blind and Visually Handicapped. Annual Reports, 1969, 1970, 1971.

National Center for Deaf-Blind Youths and Adults, Annual Report, 1973.

New Outlook for the Blind. Monthly, 1951 through 1972.

New York State Department of Social Welfare, Commission for the Blind. *1913/Now.*

Norris, Miriam. *The School Age Blind Child Project.* AFB, 1961.

Outlook for the Blind. Quarterly, 1907–1923; bi-monthly, 1924-1933; monthly, 1942-1950. Name changed to *New Outlook,* 1951.

Pierce, Robinson. *It Was Not My Own Idea.* AFB, 1944.

The Pine Brook Report: National Work Session on the Education of the Blind with the Sighted. AFB, 1954.

Proceedings of the Conference on New Approaches to the Evaluation of Blind Persons. AFB, 1970.

Proceedings of the Conference on Nine-Dot Braille. AFB, 1964.

Proceedings, National Conference on the Blind Preschool Child. AFB, Group Reports No. 1, 1951.

Proceedings of the Research Conference on Geriatric Blindness and Severe Visual Impairment. AFB, 1968.

Proceedings of the Rotterdam Mobility Research Conference. International Research Information Service, AFB, 1965.

Redkey, Henry. *Descriptions of Nine Adjustment Centers.* Washington, D.C.: Office of Vocational Rehabilitation, HEW, 1951.

Rehabilitation Centers for Blind Persons. Report of Seminar, New Orleans, La., February 1956. Washington, D.C. U. S. Department of HEW, n.d.

Rehabilitation of Deaf-Blind Persons, Vol. 1: A Manual for Professional Workers. Brooklyn, N.Y.: Industrial Home for the Blind, 1958.

Report of the Commission to Investigate the Condition of the Adult Blind in the State of New York. Albany, N.Y.: State Legislative Printer, 1904.

Report of the National Citizens Advisory Committee on Vocational Rehabilitation. Washington, D.C.: U. S. Government Printing Office, 1968.

Report of the National Study Committee on Education of Deaf-Blind Children. Watertown, Mass.: Perkins Institution for the Blind, 1954.

Report on Visual Impairment Services Teams. Washington, D.C.: Veterans Administration, 1971.

Richards, Laura E. *Laura Bridgman: The Story of an Opened Door.* Appleton, 1928.

———. *Samuel Gridley Howe.* Appleton-Century, 1935.

———, ed. *Letters and Journals of Samuel Gridley Howe.* Boston: Dana Estes, 1909.

Ritter, Charles G. *Technical Research and Blindness.* AFB, 1956.

Robinson, Robert L., ed. *Blinded Veterans of the Vietnam Era.* AFB, 1973.

Roblin, Jean. *The Reading Fingers: Life of Louis Braille, 1809-1852.* Translated from the French by Ruth G. Mandalian. Revised edition. AFB, 1955.

Rocheleau, Corinne and Mack, Rebecca. *Those in the Dark Silence.* Washington, D.C.: Volta Bureau, 1930.

Rodenberg, Louis W. *The Story of Embossed Books for the Blind.* AFB, 1955.

Ross, Ishbel. *Journey into Light.* Appleton-Century-Crofts, 1951.

Rusalem, Herbert. *Coping with the Unseen Environment.* New York: Teachers College Press, 1972.

——— et al. *New Frontiers for Research on Deaf-Blindness.* Brooklyn, N.Y.: Industrial Home for the Blind, 1966.

Rutherford, John. *Dr. W. Moon and His Work for the Blind.* London: Hodder and Stoughton, 1898.

Salaries for Selected Occupations in Services for the Blind, January, 1966. Washington, D.C.: U. S. Bureau of Labor Statistics, 1966.

Salmon, Peter J. *Out of the Shadows.* New Hyde Park, N.Y.: National Center for Deaf-Blind Youths and Adults, 1970.

Scott, Robert A. *The Making of Blind Men.* Russell Sage Foundation, 1969.

The Seeing Eye. Annual Reports, 1968, 1969, 1970, 1971, 1972.

Sizeranne, Maurice de la. *The Blind as Seen through Blind Eyes.* Translated from the French by F. Park Lewis. Putnam, 1893.

Sommers, Vita Stein. *The Influence of Parental Attitudes and Social Environment on the Personality Development of the Adolescent Blind.* AFB, 1944.

Snowman, Daniel. *America Since 1920.* Harper, 1970.

Standards for Mobility Instructors. AFB, 1962.

A Step-by-Step Guide to Personal Management for Blind Persons. AFB, 1970.

Teachers Forum. Bi-monthly, 1928–1941.

Terkel, Studs. *Hard Times: An Oral History of the Great Depression.* Pantheon, 1970.

Thomas, Mary G. *Thomas Rhodes Armitage.* London: National Institute for the Blind, n.d.

The Training and Placement of Blind Persons in Service Jobs in Hospital Settings. AFB, 1970.

Twersky, Jacob. *The American War-Blind as Aided by the Federal Government.* Unpublished manuscript, 1947.

———. *Blindness in Literature.* AFB, 1955.

Wade, William. *The Blind Deaf.* First edition, 1901; revised edition, 1904. Privately printed.

Westrate, Edwin J. *Beacon in the Night: The Story of J. Robert Atkinson.* Vantage, 1964.

Wood, Maxine. *Blindness—Ability, Not Disability.* New York: Public Affairs Committee, 1968.

Zahl, Paul A., ed. *Blindness: Modern Approaches to the Unseen Environment.* Princeton University Press, 1950. Reprinted with updated bibliography. Hafner, 1962.

Index